TEXTBOOK

of

SURGERY

TEXTBOOK

of

SURGERY

Ijaz Ahsan

King Edward Medical College, Lahore, Pakistan

harwood academic publishers

Australia • Canada • China • France • Germany • India
Japan • Luxembourg • Malaysia • The Netherlands • Russia
Singapore • Switzerland • Thailand • United Kingdom

 Printed in India

Amsteldijk 166
1st Floor
1079 LH Amsterdam
The Netherlands

British Library Cataloguing in Publication Data

Ahsan, Ijaz
Textbook of Surgery. – 2nd. ed.
1. Surgery
I. Title
617

ISBN 90-5702-140-4

Dedicated

to

my wife

Farhat Ijaz Ahsan

for

her endless patience

and moral support

during

the long years

of writing this book

Special
Acknowledgement

My parents, Mrs Rasheeda and the late Chaudhary Mohammad Ahsan, were a source of guidance by their personal conduct of the highest order. Without their training there would have been no book.

Contents

Foreword

It was a privilege to be asked to write a foreword to this superb text, but beyond this, it was a great pleasure to be able to read the book itself. It would be no exaggeration to say that this is a superb book, designed as an entry point into the broad field of surgery, and thus indispensible to medical students, to nurses who are developing their careers in the area of surgery, and to junior surgical residents in training.

The charm and appeal of this book lies in its simplicity, directness, accuracy and completeness. In distinction to much more sophisticated volumes which have been written to cover this field, sometimes in as many as five separate volumes, the scope is broad, but the text is limited. Thus, one can read it quickly, easily, with pleasure and with satisfaction. I might comment in passing on the illustrations, which are unusual, intriguing, and certainly would be fascinating for a young student entering the surgical world.

In a text directed towards this particular audience, one should not criticize the lack of depth, inasmuch as the complexity of surgical pathophysiology today is such that one could spend endless pages probing deeper and deeper into the molecular biology of each of the systems discussed. In addition, the complexity of surgical technique today is such that one could hardly be expected to pursue it with any degree of effectiveness, but again, this is hardly what one looks for as an entry point into the field.

Obviously, this book is only a preface to a career, and clearly the young student must pursue each of the areas which are covered with a broad brush, in much more depth and precision than is available in these pages. One could not, however, ask or expect this to be done at this level of simplicity, and with the objectives that the author had in mind, it would have been very unwise to extend the breadth of this volume to pursue any of the areas in further depth. All in all, I rarely encounter a text which would be more satisfactory for the individual entering into this extraordinarily broad and complicated field which we refer to, in the most general terms, as surgery. With this group in mind, I would certainly recommend this text wholeheartedly, and encourage everyone to use this as the initial step into a marvellously complex and increasingly satisfying career.

William V. McDermott, Jr., M.D.
David W. and David Cheever Professor of Surgery
Harvard Medical School, Boston, Massachusetts, USA

Preface to the Second Edition

This second edition of the book has been thoroughly updated to include the evermore rapid advances being made in the subject of surgery. Throughout the book the latest imaging methods and biochemical investigations have been included. Similarly, the new non-invasive and minimally invasive investigative procedures have been described. At the same time, the changing perspectives in the treatment of trauma, infection and neoplasia have been discussed. Most chapters have undergone extensive revision, and the subjects of Critical Care and Skin have been written in separate chapters. It is hoped that the book will continue to provide medical students and doctors with essential information about the broad field of surgery.

Preface to the First Edition

This book has been designed primarily for undergraduates. An effort has been made to avoid burdening it with too much detail, but to explain whatever is included in as simple a language as possible. The first seventeen chapters have been devoted to a discussion of general principles, because it is felt that in a book of this type a generous amount of space should be reserved for this aspect of the subject.

Postgraduates can use the book for a rapid revision of the whole subject. At the same time, in these times of over-specialization there is a need to keep in mind an overall perspective of medicine and surgery. Therefore it is hoped that clinicians not engaged in the practice of surgery, such as general duty doctors, general practitioners and consultants in other specialties, will find it useful on their bookshelves, to be consulted as and when the need arises.

Acknowledgements

My teachers of surgery, the late Professors Amiruddin, Riyaz-e-Qadeer and Sardar Ali Sheikh set me on the road leading to the production of this volume. Professor William McDermott, Professor of Surgery, Harvard Medical School provided valuable critical comments on certain chapters, and has kindly written a Foreword. Professor Rashid Lateef Khan and Dr Sajid Usman Kaul helped with numerous valuable suggestions throughout the preparation of both editions of the book.

Professor Ghazanfar Ali Shah and Dr Jawad Sajid Khan provided critical comments on chapters pertaining to their respective fields. I am also obliged to Professors Naseer Mahmood Akhtar, Ghulam Mustafa and Munir-ul-Haque, and Drs Farrukh Zaman and Nazir Qazi, the last-named from Abu Dhabi, for valuable comments and suggestions.

Professor Rashid A. Mian has kindly provided most of the radiographs, Dr Nawaz Anjum and Dr M. Younus Sheikh x-rays, CT scans and ultrasound pictures, and Professor Majid Chaudhary one of the clinical photographs. Dr Nasir Awan has prepared the index.

Dr Javed Raza Gardezi has written critical comments on each chapter of the book and two medical students have provided exhaustive comments, namely Dr Asad Ali Chaudhary and Dr Munir Aftab. I am greatly indebted to Mr Salim Parvez, Librarian, King Edward Medical College, for his help with the searching of the literature. Mr Tariq, Artist, College of Physicians and Surgeons of Pakistan, has been responsible for the artwork. My daughters, Mrs Saira Shahbaz and Mrs Amina Haque, helped with proof-reading and comments.

Last but not least the publishers have been most courteous and helpful throughout.

PART I

PRINCIPLES

1 Introduction

Surgery has been practised from time immemorial. The earliest examples of surgical work included the care of wounds, the drainage of abscesses and the splinting of fractures. Modern surgical practice has come a long way from those early days. Before he embarks upon a detailed study of the subject, the student should have a general idea of what surgery is all about, and what is its scope. At the same time he should be knowledgeable about the way in which, over the centuries, surgery has evolved to attain its present state of refinement and advancement.

The scope of surgery

Surgery can be defined as that branch of medicine which treats diseases and injuries by manual or operative methods. Let us see what this means in actual practice. If a viscus is diseased, it may be *removed* by operation, for example an appendix which is inflamed, or a testis which is the seat of a cancer. If an organ is irreversibly diseased but is vital for life, e.g. the heart or the liver, it may be *removed and replaced* by another, taken from a living donor or a fresh cadaver (transplantation). If a bone is broken, its ends are brought into alignment and held together, either in a plaster of Paris cast or by internal fixation by a nail, until they unite to each other.

Many internal organs are in the form of hollow tubes, e.g. intestines, arteries, veins, ureters, bile ducts, etc. If such a tube gets blocked the contained fluid, e.g. blood, urine or bile accumulates and stagnates in the tube, producing harmful effects on the person's health. Such a tube needs to be *unblocked*, and an important part of any surgeon's work consists of unblocking such tubes. In this sense surgeons are plumbers, or in other words biological engineers.

There are many methods of dealing with such a block in a tube. The *material* blocking the tube may be *removed* by slitting open the tube. For example a polyp in the small intestine, or deposits of cholesterol in an artery, may be removed through an incision in the wall of the intestine or artery. In other cases the narrowing may be eliminated by shifting a *flap* of the wall of the tube across the narrow area to widen it, as at the pelviureteric junction in a case of hydronephrosis. If the blockage is due to excessive hypertrophy of a sphincter it may be dealt with by *dividing the sphincter,* as in infantile pyloric stenosis.

If the block cannot be eliminated by one of the above methods, the blocked segment of tube may be *removed* and the continuity of the tube restored, as in the case of the intestine or an artery. In the case of the intestine the ends are simply brought together and joined to each other. With an artery the ends normally cannot be mobilized and brought together; therefore, the gap is usually filled either by a segment of a vein, or by a tube made of synthetic material. If the tube can neither be unblocked nor removed, the block may be *bypassed*. For example, in a case of inoperable carcinoma of the caecum the ileum may be joined to the transverse colon, bypassing the obstruction.

The job of a surgeon consists of finding out the cause of the patient's symptoms i.e. the nature of his illness, and using the appropriate operation or other mode of treatment to remedy the defect. For this he must first possess knowledge of the natural history of different surgical conditions. At the same time, he must be familiar with the different methods of examination and investigation to extract the maximum information from the patient for arriving at the correct diagnosis. Next, he must know which operation or other method of treatment suits his patient the best, and should be able to employ it. Finally, if a complication arises during the postoperative course, he should be able to deal with it.

But that is not all. The surgeon should not be a mere robot carrying out the above-mentioned functions to perfection. He should above all be a compassionate human being, pleasant and smiling. Most patients are afraid of surgical operations. If the practitioner of the art is seen by them to be friendly, their fear of the operation is considerably reduced, which makes it easier for them to withstand what they expect to be an ordeal. In cases with incurable illnesses the surgeon must utter words of encouragement, and must never let the patient feel he has been forsaken by his medical attendants.

The reader should remember that on becoming a surgeon he is going to have the privilege, but also the responsibility, of working on the most precious asset of an individual, namely his health and life, and that the patient's welfare should always be his first and foremost concern. He will be judged by how well he discharges this responsibility. Surgery offers a fascinating, although a demanding career. The author feels privileged in welcoming newcomers into this field.

The evolution of surgery

Surgery is old as mankind itself. Human skulls in which circular fragments have been removed as if by trephine have been found dating back to the Stone Age. Such operations were performed for headache and for epilepsy in order to allow the egress of evil spirits! However, apart from the splinting of fractures and the drainage of abscesses, not much of consequence was achieved in the ancient world. One of the reasons for the slow development of surgery was the severe punishments reserved for surgeons in the case of failure. For example, under the code of Hammurabi in western Asia about 4,000 years ago, if the patient died after operation, the surgeon's hands were cut off!

Even from those far-off times, examples of accurate recording are occasionally found. From the Egypt of 5,000 years ago, the Edwin Smith Papyrus describes a series of 48 cases of trauma, listed from the head downwards, and enumerated in order of increasing severity of injury, which is indeed startling for a paper written so far in the past. The value of fixation in the treatment of fractures was appreciated, and splints were made from linen bandages impregnated with resin.

The single greatest achievement in the history of medicine was the exclusion of demons, spirits and sin from the explanation of the cause of disease. Only after this was done could true cause and effect relationship be sought for and established. Darius I of Persia established at Sais around 500 B.C. what seems to have been the first school of medicine. Students were selected 'from among the sons of men of consequence, no sons of the poor were among them'.

The god of Greek medicine was Aesculapius. During the 5th century B.C. numerous temples of health were erected to him. The priests treated patients with a combination of mysticism, burnt offerings and baths. The best known pupil from one of these schools was Hippocrates. He was distinguished by his straightforward observations and logical deductions. He clearly recognized the principle of traction in the reduction of fractures and dislocations. He classified physicians into the ordinary practitioners, those of a higher class, and the intelligent ones. In those days the surgeon was usually to be found in the first category.

An opportunity for the development of physicians of the second category arose with the founding of a medical school by Alexander's successor Ptolemy Soter at Alexandria in the 4th century B.C. Scholars and books were brought here from Greece and from the whole world. Dissections of the human body were started and normal body functions studied. The pulse was counted and the flow of blood through arteries and veins noted. The lens was removed for the treatment of cataract. The library became a fabulous institution, containing 700,000 papyrus rolls; when it was destroyed by the invading armies of Julius Caesar, civilization received a very severe blow. Some of the achievements in medicine have been preserved for us by the writings of Celsus and Galen. The former's treatise *De Medicina* is a remarkable document. The last two of eight books concern surgery. The cardinal signs of inflammation are stressed, the treatment of fistulas, the drainage of abscesses, use of the ligature, and debridement of wounds is described. The removal of bladder stones is detailed.

The Romans possessed a strong antipathy to the medicine of a foreign people. For centuries the contributions of Hippocrates and the Alexandrian school were held in contempt. In its place they preferred to adhere to mysticism, and were without physicians for 600 years until, after the conquests by Pompey in the first century B.C., many Greek physicians began to migrate to Rome.

The development of medicine over the next 1500 years was to be coloured by the work of Galen. Apart from numerous anatomical dissections, he studied function. He called attention to the fact that injury to the cord between the first and second cervical vertebrae produced instant death, between the third and fourth respiratory paralysis, while below the sixth the muscles of the thoracic cage were paralysed and there was chiefly diaphragmatic respiration.

The millenium following upon the death of Galen was quite unproductive, for two main reasons. Firstly, the authority of Galen was so great that none could challenge it for many centuries after his death, and this led to intellectual stagnation. Secondly, the Christian Church took hold in the Mediterranean area, and the concept of cure by prayer and miracle was strengthened. It was believed that disease was caused by sin. Therapy was thus directed to the soul and not the body. There was an edict against dissection of the human body. At the same time the body was not to be mutilated, and therefore the making of an incision was condemned. Under such a situation surgery could not develop, and in fact rapidly declined in the Christian lands.

Fortunately the intellectual leadership, which now moved eastward to the Arabic world, carried with it the Greek achievements which were translated into Arabic, preserved and modified. The prominent names are those of Rhazes (860 to 932 A.D.) and Avicenna (980 to 1037 A.D.). One whole book in the former's *Continens* is devoted to surgery. The writings of these two dominated medicine of the Western world for centuries.

In 1092 the Pope decreed that monks were not to wear beards. A barber was therefore employed in most monasteries. It was also the custom for monks to be bled at intervals, and naturally it was the barber who performed this function also. These barber-surgeons soon started performing minor surgical procedures, first inside the monastery, but later in society in general.

In 1163 the Council of Tours declared that 'the Church abhorreth bloodshed'. Now, most educational institutions were operated by the Church, and had to respect this ban. Therefore by default surgery had to be practised by uneducated and often unethical craftsmen — the barber and the lithotomist.

During the sixteenth century impressive advances were made in the study of both the structure and function of the human body. Vesalius concentrated on anatomy. Inspired by the depiction of the human form by artists of the calibre of Raphael and Michaelangelo, he hired artists of the first rank to illustrate his dissections. William Harvey was impressed with the demonstration by Fabricius of one-way valves in veins, and deduced the system of circulation of the blood.

During the seventeenth century Malpighi in Italy demonstrated, under a microscope, capillaries and capillary circulation, the layers of the skin, nerve pathways in the spinal cord, and the glomeruli of the kidneys. It was also shown that blood contained a solid component, the red cells. Boyle showed that air was necessary for an animal to sustain life, and that the lungs provided this function. His assistant Hooke gave the concept of the cell. The same century also witnessed the performance of operations on the abdomen, including colostomy and cholecystostomy. John Hunter made important contributions in experimental surgery, including the implantation of lead pellets into the shaft of long bones of puppies to demonstrate that longitudinal growth took place at the epiphysis. His pupil Abernathy demonstrated the regeneration of peripheral nerves following neurectomy and suture.

In America, surgery hardly existed until after the revolution. The first medical school in America was started in Philadelphia in 1761. William Shippen, the first professor of surgery, had studied with Hunter at London. In Boston John Warren, also a surgeon, played an important part in the founding of the Harvard Medical School. Because of its late beginnings, surgery in America was saved the turmoil of being involved with barbers, of being controlled by the church, and of having to contend with overbearing physicians. At first American surgery represented a transfer from European centres; later it assumed a character of its own.

The discovery of anaesthesia during the nineteenth century was a quantum leap forwards. Both ether and chloroform were first used in the 1840's. Surgical operations could now take place in a calm and quiet atmosphere, and the surgeon could proceed in an unhurried manner. Before this time, the surgeon had to employ strong men to restrain the patient on the operation table, and it is obvious that only the simplest procedures had been possible under those circumstances. It is not a mere coincidence that a very large number of complicated and extensive operative procedures were first carried out during the succeeding half of the same century; anaesthesia had made the job of the surgeon much easier. Thus we notice Kocher with his thyroidectomy, Halsted and his radical mastectomy, and Billroth and Polya with their respective gastrectomies, all within the span of a few decades. By achieving these 'firsts' due to the availability of anaesthesia the surgeons of that generation assured their place in history, and appear larger-than-life even today.

From that time onwards the speed of scientific progress picked up considerably, so much so that more advancements have been made during the twentieth century than in the previous fifty centuries combined. Removal of the lung for cancer, and removal and substitution of the oesophagus by the stomach became routine procedures.

Since the Second World War, developments in the field of surgery have proceeded with mind-boggling speed. Operations like replacement of the heart, liver or kidneys, which could not even be imagined a few decades ago, are commonplace. Whereas previously surgery consisted mainly of ablative procedures, advances in surgery are more and more being made in the field of reconstruction, whether in the case of the urethra in cases of stricture, the rectum in congenital anomalies, the thumb in cases of loss due to trauma, or the mandible after its excision for malignant disease. At the same time, plastic surgeons are constantly inventing newer and better methods of correction of defects due to congenital anomalies and loss of tissues.

Finally, with the emergence of large numbers of independent states around the globe, medical schools have come up in these countries. With the numbers of physicians and surgeons multiplying with geometric progression, specialization and super-specialization is the order of the day. More and more medical schools in these countries are achieving a reputation and status unimaginable a few decades ago. Often only a year or two elapses between the introduction of a new technique in the advanced countries and its adoption in these developing countries. In this environment of intense international competition, the future of surgery is assured worldwide.

2 *Wounds*

This is one of the most important chapters in this book, because all his life a surgeon has to take care of wounds. Whether he operates upon the stomach or the kidney, the hand or the foot, a wound inevitably results. Again, he has to look after wounds sustained at home, in the factory, in traffic accidents, and due to assault by different weapons. He should thus have a very clear understanding of the process of wound healing to be able to take good care of the thousands of wounds he will come across during his surgical career.

Historical note. In ancient times wounds were taken care of gently. The principles were: removal of foreign bodies, suturing, and covering with clean materials. However, in the fourteenth century, with the increasing use of gunpowder and the frequency of bullet wounds, aggressive methods of wound care were employed. Boiling oil and hot cautery replaced simple washing. Cleanliness was forgotten. This attitude produced disastrous results. The mortality rate after amputation of the thigh ranged from 80 to 100%, mostly due to sepsis.

In the sixteenth century, during a particular battle the supply of oil was exhausted, and Ambrose Pare, the surgeon, had to treat amputation wounds without boiling oil. To his surprise, these wounds healed rapidly without the normally expected complications. From this beginning the era of gentle wound care evolved. John Hunter and others showed that minimizing tissue injury produces rapid healing. Most technical advances in wound care over the past century have been based on this concept of minimum interference. Finally the late nineteenth century witnessed the discovery of bacteria and the introduction of aseptic surgical techniques to keep those micro-organisms away from wounds. This inaugurated the modern era of wound management.

THE PROCESS OF HEALING

The inflammatory response. Inflammation, followed by repair, commences as soon as a wound is inflicted:

Coagulation. Injury causes haemorrhage from damaged vessels. Platelets derived from the haemorrhage release clotting factors to produce fibrin, which is haemostatic and also forms a mesh for the migration of inflammatory cells and fibroblasts. Platelets are also the first cells to produce several essential cytokines which modulate most of the subsequent events in wound healing.

Inflammation. Within a few hours white blood cells accumulate in the wound. At first the predominant cell is the *polymorphonuclear* leucocyte. These cells die, lyse, and release acid hydrolases. Soon the proportion of *monocytes* increases. These cells continue their activity of clearing the debris for several weeks. It is of interest to note that wound healing proceeds normally in the absence of both polymorphs and lymphocytes. In contrast to this, monocytes must be present for normal production of fibroblasts, and for invasion of the space by them. Inflammatory cells regulate connective tissue matrix repair; however, the messengers of repair are the cytokines, which in the past were called 'growth factors'.

Fibroplasia. It is at this stage of wound healing that *fibroblasts* make their appearance, and soon they start laying down collagen fibres. Most of these fibroblasts are derived from the local mesenchymal cells. As the fibroblasts and capillaries advance into an area, the previously laid fibrin strands get dissolved by the enzyme plasminogen activator produced by the endothelial cells of the capillaries. If large amounts of fibrin, blood clot or dead tissue are present, they constitute a physical barrier against fibroblast penetration. It is only after the macrophages have removed all this matter that fibroblasts can come in and start laying down collagen fibres.

Finally when the fibroblasts, with the help of nutrients brought by the capillaries, have laid down collagen, they themselves are no longer required. Both fibroblasts and capillaries now get greatly reduced in number. Collagen fibres now become the predominant feature of the wound. Quite quickly, small bundles of fibres running in different directions fill the entire wound space. These bundles enlarge gradually and produce a massive, dense collagenous structure, the scar, binding the divided tissues firmly.

Components of healing. Three separate mechanisms are involved in all healing processes:

Epithelialization is the process whereby keratinocytes migrate and divide to re-surface loss of skin or mucosa. This activity ceases when epithelial contact is re-established with adjacent epithelial cells. It proceeds most rapidly in a moist, highly oxygenated environment.

Contraction is the process which leads to spontaneous closure of full-thickness skin wounds. It is the form of migration that involves the whole thickness of the skin and subcutaneous tissues. It therefore proceeds most readily in areas where the skin is loose such as the back of the neck. It is due to forces exerted by specialized fibroblasts which contain contractile elements in their cytoplasm and are called myofibroblasts. It is the same process that leads to constriction of tubular organs such as the common bile duct or oesophagus after injury. It is a physiological process and must be distinguished from the pathological process of scar contracture or cicatrization which produces distortion and limitation of movement.

Connective tissue formation is the process whereby fibroblasts are recruited to the site of injury and produce a new connective tissue matrix. It is the mechanism by which the main body of the wound is united, and the strength of a wound following surgery depends upon it. The cross-linked collagen in the connective tissue provides strength and integrity to all the tissues. The major components of the extracellular matrix and their functions are the following:

Component	*Function*
Collagen	Strength, support and structure for all tissues
Elastin	Allows tissues to expand and contract
Fibronectin	Mediates cell-matrix adhesion
Proteoglycans	Store moisture, absorb shock
Hyaluronic acid	Provides fluid environment for cell movement

Cytokines in wound healing. A cytokine is a soluble molecule produced by a cell to induce a biological effect elsewhere. It acts as a messenger at its destination. The effect varies according to the cytokine and the cell, but typically these molecules signal certain cells to activate, divide, or home in on a particular site in the body. Some examples are given in Table 1.

TYPES OF WOUNDS

Wounds are of two types — closed and open wounds.

CLOSED WOUNDS

When a surgeon incises the skin cleanly with a sharp knife and then sutures the wound neatly, coapting the wound edges accurately, there is very little dead tissue or extraneous matter in the wound, which therefore heals very promptly. Repair in this manner is called *healing by first intention.* The duration and intensity of this inflammatory response depend upon the amount of local tissue damage. In the usual clean incision acute inflammation subsides within a few days. While dead material is being removed from the deeper areas the epidermis at the wound edges begins to thicken within a few hours of injury. If the wound has been sutured carefully, the edges are closely coapted to each other. Epithelial cells migrate across the defect and within 48 hours the entire wound surface is epithelialized, many layers of cells being produced. At the same time, the superficial layers become keratinized, as in the normal skin.

If the wound is a badly lacerated one, or has been made by the surgeon without using fine and gentle technique, extensive tissue injury may be present, which may prolong the inflammatory response for many weeks, or even months. The presence of foreign bodies or bacteria also prolongs the time taken for healing.

OPEN WOUNDS

The basic morphological and chemical processes operating in open wounds are the same as in incised and sutured wounds. However, the clinical problem presented is entirely different. Contraction takes place which distorts the wound, and epithelialization over the wound becomes a problem, specially if skin has been lost. The natural healing of an open wound is called *healing by second intention* or *by granulation.*

Open wounds without skin loss. If an incised wound is allowed to remain open it begins the healing process normally. An inflammatory exudate collects on the surface. Marginal epithelial cells mobilize, divide and migrate down the edges under the exudate. Injured venules branch and form capillary networks, and fibroblasts invade the injured area. The surface of such a wound is granular due to the looped ends of the advancing capillaries. This appearance has given it the name of *granulation tissue.* If the wound is heavily contaminated it is best left open for a few days. During this period the number of bacteria on the wound becomes greatly reduced, and the wound can be closed. This *delayed primary suture* can prevent infection from developing in contaminated wounds.

Open wounds with skin loss. If a piece of skin has been lost and the wound is left alone, it is closed by the process of contraction. The wound contracts by stretching the surrounding skin, *not by production of new skin.* In areas which are away from joints and where the skin is loose, wound contraction produces minimal deformity. However, where mobility is important, e.g. the fingers, contraction resulting even from a small wound produces serious functional impairment.

Contraction can best be eliminated or minimized by immediately replacing the missing skin. Full thickness

Table 1 Some cytokines that promote wound healing.

Cytokine	Source	Function
Platelet-derived growth factor (PDGF)	Platelets, macrophages, endothelial cells and smooth muscle cells	Fibroblast proliferation; chemotaxis; collagen metabolism; activation of neutrophils, macrophages; angiogenesis
Tumour necrosis factor (TNF)	Macrophages, mast cells, T lymphocytes	Fibroblast proliferation
Interleukins (IL-1 etc.)	Macrophages, lymphocytes, other tissues and cells	Ditto plus collagenase, neutrophil chemotaxis
Epidermal growth factor (EGF)	Platelets, saliva, urine, milk, plasma	Fibroblast & epithelial cell proliferation; granulation tissue formation

grafts or flaps work best in this respect; partial thickness grafts are less effective, because they themselves contract down to some extent. But if the areas of skin loss are large, they represent the only practical method available for replacing the loss. In areas where the tissues are fixed and there is little excess of skin (e.g. over the skull or lower leg), even maximal contraction cannot close a large defect. Sufficient skin simply cannot be pulled into the wound. The wound remains uncovered as an open ulcer, and has to be treated by a skin graft.

Open wounds are covered by a plasma protein exudate which becomes dried, and also contains dead cells. This is called a *scab.* In the case of burns the denatured collagen of the dermis may remain in place. This is called an *eschar.* In either case granulation and epithelialization occur beneath the surface of the scab or eschar.

Epithelialization. Epithelial cells can migrate up to 2.5 cm from the wound edge to close a defect. However, defects which are too large cannot be covered by this process. In such a case the wound becomes a chronic open ulcer. Adequate coverage by skin grafts can prevent this disastrous complication.

The stimulus for epithelial repair is unknown. The loss of contact between cells undoubtedly plays a part. When an area is denuded of epithelium, the marginal cells divide and migrate across the area. This activity ceases when contact is re-established with adjacent epithelial cells.

Epithelialized scar tissue is not as strong a covering as normal skin. The normal epidermis is very firmly attached to the underlying dermis by a strong basement membrane which has an undulating surface for a more secure union. The hair follicles and sweat glands also provide a strong epidermal-dermal junction. On the other hand, the junction of epithelium with scar tissue is quite weak and flimsy. Even minor shearing forces produce epithelial separation and loss. At the same time, whereas normal skin is quite thick, having many layers of cells and squames, the epithelium covering scar tissue is usually much thinner. For both the above-mentioned reasons, epithelialized scar tissue remains a poor substitute for skin.

PHASES OF HEALING

During the first few days nothing seems to be happening in the wound, and therefore this has been called the *lag phase.* It should better be called the *preparation* phase, because during this period the metabolites required for repair are being collected at the site.

During the next few weeks the cells and capillaries proliferate. Neutrophils and macrophages are prominent, and fibroblasts lay down collagen in increasing amounts. In an open wound this fibrocellular tissue is called granulation tissue, because its surface is granular due to the looped ends of advancing capillaries. This is the phase of proliferation or *fibroplasia.*

After a few weeks these activities slow down. Fibroblasts and capillaries are now fewer in number, but strength progressively increases. This third phase is called the *maturation* or *differentiation* phase, and lasts many months.

FACTORS INFLUENCING WOUND HEALING

General factors. Healing proceeds more rapidly the younger a patient, provided he is well nourished. This increased vigour of repair may explain why hypertrophic scars and keloids are more common in the young. A patient who is suffering from malnutrition is deficient in proteins, which are the building blocks for repair of damaged tissues. Therefore his wound will heal slowly. However, the wound enjoys biological priority compared to ordinary tissues. Therefore, protein depletion has to be severe before healing is affected. Similarly, deficiency of vitamin C and zinc, and administration of steroids or cytotoxic drugs delays healing. Wound healing is also impaired in the jaundiced or uraemic patient, due to disordered metabolism of the tissue cells.

Local factors. ***Blood supply***. *A good blood supply is essential for prompt healing of a wound.* The face is richly supplied with blood, so wounds in this area heal well. On the other hand, blood supply to the feet is poor, and wounds on the feet take a long time to heal. Similarly, the arterial insufficiency of arteriosclerosis and diabetes may cause tissue necrosis and delay wound healing, specially in the feet. In patients with peripheral vascular disease, sympathectomy increases the blood flow and results in improved healing.

Tension in an inflamed tissue may cause a loss of blood supply and hence hinder the process of wound healing. If gross oedema is present the wound should not be sutured, because this further increases the tension.

Infection. *It should be remembered that local infection is the most important cause of delayed wound healing and dehiscence.* Infection causes an inflammatory response which increases tissue tension. Tissue necrosis may also occur and cause wound breakdown. Collagen synthesis is depressed and collagenolysis is increased.

Oxygen. *Oxygen is the most important wound nutrient.* A wound can only heal if its cells are functioning in a healthy vigorous fashion. The delivery of oxygen to the wound is impaired by a number of local factors, such as tissue trauma and tight sutures.

COMPLICATIONS IN WOUND HEALING

In the short term a wound may get infected, and it may breakdown. In the long term, the scar tissue produced in the wound may produce problems.

Wound infection. This is the most common and troublesome disorder of wound healing. In the past it was believed that contamination was mainly a postoperative problem, and that attention to ward design and dressing care would solve the problem. However, this has not been borne out by experience.

If bacteria are swabbed on the surfaces of a number of primarily closed wounds within the first six hours, nearly all get infected. After that time it becomes increasingly difficult to infect the wounds, until at 5 days they are as resistant as normal skin. Recent work suggests that in general surgical practice the main source of contaminating organisms is endogenous.

Degrees of contamination. A *contaminated* wound is one in which there has been gross spillage from the GI tract or, in the case of the biliary or GU tracts, definite infection is present. A clean wound with a major break in sterile technique also comes into this class. The reported infection rates here are between 15 and 25%, when prophylactic antibiotics are not used. Finally, in a *dirty* wound the wound surfaces are directly contaminated by purulent material or continuing discharges from hollow viscera. Infection rates are usually in excess of 25%.

It should be remembered that *local trauma from forceful retraction, excessive use of diathermy for haemostasis, and inaccurate suture ligation nullifies the most painstaking attention to asepsis.* The presence of a single piece of sterile silk suture material has been shown to enhance the infectivity of staphylococci thousands of times.

Dehiscence. If the margins of a healing wound break apart, it is a disaster. At the very least the patient requires another operation, and his hospital stay is prolonged. At the worst, specially in a patient with cardiac or vascular complications, a fatality may result.

Although collagen is rapidly synthesized, strength is recovered quite slowly. It takes almost 3 months for aponeurosis to recover 70% of its strength. While the strength of a wound is recovering, the synthesis and lysis of collagen are delicately balanced. Wound strength is therefore adversely affected by any factor which delays its synthesis or increases its lysis.

Synthesis is impaired in long-term steroid therapy, radiation injury, uraemia, jaundice and diabetes. It is also interfered with if starvation has been severe enough to reduce the body weight by about 20%. Antimitotic drugs delay collagen synthesis by paralyzing the fibroblasts, while hypovolaemia has the same effect due to the anoxia produced by it.

Wound fibrosis. In the closure of a wound, the formation of fibrous tissue is very necessary. However, an excess of such tissue can be a nuisance, specially at certain sites. For example:

1. If fibrous tissue glues down the tendon of a finger to its sheath, the tendon may no longer be able to glide freely in the sheath, resulting in stiffness of the finger, which is a serious disability, specially in certain professions. Similarly, fibrous bands forming on the peritoneal surfaces of the intestines may constrict and obstruct the intestines.
2. Fibrous tissue formation in a hollow tube, specially if circumferential, may narrow the lumen of the tube and make the passage of the contents of the tube difficult, e.g. in the oesophagus, ureter, etc.
3. Fibrosis of the mitral valve may produce stenosis and lead to right heart failure.
4. Bands of fibrous tissue across the portal tracts in the liver may constrict the tributaries of the portal vein and produce portal hypertension.
5. Traumatic cerebral scars resulting from head injuries may pull upon and irritate the underlying brain and result in epilepsy.

Attempts are being made to control such fibrosis, both by reducing the inflammatory response and by specific antifibrotic treatment of the scar. Polymerization of protocollagen may be prevented by β-aminoproprionitrile; penicillamine has similar effects.

SCARS

A scar is defined as the mark remaining after the healing of a wound or other pathological process. Although a scar may look thick and pink in the beginning, it changes in bulk and form over a period of many years. Its colour fades, its bulk decreases, any excess of pigment is resorbed, and it becomes less conspicuous. In a few persons, however, skin wounds do not heal normally, and instead produce massive keloids or hypertrophic scars.

Wounds in the foetus heal without any scars. One reason appears to be that the levels of hyaluronic acid are higher in foetal wounds, and this allows an orderly deposition of collagen. In due course it may become possible for surgeons to take advantage of this property of foetal wounds and repair cleft lips, etc. *in utero,* for healing without scars. It would be even better if the conditions obtaining in the foetus could be reproduced in adult wounds, so that scarring could be minimized or even eliminated in all wounds.

The strength of scars. Because of the above-mentioned changes, with the passage of time wounds become stronger. At two days, bursting strength in an incised rat skin wound is about 100 gm per linear centimeter. When collagen fibres appear on the third day, bursting strength increases rapidly, and by three weeks has reached over 1 Kg per linear centimeter. It should be noted that gain in strength does not stop here. Skin wounds continue to gain strength rapidly for about four months, and then more slowly for one year. However, normal elasticity, which is important in some tissue functions, is lost in scars. Most of the strength of scars comes from the *collagen fibres* they contain. Scars gain strength in three ways:

1. The number of collagen fibres increases.
2. The strength of individual fibres increases.
3. The irregularly arranged collagen fibres are replaced by fibres which are oriented more effectively.

Scar remodelling. The appearance of a scar changes over a period of many months. This process is called *scar maturation.* The red, firm scar becomes pale and soft, and is no longer adherent to the underlying structures.

With scar formation all injured tissues get bound together in a single unit by strong collagen fibres. This has different effects at various sites. In abdominal incisions it does not matter if the peritoneum, muscles, fascia and skin are welded into one unit. However, in many situations such a result is unsatisfactory. For example if a wound of a finger involves skin, tendon and bone, all injured components are quickly united by scar. The scar becomes strong, but active movements become impossible and the finger becomes stiff, resulting in a major disability.

Abnormal collagen metabolism. *Production.* In a normally maturing scar, collagen is at the same time being synthesized and lysed. This balance may be disturbed in different situations:

1. In keloids and hypertrophic scars, there is excessive synthesis and diminished lysis of collagen.

2. In scurvy the synthesis of collagen fails due to lack of vitamin C and the wound breaks down, because in the meantime lysis is continuing normally.

Arrangement. In uninjured skin, collagen fibres are arranged in well organized bundles. In sutured wounds, they lie in a haphazard manner, later coalescing to form irregular masses. However, the normal architecture is never restored.

Hypertrophic scars and keloids. Keloids and hypertrophic scars are both abnormal healing processes that occur after trauma or surgery. However, hypertrophic scars remain within the boundaries of the original wound and regress with the passage of time. By contrast, keloids extend beyond the boundaries of the original wound and do not regress. They usually recur after excision unless additional therapy is given. Keloids are normally pink in their early stages, but become hyperpigmented later. They are most common in negroes, and occur less often in light-skinned people. The most common sites of occurrence include the sternum and shoulder. Keloids contain a significant number of mast cells and have an abnormally high histamine content. As a result, these patients often suffer severe itching.

In both keloids and hypertrophic scars there is over-abundant production as well as decreased degradation of collagen. This is probably because of an excess of growth factors. Keloid cells produce increased amounts of cytokines, e.g. the transforming growth factor TGF-b. If antibodies to TGF-b are placed in guinea pig wounds at the time of closure, the wounds heal without any scars. This suggests that in the future inhibition of this growth factor may play a significant role in the clinical control of keloids and hypertrophic scars.

Treatment. At the present time the treatment of keloids and hypertrophic scars is not satisfactory:

1. For the severe itching an oral *antihistamine* is often helpful.

2. *Triamcinolone* may be injected into the keloid or hypertrophic scar. The adult dose consists of 2 ml of a solution containing 40 mg/ml, injected every 6 weeks to avoid systemic effects. The itching and pain are often relieved. The treatment also makes the lesion softer and smaller, and may be the only therapy required for small lesions. Complications include local atrophy of the skin and subcutaneous tissues, which may be severe.

3. *Surgical* treatment should be carried out only after careful consideration, because whereas a hypertrophic scar will usually regress without operation, a keloid tends to recur after excision. The patient should be made aware of the high risk of recurrence. Triamcinolone may be used in conjunction with surgery, being injected into the wound margins at the time of closure after excision. Some start the injections at various times after surgery.

4. The pattern of formation of new collagen in a wound is abnormal. While the fibres are being formed, their molecules get cross-linked and thus irreversibly fixed. If this cross-linking could be delayed, a more normal pattern of collagen would have time to develop. β-aminopro-prionitrile and penicillamine have shown promise in this respect. Finally, compression has also been of benefit in some cases.

Radiation therapy is mentioned only to be condemned. There have been no long-term follow-ups reported, and the late development of skin cancer after radiation constitutes a potential hazard.

THE CARE OF WOUNDS

This is a very important part of a surgeon's work, and good care of wounds pays rich dividends. If an operation wound heals promptly, a satisfied patient goes home within a few days; if the wound gets septic the matter may linger on for months, causing much distress, financial loss and frustration. During the past two decades wound healing has attracted considerable attention:

1. The mechanisms of repair are being defined on a biochemical and molecular level, and advances in molecular biology are helping the development of new drugs to enhance wound healing.

2. The economic loss imposed by chronic wounds is being realized.

3. Reconstructive techniques have improved with the advent of musculocutaneous flaps and microvascular free-tissue transfers.

And yet, in this age of advanced technology, in actual practice wounds are often badly managed. First of all, aseptic technique is not strictly adhered to. It is no use our discussing the properties of the latest and most expensive antibiotic in eradicating infection, if we are not first willing to take elementary aseptic precautions.

The *after-care* of wounds is also often carried out casually:

1. A separate set of instruments is not always used for each dressing.

2. In the tropical countries ceiling fans should be switched off while dressing wounds in order to minimize the chances of cross-infection; this is not always done.

3. The number of visitors to wards is too large. They bring in bacteria.

4. Septic cases are not always properly isolated.

5. The care of even difficult perineal wounds resulting after operations on anal fistulae is handed over to the most junior member of the surgical team, without much supervision.

Conversely, attention to all the above points leads to prompt wound healing.

Antiseptics. Antiseptics are chemicals which are capable of killing free-living organisms. Unfortunately, many also have a corrosive action, and leave stains. At the same time only a few kill spores. Thus in this respect they are inferior to steam sterilization or the hot air oven. The common antiseptics employed in surgical practice include the following:

For the skin. *Alcohol.* This is the cheapest and best chemical available for the routine cleansing of the skin around wounds, and allows removal of grease, dirt, etc. It is used in the form of *methylated spirit*; the methyl alcohol is added to make it poisonous, so that it cannot be misused by being drunk as an intoxicant.

Ether. Ether is a strong solvent of fats. A gauze swab soaked in ether solution removes particularly sticky grease, dirt, dried up discharges and marks of adhesive plaster in a most efficient manner. This solvent property of ether is not widely appreciated; it should be available on every dressing trolley for this purpose.

Povidone iodine solution has completely displaced tincture of iodine, which consisted of alcohol with the addition of 2% iodine. With the latter, cases of sensitivity to iodine were numerous. When combined with povidone, iodine is free of this toxicity. Its antiseptic effect, when applied and left on an area of skin, is considerable. Because of its bland nature, it can also be applied to wounds.

Cetavlon, diluted 1 in 40 or 1 in 100, is a mild antiseptic as well as detergent. It is used for cleansing wounds during dressings.

Chlorhexidine in a soapy solution is widely used by surgeons for washing their hands and forearms during scrubbing up.

For the wound. *Sodium hypochlorite.* This solution looks and smells like lime water. The wound is lightly packed with gauze soaked in this liquid. It clears up dirty wounds, helping greatly in the removal of sloughs. It comes under the label of Eusol.

Hydrogen peroxide solution is useful in wounds infected with anaerobic organisms.

Mercurochrome. This solution is applied to a wound for its continuing effect, and is probably useful. However, it stains the wound and surrounding skin red, and it becomes difficult to judge whether this is due to inflammation or to the colour of the solution. It is therefore no longer very popular. *Acriflavine* has similar properties but again, because it colours everything yellow, has lost some of its popularity.

For instruments. *Pure phenol* and *cresol* are very strong antiseptics and are suitable for immersion of sharp instruments for sterilization.

Glutaraldehyde 2% solution is effective, and is gentle to delicate instruments like cystoscopes. Spores require 10 hours of immersion for destruction.

CARE OF DIFFERENT KINDS OF WOUNDS

Surgical wounds. Most clean and sutured operation wounds require very little care. Because they have been made under aseptic conditions infection is not a problem. Because a minimum of trauma has been inflicted by using a sharp knife and gentle dissection, there is not much debris to be removed. Because absolute haemostasis has been achieved, there is no haematoma. Because the wound margins and edges have been accurately brought together, there is no dead space where serum could collect and become infected. All that is required in most cases is a *dry gauze dressing,* specially for the first day or two, until the wound becomes sealed off by coagulated serum.

Cotton-wool gauze is the best material for this purpose. It conceals the wound from view, protects it from dust, flies and knocks, and gently splints it. It soaks up any slight discharge, but very importantly, it allows free evaporation of sweat etc., and prevents the accumulation of moisture. Only if a complication e.g. haematoma or infection arises does the treatment have to vary from this simple routine.

Incised wounds. Incised wounds are inflicted by pieces of glass or by knives. In these wounds damage to the tissues is minimal. They may be closed by primary suture. Divided tendons, nerves and major vessels should be repaired at the same time. Penetrating wounds can damage important structures. This is the reason for the rule that all stab wounds of the abdomen must be explored.

Lacerated wounds. These commonly follow road traffic accidents. They are often contaminated with dirt and organic matter. If crushed and dead muscle is present, the risk of infection is increased. *Dead tissue must be removed thoroughly.* After this some of these wounds can be sutured primarily. However, the stitches should be applied loosely, in order to avoid tension and to allow any excessive exudate to discharge between them. Many lacerated wounds are so contaminated that after debridement they are best left open, being closed about a week later by the method of *delayed primary suture.* Repair of tendons and nerves is usually postponed for 4 to 6 weeks in these irregular wounds.

Crushed wounds. These commonly occur in severe industrial or road traffic accidents. *The main danger is from dead tissue,* all of which must be removed. At the same time, marked inflammatory oedema occurs in the injured tissues. If such a wound is sutured, tissue tension increases further and may cause more necrosis. All tension must be relieved by longitudinal incisions into the deep fascia. After this the wound must be left open.

When oedema has subsided in 4 to 6 days, and if infection has not occurred, *delayed primary suture* of the wound can be carried out. If the wound is still infected, it should be left open until infection is controlled, and then closed by *secondary suture.*

Open wounds. Open wounds require much more detailed care, and for much longer, than closed wounds. The dressing should be such which will not adhere to the granulation tissue, otherwise each time it is removed this tissue is damaged. Gauze impregnated with vaseline is commonly used. The amount of vaseline should not be excessive, otherwise it prevents the serum or other discharge from escaping into the overlying cotton wool. The cotton wool is held in place by a gauze bandage.

It is very bad practice to seal a dressing overlying a septic wound with sticking plaster. In fact by sealing even a clean sutured wound with adhesive plaster one creates a humid environment by preventing evaporation of perspiration from that portion of the skin. This excessive humidity can encourage infection. Therefore, even clean sutured wounds should not be sealed by adhesive plaster.

Specially when on the limbs, open wounds may be treated by *warm sitz baths.* Normal saline is the most physiological fluid for this purpose. It can easily be prepared by adding two teaspoonfuls (9–10 gm) of table salt to every liter of water. This method is usefully employed in perineal wounds. The patient is asked to sit in a basin of warm normal saline once or twice a day for a few minutes. This causes both irrigation and fomentation, and expedites wound healing.

The value of fomentation. Before the advent of antibiotics, hot fomentation was the only available method of management of inflammation and infection, and it was very useful. Nowadays an excessive amount of reliance is placed on antibiotics. They are sometimes used even when there is no infection but only inflammation, following trauma. Certainly, antibiotics have a place in the treatment of infection, but fomentation has an action complementary to that of antibiotics. Hot fomentation causes marked vasodilatation, so that many times more blood circulates through the inflamed tissues. Not only does this blood bring in more oxygen and nutrients, it also helps to promptly remove the waste products of inflammation, so that they do not accumulate in the tissues and produce deleterious effects. In short, the vasodilatation produced by fomentation greatly accelerates the process of inflammation and repair, resulting in earlier wound healing; therefore, fomentation should be employed more often. Even if antibiotics are employed, fomentation does no harm. The vasodilatation produced by fomentation allows larger quantities of antibiotics to be brought into the inflamed tissues, with beneficial effects.

Treatment of oedematous granulations. An infected wound often shows pale, oedematous granulations. These can be made more firm and pink by extracting fluid from them. For this purpose *magnesium sulphate glycerine paste* is very useful. Because it is strongly hypertonic, it extracts fluid due to its very high osmotic pressure. The hypertonicity also destroys bacteria. This paste should never be used on a fresh wound, because at that time the ends of severed nerves in the tissue are exposed, and mag. sulph. paste would cause intense pain. However, in a few days the nerve ends have been covered by a layer of granulations. Although the paste can cause the patient some discomfort this is short-lived, as it quickly becomes diluted. Improvement in the condition of the wound is usually very rapid.

If a small area of the wound shows excessive granulations, a 10 to 15% *solution of silver nitrate* can be applied. The caustic effect makes the granulations more firm. Alternatively, the surface of the wound may be touched by a crystal of silver nitrate. This has a very good astringent effect. If a silver nitrate crystal is used, care should be taken to remove it after touching the wound surface with it, as otherwise it can cause a burn. For the same reason silver nitrate powder should not be used, as it can spill over and cause a burn. To minimize the pain resulting from touching with silver nitrate, xylocaine jelly may be applied to the wound surface a few minutes in advance of the treatment. If sloughs are present in the wound, *Eusol* solution (a transparent solution containing sodium hypochlorite) can be used to help them separate. Gauze dipped in Eusol is used to dress the wound.

The importance of rest. For prompt healing of the wound it is extremely important to give rest to the injured part. This is specially important for wounds overlying joints, e.g. elbow or knee. Each movement of a joint stretches the wound and tears and damages the delicate granulation tissue which is being gradually built up by the microscopic processes of repair. Because movement of every joint takes place many times a day, the granulation tissue never gets an opportunity for uninterrupted healing, and the wound may become a chronic ulcer. Rest to the part, by bed rest or by splinting the limb, helps the same wound heal within a matter of weeks. In such a wound any number of antibiotics cannot achieve what simple rest can.

In the upper limb, rest can be provided quite simply by placing the limb in a sling. In the lower limb, the patient cannot hop around with one leg in a sling; so bed rest has to be enforced. Neglect of such a precaution leads to greatly delayed healing in the wounds resulting from even straightforward minor operations on the feet. This can best be explained to the patient by reminding him that if he were to walk about, he would be placing the weight of the whole body on the wounded part hundreds of times a day.

In the case of *abdominal operations,* if the only consideration was prompt wound healing one would advise absolute bed rest. However, this type of rest produces its own problems. Immobility after a major abdominal operation can result in hypostatic pneumonia. It can also produce deep vein thrombosis, which may lead to pulmonary embolism and death. Therefore one has to work out a compromise between the requirements of the wound and of general care of the patient. Early gentle but not excessive mobilization of the patient is advised, followed by gradual return to activity over a period of a few weeks.

BANDAGES AND DRESSINGS

A firm bandage applied properly over a pad of cotton-wool benefits a wound in many ways. By exerting firm and even pressure on the wound it discourages excessive oedema formation, collection of serum and the formation of a haematoma. If the wound is near a joint the bandage, by splinting the part, discourages movement and reduces the resultant pain. The cotton wool serves to absorb any discharge that may come out from the wound. *Every medical student should be taught to apply a well-fitting bandage to any part of the body.*

The importance of cotton wool as a dressing material. During the different ages cotton wool has remained the best material for the dressing of wounds. The important feature of cotton is its absorbent property. Unlike silk or nylon, it soaks up a large volume of fluid. Thus, it removes the fluid from immediate contact with the surface of the wound, where it would have caused maceration of the tissues. At the same time, being freely water-miscible, it allows fluids to seep through it and evaporate, producing a dry environment, in which bacteria cannot grow.

Role of different parts of a dressing. The surgeon must have a clear concept of the purpose of each of the different components of a dressing. If the wound is a *clean sutured incision,* commonly a small amount of sterilized gauze is placed to cover the wound, and is held in place by adhesive plaster. The gauze serves to conceal the wound from view. It also absorbs any small quantity of serum that may seep through the wound. Finally, if the environment is unhygienic it prevents dust and flies settling on the wound.

If the wound is clean and dry but needs some support and splintage, the gauze is covered by pads of cotton wool, and the whole is held in place by a bandage. The bandage is applied firmly (though not tightly), and helps to exert gentle pressure on the wound, which reduces the tendency to oedema formation and minimizes the pain. The cotton wool helps to distribute the pressure of the bandage evenly and makes the dressing more comfortable.

Table 2 Wound dressings.

Class	Composition	Properties	Indicated in wounds with..
Films	Semiocclusive polyurethane	Provides moist environment	Nil or minimal exudate
Impregnates	Fine mesh gauze with antibacterials	Does not adhere, promotes epithelialization	Moderate exudate
Calcium alginate	Fibres of calcium alginate	Highly absorbent, facilitates moist healing	Much exudate
Foams	Polyurethane film coated, absorbent	Absorbs fluid, debrides, vapour permeable	Much discharge, sloughs
Hydrocolloids	Hydrophilic colloid	Absorbs fluid, promotes granulation, epithelialization	Partial thickness wounds, pressure ulcers

If the wound is an *open* one, the gauze may adhere to the granulation tissue and make the change of dressing a painful experience. Therefore a layer of vaseline gauze is applied to the wound surface first, followed by dry gauze, cotton wool and bandage. Here the cotton serves a dual purpose. Not only does it help distribute the pressure of the bandage evenly, but it also soaks up any discharge of serum, pus or blood etc. If the discharge from a wound soaks the dressing, it is important to change the dressing promptly, otherwise the skin exposed to the discharge becomes macerated and irritated. At the same time, the moist external surface of the dressing allows the spread of the infection to the patient's bedclothes and thence further afield. This is the reason for the frequent change of dressings in discharging wounds, otherwise in clean incised and sutured wounds the dressing can be left in place for many days.

Modern dressings. During the last decade many new 'active' dressings have become available; some of them with their properties and uses are listed in Table 2. A good material for use as dressing for the deeper wounds is *silastic foam*. Two solutions are provided. These are mixed and poured into the wound. The silastic foam which forms quickly sets to produce a sponge, which conforms to the contours of the wound and provides an exact fit. It can be removed from the wound, washed and used again. It is inert and non-adherent.

3 *Trauma*

Trauma is defined as damage inflicted upon the body by an external force. About two centuries ago trauma was rarely a cause of death or serious disability. There were very few roads, and the horse-driven carriages of those days were slow. The arrival first of the railways and then of automobiles and aircraft changed all that. Today travellers move at speeds unimaginable in those days, and when a collision takes place the injuries inflicted on the body are proportionately severe. At the same time the number of automobiles has increased to millions. It is therefore not surprising that trauma counts as one of the major killers today. In order to understand how to look after a patient who has undergone a surgical operation or other kind of trauma, one must be familiar with the manner in which his body normally responds to injury, i.e. the changes which occur in the post-traumatic state, and how they are produced.

Metabolic response to trauma

After major trauma the body responds in a well-organized manner to the injury, conserving fluids, providing energy, if necessary at the cost of the body cell mass, etc.

CIRCULATORY FLUID VOLUME

One of the most important effects of trauma is a loss of circulating body fluids. Before discussing the effects of such a loss it is necessary to consider why it is important to maintain a normal blood volume, and to see how it is maintained during health.

Importance of maintenance of normal blood volume. In order to sustain life and health it is essential firstly that oxygen and nutrients be supplied to the cells of the different organs, and secondly that waste products be carried away from them. These two processes require perfusion of a sufficient amount of blood through the capillaries passing adjacent to the different cells. This perfusion in turn depends upon an adequate cardiac output, which is maintained by a sufficient blood volume and venous return. Therefore, for normal function of the cells of the different organs it is important that blood volume be maintained within normal limits.

Trauma lowers the blood volume. This is brought about in two ways:

1. From direct loss of blood.
2. From loss of fluid in the form of an exudate.

This fluid is sequestrated in the injured organ, so that a '*third space*' is formed. The result is that it is no longer available for exchange, and if a large quantity of fluid is thus lost, hypovolaemia ensues.

Response to reduced blood volume. When the blood volume falls the stimulation of the baroreceptors is reduced. Therefore the *nervous system is no longer inhibited to the same extent* as before. This loss of inhibition has the following important effects:

1. There is increased sympathetic activity. The adrenal medulla secretes more epinephrine and norephinephrine which constrict the arteries except those of the heart and brain. This helps in restoring the blood pressure to normal.
2. The kidney secretes more renin, which leads to the formation of angiotensin. The latter is a peptide having vasoactive properties. It constricts the arterioles and veins, thus reducing the vascular bed. It also constricts the renal arterioles, causing the kidney to conserve water and salt. In this manner it leads to an increase in the body fluid volume, which helps in raising the arterial blood pressure.
3. The secretion of ACTH and ADH from the anterior and posterior pituitary is reflexly increased.

In this way a decrease in blood volume causes a compensatory build-up of body fluids as well as an increase in blood pressure, thereby compensating for the original deficit and restoring the internal environment to normal.

BIPHASIC RESPONSE

The metabolic response to trauma manifests itself as a biphasic response, consisting of the ebb and flow phases. The *ebb* phase begins immediately after injury and is accompanied by hypotension, decreased intravascular volume, decreased cardiac output, poor tissue perfusion and haemodynamic instability. Loss of intravascular volume is an important factor in its development. However, the initial fall in cardiac output takes place before major loss of vascular volume, and is produced by neurohumoral mechanisms including histamine, activated complement factors, oxidants and prostanoids. Metabolic expenditure at this time shows a hypometabolic state, with a decrease in oxygen consumption.

If successful resuscitation takes place, the *flow* phase of the physiological response to trauma sets in. Cardiac output is restored to normal and later rises to more than *twice* the resting state for uninjured individuals. The accompanying hypermetabolic response is characterized by a large increase in metabolic expenditure, increased heat elimination, erosion of body cell mass and weight loss. The magnitude of this response is proportional to the size of the injury. The patient remains hypermetabolic as long as wound healing continues; this persists as long as the wound is hyperaemic and immature and only declines to normal values when the wound is fully mature.

ACIDOSIS

In low flow states and in cardiovascular collapse, large quantities of lactic acid accumulate and acidosis results. This acidosis is the *result* of the hypoperfusion and anaerobic metabolism, and not the cause of it. Acidosis interferes further with cellular function. It has profound effects on the cardiovascular system:

1. It reduces myocardial contractility.
2. It decreases the response of the myocardium and peripheral vessels to catecholamines.
3. It predisposes the heart to the development of arrhythmias.

If compensatory mechanisms are blocked or the change occurs too rapidly, death may result.

THE CENTRAL NERVOUS SYSTEM AND ENDOCRINE CHANGES

The main stimuli which activate the endocrine response to injury are hypovolaemia and pain. The hormonal response is diffuse, including increased release of ACTH, cortisol, growth hormone, epinephrine and norepinerphrine, glucagon, renin and aldosterone. *The hypothalamus controls these responses.* The afferent pathways are shared to a considerable extent. The result of this sharing is that the neuroendocrine response to injury is well coordinated.

THE HORMONES TAKING PART IN THE NEUROENDOCRINE RESPONSE

A large number of hormones take part in the response to trauma:

Epinephrine and norepinephrine. These are both secreted in response to trauma. *The secretion of these two hormones is the most basic of all post-traumatic hormonal responses.* This is so firstly because they are stimulated by all forms of trauma and stress. Secondly, they produce widespread effects on the circulation, on metabolism, and on the activity of other hormones. They increase the cardiac output and raise the blood pressure. They produce vasoconstriction in the skin, gastrointestinal tract, kidneys etc. to conserve blood for the essential organs, namely the heart and brain. Epinephrine stimulates glycogenolysis and lipolysis and inhibits the release of insulin. The increased secretion usually lasts only a day or so, unless the injury is a severe and persisting one.

If, however, because of continuing trauma, or because of the mistake of over-administration by the surgeon, the levels of these hormones remain high for a prolonged period, their effects on the body are harmful due to two reasons:

1. The energy stores (e.g. glycogen stores in the liver) become exhausted.
2. *Prolonged peripheral vasoconstriction produces ischaemia of cellular tissues.* Thus in the kidney ischaemic damage produces oliguria or anuria; in the stomach it results in acute gastric erosions, leading to haematemesis and/or melaena.

Cortisol. Injury leads to an increased secretion of ACTH and therefore of cortisol. In the presence of significant hypovolaemia ACTH secretion will persist until blood volume is restored.

In patients who have been on steroids for a long time the adrenal cortex undergoes atrophy. If they are not given steroids during an operation they may sometimes die because of failure of cortisol release from an adrenal rendered inactive by atrophy. Thus cortisol is necessary for the normal response to trauma, and it is very important to ask for a history of corticosteroid administration during the preoperative work-up of the patient.

Renin. In most cases of trauma there is increased secretion of renin by the cells of the juxtaglomerular apparatus of the renal afferent arterioles. Renin secretion is increased by sympathetic stimulation of the juxtaglomerular apparatus, by lowered renal arterial pressure, and by decreased delivery of sodium to the distal tubules. Renin converts angiotensinogen to angiotensin I. The latter is converted by an enzyme to angiotensin II. This substance stimulates the adrenal cortex to secrete aldosterone. It also increases the secretion of ADH and of ACTH from the pituitary.

Aldosterone. This hormone acts on the distal nephron to increase reabsorption of sodium, partly in exchange for potassium and hydrogen. *This effect is critical for life.* It is the main mechanism by which the kidney can excrete the potassium and acid which builds up in severe trauma, and thus prevent a dangerous degree of hyperkalaemia and acidosis, which could be fatal.

Antidiuretic hormone (ADH). In most cases of trauma there is an increased secretion of ADH due to afferent stimuli acting on the hypothalamus. Hypovolaemia also stimulates ADH release. This hormone acts on the distal tubule to increase water reabsorption. In the presence of ADH, if water is given without salt, sodium gets diluted and hyponatraemia results. If administration is continued, water intoxication may result, which produces disorientation, or even coma.

Glucagon. This is a diabetogenic hormone produced by the alpha cells of the pancreatic islets. Secretion is increased by hypoglycaemia and by sympathetic stimulation acting on the alpha cell. The main result of glucagon secretion in trauma is an *increase in blood glucose.* This is brought about by stimulation of glycogenolysis, gluconeogenesis and lipolysis.

Insulin. Secretion of insulin is never increased in response to trauma. In fact in the immediate post-traumatic period there is a relatively diabetic glucose tolerance curve, due to increased levels of epinephrine, ACTH, cortisol and glucagon, and reduced levels of insulin.

METABOLIC CHANGES AFTER INJURY

After a severe injury there is marked tissue wasting and weight loss. This is due partly to semistarvation and partly to the greatly increased catabolism following injury. *After injury the basic fact which stands out is that the body cell mass is sacrificed, while the extracellular volume is preserved.*

BODY CELL MASS

When cells are destroyed the products of cellular lysis are released into the extracellular fluid. Some of these compounds are converted into glucose and burned for energy. Most of the nitrogen is excreted in the urine as urea.

Skeletal muscle is the worst sufferer. The tissue most affected is skeletal muscle. This is shown by the visible and rapid decrease in bulk of the palpable muscles. The caloric requirements are increased to 5,000–6,000 per day. Relative starvation is the rule, and is the cause of the negative nitrogen balance. This release of the products of cellular protoplasm to the extracellular fluid and their excretion produces the following effects:

1. A negative nitrogen balance.
2. The loss of intracellular electrolytes (particularly potassium, phosphate and sulphate) into the extracellular fluid and thence to the urine via the kidneys.

Little effect on viscera. Whereas skeletal muscle mass is rapidly reduced, this catabolism of the post-traumatic state does not have much impact on the cell mass of *visceral* organs such as brain, heart, lungs, kidneys, gastrointestinal tract and liver. At the same time, even muscle recovers completely without any residual weakness. This suggests that each muscle cell is maintained intact in spite of severe reduction in its protoplasm.

Transient loss of tissues. Medium grade injury in the adult causes a loss of approximately 1 kg of wet lean muscle. At the same time body fat is lost. There is no evidence that this transient drain on muscle cells and fat after injury has any harmful effects on the healing of wounds and fractures, or the later achievement of a positive nitrogen balance.

Prolonged starvation. On the other hand *prolonged* starvation, either before or after injury, has clearly adverse effects upon all aspects of wound healing and bodily function, and is favourably affected by increased nutritional intake.

The importance of protein. It must be remembered that body protein is not designed primarily as a source of fuel, but performs other important functions in the form of enzymes, plasma proteins, structural protein, cardiac and skeletal muscle etc. During starvation man attempts to conserve protein by burning fat instead.

The need for alimentation. In short-term starvation the body is able to replenish protein at a rate equal to its degradation. However, with prolonged fasting in the presence of marked catabolism due to trauma, endogenous plasma proteins are burned. In this situation the liver cannot synthesize albumin at a rate equal to its loss. Therefore it becomes necessary to replace plasma proteins from exogenous sources. *Thus it is very important to administer amino acids, albumin or plasma to surgical patients who are in a catabolic state and unable to eat.* This is necessary not only to replace the plasma protein which has been lost externally or into the third space, but also that which is burned as fuel.

EXTRACELLULAR FLUID VOLUME

While the body cell mass is being reduced by lysis of protoplasm, the body devotes several active mechanisms to the conservation of extracellular fluid, and thus to the maintenance of plasma and blood volume.

Firstly, the level of sodium in the urine, sweat and saliva falls, preserving this ion.

The importance of sodium. The question might be asked: why is it so important to conserve sodium? The answer is that the *total osmolality* of extracellular fluid (and therefore its total volume) is largely determined by the sodium content. Sodium is the *water-holding* ion of the extracellular fluid. After injury a mechanism for conservation of fluid comes into play. There is a sharp restriction in the excretion of free water (antidiuresis). This is shown by a rising urine osmolality due to reabsorption of water in the distal tubules. In spite of the fact that it contains a reduced amount of sodium, the *osmolality of the urine is high.* This is due to the raised concentrations of the waste products of cellular lysis, namely phosphate, potassium and urea. Large water loads should therefore not be given to the postoperative patient. He is more apt to retain this water than the normal person. After injury patients are more easily swamped with sodium and water loads than in the normal state.

The plasma protein level falls due to dilution. This produces a tendency towards tissue oedema, specially of the lungs and brain.

CARDIOVASCULAR FUNCTION

High cardiac output. In the post-traumatic patient or after a low-flow state, elevated cardiac output is usual. This is due to two factors:

1. The effect of catecholamines, which stimulate the heart.
2. The shift of the oxyhaemoglobin dissociation curve to the left. The oxyhaemoglobin does not give up its oxygen to the tissues easily. Therefore in order to supply sufficient oxygen to the tissues an increased cardiac output is required.

In heart disease. In persons with heart disease who cannot support a high cardiac output the following undesirable effects can result:

1. *Cardiac* arrhythmias and congestive cardiac failure.
2. Peripheral *tissue* anoxia with lactic acidosis.
3. *Organ* failure (brain or kidneys).

RENAL FUNCTION

Post-surgical renal damage. Any significant reduction of blood volume produces renal vasoconstriction with hypoperfusion of the kidneys. When glomerular filtration rate falls below 20 ml per minute the kidney becomes very vulnerable to nephrotic damage from porphyrin pigments, drugs or chemical poisons. It is this combination of factors which results in post-traumatic renal insufficiency.

When there is decreased perfusion pressure at the afferent arteriole of the glomerulus, the juxtaglomerular apparatus interprets it as volume deficiency, and stimulates the production of renin, angiotensin and aldosterone. The result is a rise in blood pressure, retention of sodium and an alkalotic trend. If hydration and an osmotic load (in the form of mannitol, glucose or salts) are maintained, the result is well-filled renal tubules and high glomerular filtration rates. This is how adequate hydration and solute loading protect the kidney.

GASTROINTESTINAL TRACT

Reduced gut function. After severe injury anywhere in the body both absorption and motility of the gastrointestinal tract are reduced. If the injury involves the peritoneal cavity this reduction in gastrointestinal function is much more severe and prolonged. If efforts are made to feed the patient at this time the result is abdominal distension, severe peristaltic abdominal pain, and vomiting. It is in such a situation that special diets are particularly useful.

Special diets. The slow infusion of a *hydrolysed diet* into the small bowel (e.g. through a feeding jejunostomy), may be well absorbed and provide satisfactory nutrition in the post-traumatic patient, even though peristalsis is slow and the patient unable to hydrolyse and absorb a full protein-starch diet. When the total surface of available gastro-intestinal tract is inadequate, e.g. after massive resection of small bowel, the use of diets containing the basic elements of food, e.g. amino acids, glucose, etc. *('elemental diets')* helps convalescence greatly, as these diets do not have to be digested before absorption.

LUNGS

A variety of mechanisms can damage the lungs after trauma. They may arrive at the lungs by the airway, by the bloodstream, or by direct trauma:

Airway

– Aspiration of gastric contents.

– Inhalation of smoke chronically (heavy smoking) or acutely (burns).

– Prolonged mechanical ventilation.

– Prolonged immobilization in one posture, allowing secretions to collect and become infected.

Blood stream

– Fluid overload with osmotic dilution and pulmonary oedema.

– Multiple small platelet emboli from the area of trauma.

– Micro-organisms from peripheral infection.

– Vasoactive substances affecting pulmonary circulation: serotonins, catecholamines, and the kinins.

– Microemboli of transfused blood.

Direct trauma to chest and lungs

– Unstable rib cage, e.g. crushed chest.

– Prolonged open chest with collapsed or underperfused lung tissue.

When the combined effect of these different factors is great, post-traumatic pulmonary insufficiency results. The most common conditions predisposing to pulmonary insufficiency are a history of heavy smoking, chronic asthma, emphysema and bronchiectasis.

BRAIN

When arteriosclerosis is present, as in older people, cerebral function is very sensitive to poor perfusion. The left-shifted oxyhaemoglobin dissociation curve of alkalosis further reduces cerebral function. The symptoms produced by cerebral dysfunction are: disorientation, hallucination, extreme restlessness and coma.

Hypocarbia and alkalosis reduce cerebral function by producing cerebral vasoconstriction, and may lead to loss of consciousness. *This is a very bad sign in a surgical patient.* The brain needs an adequate supply of well-oxygenated blood with normal levels of glucose.

COMPONENTS OF ACUTE INJURY

Acute trauma commonly has three components: the local tissue wound, the volume reduction produced, and the catabolic state induced by the injury.

The tissue wound. Every wound initiates catabolism, and a continuously open wound inhibits anabolism. It fills up with a coagulum of albumin, globulin and mucopolysaccharides. This is changed to procollagen, and with the invasion of fibroblasts collagen is formed and tensile strength is gradually resumed.

Interestingly, this early and most significant phase of wound healing is completed during the period of negative nitrogen balance. Restoration of nitrogen anabolism is not necessary for wound healing. However, it is important for regaining muscular strength and vigour. The only substance required from outside the body for wound healing is ascorbic acid. Even here, deprivation of this substance for up to a month has no effect on wound healing if the patient has normal stores to begin with.

Haematomas in the tissue are a common result of injury or surgical operation. The blood undergoes haemolysis, and presents the kidney with a load of porphyrin pigments to excrete. If kidney function is impaired, these pigments (haemoglobin, methaemoglobin or myoglobin) can be nephrotoxic.

In the body's economy the wound has a high priority in its demand on building materials. Even in emaciated patients with advanced cancer undergoing palliative surgery one commonly finds strong healing and a firmly cicatrized wound. Conversely wound dehiscence, in which there is almost complete absence of fibroplasia, is as likely to occur in the previously healthy person as in the nutritionally depleted patient.

Burns provide an example of wounds that cannot be closed for many weeks or months; they are chronically colonized and infected. As long as a burn or other wound remains open, it inhibits protein anabolism and the resumption of growth. The patient remains ill and in negative nigrogen balance. As soon as the wound is healed or grafted the nitrogen balance becomes positive even on a low intake of calories and nitrogen, either by mouth or by the intravenous route.

Volume reduction, hypoperfusion and the low flow state. The confusion between injury and shock causes a great deal of difficulty. It is better to avoid the term shock altogether. It is preferable to use the terms 'volume reduction' and 'low flow state'.

Volume reduction. The term volume reduction means any reduction in the *effective* circulating volume of the blood.

This may be due firstly to simple haemorrhage. Secondly, it may be the result of acute desalting water loss, as in vomiting, diarrhoea, pancreatic fistula, intestinal obstruction etc.

Low flow state. The low flow state is defined as a situation in which *hypoperfusion of tissues passes the boundaries of physiological compensation* with disordered metabolism of all tissue cells as a result of anoxia. In other words *volume reduction, if severe and prolonged, leads to a low flow state.*

The key to differentiation between volume reduction and a low flow state lies in the occurrence of *cellular deterioration.* This can be measured in many ways:

1. By the deterioration of function of specific organs e.g. brain and kidney, whose function is obvious clinically.
2. By the accumulation in the blood of those electrolytes which are normally present *intracellularly,* and their excretion in the urine.
3. By the temperature and pulse rate.
4. By the raised blood levels of catecholamines.
5. By the production of prolonged severe tissue acidosis.

The presence of the above indicators of a low flow state indicates the existence of a *very critical situation.*

Catabolic state. The catabolism occurring after trauma shows a number of differences from simple starvation:

1. In simple starvation the maximum rate of nitrogen loss is 5 to 7 gm of nitrogen per 70 kg per day; in post-traumatic catabolism this figure lies in the range of 15 to 25 gm.
2. In starvation the blood sugar level falls and remains low; after severe trauma it rises.
3. The blood urea nitrogen level falls in starvation but rises after major injury.
4. In starvation urinary excretion of creatinine is very gradually reduced as the body cell mass falls; after severe injury it rises sharply.

In spite of these clear differences, starvation contributes an important component to post-traumatic metabolism, specially when it is continued for more than a few days after injury or operation.

Management. Predigested foods and balanced intravenous feeding mixtures are important in damping out the starvation component in the post-traumatic period. This is specially important in chronically ill patients with intestinal diseases, wounds, burns or chronic sepsis.

THE PHASES OF CONVALESCENCE

Four phases of convalescence are commonly recognized:

Acute injury phase. The patient has a rapid pulse with elevated cardiac output. He feels ill, desires to sleep, requires analgesics, does not wish to be disturbed, and wishes to remain immobile. *If the operation is smoothly performed with a minimum of tissue trauma and body fluids are restored to normal, both pain and the endocrine response to injury are minimized.* Body temperature is usually elevated after injury. Excellence of surgical and anaesthetic technique reduces this fever to a minimum. In two to five days this phase draws to a close. The patient looks brighter, the pulse rate and temperature are reduced, and he enters the turning point phase. Catecholamine responses have ceased.

Turning point phase. In this phase persistalsis returns, flatus is expelled, appetite improves, and diuresis occurs. The patient desires to see visitors and to 'return to living'. Food is assimilated easily as in simple starvation. Muscle protein synthesis occurs rapidly. The young woman again applies her lipstick and powder.

Anabolic phase. There is increasing strength, appetite, and food intake, normal absorption and a positive nitrogen balance. Most patients are returned home. Both growth hormone and insulin are active, restoring nitrogen compounds to the synthesis of actin and myosin in muscle.

Most surgical *complications* inhibit normal nitrogen anabolism. The most common of these are *prolonged wound sepsis, unhealed wounds, septic fractures and intestinal fistulae.* The condition of such a patient does not improve. He remains hospitalized or is discharged home to remain in bed.

As stated above, positive nitrogen balance is not required for the healing of the wound. However, it is essential for gain in strength and for the social rehabilitation of the patient.

Fat gain phase. When nitrogen balance returns to zero balance (indicating that muscle mass has been restored) the patient continues to gain weight and remains in positive caloric balance. Nearly all of this additional weight is due to the deposition of fat.

In conclusion, it will be seen that the body responds to trauma by a series of well-coordinated changes. A breakdown occurs only if a compensatory mechanism is overstretched.

GENERAL CONSIDERATIONS IN TRAUMA

Even today one-third of the patients who reach hospital die of surgically remedial causes. This percentage can be reduced by providing the necessary facilities as well as trained manpower.

Deaths from trauma. When one considers patients dying of trauma:

1. Approximately 50% die *instantaneously* or within a minute or two after trauma, generally due to an injury or a combination of injuries considered to be fatal, e.g. brainstem laceration or a ruptured heart. Only measures aimed at preventing accidents or decreasing the severity of the injury, e.g. motor vehicle safety restraints, can help reduce mortality from this cause.
2. About 30% patients die *within the next few minutes to hours* following injury, usually due to severe haemorrhage. *This period includes the '**golden hour**' which affords the clinician the best opportunity to safeguard the patient's life by high-quality pre-hospital care and prompt conveyance to a well-equipped hospital.*
3. The remaining 20% deaths occur *days or weeks* after injury, usually from complications, e.g. infection and multiple organ failure. A better understanding of immune depression can help prevent some of these deaths.

Facilities. The facilities for undertaking the care of victims of trauma at the site of the accident, at the hospital, and at a specialized trauma centre, should include the following:

1. Well-equipped ***ambulances*** with staff trained in the care of trauma victims.
2. Emergency rooms in hospitals, each provided with a ***'trauma area'*** equipped for emergency resuscitation. This room should contain such items as overhead operating room lights, oxygen, cardiac monitors and a defibrillator. A cabinet in the room should contain the following items:
    1. Laryngoscopes with different-sized blades.
    2. Endotracheal tubes of different sizes.
    3. Tracheostomy tray.

4. Closed chest drainage tray and different-sized tubes.
5. Venesection tray.
6. Central venous catheters.
7. Syringes for abdominal paracentesis.
8. Pericardiocentesis and peritoneal lavage catheters.
9. Intravenous fluids with tubing.

The cabinet shelves should have clearly visible labels under each tray or set of instruments. The trays should be kept in this trauma room and not in central supply, as a delay of even a few minutes may prove fatal in the very urgent case.

3. A ***trauma system*** operates within a city or province, and provides for rapid transport of victims of major trauma to specified hospitals (called trauma centres above), because they have concentrated resources and expertise to treat severely injured patients immediately and effectively. The integration of pre-hospital care, rapid transport and immediate surgical treatment within a trauma system *reduces preventable deaths* from this cause from nearly 25% to about 5%.

Priority by type of injury. There are three groups of patients according to the urgency of the case:

1. Injuries *immediately threatening life,* by interfering with vital physiological functions, e.g. obstruction of an airway or excessive bleeding from a wound. The primary treatment is to establish an airway and control the bleeding. Such a patient may require operation e.g. laparotomy or thoracotomy within a few minutes, for occluding major vessels to control massive internal bleeding.

2. Injuries posing *no immediate threat to life.* These include patients with either blunt trauma or gunshot or stab wounds to the chest or abdomen, but where the vital signs are stable. Most patients with trauma belong to this category. They usually require surgical procedures within 1 or 2 hours. X-rays may be obtained to determine the course of the missile and the extent of the possible associated injuries, such as fractures. *A doctor must be constantly in attendance*, because such a patient may develop shock (e.g. from internal haemorrhage) at any moment; if this happens he must be taken to the operating room immediately.

3. Injuries *producing occult damage.* These are patients in whom the exact nature of the damage is not apparent. Surgical exploration may be delayed for hours or days, as with delayed rupture of the spleen.

The management of trauma

Complete trauma care should consist of five phases: prehospital phase, resuscitation, operation, intensive care and rehabilitation.

Prehospital phase. As mentioned above, prehospital care helps most in patients belonging to the second group listed above, who can be saved if medical care is provided early. Prehospital care can be divided into basic life support and advanced life support.

Basic life support. Basic life support includes the following skills, *in which all prehospital personnel, e.g. ambulance drivers, should be adequately trained.* This can save lives:

1. *Extrication*, i.e. removing the victim from the site of the accident while providing immobilization of the spine and extremities to prevent further injury.

2. *Spinal protection*, including strapping the patient to a back board and immobilizing the head with sandbags and tape.

3. *Immobilization* of the extremities with splints: this prevents further damage to vessels, nerves and soft tissues and reduces the extent of haemorrhage around the fracture.

4. *Control* of external *bleeding*: this can be achieved by firm pressure over the wound.

5. Cardiopulmonary *resuscitation* if required. An adequate airway must be ensured and ventilation provided first, because without it cardiac massage is of no use.

Advanced Life Support. *Airway.* A patient who answers when questioned has an adequate airway and can be assumed to be able to protect that airway from aspiration. On the other hand a patient who is unconscious whether due to head injury or hypovolaemia is at risk for aspiration, and requires control of the airway. In comatose patients an endotracheal tube should be passed. This protects the patient from aspiration. It also enables gas exchange to be controlled. Further, the patient can be hyperventilated to control intracranial pressure.

Circulation. The *blood pressure* is assessed by palpation. If the radial pulse cannot be palpated, the arterial pressure is probably less than 80 mm Hg. *Peripheral perfusion* is estimated by evaluating the time required for capillary refilling. Delayed capillary filling (determined by compressing the capillary bed and watching for filling in less than two seconds) is a good clinical indicator of shock. If a patient has peripheral evidence of hypoperfusion and a blood pressure less than 90 mm Hg, he has lost 20–40% of blood volume, i.e. in the adult about 1–2 liters.

Catheters should be inserted into peripheral veins and isotonic crystalloid solution i.e. Ringer's lactate administered. Haemorrhage should be arrested by direct pressure and fractures splinted before or during transport.

Brain. In severe head injury a patent airway must be established and hyperventilation initiated as first line therapy and mainstay of treatment. In addition, circulating volume must be restored, to maintain cerebral perfusion pressure.

Resuscitation. ***Primary survey.*** At the hospital a primary survey is carried out to identify life-threatening conditions and management is begun immediately:

1. The *airway* is reassessed and cleared of blood, vomit and foreign body. The lungs are auscultated to assess the adequacy of ventilation. If this is inadequate (i.e. respiratory distress or respiratory rate greater than 35), the patient should be ventilated by a bag valve device (e.g. Ambu bag) connected to a mask until definitive airway control can be obtained with an endotracheal tube. Injuries which can compromise ventilation and perfusion, and require definitive airway management include: open pneumothorax, tension pneumothorax, massive haemothorax and a massively crushed chest.

2. *Haemodynamic status* is next assessed; useful indicators of the same include blood pressure, pulse, skin perfusion, urine output, mental status, and central venous pressure.

4 *Burns and grafts*

A major burn is one of the most severe injuries which can be suffered by man. Around the world millions of people suffer burns every year and tens of thousands die, resulting in great economic and social loss. Proper treatment requires understanding not only of the local injury but also of the haematologic, nutritional, immunological and psychological derangements that occur. The patient must be treated and rehabilitated as a whole person. In 1945 the United States army introduced the concept that major burns were best cared for in a 'burn centre'. This resulted in rapid improvement in survival and a reduction of morbidity of burned patients. Further, it led to the emergence of regional specialty treatment centers in other disciplines.

INCIDENCE

The largest group of burned patients are children under the age of 6 years, specially those less than 2 years old, the vast majority suffering from scald burns. A secondary peak incidence is seen between the ages of 25 and 35 years because of occupational injuries. Burns are more common among less advantaged persons due to overcrowding, faulty electrical systems, open-flame heating equipment, etc. Occasionally, inhabitants of cold climates sustain extensive superficial body burns from the misinformed practice of sunbathing in summer in the tropics. At the same time, severe friction can result in a burn (Fig. 1).

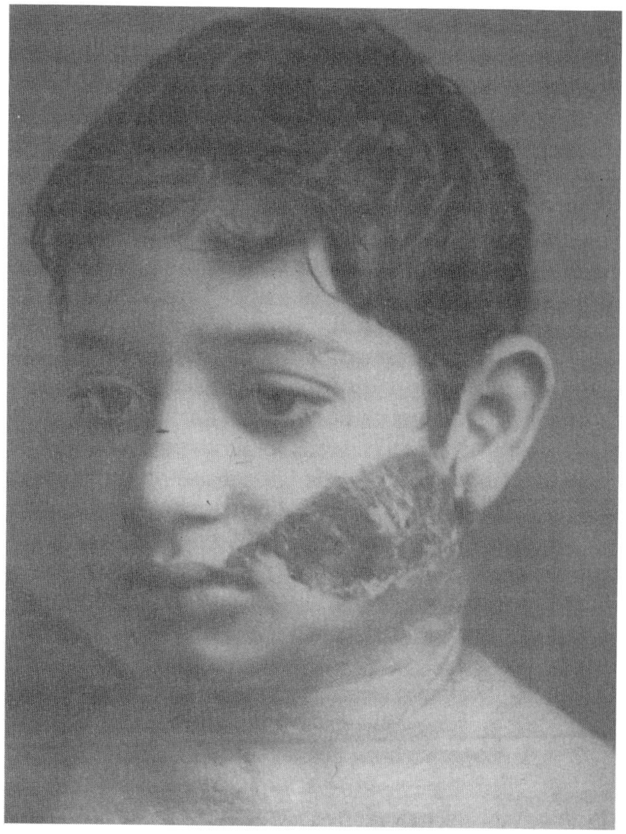

Fig. 1 Friction burn. The young boy's face was rubbed against the concrete of the road during a road traffic accident.

EVALUATION

The severity of a burn depends upon the following factors:

1. The age of the patient.
2. The extent of the burn.
3. The depth of the burn.
4. The actual site involved.
5. Whether an inhalation burn has also occurred.
6. The presence of coexisting disease states.

The *age* of the patient is important; burns in persons below the age of 3 years and over 60 years have more serious consequences for the patient than at other ages.

The *extent* of the burn is recorded in terms of percentage of body surface area burned. A *burn diagram* should be used, the exact location and extent of the burn being drawn on the body diagram. A rough estimate can be made in adults by using the Rule of Nine (Table 1), which indicates the area of each limb or part of the trunk as 9% or a multiple of 9% (See also Fig. 2). In small infants the head and neck as well as the trunk are relatively larger then the limbs, so the Rule of Nine is not applicable and other more detailed formulae have to be used. For small burns an area equivalent to the patient's hand approximately equals 1 percent of the body surface.

The *depth* of a burn is difficult to estimate. Generally, scalds tend to be superficial, and chemical and electrical burns are deep. Redness of the skin and thin water blisters generally occur in superficial burns, and thick blisters and

Table 1 Rule of nine.

Head and neck	9%
Right upper limb	9%
Left upper limb	9%
Front of chest and abdomen	18%
Back of chest and abdomen	18%
Right lower limb	18%
Left lower limb	18%
Genitals	1%
Total	100%

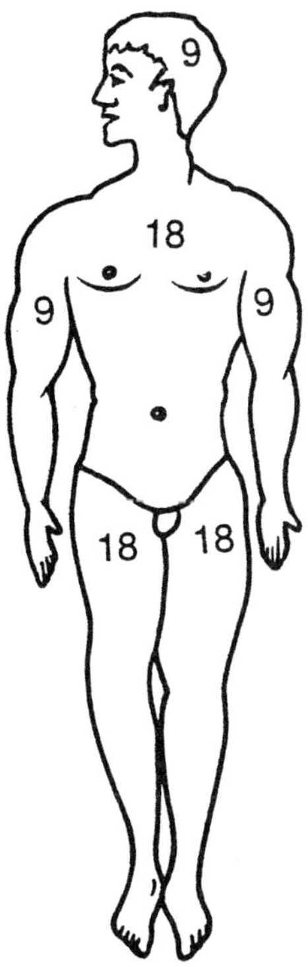

Fig. 2 Rule of nine.

leathery eschar in deep burns, but appearances may be deceptive. Sensation is not as helpful for estimating the depth of a burn as was once thought. In deep burns pinprick sensation is absent, but it can also be absent in burns of moderate depth. However, for the initial treatment of burns it is only necessary to separate those injuries which are clearly superficial and will heal rapidly from those which are deeper and will require hospitalization and specialized care. Accurate differentiation between superficial and deep burns becomes possible by the second week after the burn. During the first few days the extent of the burn is more important than its depth, for estimating fluid requirements and directing care. Later, when the question of skin grafting arises, burn depth assumes more significance.

Burns of the face and neck, hands, feet and perineum pose special problems in their reconstruction and rehabilitation. A common cause of instability and increased mortality in burn patients is severe *inhalation* injury producing extensive damage to the airways with pending obstruction, and this should be detected during the primary survey. Burnt nasal hair, conjunctivitis, hoarseness, bronchitis and carbon particles in the sputum should raise suspicion of inhalation injury.

A secondary survey should detect *associated* injuries such as head injuries, fractures, etc. *Coexisting disease,* whether cardiovascular, respiratory, renal or metabolic, can complicate the care of a burned patient and increase the mortality. On the other hand epilepsy and alcohol or drug abuse tend to predispose patients to burns. *Laboratory* studies should include blood count, electrolytes, biochemistry profile and blood gases, as well as carboxyhaemolobin concentration if indicated.

PATHOLOGY

THE LOCAL INJURY

Human skin can tolerate temperatures upto 40°C for brief periods of time. Temperatures above this result in increasing tissue destruction. Three zones of injury have been described. At the centre of the injury the cells are *coagulated.* Outside this is a zone of injured cells which *can survive* under ideal circumstances, but usually progress to tissue death. This area has been called the zone of *stasis.* Further out lies the zone of *hyperaemia* which recovers over a period of a week or so.

CLASSIFICATION OF BURNS BY DEPTH

Considering their depth, burns can be classified into the following categories:

1. Superficial (first-degree) burns. There is only erythema and discomfort. Within a few days the outer injured cells peel off, leaving no scarring.

2. Partial-thickness (second-degree) burns. These can be further subdivided into two types:

i. *Superficial partial-thickness burns.* The characteristic features in this type of burn are the blisters which form on the surface of the skin, and the exquisite sensitivity to stimuli, even a current of air. Since the basal layers of the skin are not destroyed, regeneration occurs promptly and these burns usually heal spontaneously in two or three weeks without infection (Fig. 3).

ii. *Deep partial-thickness burns.* These burns are more severe, with many areas of marginally viable tissue. They

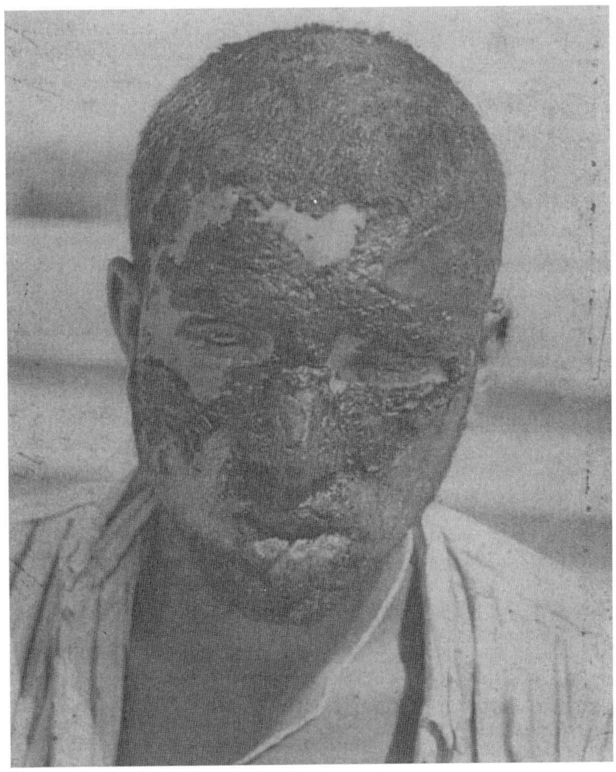

Fig. 3 Superficial partial-thickness burns face, 2 weeks old. The scabs are separating; underneath, the skin is intact.

show a decreased sensitivity to stimuli, e.g. pinprick. They can be defined as burns that take longer than 3 weeks to heal; this prolonged healing often results in hypertrophic scar formation. The skin only survives and heals under the most optimal conditions, otherwise it gets converted into a full-thickness burn. Only after 10 to 14 days can it be predicted accurately whether excision and skin grafting would give results better than natural healing. Many techniques have been tried with partial success to determine burn depth. These include thermography, fluorescein flowmetry, ultrasound, MRI, etc. However, *clinical observation remains the most reliable method* of assessing the need for grafting.

3. Deep (third-degree) burns. These burns contain totally destroyed skin. They are readily recognized. They appear white, charred, or parchment-like, and thrombosed veins can be seen through the dead tissue. These lesions are insensitive to pinprick. Fluid and cellular infiltrate accumulate in the margins of the wound. Whereas in the more superficial burns the vascularity of the skin is increased, this full-thickness burn is an avascular injury. It cannot heal by itself. Total-thickness skin loss can only be restored by ingrowth from the margins of the wound, or by application of skin grafts from the non-burned portions of the body.

4. Fourth-degree burns. These burns involve death or injury to subcutaneous tissues, such as fat, fascia, muscle or bone. After a burn is sustained oedema, decreased blood supply or bacterial invasion may further injure or destroy cells that have survived the initial thermal insult.

Burn oedema. A great deal of fluid accumulates in the burn area, due firstly to increased capillary permeability, and secondly to the breakdown of the cell membrane which damages the sodium pump. This causes an increase in intracellular sodium and water and an efflux of potassium. Neutrophils and monocytes also migrate into the area.

THE SYSTEMIC RESPONSE

Each one of the different organ systems of the body responds to the trauma of a major burn.

The circulation. In a major burn as much as 60% of the extracellular fluid may be lost, due firstly to excessive evaporation following destruction of the skin barrier, and secondly to fluid moving into those cells which have been injured by heat. Most of this loss occurs during the first 8–12 hours, but massive fluid losses continue for upto 48 hours after the injury.

The red cell mass is also reduced. This reduction is brought about by many factors, including the following:

1. Red cell destruction by heat.
2. Red cell trapping by the macrophage-phagocyte system.
3. Losses through capillary permeability and thrombus formation.

These losses of extracellular fluid and of red cell mass lead to a reduced blood and plasma volume, which causes a reduction in cardiac output. If episodes of hypovolaemia and reduced cardiac output occur, blood flow to the wound is diminished, predisposing the healing wound to necrosis of poorly perfused tissue and infection.

The lungs. In a patient with a major burn the function of the lung can be impaired by the following factors:

1. An unyielding leathery eschar may be present around the thorax, which limits respiratory excursions and hinders ventilation.
2. The large volumes of salt-containing solutions infused may lead to considerable weight gain, making the chest wall heavy and hard to move.
3. Toxaemia affecting the gut may produce reflex ileus which elevates the diaphragm, further reducing the vital capacity.
4. An inhalation burn may result in gross oedema of the respiratory passages.

All the above factors combine to produce an impairment of ventilation and of effective coughing which predisposes the patient to the development of collapse of the lung, bronchopneumonia and other pulmonary complications.

The kidneys. In cases with very extensive burns renal damage sometimes occurs. The events leading to a harmful effect on the kidney occur in the following sequence: in response to the trauma and hypovolaemia of the major burn the posterior pituitary releases antidiuretic hormone and the adrenals release aldosterone, so both water and salt are maximally reabsorbed from the tubules. Thus a greatly reduced volume of concentrated urine with a small amount of sodium is passed. The injured cells in the burned area release myoglobin and haemoglobin besides other waste products. If an adequate glomerular filtration rate is not maintained, or if renal ischaemia occurs due to severe hypotension, these products cannot be effectively removed, and *acute tubular necrosis* occurs. This is the basis of the renal failure which was previously a common event in burn shock. If volume losses are replaced by similar fluid, renal blood flow is maintained, a good urinary output (30–50 ml/hr in an adult) is ensured, and damage to the kidney is prevented.

The gut. *Stress ulceration* often occurs in a major burn. This can take one of two forms. The first type is the acute duodenal ulcer which can occur in any extensive burn and is called a *Curling's ulcer.* Secondly, *acute gastric erosions* can occur due to the stress associated with a major burn. These are multiple tiny erosions in the gastric mucosa, and are found in the fundus and body of the stomach.

Either of these two forms of ulceration present with haematemesis and melaena, which may be massive. Their incidence after major burns can be reduced by the prophylactic use of antacids. If haemorrhage does occur, ice-cold saline lavage of the stomach is started and blood transfusion given if necessary. Surgery is only rarely required. At operation the bleeding is arrested by undersewing the bleeding vessel at gastrotomy or duodenotomy, and then vagotomy and antrectomy is the procedure of choice.

Reflex *ileus* may occur due to intestinal paralysis probably from the toxins of bacteria infecting the burn. This delays the onset of oral feeding. At the same time the resulting abdominal distension splints the diaphragm, impairs ventilation, specially in the lower lobes of the lungs, and predisposes the patient to the development of respiratory infections.

Metabolism. In a major burn, due to loss of the skin barrier over a large area of the body surface, fluid losses from evaporation are greatly increased. The resultant cooling causes shivering, leading to a markedly elevated metabolic rate and much loss of energy. This hypermetabolic state leads to severe catabolism and rapid loss of weight. It can be corrected by early closure of the burn wound by skin grafts.

Immunity. As a major burn is a very extensive wound, it produces deficiencies in both cellular and humoral defences. There is lymphocytopenia, with delayed rejection of allograft skin. The level of immunoglobulins is depressed, as is the inflammatory response. *This reduced immunity predisposes the patient to septic complications* both locally in the burn wound and at distant sites, as explained later.

THE TREATMENT OF BURNS

EMERGENCY TREATMENT

The burning process should be stopped as rapidly as possible by extinguishing the flames and *pouring cold water on the burnt area to terminate the continuing heat damage to the skin,* removing the patient from contact with an electric current, or washing away any chemicals. In the case of electric burns, the rescuer must avoid becoming a part of the circuit himself. If the patient has suffered injury from high voltage, cardiopulmonary resuscitation as well as subsequent ventilatory support may be necessary, and should be instituted immediately. If the patient got burned in a confined space, carbon monoxide poisoning may be present, and 100% oxygen should be administered.

Minor burns. These can be treated as outpatients. Their management consists of tetanus prophylaxis, analgesia and prevention of burn wound infection. If the patient has had tetanus immunization during the preceding five years a tetanus toxoid booster should be administered. If not, human antitetanus immune globulin should be given for passive immunization, and active immunization started. In the minor burn the only sepsis likely is that due to the beta-haemolytic streptococcus; therefore only systemic penicillin during the 72 hours of burn oedema is necessary. The wound can be dressed by a non-adhering gauze covered by a bulky absorptive dressing. The part should be immobilized in a functional position. The wound is inspected at 24 hours and then regularly until healing occurs. Superficial burns are quite painful, therefore analgesics should be prescribed liberally.

Moderate-sized and major burns. These require hospitalization. A *large bore needle* or plastic cannula is immediately introduced into a peripheral or central vein so that fluids can be run in to prevent vascular collapse. An infusion of *buffered electrolyte solution*, e.g. Hartmann's, is begun at a rapid rate. An indwelling urinary *catheter* is inserted *with full aseptic precautions* and connected to a closed system, to monitor the hourly urinary output which indicates adequacy of the circulation. If *respiratory distress* is present it can be due to a leathery eschar encircling the chest. If so, an escharotomy should be performed to release the restriction of rib motion and improve ventilatory function. Inhalation of noxious gases can cause *oedema of the pharynx or glottis.* This may produce upper airway obstruction requiring *endotracheal intubation.*

In the extremities an *encircling eschar* can impair circulation due to oedema in the deeper tissues; surgical *escharotomy* may be required. *Pain and anxiety* must be relieved. Analgesics should be given intravenously, because intramuscular absorption is unpredictable due to the decreased cardiac output and massive fluid shifts. A nasogastric tube is used for gastric decompression until the ileus regresses. Tetanus and streptococcus infection are prevented as outlined for minor burns.

DEFINITIVE TREATMENT

Definitive management of the patient with a major burn resolves itself into the following parts:

1. Fluid replacement.
2. Monitoring.
3. Nutritional care.
4. Care of the burn wound.
5. Rehabilitation.

FLUID REPLACEMENT

Many liters of fluid are lost from the surface of a major burn, specially during the first 48 hours. While replacing these losses the appropriate types of fluid must be administered in the correct quantities.

Type of fluid. 1. During the first 24 hours the capillaries are extremely permeable, and if colloid is administered, e.g. in the form of plasma, it will leak out. Therefore during this period an electrolyte solution should be used. The best solution is a buffered *salt* solution, e.g. Ringer's lactate solution. Normal saline contains too much chloride, whereas in the buffered salt solution some of the chloride is replaced by lactate, so that this solution very closely approximates in composition the extracellular fluid which is being lost.

2. After the first 24 hours capillary integrity returns. Therefore *colloid* does not any longer leak out of the capillaries, and can be used to replete the plasma volume. If this is done, in a few more hours both cardiac output and plasma volume return to normal, or in other words resuscitation is complete.

3. Further administration of salt only aggravates the oedema, so from now onwards *water* is given in the form of 5% glucose in water.

Volume of fluid. The greater the body weight and the more extensive the burn, the larger the volume of fluid required for replacement of the losses.

First 24 hours. If, as recommended above, *buffered salt solution,* i.e. Ringer's lactate, is used during the first 24 hours, 4 ml of the solution is required for every one percent of body surface burnt per kilogram body weight during the 24 hours. Thus the volume is:

4 ml/kg body weight/% body surface area burnt.

However, if *colloid* is used, less than half the above amount is required, and only 1.5 to 2 ml per kg per one percent body surface burnt is given in the 24 hours. Thus the volume administered is:

1.5 to 2 ml/kg body weight/% body burnt.

Examples of colloid solutions include human plasma protein fraction, human albumin 4.5%, or a synthetic plasma expander like Dextran 110.

Speed of administration. Whichever of the above two types of fluids, i.e. salt solution or colloid, is chosen for administration, 1/2 of it is given in the first 8 hours, 1/4 in the second 8 hours, and the remaining 1/4 in the third 8 hours. This is because the loss of fluid is greatest in the first 8 hours, and slows down later.

Urine output. In major burns the urine output should be closely monitored, as it indicates whether replacement of fluid has been adequate or not. An output of 30–70 ml of urine per hour is required. If this much urine is passed, it indicates that the fluid losses are being satisfactorily replaced, and that sufficient fluid is being provided to help excrete the increased quantities of waste products resulting from the raised level of catabolism due to the major burn.

Second 24 hours. During the second 24 hours after the burn approximately half the above amounts will be required, as the losses of fluids from the burn are gradually decreasing in amount.

Fluid replacement in children. Small-sized objects have a larger surface area per kg of weight. Children are smaller in size than adults, therefore this rule applies to them also, i.e. compared to their weight, their surface area is greater. Now, the larger the surface area the greater the fluid loss per kg, and a similarly large volume of fluid is required for replacement. In actual practice it works out like this: when Ringer' lactate solution is used, instead of the 4 ml/kg body weight/1% body burnt recommended above for adults, 5 ml is used. Similarly, when colloid is used, instead of the 1.5 to 2 ml/kg body weight/1% body burnt, 2.5 ml is used. Except from this difference in the volumes used, fluid replacement in children is carried out on the same lines as in adults.

However, it should be remembered that even if a clinician follows a particular formula very carefully, he cannot be sure that the fluid and electrolyte requirements have been correctly met. It is only by repeated clinical observation that one can be certain in this respect. The patient with a major burn should have his fluid requirements evaluated and the necessary adjustments made, not on a daily but an hourly basis!

Indicators of adequate fluid replacement. The parameters to watch, in assessing the adequacy of the circulation, are the following:

1. The patient should be mentally alert.
2. The pulse rate should be below 120/min.
3. The urine volume should be at least 30 ml/hr in the adult and 1.2 ml/kg/hr in the child.
4. If a central venous line has been passed, the central venous pressure should be between 2 and 8 cm of water.
5. The haematocrit value should be less than 60%.

MONITORING

All major burn victims require cardiac monitoring, preferably with periodic arterial blood gas determinations, at least during the first 24 hours after the burn is sustained.

NUTRITIONAL CARE

In every major injury, including any extensive burn, the metabolic rate is greatly increased, with a marked catabolic response, so that there is weight loss, a negative nitrogen balance, and retarded wound healing. During the catabolic phase the levels of the catabolic hormones (glucagon and catecholamine) in the plasma are elevated, whereas the level of the anabolic hormone (insulin) is lowered. Protein catabolism does not proceed uniformly in all tissues; muscle protein is sacrificed to save the structural and functional integrity of vital organs such as the heart and liver, so muscle wasting is a marked feature. The negative nitrogen balance can be corrected if a sufficient caloric and nitrogen intake is provided (about 20 grams of nitrogen per square meter of body surface per day). If this is not done the patient becomes severely malnourished. If fat is omitted from the enteral and parenteral solutions, essential fatty acid deficiency may develop after prolonged nutritional therapy. The patient develops dermatitis, thrombocytopenia, impaired wound healing and loss of hair. This can be prevented by weekly parenteral administration of a liter of lipid emulsion, or by the addition of safflower oil to the enteral solutions. Water-soluble vitamins (B complex and C) are depleted rapidly, and 250 to 500 mg vitamin C should be administered daily. The fat-soluble vitamins (A, D, E and K) are depleted more slowly, and need replacement only after prolonged parenteral feeding. Frequent determinations of calcium, magnesium and phosphorus levels should be carried out, apart from electrolytes. Finally, zinc is an important co-factor in wound healing, and periodic measurements of zinc, copper, manganese and chromium provide guidelines for replacement.

Consequences of malnutrition. Inadequate nutritional replacement produces the following serious consequences:

1. Profound weight loss.
2. Decreased immunological response.
3. Decreased leucocyte function, and therefore reduced host resistance.
4. Impaired wound healing.
5. The superior mesenteric artery syndrome: in the emaciated supine patient the acute angle between the aorta and the superior mesenteric artery is further reduced so that the third part of the duodenum is compressed between these two structures. This leads to anorexia, nausea and vomiting, and results in poor food intake and further malnutrition.
6. In the bedridden supine patient most of the energy utilized is spent on maintaining normal respiratory function. When the energy available becomes insufficient even for this activity, ineffective respiratory effort causes *atelectasis,* and lung infection by opportunistic pathogens supervenes. The most common cause of death in these patients is pulmonary sepsis.

Although the effects of severe malnutrition have been described above in the case of a major burn, *a similar situation arises in a major injury of any type*, specially one complicated by infection.

Remedial measures for malnutrition. The consequences of severe malnutrition can be minimized by paying attention to the following aspects of patient care:

1. *Control of heat loss.* In major burns, a great deal of heat is lost due to evaporation from the extensive burn surfaces. If the patient is treated without dressings, radiation also plays a part in heat loss. As a response to this heat loss, the metabolic rate is greatly increased in order to maintain the body temperature, but this leads to rapid loss of weight. This hypermetabolic state can be controlled by insulative occlusive dressings. If the patient is being treated without dressings, electric heaters may be used to keep the environmental temperature at 31°C.

2. Apprehension and *pain* potentiate the release of catecholamines; they are controlled by analgesics and tranquilizers.

3. *Infection* is prevented by isolation, careful nursing and the judicious use of antibiotics.

4. The burn wound is *closed early,* as this step alone greatly reduces the catabolic state.

5. However, the most important aspect of the nutritional management of the burn patient is the provision of an *adequate number of exogenous calories* and nitrogen. Extensive tissue breakdown in major burns results in protein catabolism. Nitrogen is produced, and appears in the urine as urea. If nutritional support is not provided, protein catabolism is further increased in order to provide energy. This results in a decrease in lean body mass and loss of weight. With small burns this weight loss is minor, e.g. about 5% of body weight for a 10% burn. However, if nutritional support is not provided in cases of burns exceeding 40% of body surface, upto 30% of body weight can be lost. Whenever possible the gastrointestinal tract should be used for providing nutrition; this is not only the best method but also very much cheaper. Parenteral nutrition should be reserved only for those patients where the gut cannot be employed. Complete homogenized diets are well tolerated by the patient with a major burn. On the other hand partially digested diets have a high osmolality, and may cause diarrhoea and dehydration. The advantages of enteral feeding are many:

1. Enteral nutrients maintain the integrity of the digestive tract and minimize the chances of bacterial translocation from the gut, which could result in the sepsis syndrome.

2. An oral diet preserves the gut mucosa and the output of enzymes by it.

3. Oral feeding stimulates the elaboration of trophic hormones, e.g. gastrin.

4. Enterally administered calories stimulate release of insulin, which promotes anabolism.

Additional measures. 1. Low environmental temperatures increase the metabolic expenditure and lead to loss of weight. This tendency can be eliminated by keeping the ambient temperature at 31°C, i.e. four degrees higher than the neutral temperature for normal subjects.

2. *Pain* on dressing and other procedures increases metabolic expenditure. This can be reduced by analgesics and sedation.

3. Physical exercise promotes preservation of muscle bulk, and supervised physical therapy should be provided to all patients requiring prolonged hospitalization from any cause.

4. Expeditious wound closure is the most effective measure for minimizing the loss of energy from the wound.

CARE OF THE BURN WOUND

The aims of the local treatment of the burn are three:

1. Avoidance of further damage to cells already injured.
2. Prevention of infection.
3. Early closure of the burn wound.

In a small burn wound full-thickness excision and grafting can be carried out if necessary. However, in the more extensive burns this is not possible, because as the area to be excised increases, the available donor sites decrease. As large scale excision cannot be carried out the wound has to be supported while the reversibly injured cells heal. This demands protection from bacterial invasion.

Protection from infection. The skin is not sterile. It contains many bacteria in the hair follicles and sweat glands. The surgeon's aim is to prevent an increase in these exogenous bacteria to levels sufficient to cause burn wound sepsis. Historically, the local care of burns has evolved through three stages:

1. *Occlusive dressings*. Classically, burns were treated locally by occlusive dressings. After cleansing and debridement an inner layer of gauze impregnated with vaseline etc. was covered by a layer of absorptive cotton wool and held in place by a gauze bandage. This dressing remained intact until exudate soaked through it, or odour, pain or fever made inspection of the wound necessary. The idea behind these dressings was to protect the wound from bacteria, which were supposed to come from the environment. However, in due course it was shown that normal skin contains upto 10 organisms/gm of tissue (in the hair follicles and sweat glands as mentioned above). It was thus realized that not only was the main threat from within the skin, but also occlusive dressings, by providing a warm and moist environment, actually *encourage* the multiplication of bacteria and pave the way for invasive infection.

2. *Exposure treatment*. To overcome this problem exposure treatment was introduced. In this method a dry eschar forms over the burn wound and acts as a physiological dressing. This prevents the access of exogenous bacteria.

However, even this exposure treatment has its limitations. As with occlusive dressings, the only organisms from which the patient is protected are the exogenous bacteria, and these are not the major offenders. At the same time the drying up of the injured cells damages them further and burn wounds treated by exposure become deeper.

3. *Semi-open technique*. Because of dissatisfaction with both open and closed methods the semi-open technique has been evolved. In this method an ointment or solution containing a chemotherapeutic agent is applied to the wound surface. The three most commonly used agents are the following:

1. Silver sulphadiazine cream.
2. Silver nitrate solution.
3. Mefenide acetate.

This is the only method by which the multiplication of endogenous bacteria can be prevented. The effectiveness of these agents can be monitored by quantitative analysis of biopsies taken from the burn wound.

Debridement. In a partial thickness burn some of the cells in the superficial layers of the skin are dead. As they separate from the deeper layers of viable cells they need to be trimmed away. This debridement is best carried out daily by the patient soaking in a tub of warm normal saline, which can be easily prepared by making a 1% solution of common salt (1% NaCl is very close to 0.9%, which is isotonic saline). The eschar becomes softened and can be gently cut away. The method is relatively painless and helps avoid repeated sessions of anaesthesia. In those countries where bath tubs are not common, a series of showers arranged longitudinally, over a specially designed sterilizable stretcher is an excellent, and perhaps even better, substitute for a tub bath.

Closure. Once the necrotic tissue has been removed, closure can follow. In *partial-thickness* burns closure occurs spontaneously by regeneration from the surviving epidermal elements in the dermis. The *full thickness* burn requires closure by skin grafts.

Temporary coverings. When the burn is very extensive, the available donor sites cannot provide enough skin grafts. In such a case temporary closure can be achieved by *biological dressings*, which may take one of the following forms:

1. Skin from other persons (homografts).
2. Skin from animals (heterografts).
3. Amniotic membranes.
4. Synthetic dressings, e.g. nylon mesh with a collagen peptide coating.

These dressing are only temporary, and permanent closure with the patient's own skin (autografts) remains the goal of treatment. When skin grafting large areas priority should be given to the face, the neck, and the various flexion creases of the body.

Physical therapy. If a burn destroys skin over the flexor aspect of a joint, skin grafting must be carried out as early as possible. As soon as the grafts have taken, movements at the joint should be encouraged, and carried out daily. For about six months splints must be worn at night to maintain anti-contracture postures during sleep.

Rehabilitation. Rehabilitation should start the moment a burn is sustained. From the beginning burned limbs are elevated and *exercised* to minimize the oedema and reduce the need for escharotomy. The burn team should include a play therapist, who encourages children to take part in games where they are not conscious of the active exercises they are performing.

Hypertrophic scarring is a very troublesome sequel of a burn. Certain patients are prone to severe hypertrophic scar formation. Scar hypertrophy can be reduced by carefully fitted pressure garments over healed scars, which should be worn for about 6 months.

Apart from physical measures *psychological* rehabilitation is of the utmost importance. Words of encouragement should be spoken throughout the patient's convalescence. If the face is disfigured by the burns, skilful plastic surgery helps greatly in physical as well as psychological rehabilitation.

COMPLICATIONS OF BURNS

Uptil now we have described the usual course of a burn and its management. However, different complications can arise and render the treatment more difficult. The most important ones are burn wound sepsis, distant septic complications, the smoke inhalation syndrome, and complications involving the gastrointestinal tract. Marjolin's ulcer is a squamous cell carcinoma which occurs as malignant degeneration in longstanding chronic ulcers in burn scars.

Burn wound sepsis. The most important cause of death after massive burns is burn wound sepsis, when microorganisms invade subeschar tissue and bacteraemia results. The burnt skin being avascular, systemic antibiotics cannot affect bacterial growth. Moreover, host resistance is very low due to reduction in the amounts of complement and gammaglobulins available, and impairment of the activity of neutrophils and monocytes. If local antibiotics are not used, rapid bacterial colonization can occur.

Uptil now local antibiotic *creams* have been applied to the surface of the burn. These have reduced the incidence of bacterial colonization of the subeschar tissue considerably, but still not sufficiently often. If wound biopsy shows the presence of over 10^4 organisms per gram of tissue it means that bacteria have escaped control. In such cases antibiotic solutions have recently been *infused* deep to the eschar. The entire daily dose, usually of carbenicillin, is dissolved in normal saline and distributed under the eschar. This practice has considerably improved the outlook in Pseudomonas septicaemia, which used to be uniformly fatal. *Cultures* of wound, sputum, urine and blood should be obtained from all patients of major burns twice a week. The same organisms are likely to be involved in later life-threatening infections, and selection of antibiotics is made easier by reviewing these earlier reports.

Stimulation of immune mechanisms. Recently, monoclonal antibodies have been produced against endotoxin, and they have improved the survival of patients with gram-negative bacteraemia and shock. It is likely that monoclonal antibodies to cytokines will shortly prove to be effective for treating patients with life-threatening infections.

Control of infection. The following measures should be taken in this connection:

1. Patients with major burns should be isolated in single rooms, which should be closed for decontamination regularly. The rooms should be ventilated with non-recirculating air exchange systems.
2. Each room should be provided with its own wash-basin, and the personnel of the burns unit should wash their hands each time before handling the patient or carrying out any procedure. Chlorhexidine gluconate is probably the most effective cleaning agent for reducing the incidence of nosocomial infections.
3. Patients should not return from convalescent floors to visit patients in the critical care burns unit, as they are sometimes carriers of serious nosocomial infections.

Distant sepsis. In patients with extensive burns the resistance of the host is reduced, therefore distant septic complications are common. The usual sites of such complications are the lungs, the veins, and the urinary tract.

Bronchopneumonia is the most common complicating infection in cases of severe burns. Air infected with organisms from the burn is probably inhaled, because sputum cultures show the same organisms as have colonized the burn.

Suppurative thrombophlebitis occurs quite commonly in cases with massive burns. It usually follows prolonged venous cannulation. Local physical signs e.g. calf tenderness and oedema may be absent, so detection is difficult. The patient may present with bacteraemia of unknown origin, when blood cultures often yield staphylococci. The diagnosis may be confirmed by surgical exploration of all peripheral veins which have been cannulated. If pus is found, the entire offending vein or veins must be excised, otherwise fatal septicaemia could result.

Urinary tract infections. Most patients with major burns require indwelling urinary catheters to guide fluid administration during resuscitation. Such catheters should be removed as early as possible, as with increasing duration of catheter placement the likelihood of infection increases, so that *after 7 to 10 days most patients will have positive urine cultures*. The causative organisms are usually the same as in the burn wound.

Smoke inhalation syndrome. If smoke is inhaled in sufficient quantities progressive bronchospasm can develop within 24 hours, with expiratory wheezes, rales, tachypnoea and respiratory failure. Bronchopneumonia often develops due to bacterial growth distal to the occluding plugs of mucus. X-ray changes are seen only 72 hours after the injury.

Treatment includes rapid fluid resuscitation, performance of escharotomies over the chest, and monitoring of respiratory function. Humidified air and oxygen should be provided as required. If respiratory failure threatens, an endotracheal tube should be passed and mechanical ventilation carried out. Antibiotics are given parenterally. The routine use of steroids should be avoided, as they result in higher morbidity and mortality.

Gastrointestinal complications of large burns include Curling's ulcer, acute cholecystitis, acute pancreatitis, and superior mesenteric artery syndrome.

Curling's ulcer *(stress ulceration of the stomach and duodenum).* Mucosal erosions are seen in over three-fourths of patients with burns of over 35% of the body surface, and one-fifth of these progress to frank gastric or duodenal ulcers. Keeping the pH above 5 with antacids or H_2 blockers has proved effective in preventing these lesions. Rarely, surgery may be required for severe haemorrhage or perforation of a Curling's ulcer; in that case vagotomy and gastric resection has produced the best results.

Acute pancreatitis is seen in one-third of the patients in critical care burns units. Treatment consists of supportive measures, nasogastric suction and parenteral nutrition.

Acute cholecystitis may be seen from time to time, either due to haematogenous spread from a primary focus in the septic patient, or in patients with marked dehydration, ileus or pancreatitis. Physical examination is difficult and ultrasound or CT examination should be employed. Once the diagnosis is made, cholecystectomy is indicated to avoid perforation of the gallbladder. In an unstable critically ill patient tube cholecystostomy may be carried out at the bedside.

Superior mesenteric artery syndrome has been described above as one of the manifestations of advanced malnutrition.

Marjolin's ulcer. Marjolin noted that chronic ulcers in old burn scars often resulted in malignant degeneration, commonly in the form of a squamous cell carcinoma but occasionally as a basal cell carcinoma. Therefore, malignant degeneration should be suspected in any healed burn scar which exhibits chronic breakdown. If biopsy shows malignancy, wide excision should be carried out. If cancer is not present, an unstable burn scar should still be excised and resurfaced.

Oil stove deaths. In some underdeveloped countries young women cooking the family meals over kerosene oil stoves sometimes die from severe burns. The mother-in-law is often blamed; at other times it is thought that the stove bursts. The truth is otherwise. The mother-in-law does not kill, as suggested by the fact that one-third of the young girls dying are unmarried. The stove does not burst; not a single piece of metal from a stove has ever been recovered from any young girl's body. At the same time, researchers from the author's clinical unit recovered the suspected stoves; none of them had burst. The real cause is carelessness in the use of these rather imperfectly made stoves. A set of instructions, on the lines of the following, broadcast on the radio helps reduce the incidence of these tragic accidents:

Do not pour kerosene oil into a lighted stove; do not carry a lighted stove; do not wear synthetic clothes: if you have to, wear a canvas apron over them, etc. etc.

Skin grafts and flaps

Introduction. If an area of skin is destroyed, the defect has to be filled in by skin brought from outside in the form of a graft. If this is not done two problems arise: firstly, the raw area takes a very long time to heal, with infection and a purulent discharge continuing in the meantime. Secondly, and specially if the area of skin loss lies over the flexor aspect of a joint, a contracture results. This produces an unsightly deformity, and at the same time limits joint motion, sometimes resulting in considerable disability. The skin defect can be filled either by free skin grafts or skin flaps.

SKIN GRAFTS

A skin graft is a segment of skin which has been totally separated from its normal bed (donor site) and is transplanted to a new area (recipient site).

Sources of grafts. An *autograft* is a graft transplanted from one area to another in the same individual. A *homograft (or allograft)* is transplanted from one individual to another in the same species. A *heterograft (or xenograft)* is transplanted from one individual to another of a different species.

Thickness of grafts. A partial-thickness skin graft includes epidermis but not the whole dermis. A full-thickness graft includes epidermis and full thickness of dermis, sometimes with portions of underlying tissues e.g. muscle, cartilage or bone.

Partial-thickness grafts. These are commonly taken from the outer side of the thigh. They may be cut thin, medium or thick. The thicker grafts have the following characteristics:

1. They look better.
2. They contract less.
3. Their chances of survival are somewhat less than those of the thinner grafts, because they have more cells to be nourished before a blood supply is established.

When partial-thickness grafts are taken, the deeper layers of skin are left behind, and the donor area heals spontaneously within about a fortnight. Therefore even very large skin defects can be covered by this method, and partial-thickness grafting is the standard method for resurfacing extensive burns.

Full-thickness grafts. These grafts give the best colour match, the most padding, and the least contraction. However, they can survive only over very vascular recipient sites. Further, the donor sites cannot heal spontaneously, because the whole thickness of skin has been removed. Therefore only relatively small-sized grafts can be taken, so that the resultant skin defect can be dealt with by primary closure. For example, if a small skin tumour is removed from the face and a skin defect results, an elliptical segment of skin can be taken from the retroauricular or supraclavicular regions to repair it (Plate VII–I). The segment should be cut to the exact size and shape of the defect for best results.

Composite grafts. Due to trauma, or after removal of a small skin tumour, there may be loss of an ala of the nose. The ideal tissue for replacement of the defect is a piece of cartilage covered on both sides with skin. This can be obtained by excising a triangular segment from the middle of the margin of the pinna. This contains two layers of skin with cartilage in between. The defect in the helix can be closed by direct suture using fine suture materials. Such a transplant is an example of a composite graft.

SKIN FLAPS

A skin flap is a segment of skin and subcutaneous tissue which is transferred from its original position to another site while maintaining its own blood supply through a 'pedicle'.

Advantages of skin flaps. The cosmetic and functional result after skin flaps is better than after skin grafts:

1. The original colour and texture of the skin is usually maintained.
2. Hair growth, sweating and sensation are at least partly preserved.
3. Flaps are more durable, specially over pressure points.

Indications for use of flaps. Reconstruction by a flap may be required in any of the following situations:

1. If the recipient area lacks the vascularity required to support a skin graft.
2. If padding is required over a bony prominence.
3. If a good aesthetic result will be achieved by a skin flap.
4. If further surgery will be required beneath the reconstructed area.

Causes of failure of skin flaps. If a skin flap fails it is commonly due to an error of technique. Some examples follow:

1. Suturing a flap under tension may cause necrosis by interfering with the venous or arterial flow.
2. Pressure on the flap by a tight constricting dressing may similarly compromise the circulation.
3. If haemostasis is imperfect a haematoma may form and cause considerable damage to the flap.
4. Infection is not common, but can severely damage a flap when it does occur. In flaps with a poor blood supply the organisms are mostly anaerobic. With well-vascularized flaps, infection is usually due to the beta-haemolytic streptococcus.

CLASSIFICATION OF SKIN FLAPS

Skin flaps may be classified as follows:

1. Arterial pattern flaps.
2. Random pattern flaps.

i. Local flaps:

(a) Advancement flap (Fig. 4).

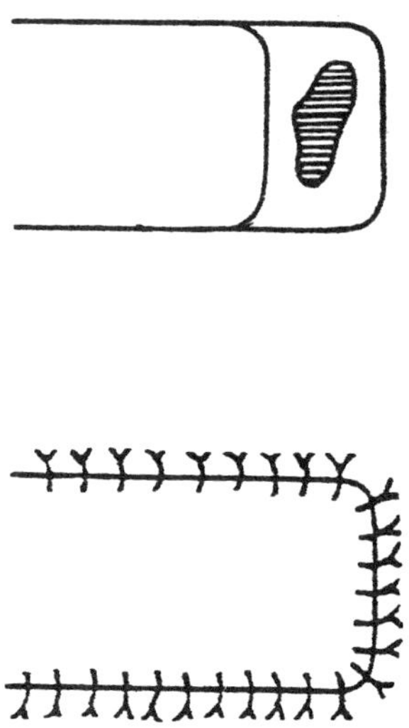

Fig. 4 Advancement flap.

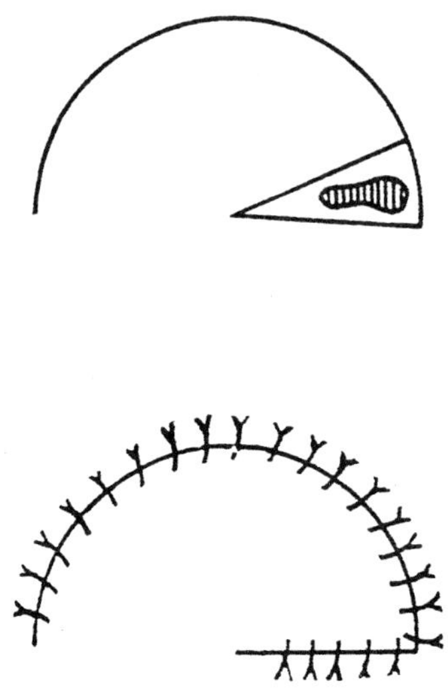

Fig. 5 Rotation flap.

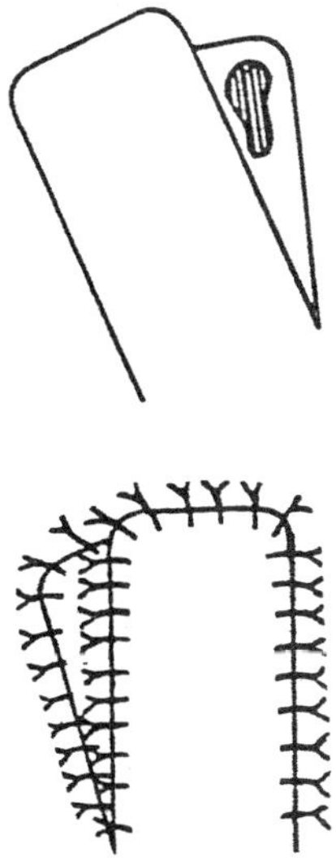

Fig. 6 Transposition flap.

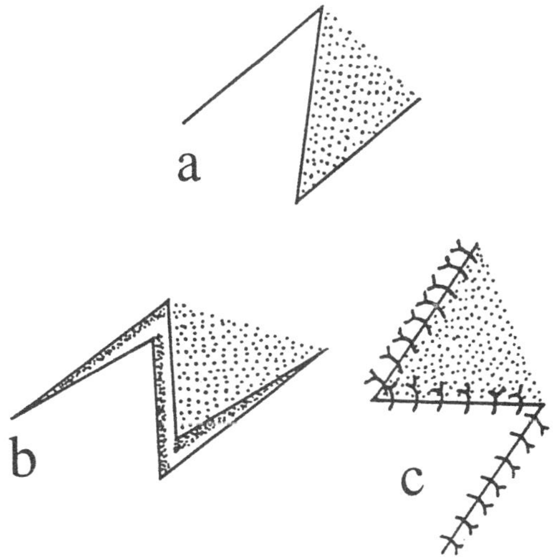

Fig. 7 Z-plasty.

(b) Rotation flap (Fig. 5).
(c) Transposition flap (Fig. 6).
(d) Z-plasty (Fig. 7).
ii. Flaps from a distance, e.g. tubed pedicle flap.
3. Myocutaneous flaps.
4. Free flaps.

Arterial pattern flaps. An arterial pattern flap carries with it a cutaneous artery which enters its base and runs longitudinally within the flap. Such a flap can be fairly long because of its feeding artery. One example is the long flap of the forehead containing the anterior branch of the temporal artery (Figs. 8 and 9).

Random pattern flaps. These flaps lack an anatomically recognized artery. Therefore there are strict limitations on their length, which should usually not be more than twice their width, otherwise blood supply in the distal part may be insufficient, leading to necrosis of that part. These flaps may take the following forms:

1. *Local flaps.* i. *Advancement flaps.* In this variety of local flap a quadrangular area of skin is stretched forwards to cover an adjacent defect.

ii. *Rotation flaps.* Here a semicircular segment of skin rotates and stretches to fill a defect.

iii. *Transposition flaps.* In this type a quadrangular piece of skin hinges laterally to resurface an adjoining area.

iv. *Z-plasty.* In this technique two triangular skin flaps are interchanged in position to gain length along a scar at

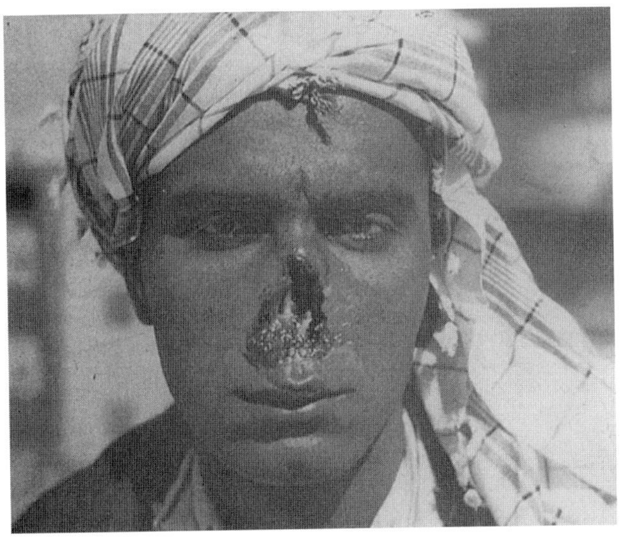

Fig. 8 Nose cut off for alleged adultery.

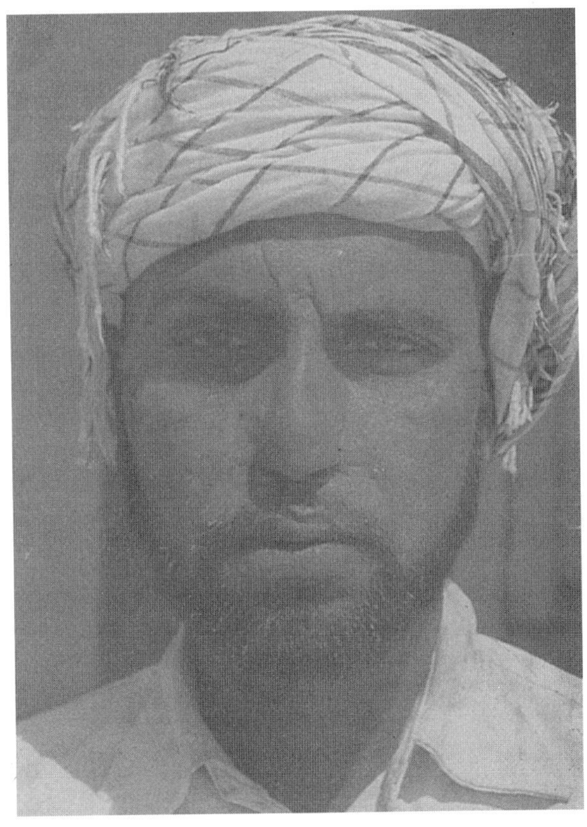

Fig. 9 Nose repaired by 'scalping' flap.

the expense of adjacent tissues. This method enables a surgeon to lengthen a contracted scar or to treat a web contracture.

2. *Flaps from a distance.* Examples of such flaps include an arm flap which is brought directly to the nose. When a flap is brought over a distance e.g. from the abdominal wall to the hand, its pedicle is usually 'tubed'. It is therefore called a tubed pedicle flap.

3. *Myocutaneous flaps.* At many sites in the body a muscle can be elevated with its longitudinal segmental blood supply, carrying its overlying skin with it. Such a flap is called a myocutaneous flap. It helps not only in providing good full-thickness skin for resurfacing a defect, but also in filling irregular defects of body contour. An example of such a flap is the use of the latissimus dorsi muscle during the operation of mammoplasty following a mastectomy for breast cancer.

4. *Free flaps.* The use of extremely fine instruments and suture materials, with the help of mangification *(microvascular techniques),* has enabled anastomoses of arteries and veins of less than 1 mm diameter to be carried out satisfactorily. This has allowed free-flap transfers, the vessels of the graft being anastomosed to the vessels of the recipient site, with high success rates. Because a specially tailored composite mass of tissues can be transported to a distant site in just one step, these techniques have quite a wide applicability.

Microvascular techniques need very lengthy operating sessions. However, sometimes they represent the only solution to a complicated reconstructive problem.

5 Shock

In order to live and function every cell in the body requires that oxygen and nutrients be supplied to it, and waste products be carried away from it. Both these processes depend upon an adequate circulation of blood. Any serious interference with circulation therefore causes disordered function of all the cells in the body.

The term 'shock' has been used for two centuries to describe a progressive but gradual collapse of vital organ function after injury or surgery. Upto the 1960s shock was defined as 'decreased blood flow to vital organs'. However, during the 1970s it was found that in shock due to sepsis a high cardiac output and low peripheral resistance is present. Therefore the old definition of shock as decreased blood flow to vital organs is not valid. Shock should be defined as a state of inadequate tissue perfusion.

CLASSIFICATION OF SHOCK

Shock can be classified into the five types shown in Table 1. In the first two types, the problem is a falling cardiac output, which may be due to insufficient blood volume (hypovolaemic shock) or inefficient working of the heart as a pump (cardiogenic shock). The last three types can be grouped together as *distributive circulatory failure* i.e. a condition in which, although the cardiac function is adequate, the blood is distributed improperly, mainly due to excessive vasodilatation in the skin and splanchnic bed. The common example of distributive circulatory failure is septic shock, the others being neurogenic shock and anaphylactic shock.

MONITORING THE PATIENT IN SHOCK

Nine primary measurements are useful in the initial assessment and follow-up of patients in shock (Table 2).

Table 1 Classification of shock.

Type	Examples
I. Hypovolaemic	Haemorrhage Burns Vomiting, diarrhoea
II. Cardiogenic	Myocardial infarction Arrhythmias Cardiac tamponade Cardiac surgery Pulmonary embolism
III. Peripheral pooling	Spinal anaesthesia
IV. Septic shock	Peritonitis, major burns
V. Anaphylactic shock	Penicillin, dextrans, serum injections

Table 2 Haemodynamic and metabolic monitors in shock.

Measurements values	Average normal
1. Arterial blood pressure	120/80 mm Hg
2. Pulse rate	70 per minute
3. Central venous pressure	5 ± 2 cm H_2O
4. Cardiac output	5.8 litres/min
5. Arterial PO_2 tension	85 – 100 mm Hg
6. Arterial PCO_2	40 mm Hg
7. Haemoglobin concentration	14 ± 1 gm/100 ml
8. Urine flow	50 ml/hour
9. Arterial blood lactate	5 – 8 mg/100 ml

Eight of these can be readily determined; only cardiac output is difficult to measure accurately.

THE IMPORTANCE OF THE VARIOUS PARAMETERS

Pulse and blood pressure. A rapid pulse and low blood pressure are cardinal signs of shock and should be carefully monitored in all seriously ill patients. Decreased blood pressure is always significant, but the pressure may be normal or nearly normal until marked depletion of vascular volume occurs. This happens because hypovolaemia results in severe vasoconstriction, which reduces the capacity of the vascular bed. In such a situation the cardiac output may be low and yet the blood pressure may be maintained. In spite of these limitations, however, the level of blood pressure is a useful guide.

Pulse pressure, i.e. the difference between systolic and diastolic pressures, is related to cardiac output and normally is about 40 mm Hg. If this decreases to 20, then even if systolic pressure is normal, blood flow is probably inadequate. On the other hand if the pulse pressure is near 40 mm Hg, flow is likely to be adequate even though the systolic pressure is only 80 or 90 mm Hg. Thus, one should be interested in finding out not only whether the systolic pressure is maintained, but also whether *pulse* pressure is adequate. Continuous monitoring of the pulse is now used in most recovery rooms for seriously ill patients and for all patients after general anaesthesia. It is useful to have warning devices that alert one if any arrhythmia arises.

Central venous pressure (CVP). During critical illness the central venous pressure is an important guide to the adequacy of the circulation. *The CVP reflects the volume of blood returning to the heart and the ability of both the right and left ventricles to propel it.* It is therefore a good guide, during volume replacement, about the quantity of fluids to be administered. If the CVP is low, it means more fluid is required; if high, it shows that fluid should be restricted.

Cardiac output. The ultimate aim of the circulatory system is to maintain a good cardiac output, to enable oxygen and nutrients to be carried to the different organs and tissues and for waste products to be carried away from them. Thus if cardiac output can be determined, we have the most direct evidence of the adequacy of the circulation.

Arterial blood gases and pH. An arterial oxygen tension (Pa_{O_2}) of between 80 and 100 mm Hg is normal, depending upon the age of the patient. A tension below 60 mm Hg indicates a marginal respiratory reserve, and an increased concentration of oxygen in the inspired air is required. The main causes of a reduced PO_2 in the arterial blood are the following:

1. *Hypoventilation.*
2. *Impaired diffusion.* This occurs in some disease states where the blood gas barrier is thickened. The hypoxaemia resulting from this cause can be corrected by administering higher concentrations of oxygen to the patient.
3. *Shunt.* This occurs when some blood reaches the arterial system without passing through ventilated portions of the lung. Examples include cases of Fallot's tetralogy. Also, a consolidated pneumonic lobe contains a perfused but completely unventilated area of lung, and acts as a shunt.

Most patients suffering from shock or sepsis hyperventilate. This has two harmful effects:

1. The strenuous muscular exercise involved in hyperventilation causes exhaustion.
2. The alkalosis resulting from hyperventilation shifts the oxyhaemoglobin dissociation curve to the left. Thus haemoglobin does not easily give up its oxygen, and the supply of oxygen to the tissues suffers.

Haemoglobin concentration. Haemoglobin concentration is of fundamental importance in oxygen transport to the tissues. If the oxygen content of the inspired air is increased to 100%, this raises haemoglobin saturation only from 97 to 100%. On the other hand even moderate changes in haemoglobin concentration or cardiac output have a strong influence on oxygen transport. If haemoglobin concentration falls from 15 gm/dl to 10 gm/dl, the oxygen carrying capacity of blood is reduced by one third. If at the same time cardiac output falls to half (from 6 to 3 liters per minute) oxygen consumption will fall very markedly, from 300 to as little as 100 ml per minute, which is a serious matter.

Urine flow. In hypovolaemic shock cardiac output falls, renal vessels constrict, and renal blood flow diminishes. *In all patients under treatment for shock the urine flow should be measured every hour.* This should be at least 30 ml per hour in an adult. However, in sepsis and trauma there is an increased osmolar load due to increased breakdown of cellular proteins; therefore a urine volume of at least 1,000 ml per 24 hours is required.

Acute renal failure usually occurs as follows:

1. A period of decreased rate of urine flow sets the stage for renal injury.
2. Obstruction of tubules may result from precipitation of casts from a concentrated urine.

Arterial blood lactate level. In shock the perfusion of tissues with blood is inadequate, and this produces a decreased tissue pO_2. The result is that the breakdown of glucose is partially arrested at the anaerobic phase, with accumulation of lactate and other ions. The raised level of lactate in the arterial blood can be estimated, and is an indicator of the severity of shock.

HYPOVOLAEMIC SHOCK

In this condition the cause of shock is a reduced circulating blood volume (hypovolaemia). The patient has a low blood pressure (below 90 mm Hg), rapid pulse (above 100), a low central venous pressure, and a low urine output (under 20 ml per hour), with high urinary osmolality. There is usually a dramatic response to rapid volume replacement. The haematocrit is a guide to the type of fluid required. In hypovolaemic shock due to pancreatitis the haematocrit may be as high as 60, due to loss of fluid leading to haemoconcentration. Plasma and physiological saline i.e. Ringer's lactate solution should be given. This has two effects. Firstly, it restores the blood volume. Secondly, it reduces the haematocrit and therefore the viscosity to normal. The less viscous blood passes through the capillaries more easily, so that the cardiac output, urine flow and blood pressure are all increased. At the same time the pulse rate falls towards normal. On the other hand the patient in shock with a bleeding duodenal ulcer who has a very low haematocrit, e.g. 20, will require blood.

The peripheral vessels are severely constricted in hypovolaemic shock. This is best dealt with by volume replacement. Vasodilator drugs should not be used, because the little blood that is available will be pooled in the dilated vessels, reducing the venous return and cardiac output even further.

RESPONSE TO HYPOVOLAEMIA

The response of the body to hypovolaemia may be considered under three headings, namely cardiovascular, endocrine and metabolic responses.

Cardiovascular responses. A fall in blood pressure acts through the stretch receptors in the carotid sinus and the aortic arch. The sympathetic nervous system is reflexly stimulated. This increases the peripheral resistance by arteriolar constriction, and raises the cardiac output by increasing the rate and force of cardiac contraction. At the same time the *effective* blood volume is increased by enhanced vasomotor tone in the veins which squeezes blood from the large venous reservoirs into the great veins. Thus blood is diverted from the extremities, bowel and kidneys to more vital areas of the heart and brain, the vessels of which constrict little even under intense sympathetic stimulation. When capillary pressure falls there is a net movement of extracellular fluid into the capillary, restoring plasma volume. This is seen after moderate blood loss (upto 1,500 ml). This capillary refilling occurs at a rate of about 70 ml per hour until plasma volume is restored.

Endocrine responses. *Catecholamines.* An acute reduction of blood volume stimulates the production of *epinephrine* and *norepinephrine* from the adrenal medulla and nerve endings. Some other conditions stimulating release of these hormones include acidosis, sepsis and prolonged low-flow states. These catecholamines increase the rate and force of cardiac contraction and dilate the arteries in the myocardium and skeletal muscles. At the same time they constrict the arteries in the skin, kidneys and viscera. They also stimulate the production of glucagon and inhibit the production and peripheral action of insulin.

Antidiuretic hormone and *aldosterone*. Hypotension results in increased firing by baroreceptors, which causes increased secretion of *antidiuretic hormone* by the posterior pituitary. This hormone helps restore plasma volume by retention of water. Diminished renal blood flow activates the renin-angiotensin system, which promotes the elaboration of *aldosterone*; this hormone also helps preserve plasma volume by retention of salt.

Maximal cardiovascular and endocrine responses occur when the effective circulating volume has been decreased by 30 to 40%. Further reduction in the circulating volume cannot be adequately handled by compensatory mechanisms, and shock follows.

Metabolic responses. In the shock state catecholamines enhance glycogen and protein breakdown but are ineffective in stimulating the breakdown of fats (lipolysis). With the decreased availability of fat as fuel, the body becomes dependent on the oxidation of carbohydrate reserves, and increased formation and deamination of amino acids are characteristic of the shock state. In shock the rate of urea production is elevated, indicating faster protein breakdown. Skeletal muscle is the major tissue supplying amino acids as fuel.

Viscosity. When flow rates are slow as in shock, the viscosity of normal blood in small vessels can itself be a factor impairing tissue perfusion. Anything that decreases the haematocrit and fibrinogen concentration will decrease viscosity and improve perfusion. For this purpose low molecular weight dextran can be used, but equally effective are those fluids that simply decrease haematocrit and fibrinogen concentration, e.g. saline or Ringer's lactate.

TREATMENT OF HYPOVOLAEMIC SHOCK

The nine parameters listed in Table 2 should be measured at the outset, and the response to therapy observed. If prompt infusion of the appropriate fluids restores the parameters to normal the problem is under good initial control. In the collapsed patient a Ryle's nasogastric tube, quickly inserted by cutting down into an antecubital vein and passing it into the superior vena cava, is excellent for rapid transfusion, venous pressure measurement and repeated venous sampling. *Failure to achieve haemodynamic and metabolic stability promptly is dangerous.* The chronic low flow state promotes vital organ failure of the kidneys, liver and heart. In the hypovolaemia of trauma crystalloids must be used in addition to blood. There are at least two reasons for this:

1. Fluid is lost into the injured or operated area, which must be replaced.

2. It is desirable to reduce the haematocrit and fibrinogen concentration in small vessels to decrease viscosity and promote flow in the vessels. In the low flow state better oxygen transport is achieved if the blood is less viscous, e.g. with a haematocrit of 30% rather than 50%.

Blood pressure. Arterial pressure is a good guide to therapy. The blood volume must be reduced by 15 to 25% before systolic pressure falls below 80 to 90 mm Hg. If a patient is alert, has a normal ECG, and a urine flow of 50 ml per hour, the systolic pressure is probably adequate even if it is only 80 mm Hg. The pulse pressure is helpful as a guide to volume replacement. In shock a higher diastolic pressure is usually seen due to severe arteriolar vasoconstriction. Thus a blood pressure of 80/40 mm Hg is preferable to one of 120/100.

Composition of fluid. The best fluid to start on all patients in shock or with trauma is *Ringer's lactate.* Equally effective is 5% glucose in normal saline with 2 ampoules (90 meq) of sodium bicarbonate added to each liter to buffer the solution to pH 7.4. The reason why Ringer's lactate is best is that it closely resembles tissue fluid in composition. During trauma tissue fluid is lost and therefore Ringer's lactate is its best replacement. Recent work has shown, however, that it is the volume and speed of replacement that determines outcome more than the type of fluid. Further, that a liter of a hypertonic solution is desirable as the initial infusion because, apart from providing fluid, it draws fluid from the tissues into the vessels.

If hypovolaemic shock is due to haemorrhage, transfusion of *blood* is carried out, using the appropriate number of units of blood. When massive transfusion is required, blood should always be warmed. At the same time clotting factors should be replaced continuously. In conditions in which there is excessive loss of plasma proteins, as in acute pancreatitis, peritonitis or burns, the use of plasma, or electrolyte solutions to which albumin has been added, is of great value.

The difficulty of achieving a balance between undertransfusion and overtransfusion should not be underestimated, even with all monitoring facilities. It should be remembered that prolonged hypoperfusion carries the risk of organ tissue damage, whereas if supervision is close, fluid overload can be reversed with diuretics or haemofiltration.

Ventilation. All patients in shock should receive oxygen by mask. Respiratory failure may require further measures, e.g. ventilation.

Diuretics. If hypovolaemia has been corrected but oliguria (a urine flow of less than 20 ml per hour) persists, the use of diuretics should be considered. Urine output should be monitored hourly with an indwelling catheter. *However, it is no use placing an indwelling catheter and then forgetting to record the output every hour!*

The two diuretics in common use are mannitol and furosemide. *Furosemide* is a loop diuretic. It produces diuresis by blocking sodium reabsorption in the loop of Henle. It may cause increased loss of sodium and water in spite of a lowered serum sodium and reduced intravascular volume. In this way it can aggravate renal ischaemia. Therefore it is *contraindicated* in oliguria of hypovolaemic origin.

Mannitol is an osmotic diuretic. It produces diuresis because it is filtered by the glomerulus but not reabsorbed by the renal tubules, thus obligating the excretion of water. At the same time its administration results in an increase in intravascular volume. Therefore, if a diuretic has to be used in a patient recovering from hypovolaemic shock, it should be mannitol. It is given as 25 gm in 100 to 500 ml of 5% glucose in water over a period of 15 to 30 minutes. If there is a good response the dose may be repeated.

Vasodilators. If pre-load and contractility have been optimized but cardiac output still remains inadequate, reduction of ventricular after-load may be useful. This is achieved by the use of vasodilators, which may be divided into the direct-acting and the indirect-acting drugs.

Direct-acting. *Sodium nitroprusside* acts directly on arterioles and to some extent veins. It produces a fall in the peripheral resistance and venous return, thus reducing ventricular pre-load. *Nitroglycerine* acts directly and causes predominant venous dilatation, thus reducing pre-load. It also reduces after-load by relaxing arteriolar smooth muscle. *Hydralazine* given by i.v. bolus in a dose of 10–20 mg may be used to reduce after-load.

Indirect-acting. The alpha-blocking drugs, such as phentolamine and chlorpromazine, reduce after-load, as do beta-2 agonists such as salbutamol. These are now rarely used.

Acid-base correction. The best way to correct metabolic acidosis in shock is by restoring adequate tissue perfusion, by fully restoring the circulating volume. However, sodium bicarbonate may be required in addition. The dose may be roughly determined by the following method:

1. Multiply the body weight (in kg) by 0.2, to obtain the volume of extracellular fluid.
2. Now find out the deficit of sodium bicarbonate in each liter. This value is obtained by subtracting the level in the patient's serum from the normal level, (27 meq/l minus the value of sodium bicarbonate in meq/l in the patient's serum).
3. Now multiply the deficit in meq/l with the number of liters in the extracellular fluid. In other words multiply 1 with 2. Thus:

Dosage of sodium bicarbonate required, in meq = 0.2 × body weight × (27 minus sod. bicarb. in meq in the patient's serum).

In low flow states the ability to buffer the acidity in banked blood is reduced, so when rapid massive transfusions are required, an ampoule (45 meq) of sodium bicarbonate should be given with every 2 to 3 units of blood.

CARDIOGENIC SHOCK

Cardiogenic shock may be defined as 'inadequate blood flow to vital organs due to insufficient cardiac output in spite of a normal cardiac filling pressure'. It is seen in a wide variety of surgical patients and may be due to:

1. Myocardial infarction.
2. Arrhythmias.
3. Cardiac tamponade.
4. Delayed and inadequate volume replacement in hypovolaemia.
5. Inappropriate volume replacement in hypovolaemia with creation of a high haematocrit.
6. Pulmonary embolism.

As the heart is not functioning properly blood is dammed in the veins so that the central venous pressure is raised. However the blood pressure, arterial pO_2 and urine output are lowered. The blood lactic acid level is raised. The important haemodynamic abnormalities in cardiogenic shock are: low systolic blood pressure (80 mm Hg or less); low cardiac output (2.0 liters per minute per square meter); and a normal or raised peripheral vascular resistance.

The initial clinical evaluation of cardiogenic circulatory failure should determine the nature of the failure, the underlying cause and the severity of the problem. A full clinical history should be taken and physical examination carried out to detect ischaemic, valvular or congenital heart disease, or hypertension. An ECG will identify acute myocardial infarction, left ventricular hypertrophy, heart block or arrhythmias. Chest x-ray is required for the assessment of heart size, pulmonary markings and pleural effusion. If pulmonary oedema or cardiogenic shock is present, treatment should begin immediately. If there is less urgency, an echocardiogram provides information about the size, thickness and performance of the heart.

The treatment of cardiogenic shock consists of the following:

1. Improvement of *myocardial contractility* by inotropic drugs (e.g. dopamine 0.5 to 5 mg/kg/min).
2. The reduction of cardiac *preload* by diuretics (e.g. furosemide 10 to 100 mg intravenously).
3. The reduction of *afterload* by vasodilators (e.g. sodium nitroprusside infusion of 10 to 15 mg/min, increasing by 10 mg/min every 5 to 15 minutes).

The success or failure of therapy should be measured against clear endpoints, such as doubling of cardiac output, or a 25% reduction in pulmonary artery occlusion pressure. The ECG, arterial pressure, cardiac output, and pulmonary artery occlusion pressure should be monitored throughout the period of therapy. An arterial catheter is essential for monitoring patients receiving vasodilator or inotropic therapy, particularly when the blood pressure is labile.

DISTRIBUTIVE CIRCULATORY FAILURE

The remaining three forms of shock, namely septic, neurogenic and anaphylactic shock, can be grouped together under the heading of 'distributive circulatory failure.' In each of these types, the precapillary smooth muscle sphincters in the skin and splanchnic circulation undergo relaxation, resulting in a marked increase in the capacity of the vascular bed in these organs. Diversion of blood supply to these non-essential organs results in insufficient oxygen delivery to the vital organs, and shock results.

SEPTIC SHOCK

In septic shock the cardiac output is adequate but blood is distributed improperly to different parts of the body. This is mainly due to excessive vasodilatation in the peripheral vascular system, including the skin and splanchnic bed. This is brought about as follows: with the lysis of white cells, mediators like cytokines are liberated in the form of a cascade. These produce relaxation of precapillary sphincters in the skin and splanchnic circulation, diverting blood supply to those non-essential organs, and resulting in insufficient oxygen delivery to the vital organs.

Sepsis syndrome. The sepsis syndrome, and associated multiple organ dysfunction syndrome, is the most common cause of death in patients in critical care units. The cardiac function is normal while the peripheral vascular resistance is low, therefore the cardiac output is high. But in spite of this the filling pressures are low (high output failure). At a later stage, cardiac output along with the function of other organ systems may be greatly impaired. Those patients who do not generate high cardiac outputs in the face of a septic insult have a poor prognosis.

The patient is commonly over 45 years of age, and the genitourinary and gastrointestinal tracts are the most common sites of invasion. Several factors predispose to sepsis. These include: diabetes mellitus, steroid therapy, immunosuppressive therapy, indwelling urinary or intravenous catheters, excessive use of antibiotics, cancer chemotherapy and radiation therapy.

Clinical features. There is a hyperdynamic circulation. This is manifested by a high cardiac output, warm and dry extremities and a raised central venous pressure. As mentioned above, this is probably in an effort to supply oxygen to the deficient cells. However, in spite of this there is profound hypotension and oliguria. Hyperventilation is specially valuable as an early sign of septic shock. After operation hyperventilation can be due to pneumonia, atelectasis, pulmonary embolism or myocardial infarction. However, it should be remembered that it can also be due to septic shock.

The clinical features of sepsis syndrome include the following:

Fever > 38.5°C or < 36°C
Tachycardia > 100/min
Tachypnoea > 20/min
Hypotension, systolic BP < 90 mm Hg
Evidence of localized septic focus

Evidence of toxicity or end-organ failure
Metabolic acidosis, pH < 7.2
Arterial hypoxaemia Po_2 < 10kPa
Increased plasma lactate
Oliguria < 0.5 ml/kg/hour for 1 hour
Coagulation defect
  Prothrombin level 1.5 times control
  PTT 1.5 times control
Thrombocytopenia < 80000/cu mm
Acute deterioration in mental status
Any other sign of organ system failure

Sepsis syndrome is the pathophysiological response to systemic infection or endotoxaemia. It can be produced by a wide range of organisms including Gram-positive and Gram-negative bacteria, protozoa, viruses, and fungi. In a significant number of cases an infective organism is never isolated. Endotoxaemia, though not invariable, is usually present in severe sepsis syndrome with multiple organ dysfunction syndrome, and is associated with a poor prognosis.

MULTIPLE ORGAN DYSFUNCTION SYNDROME

The intestine contains very large numbers of bacteria in its lumen, and in the normal state of health its mucous membrane acts as a barrier between these bacteria and the host circulation and tissues. Food within the lumen of the gut is the most important stimulus for mucosal growth. When, as in cases on intravenous alimentation (usually in patients under critical care), enteral feedings are impossible or inadequate, the intestinal mucosa may atrophy. In such cases bacteria pass across the mucosal barrier and enter the tissues and the circulation. The presence of micro-organisms and their toxins triggers an immunological and inflammatory cascade. Complement is activated and a number of host-derived mediators released, including tumour necrosis factor, interleukins, and myocardial depressant factor. These and other mediators are responsible for vasodilatation, hypotension, and multiple organ dysfunction syndrome (MODS). This process is more likely to take place in inflammatory bowel disease and in obstructive jaundice, where endotoxin can spill over into the circulation.

Early *warning signs* include mental status changes, and increases in the respiratory rate, pulse, temperature and white blood count. Later hypoxia, hypocarbia, and x-ray findings of ARDS make their appearance. Once this happens, the associated mortality escalates. Increasing encephalopathy accompanies progressive respiratory failure. The onset of renal failure, usually due to acute tubular necrosis, increases the mortality rate greatly. Upper gastrointestinal bleeding, bacteraemia, and severe malnutrition are seen. As the number of failing organ systems increases, the associated mortality rises. Once four organ systems are involved, the mortality is virtually 100 percent. In the final stages coagulopathies and wound breakdown develop along with hepatic failure, most patients dying of hepatic and oliguric renal failure.

How do so many different organ systems fail together? It is probable that MODS is a summation of the effects of different humoral mediators, which are all triggered by uncontrolled infection. Vasodilatation is presumably mediated by prostaglandins, kinins, serotonin and histamine; hypermetabolism by corticosteroids and norepinephrine; membrane damage by oxygen free radicals; tissue injury and shock by tumour necrosis factor; and protein breakdown and fever by interleukin-1. Thyroid and growth hormones produce acute catabolism, while complement is responsible for damage to the microcirculation.

Bacterial translocation. Many patients succumbing to MODS show no evidence of a septic focus even at autopsy. In these, it is felt that micro-organisms enter the circulation by migrating across the gut mucosal barrier, begin the septic cascade, and perpetuate MODS. This transmigration of living bacteria or their endotoxins from the lumen of the gut, across the epithelium, to its immediate environment (including the mesenteric lymph nodes, spleen and peritoneum) and into the blood, is called bacterial translocation. This has been shown to occur in a number of conditions including haemorrhagic shock, burns, malnutrition, sepsis and jaundice.

Diagnosis. The presence of multiple organ dysfunction syndrome is clinically obvious, diagnostic criteria being as below; the greater the number of organ systems involved the worse the prognosis:

Circulatory failure
Pulse < 40/min
Mean BP < 50 mm Hg
Ventricular tachycardia or fibrillation
Metabolic acidosis, pH < 7.2
Respiratory failure
Respiratory rate < 5 or > 40/min.
$Paco_2 > 50$ mm Hg
Po_2 gradient > 350 mm Hg
Haematological failure
White cell count < 1000/cu mm
Platelets < 20000/cu mm
Haematocrit < 20%
Evidence of disseminated intravascular coagulation
Neurological
Glasgow coma score < 6
Seizures
Gastrointestinal failure
Ileus
Haemorrhage
Acute renal failure
Urine output < 400 ml/24 hours
Hepatic failure
Coagulation defects
Rising hepatic enzymes
Rising alkaline phoshatase

Management. *Prevention.* Treatment of septic shock is properly based on *prevention of the septic conditions leading to it.* Antibiotic therapy has not reduced the incidence of infection with complicating septicaemia. Further, *prolonged antibiotic therapy permits the development of antibiotic resistant strains of Gram-negative bacteria and their invasion of the bloodstream.* If a prophylactic antibiotic is used, as in a patient undergoing elective surgery on the gastrointestinal tract, it should be started before the operation or not given at all. It has been shown conclusively that if an antibiotic is started after the operation it is quite ineffective in preventing infection.

The antibiotic should either be administered intramuscularly when the patient is called to the operation theatre or intravenously with induction of anaesthesia, and then 4 hours and 12 hours after operation. This type of short course avoids toxicity, provides a high blood level at the time of risk, does not lead to the development of resistant strains, and greatly lowers the infection rate in clean contaminated cases. Prolonged courses of prophylactic antibiotics should be avoided, as they do not lead to any further reduction in the rate of infection.

Catheters. Intravenous, intra-arterial and urinary catheters are frequent sources of infection and septicaemia. *They should be used sparingly, and removed as soon as possible.*

Treatment. *Early recognition* of septic shock is important, and hyperventilation is a particularly valuable warning sign. Management aims at organ system support where required, suppression or amelioration of the toxic effects of the septic process, and identification and eradication of the septic focus. Some forms of organ system support, such as mechanical ventilation and haemofiltration are readily available. Others, such as the support of the brain, circulation and gastrointestinal tract, have to be approached indirectly by trying to attain supranormal levels of oxygen delivery. Appropriate antibiotics are selected, but these will prove ineffective unless surgical drainage of the focus of infection is undertaken.

Antibiotics. These have to be given intravenously because if administered orally or intramuscularly they would not be absorbed due to inadequate tissue perfusion. Treatment is usually started with one of the aminoglycosides (gentamycin or kanamycin), but when culture and sensitivity tests are available, a less toxic but effective drug should be substituted. If the infection is by gram-positive cocci, a synthetic penicillin is used. In anaerobic infections bacteroides are frequently seen. A commonly used combination consists of 10 million units of penicillin, 4 mg per Kg per day of gentamycin and 500 mg 8 hourly of metronidazole. If gram-positive bacilli are present they are most likely clostridia, and penicillin only is required.

Haemodynamics. A higher than normal cardiac output is required. This may require administration of blood, saline, isoproterenol or all three.

Drainage of abscesses. Patients in whom a septic focus is drained have a very much better prognosis than those where this is not done.

Corticosteroids. This therapy is not of proven value; however it is widely used. Large doses are used (50–150 mg per kg of hydrocortisone in a single bolus). The benefits are stated to be three-fold: firstly, the function of the lungs and the kidneys is improved. Secondly, steroids stabilize cellular and subcellular membranes. Thirdly, they stabilize the membranous portion of the microcirculation.

Immunotherapy. Many attempts have been made to interrupt the inflammatory cascade of sepsis. Recently, antibodies against the lipopolysaccharide part of endotoxin have been used in cases of Gram-negative sepsis, with significant reduction in overall mortality, particularly in those presenting in shock. Such immunotherapy may, in time, become the standard treatment for sepsis.

'*Selective decontamination*' of the gut has been attempted, in patients with major trauma or granulocytopenia and those receiving liver transplants, by the use of nonabsorbable antibiotics selected to decrease enteric flora. Combinations of these antibiotics include oral polymyxin, amphotericin and gentamycin with a systemic b-lactam like ceftazidime. A decrease in the incidence of nosocomial lung infections has been reported, although mortality has not been affected.

Both *selective decontamination* and *early enteral feeding* hold out hope for the future. To conclude, different steps in treatment of multiple organ dysfunction syndrome are as follows:

Circulatory failure
Optimize cardiac preload
Inotropes, vasopressors

Correct anaemia, treat arrhythmias
Respiratory failure
Oxygen, mechanical ventilation, PEEP
Extra- and intracorporeal gas exchange
Haematologic failure
Red cells, platelets, fresh frozen plasma
Correct antithrombin III deficiency
Neurological failure
Control seizures
Gastrointestinal failure
Parenteral nutrition
Stress ulcer prophylaxis
Selective decontamination
Acute renal failure
Haemofiltration/haemodialysis or:
Restrict fluids & potassium
Reduce nitrogen intake
Adjust drug dosages
Hepatic failure
Fresh frozen plasma, albumin
Nutritional support.

NEUROGENIC SHOCK

Neurogenic shock is that type of shock which follows serious interference with the balance of vasodilator and vasoconstrictor influences to both arterioles and venules. It is seen in clinical syncope, as with sudden exposure to unpleasant events such as the sight of blood, the hearing of bad tidings, or the sudden onset of severe pain. It is also seen in serious paralysis of vasomotor influences, as in high spinal anaesthesia.

The clinical picture in neurogenic shock is different from that seen in hypovolaemic shock. Although the blood pressure can be very low, the pulse rate is usually slower than normal, and the skin is warm. Not only is the cardiac output reduced but also the resistance of the arterioles and the tone of the veins is diminished. The blood volume is normal. However, as the reservoir capacity of both arterioles and venules is greatly increased, there is a decreased venous return leading to a reduction in the cardiac output.

Treatment. If neurogenic shock is not corrected, the blood flow to the kidneys is reduced and damage to the brain results as well. Subsequently, all the harmful effects of hypovolaemic shock appear. Fortunately the treatment is simple. Shock in high spinal anaesthesia can be treated by a vasopressor such as ephedrine or phenylephrine, which increases cardiac output and at the same time produces peripheral vasoconstriction. In mild cases of neurogenic shock such as fainting, simply removing the stimulus or relieving pain will be adequate treatment, so that the vasoconstrictor nerves can regain the ability to maintain the normal resistance of arterioles and venules. At the same time, *the patient should immediately be placed in a recumbent position* to facilitate venous return and increase cardiac output. In cases of spinal cord transection there may be a great deal of loss of blood and extracellular fluid into the area of injury. It may be difficult to decide about the relative need for fluid replacement and vasopressor drugs. Central venous pressure measurements are of great help in such a situation. It is better to slightly overexpand the volume than to give an excessive amount of vasopressors.

ANAPHYLACTIC SHOCK

Anaphylaxis is defined as an unusual or exaggerated reaction to a foreign protein or other substance. The antigen combines with IgE on the mast cells, releasing large amounts of histamine and slow release substance-anaphylaxis (SRS-A). These chemicals produce bronchospasm, laryngeal oedema, and respiratory distress. Due to the resulting massive vasodilatation and hypoxia, the patient ends up in hypotension and shock. The drug most often responsible for anaphylactic shock is penicillin. Other agents include dextrans and serum injections. The mortality is around 10%.

Treatment. The aims of treatment in severe allergic reactions are three: to correct arterial hypoxaemia, to restore intravascular fluid volume, and to inhibit further release of chemical mediators. The administration of antigen is stopped. An adequate airway is ensured, and oxygen is added to the inspired air. Adrenaline is given intravenously, intramuscularly or via the endotracheal tube: 4–8 mg i.v. for hypotension, 0.5 ml of 1:1000 (0.5 mg) for cardiovascular collapse. Fluids are given in sufficient quantity, both crystalloids and colloids. If there is bronchospasm, aminophylline or adrenaline are used. In cases with pulmonary oedema positive pressure ventilation is provided. For inotropic action adrenaline or noradrenaline may be employed in a dose of 2–4 mg/min. Acidosis may need to be corrected. It should be remembered that steroids produce no benefit in the acute phase, and antihistamines are useful only in angioneurotic oedema.

6 Haemorrhage, haemostasis and blood transfusion

Haemorrhage

Haemorrhage is normally a serious matter, and its control is one of the important duties of a surgeon. He should be able to detect the source of the bleeding and to estimate its amount. Further, he should know how to stop the bleeding.

Source of the haemorrhage. Haemorrhage may occur from an artery, from a vein, or from capillaries:

1. If an *artery* is bleeding the blood is bright red and comes in spurts, in time with the pulse. If the bleeding continues for a long time, and specially if replacement of blood loss has been carried out with electrolyte solutions, the blood may be quite watery.
2. If the blood is coming from a *vein* it is dark red, and flows steadily without spurts. The beginner might imagine that bleeding from veins ought to pose a lesser problem than haemorrhage from the high-pressure arteries. However, such is not always the case. Haemorrhage from large, and specially deep-seated, veins can tax the ingenuity of the most experienced surgeon, and therefore should not be taken lightly.
3. *Capillary* haemorrhage is bright red, and may be quite a rapid ooze. In certain blood disorders it may continue for many hours, and the blood loss can become quite serious.

Haemorrhage from a wound. When a wound is sustained, either due to operation or trauma, haemorrhage may take place either immediately, after a few hours, or after a few days. Depending upon the time at which it occurs, it is classified as follows:

1. *Primary* haemorrhage is that which takes place at the time of the injury or operation.
2. *Reactionary* haemorrhage usually occurs within a few hours, and is most commonly due to slipping of a ligature or dislodgement of a clot. Alternatively, it may occur due to the fact that the artery went into spasm at the time of the injury but later the spasm passed off, with resulting haemorrhage.
3. *Secondary* haemorrhage takes place one or two weeks after the injury or operation. It occurs from sloughing of the wall of the artery, often due to infection. Other causes of erosion of the arterial wall include pressure from a drainage tube or a fragment of bone, and infiltration by a cancer. Secondary haemorrhage can also follow ligation and division of an artery, and arterial operations. There may be 'warning' haemorrhages in the form of bright red stains on the dressing, followed by a sudden severe haemorrhage.

Secondary haemorrhage is specially common after anorectal operations. This is due to the presence of a certain degree of infection along with moisture which causes maceration of the tissues. Haemorrhoidectomy wounds are specially prone to this complication, because they involve division and ligation of the arteries supplying the piles.

External and internal haemorrhage. *External* haemorrhage takes place onto an external surface of the body, for example when the femoral artery is cut across. The quantity of blood lost is easy to estimate, as it is all visible.

Internal haemorrhage is invisible, or *concealed* haemorrhage, as in the case of rupture of the spleen, ruptured ectopic gestation, or fracture of the femur. In certain cases concealed haemorrhage can become revealed, as in haematemesis or melaena from a peptic ulcer, or haematuria following blunt trauma to the kidney.

Clinical features of haemorrhage. When external bleeding takes place it is visible. Apart from this, the signs and symptoms of blood loss are as follows: there is increasing pallor and a rising pulse rate. The patient is restless, and in advanced cases there are deep sighing respirations, a condition which is called *air hunger.* The skin is cold and moist, the veins are empty, and there is thirst.

The *pulse* and *blood pressure* should be recorded every 15 or 30 minutes. When they stabilize, they can be recorded every 2 to 4 hours. The blood pressure is normal at first, and falls only after a good deal of blood has been lost. Therefore, even if the blood pressure is normal, it is possible that severe hypovolaemia may be present. In such a situation the blood pressure is being maintained by shutting off large parts of the vascular bed by vasoconstriction in the non-essential organs. Any further loss of blood volume can lead to sudden collapse and even death. It is therefore important to *palpate the hands and feet* to see if they are warm or cold. If they are warm, it means there is no vasoconstriction, and implies that the blood volume is sufficient. On the other hand cold extremities indicate serious hypovolaemia. With respect to the volume of blood lost, haemorrhage can be *classified* as follows:

Class I haemorrhage, with loss of less than 15% of total blood volume (TBV): this produces very little effect on pulse or blood pressure.

Class II haemorrhage, with loss of 15 to 30% of TBV, produces tachycardia and decreased pulse pressure.

Class III haemorrhage, i.e. loss of more than 30% of TBV, with tachycardia, tachypnoea, hypotension, oliguria and impaired mental status.

Replacement. Blood loss of upto 20% of total blood volume should be replaced with crystalloid solutions; 20 to 50% loss with crystalloids and red blood cell concentrates; and loss greater than 50% with crystalloids, red blood cells and albumin or plasma.

ESTIMATING THE SIZE OF A HAEMORRHAGE

Before the blood lost during a haemorrhage is replaced the clinician should arrive at a rough estimate of the amount of blood lost. In a severe haemorrhage the haemoglobin level, haematocrit, central venous pressure, cardiac output and urine output are all reduced, and the extent of their fall can give some idea of the amount of blood lost.

Haemoglobin level. Immediately after haemorrhage there is no change in the haemoglobin level. However, within a few hours the blood is diluted by the movement of extracellular fluid into the blood vessels, and the haemoglobin level falls.

Packed cell volume or haematocrit. As in the case of haemoglobin, the packed cell volume also falls due to haemodilution.

Central venous pressure (CVP). If the blood volume is low the veins are not well filled, and the hydrostatic pressure in the major veins (central venous pressure) is low. Conversely, if the blood volume is excessively high, the CVP is raised. The normal lower and upper levels of CVP, measured at the level of the midaxillary line, are 4 and 10 cm of water respectively. If measured at the sternal angle the readings are 3 to 4 cm lower.

For the purpose of measurement of the CVP, an intravenous catheter is passed either into the internal jugular vein in the neck, or into the subclavian vein through the infraclavicular route. A chest x-ray is taken to ensure that its tip is lying at the lower end of the superior vena cava or in the upper third of the right atrium. A saline manometer is connected to the catheter through a 3-way stopcock. If the CVP is low the venous return should be supplemented by intravenous infusion; if it is high the amount of fluid given should be restricted. Single measurements of CVP are in fact less useful than serial measurements. At the same time, the response of the CVP to a fluid challenge (a rapid infusion of 100 to 200 ml) is a good indicator of circulatory status and right ventricular function.

It is better to measure the CVP with an electronic pressure transducer. Not only are the readings more accurate, they are available continuously. Transducers show readings in mms Hg (1 cm H_2O = 1.36 cm Hg).

Cardiac output. In hypovolaemia it is particularly important to maintain a good cardiac output. Before a commonly used method of estimating cardiac output is described, a few points may be mentioned:

1. Cardiac output is the product of the pulse rate and stroke volume (cardiac output = pulse rate × stroke volume).
2. Pulse rate is easy to measure, stroke volume is not; it requires elaborate equipment.
3. Pulse pressure (systolic minus diastolic pressure) is easy to estimate, and *is a good measure of stroke volume.*
4. Thus if the pulse rate and pulse pressure are known, a rough estimate of cardiac output can be arrived at.

Simple method of estimating cardiac output. If the pulse rate and pulse pressure are measured and both are found to be reduced, the cardiac output must be low. This should alert the clinician so that he can take remedial action. In a situation where even a blood pressure apparatus is not available, the pulse pressure can be roughly estimated by feeling the pulse. If the pulse pressure is low the pulse is 'thready' or of 'low volume'. *Thus if the pulse is not only slow but also thready, it means the cardiac output is low.*

Urine. The urine output is a good indicator of renal blood flow, which is determined by the cardiac output. Therefore, the amount of urine passed should be carefully monitored in every case of severe haemorrhage. The level in the urine bag should be read every hour and the urine output recorded, which should be above 25–30 ml per hour at the very least.

Measurement of blood loss. It is not always easy to estimate the exact amount of blood lost during trauma or operation. However, a few guidelines may be of some help. If *blood clot* is found around the site of injury it is helpful to remember that clot which is of the size of a closed fist is about 500 ml in volume. In a *fracture* of the tibia if a moderate degree of swelling is present, 500 to 1,500 ml of blood may have been extravasated into the muscles. In a fracture of the femur as much as two liters of blood may be lost into the tissues.

Perhaps the best method of estimating blood loss during operations is to *weigh the swabs* used to mop up the blood, and to deduct their preoperative weight from this weight. A delicate weighing scale is required for this purpose, but it is much better than pure guess-work. In extensive operations such as partial gastrectomy the figure obtained this way should be multiplied by one and a half, and for even more extensive operations like abdominoperineal resection of the rectum, by 2.

The aim of familiarization with the amount of blood lost during operation can also be achieved in a different manner. Drapes can be arranged as in an operation, known volumes of blood, e.g. from 10 ml to 200 ml, spilt onto the drapes, and the size and disposition of the blood-stains noted. This can help estimate the amount of blood when it is actually lost during an operation.

THE TREATMENT OF HAEMORRHAGE

The treatment of haemorrhage resolves itself into two parts:

1. The arrest of bleeding *(haemostasis).* This is discussed in the next part of this chapter.
2. The replacement of the blood lost. This is carried out by *blood transfusion* or by infusion of plasma substitutes. This subject is discussed in the third and last part of this chapter.

Haemostasis

Haemostasis is defined as the arrest of haemorrhage, either by the physiological processes of vasoconstriction and coagulation, or by surgical means.

PHYSIOLOGICAL METHODS OF HAEMOSTASIS

The process of haemostasis begins immediately after injury. It is a complex process which prevents or terminates blood loss, provides a fibrin network for tissue repair, and ultimately removes the fibrin when it is no longer required. On the other hand endothelial cells 'do their best' to keep the vessels open by preventing clotting. They inactivate adenosine diphosphate, thus interfering with platelet recruitment. They provide an environment in which thrombin is inactivated by complexing with antithrombin III. Finally, they release thrombomodulin that downmodulates the coagulation process.

Four major events take part in the process of haemostasis, both simultaneously and consecutively. They are: vascular constriction, platelet plug formation, fibrin formation and fibrinolysis.

Constriction of vessels. Vasoconstriction is the initial vascular response to injury. It is dependent upon local contraction of smooth muscle that provides a reflex response to various stimuli including sympathetic nerve stimulation and circulating norepinephrine. A powerful constrictor of smooth muscle, thromboxane, is also released by platelets. Serotonin, bradykinin and fibrinopeptides are also capable of contracting smooth muscle.

Mechanical factors play an important part in the arrest of haemorrhage. Of these, two are particularly important: the manner of division of the artery, and the size of the cavity into which bleeding is taking place.

Manner of division of the artery. If a medium-sized artery is cut right across it can retract very well. At the same time it can contract down fully, so that haemostasis can take place. On the other hand if the same artery is incompletely divided the elastic fibres and smooth muscle in its wall contract, and the lateral tear in the artery tends to gape open and enlarge in size. Thus blood continues to flow, resulting in severe haemorrhage. Therefore, a lateral tear is far more dangerous than a complete transection.

Size of the cavity. The size of the cavity into which bleeding takes place is important in haemostasis. If bleeding takes place into a cavity which is *small* in size, it quickly fills up until it can accommodate no more blood, and haemorrhage stops. On the other hand bleeding into one of the *major* body cavities namely the peritoneal or pleural cavities is dangerous, because very large quantities of blood can be accommodated in those spaces without tamponade, so that arrest of bleeding does not take place. At the same time in the case of the pleural cavity the accumulating blood reduces the vital capacity and interferes with ventilation. Finally, when there is *low perivascular pressure*, as with the muscle atrophy of old age, in prolonged steroid therapy, and in the Ehlers-Danlos syndrome (defective conversion of procollagen to collagen), bleeding tends to be more persistent.

Function of platelets. Platelets are 2-micron fragments of megakaryocytes, numbering 200,000 to 400,000 per cu mm in the circulating blood, with a life span of 7 to 9 days. They play a very central role in coagulation and haemostasis. Normally they do not adhere to each other or to the vessel wall. However, when a vessel is disrupted, platelets form a plug which stops bleeding. Injury to the intima exposes subendothelial collagen to which platelets adhere within a few seconds. This requires von Willebrand factor, a protein that is lacking in patients with von Willebrand's disease. The platelets then develop pseudopodial processes and also initiate a release reaction that recruits other platelets from the circulating blood. As a result a loose platelet aggregate forms, sealing the disrupted blood vessel.

Platelets provide coagulation factors to most steps of the coagulation cascade. When platelets come across damaged tissues with their exposed collagen, they aggregate and release thromboxane A^2 and serotonin, which promote the contraction of divided vessels and the further aggregation of platelets. They also provide platelet factor 4, platelet-derived growth factor and adenosine diphosphate (ADP), which help in compaction of the platelets and the formation of an amorphous plug. The lipoprotein surface provided by the platelets catalyses the conversion of prothrombin into thrombin. Again, platelet factor 3 promotes coagulation by providing phospholipid to several stages of the coagulation process such as the activation of factors X and II, while platelet factor 4 inhibits heparin.

The mass of fused platelets forms a plug in the damaged vessel. The platelet plug contracts, reinforcing the contraction of the vessel. At the same time thrombin, which itself is a product of coagulation, helps the aggregation and fusion of platelets. Finally, platelets also play a role in fibrinolysis by releasing an inhibitor of plasminogen activation.

Fibrin formation (coagulation). The next important step in the process of haemostasis is the formation of a fibrin clot. Before this can take place a series of reactions occurs, involving about a dozen different coagulation factors acting one after the other. There are two initiating pathways, the 'intrinsic' and the 'extrinsic'. The *intrinsic* pathway involves components normally present in the blood, and comes into play in intact blood vessels. The *extrinsic* pathway is initiated by tissue proteins; this happens when a vessel is damaged and blood spills into the tissues or onto the exterior. At every step of each of the pathways there is an increase in effect, so that the whole acts as an amplification system. The series of steps is shown in schematic form in Fig. 1.

Fibrinolysis. If fibrin was formed in excess, or in areas where it was not necessary, it would have disastrous results. An efficient system for dissolving excessively formed clot is therefore required. This is provided by *plasmin* (also called fibrinolysin). This is a strong proteolytic enzyme that breaks down fibrin into much smaller soluble fragments, thus dissolving excessive amounts of clot. It is derived from a precursor plasma protein (plasminogen). Fibrinolysis is initiated at the same time as the clotting mechanism under the influence of circulating kinases, tissue activators, and kallikrein present in many organs including vascular endothelium.

SURGICAL METHODS OF HAEMOSTASIS

In a first-aid situation away from hospital, the following methods may be employed for controlling haemorrhage:

1. *Packing.* The wound may be packed with gauze, or with any clothing material available. This is held in place by a bandage applied firmly. Unfortunately, laymen are often not aware of the fact that this simple step can be life-saving.

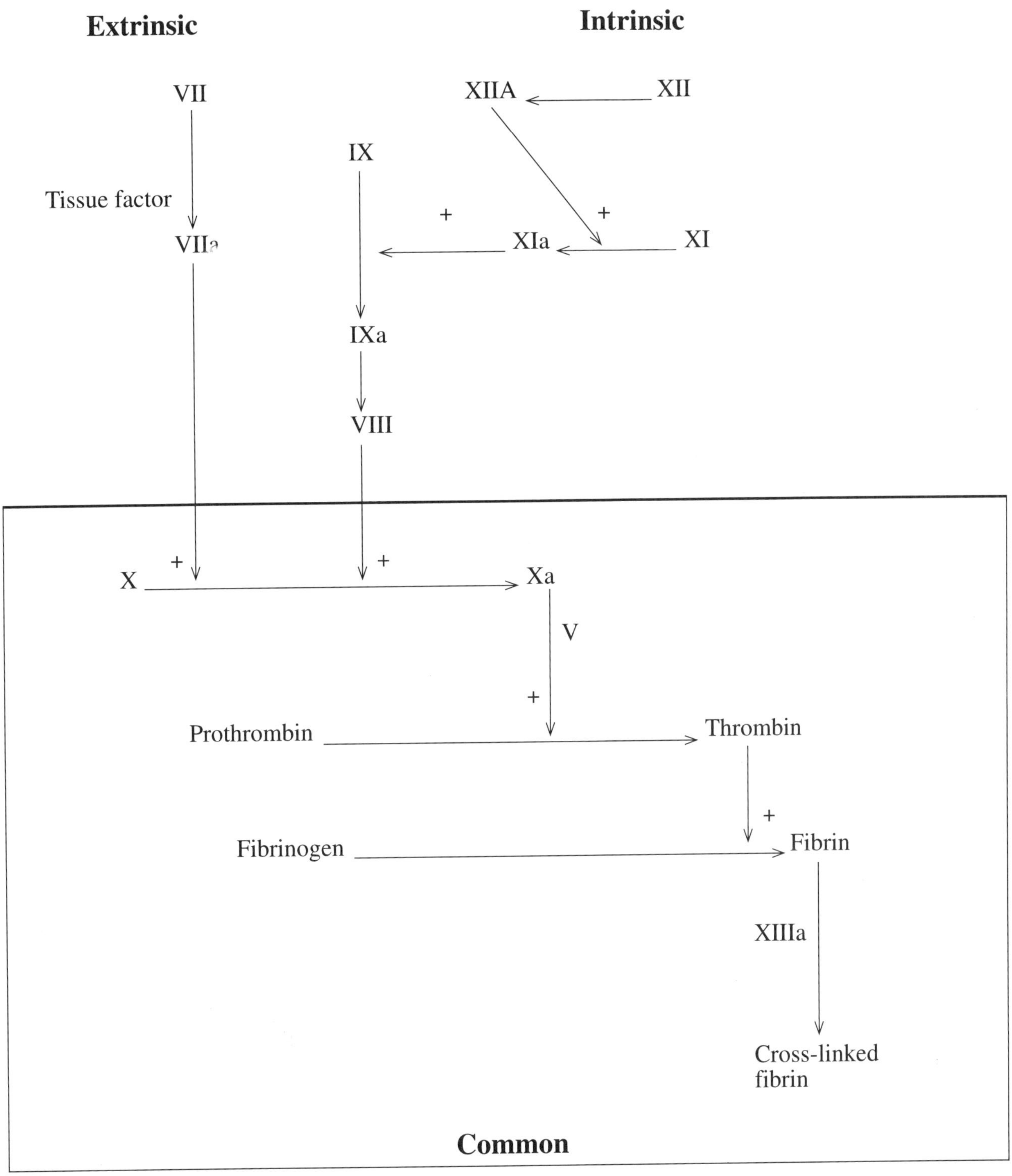

Fig. 1 Schematic version of the coagulation system.

2. *Tourniquets*. The cord-like Samway's tourniquet can be used to stop bleeding from a limb. However, there are many disadvantages associated with its use:

i. There is no way of regulating the pressure, so that very excessive pressure may be applied.

ii. The pressure is applied through a narrow rubber cord i.e. it is not distributed over a wide area, so that its harmful effect is further increased. The result is that damage to nerves and traumatic spasm of the arteries can occur.

The cuff of a blood pressure apparatus is free from both these defects. The pressure can be controlled to be just a little higher than the systolic pressure. Further, this pressure is distributed over the much wider area of the broad sphygmomanometer cuff. For these reasons damage to nerves or arteries is much less common with its use.

If a tourniquet is not tied tightly enough, it may occlude only the veins and not the arteries, and may encourage bleeding instead of stopping it. If a tourniquet after being applied is forgotten and is not removed, disastrous consequences may result, including gangrene requiring amputation of the limb. Various expedients have been employed to avoid such a major tragedy. For example, the letter 'T' may be written on the patient's forehead. Alternatively, the tourniquet may be attached to the operating table, so that the patient cannot be lifted off the table and onto the trolley without releasing it. This latter is probably the better method. A tourniquet should not be left on for longer than about 45 minutes. If it has to be employed for a longer period, it should be released for a few minutes at the expiry of this period, and then reapplied.

At the hospital. The following methods may be employed to arrest bleeding:

1. The most common method is to grip the bleeding point in the jaws of an *artery forceps.* The blood vessel is now *ligated* by catgut etc. If it is a small vessel it can also be sealed off by diathermy. A *diathermy machine* (dia = through; therm = heat) passes electric current through the body. One electrode, which is applied at an area away from the site of the operation, has a large surface. The second electrode is applied to the artery forceps which is holding the bleeding vessel. This electrode is nearly pin-point. The result is that the current passing through the body converges at this point, so that the spot becomes greatly heated and the tissue is coagulated, resulting in arrest of bleeding.

2. *Packing.* In the operation theatre the need for employing this method should be exceptional, because in most cases the bleeding points can be accurately localized and ligated or dealt with by diathermy. But in the ward this is a useful temporary expedient before the patient is taken to the operation theatre.

3. *Fibrin foam or gelatin sponge.* These can be applied to an area from where persistent capillary oozing is occurring. The sponge is in due course absorbed and replaced by granulation tissue.

4. *Haemorrhage into viscera.* If severe haemorrhage starts from an artery supplying a viscus, there are many methods of dealing with it:

i. The bleeding viscus may be *excised*, as in splenectomy.

ii. The artery supplying the bleeding viscus may be *ligated.* For example, in a case of persistent profuse haematuria after prostatectomy, or when an inoperable cancer of the uterine cervix continues to bleed furiously, the *internal iliac arteries may be ligated* on both sides, and the bleeding usually stops.

iii. If bleeding is occurring into the lumen of a hollow viscus, *endoscopy* may be carried out and the bleeding point dealt with. Two examples follow:

(a) In bleeding from oesophageal varices, a *sclerosing agent* is injected into the varices.

(b) In the case of a bleeding artery in the base of a peptic ulcer, *diathermy or laser coagulation* of the bleeding point is carried out.

iv. *Therapeutic embolization.* If the lumen of a bleeding artery could be filled with small artificial emboli, it would get occluded and the bleeding would stop. This is the basis of this recently introduced method. A Seldinger catheter is passed up into the aorta, usually from the femoral artery. This catheter has a fine angulated tip, which is positioned into the origin of the concerned visceral artery. Artificial emboli consisting of blood clot or plastic microspheres are injected into the bleeding artery. This usually helps control the bleeding. Examples of the use of this technique include embolization of the following arteries:

(a) The gastroduodenal artery, to treat a bleeding duodenal ulcer.

(b) The hepatic artery, to relieve the pain of a cancer of the liver, by causing it to shrink in size due to reduced blood supply.

(c) The renal artery, to arrest persistent haemorrhage from an inoperable tumour of the kidney.

Because it is a relatively minor procedure, therapeutic embolization is specially indicated in cases of advanced malignancies for palliation.

ABNORMALITIES OF COAGULATION

CONGENITAL DISORDERS OF COAGULATION

Haemophilia. The most common congenital abnormality of haemostasis is *haemophilia A.* It arises due to lack of factor VIII activity. This is a sex-linked inherited disorder in which males exhibit the disease and females act as carriers. The condition can also occur without any family history, suggesting that spontaneous mutation can also occur.

The main problem is bleeding, both spontaneous and after even slight trauma. The most common surgical problems are orthopaedic. Repeated haemorrhages occur into joints, leading to severe disabilities. At the same time, spontaneous retroperitoneal bleeding may occur, causing severe abdominal pain, tenderness and paralytic ileus. The clues to diagnosis are: a falling haematocrit value, laboratory evidence of poor control of the disorder, and sometimes other evidence of spontaneous bleeding. Death usually results from haemorrhage into the central nervous system.

The *treatment* of haemophilia aims at maintaining factor VIII levels by repeated infusions to prevent spontaneous bleeding. If operation is to be carried out or active bleeding is occurring, higher levels of factor VIII are maintained. However, it is generally better to tide the patient over without operation. It should be mentioned that preparations of factor VIII are extremely expensive.

Haemophilia B (Christmas disease). This is a congenital deficiency of factor IX. It is less common than haemophilia A, and the clinical manifestations are usually milder. Patients with the severe form of the disease require substitution therapy to prevent spontaneous bleeding. Even those with minor disease require substitution therapy whenever major or minor surgery is performed. During severe haemorrhage, treatment should aim to achieve plasma factor IX levels of 20 to 50 percent of normal for about 5 days, and then at 10 to 20 percent of normal for another 10 days. When an operation is required, plasma levels of 50 to 70 percent of normal should be achieved.

ACQUIRED DISORDERS OF COAGULATION

Platelet abnormalities. Thrombocytopenia is the most common abnormality of haemostasis that results in bleeding in the surgical patient. It may be due to:

1. Idiopathic thrombocytopenic purpura (ITP), systemic lupus erythematosus (SLE), or the secondary hypersplenism and splenomegaly of sarcoid, Gaucher's disease, lymphoma and portal hypertension. The marrow shows a normal number of megakaryocytes.
2. Leukemia, uraemia or cytotoxic therapy: the number of megakaryocytes in the marrow is generally reduced.
3. Massive blood loss with replacement by stored blood.

Thrombocytopenia is often accompanied by impaired platelet function. A variety of drugs also interfere with platelet function. These include aspirin, ibuprofen, indomethacin, lignocaine and penicillins.

In general 60,000 platelets per cu mm are adequate for normal haemostasis. If an elective operation is planned, a count greater than 50,000 per cu mm requires no specific therapy. Occasionally, thrombocytopenia may be seen due to vitamin B_{12} or folic acid deficiency, after total gastrectomy or in cases of severe intestinal malabsorption. Supplying the appropriate nutrient corrects the thrombocytopenia in 2 or 3 days. If the patient has ITP or SLE and a low count, steroids generally help to raise it to more normal levels.

In massive blood transfusion, prophylactic administration of platelets is not recommended. However if required, 4 to 8 platelet packs raise the circulating platelet count sufficiently. If the patient is refractory to standard platelet transfusions, human leucocyte antigen-compatible platelets have proved effective.

Liver disease. Liver disease has multifarious effects on coagulation:

1. All the prothrombin-related factors are produced solely in the liver (factors II, VIII, IX and X), and all may be depleted if the liver is diseased.
2. Factor V is manufactured only in the liver and does not store well in banked blood. Deficiency of this factor is often the major clinical defect.
3. Factor I (fibrinogen) is also produced only in the liver. However, dangerously impaired synthesis seems to occur only in the advanced stages of liver disease.
4. The liver produces antiplasmins, clears plasminogen-activators and removes circulating products of fibrinolysis. Thus, in serious liver disease fibrinolysis escapes control and becomes excessive, producing bleeding.
5. The indirect effects of liver disease add to the problem. Destruction of liver tissue produces fibrosis around portal tracts and results in portal hypertension. This causes passive enlargement of the spleen with excessive destruction of platelets, which produces thrombocytopenia. Portal hypertension also produces oesophageal varices which can bleed. If the cirrhosis is due to alcoholism there may also be gastritis or duodenal ulcer, either of which can also bleed.

Thus it will be seen that due to a combination of all the above factors, in advanced liver disease there is a marked tendency to bleed.

Drugs. Perhaps the most common cause of acquired coagulation disorders today are drugs, and a history of intake of such drugs should be carefully elicited in all cases of bleeding disorders. *Aspirin* causes impairment of the function of all platelets circulating at the time of exposure. Similarly, *antitumour agents* impair the production of platelets.

Anticoagulants. Spontaneous bleeding may be a complication of anticoagulant treatment with either heparin or the vitamin K antagonists (warfarin-like drugs), and can result in a rectus sheath haematoma simulating appendicitis. The incidence of bleeding complications with heparin is reduced with a continuous infusion technique, regulating the partial thromboplastin time.

Certain surgical procedures should not be carried out in the presence of anticoagulation:

1. Prostate surgery, because of the additional problem of local fibrinolysis.
2. Blind needle aspirations.

If a patient on heparin requires an emergency operation, heparin should be discontinued; the operation can then be carried out safely after a few hours. If more rapid reversal is required, 1 mg of protamine sulphate for every 100 units of the last dose of heparin is effective.

Disseminated intravascular coagulation. Normally, coagulation is initiated locally as a reaction to local vascular injury. On the other hand in disseminated intravascular coagulation (DIC) there is an explosive activation of the coagulation cascade throughout the vascular tree. Interestingly, this results not in vascular occlusion but a bleeding tendency. This is because the initial thrombus formed undergoes very rapid lysis. Further cycles of coagulation and instantaneous lysis result in the depletion of coagulation factors including fibrinogen, and consumption of platelets. The principal causes of DIC are as follows:

- Severe infections (e.g. septicaemia).
- Malignant disease (metastatic carcinoma, leukaemia).
- Shock.
- Severe burns.
- Snake bite.
- ABO incompatible transfusion.
- Obstetric disorders:
  - Eclampsia.
  - Amniotic fluid embolism.
  - Retained dead foetus.
- Intravascular haemolysis (e.g. after systemic absorption of hypotonic fluids during transurethral prostatectomy).

Most cases of DIC are triggered by septicaemia, particularly that due to Gram-negative organisms. Malignant disease, specially in the presence of multiple metastases, is also an important cause. There is widespread bruising and extensive purpura, with persistent oozing of blood from surgical wounds and venepuncture sites. Epistaxis is common. There may be signs of vascular occlusion in the distal limbs.

Laboratory tests. In fulminant cases the blood is incoagulable. Both the cephalin kaolin clotting time and prothrombin time are greatly prolonged, but are corrected by adding normal plasma to the patient's plasma. The thrombin time is also prolonged, the fibrinogen level being below 1.0 g/l (normal 2–4 g/l). Fibrinogen degradation test levels in the blood are very high, reflecting hyperfibrinolysis. The platelet count is reduced.

Treatment. The underlying cause must be identified; its treatment removes the stimulus for further consumption of coagulation factors. Fresh frozen plasma should be infused, being a good source of coagulation factors, including fibrinogen. Cryoprecipitate is a concentrate of fibrinogen, so that volume overload is avoided. This should also be given, as well as platelet concentrates. Patients often need blood in addition to plasma products. Inhibitors of fibrinolysis, e.g. tranexamic acid are useless and may precipitate thrombosis. Low-dose heparin is also not widely advocated any longer.

Investigation of bleeding disorders. A carefully taken history and physical examination help in determining the following:

1. Whether there is a *generalized* haemostatic defect. This may be suggested by bleeding from multiple sites, spontaneous bleeding and bleeding into the skin.
2. Whether the defect is *inherited* or *acquired.* A family history of a bleeding disorder should be sought. Severe inherited defects become apparent in infancy, while mild inherited defects come to light only later, for example after surgery, childbirth or trauma.
3. Whether the bleeding suggests a *coagulation* defect or a *vascular/platelet* defect. Coagulation disorders are typically associated with haemarthroses and muscle haematomas. On the other hand vascular/platelet bleeding is characterized by easy bruising and spontaneous bleeding from small vessels. The bleeding is mainly into the skin and from mucous membranes, often from the nose and mouth. The term purpura includes:

1. *Petechiae*, which are small skin haemorrhages varying from pinpoint to a few millimetres in diameter, and which do not blanch on pressure.
2. *Ecchymoses*, which are small bruises.

LABORATORY TEST FOR DISORDERS OF COAGULATION

The common tests utilized are the following:

Whole blood clotting time measures the intrinsic coagulation system, but is insensitive and variable.

The one-stage prothrombin time (PT) reflects the extrinsic clotting system i.e. factors II, V, VII and X, but is most sensitive to deficiencies of factor VII. Therefore it is the standard method for monitoring patients receiving vitamin K antagonists.

The activated partial thromboplastin time (APTT) also measures the intrinsic clotting mechanism, but unlike the whole-blood clotting time the results are very reproducible and fairly sensitive. It is sensitive to factors VIII, IX, XI and XII, as well as the factors normally detected by the one-stage prothrombin time. It is useful for screening haemophiliacs, for assessing coagulation in patients with liver disease before surgery, for regulating the dose of heparin, etc.

Tests of fibrinolysis. *Fibrin degradation products* can be measured by immunological methods. The euglobulin clot lysis time is a rapid and sensitive test of fibrinolysis.

The *platelet count* can be measured. However, a great deal depends upon the functional state of the platelets. One of the best tests of platelet function is a very carefully performed *bleeding time.* Tests for provoked petechiae are less sensitive and less reproducible.

To conclude, it must be emphasized that in the care of the bleeding patient the various laboratory tests are less important than careful history-taking and clinical examination, past history of bleeding and response to trauma, recent history of ingestion of drugs, knowledge of the functional state of the liver, and an enquiry for the presence of malignancy, dead tissue, uncontrolled infection and areas of poor perfusion. To order laboratory tests or to commence treatment without thorough investigation into these factors is like putting the cart before the horse. A questionnaire can be designed to ask about:

Prolonged bleeding after biting the tongue or after dental extraction.

Bleeding problems after minor and major operations.

Bruising without injury.

Excessive menstrual bleeding.

Aspirin taken during the preceding week.

The *further course* to be followed depends on the results of the tests:

1. If the history is *negative.* If the operation is minor, no tests are required. In the case of a major operation, platelet count, blood smear and PTT should be carried out.
2. If the history *suggests defective haemostasis* and the operation is major, bleeding time and APTT should be carried out in addition to the above tests.
3. If the history is *strongly suggestive,* the above tests should be carried out. At the same time the bleeding time should be tested 4 hours after 600 mg of aspirin. Further, operation should not be carried out for 10 days after the test.

Excessive bleeding during or shortly after operation may occur due to ineffective local haemostasis, an undetected haemostatic defect or consumption coagulopathy, or as a complication of blood transfusion. Excessive bleeding at operation without bleeding from other sites suggests *inadequate local surgical control* of haemorrhage. However, operations on the prostate, pancreas and liver may be followed by excessive bleeding even after careful haemostasis, because operative trauma may *activate plasminogen* and cause fibrinolysis on the raw areas. Interruption of plasminogen activation by administration of epsilon aminocaproic acid for a day or two usually proves effective for haemostasis.

A *haemolytic* transfusion reaction in a patient under anaesthesia may manifest itself by diffuse bleeding in a previously dry operative field. The haemolysed red cells release adenosine diphosphate which causes platelet aggregation, the platelet aggregates being swept away by the blood.

During biliary tract surgery in cirrhotic patients diffuse bleeding may occur due to portal hypertension and coagulopathy. Vasopressin is used intravenously to reduce the portal hypertension, while epsilon aminocaproic acid (EACA) can be employed to control the increased fibrinolysis.

Blood transfusion

Blood transfusion can be a life-saving procedure. However, it can also be followed by serious reactions due to incompatibility and otherwise. Therefore, blood should be transfused only when really indicated, and stringent precautions should be taken before and during the transfusion. This is all the more important because of the rising incidence of AIDS and hepatitis along with intravenous drug abuse.

INDICATIONS FOR BLOOD TRANSFUSION

Some of the important indications for blood transfusion are as follows:

1. Following *haemorrhage*, which may be due to:

i. Trauma with severe blood loss.

ii. Bleeding from pathological lesions, e.g. from the gastrointestinal tract.

iii. Major operative procedures with extensive dissection, in which a fair amount of blood is lost.

2. After extensive *burns*, where a good deal of blood is destroyed in the burnt skin.

3. *Before operation*, in a case of chronic anaemia, where surgery is indicated urgently and there is insufficient time for iron therapy. However, recently this indication has been questioned, and the teaching that a haemoglobin value of less than 10 g/dl mandates preoperative blood transfusion has been challenged. The cardiac output does not rise until the haemoglobin value falls to 7 g/dl. According to this view, even patients with a haemoglobin value below this figure in whom significant bleeding during operation is not expected are not considered candidates for preoperative transfusion.

4. *Postoperatively*, in a patient where severe anaemia has resulted from infection.

5. In a patient with a *bleeding disorder*, e.g. haemophilia or thrombocytopenia, either to prevent haemorrhage or to arrest it.

Massive transfusion is defined as a single transfusion greater than 2500 ml, or 5000 ml transfused over a period of 24 hours. The problems which can arise include circulatory overload, DIC, dilutional thrombocytopenia, impaired platelet function and deficiencies of factors V, VIII and XI. The routine use of sodium bicarbonate is not recommended, as it shifts the oxyhaemoglobin dissociation curve to the left, and also presents a sodium load to a compromised patient. The risk of haemolytic transfusion reaction due to incompatibility can be reduced by screening each donor. Similarly, the risk of infection increases with each additional unit. If diffuse bleeding takes place, coagulation tests and platelet counts should be carried out and deficits corrected with platelet packs and fresh frozen plasma.

BLOOD COMPONENTS AND PRODUCTS

Specially in the advanced countries, most blood collected from donors is processed into blood components and products. It is normally preferable to transfuse only the component or product required by the patient rather than whole blood. Not only is this the most effective way of using donor blood which is a scarce source; it also reduces the risk of complications from transfusion of unnecessary components of the blood.

Whole blood should be reserved for acute blood loss; even here *packed cells* or *red cell concentrates* plus crystalloid or colloid solutions are acceptable alternatives.

Fresh frozen plasma contains most of the coagulation factors in concentrations approaching those in normal plasma. It is a very good source of coagulation components, but quite large volumes are required for clinical effect. It has an important role in the following conditions:

1. In patients with multiple coagulation defects resulting from hepatic insufficiency.
2. In disseminated intravascular coagulation.
3. Where labile clotting factors have been depleted by the transfusion of very large volumes of old stored blood.

Cryoprecipitate (cold precipitate) was developed when it was found that a cold precipitate of plasma was rich in antihaemophilic globulin (AHG) i.e. Factor VIII. It also contains von Willebrand factor along with some fibrinogen. It is no longer used for the treatment of Haemophilia and von Willebrand's disease because of the greater risk of virus transmission compared to virus-inactivated coagulation factor concentrates.

Factor VIII and IX concentrates are freeze-dried preparations obtained from large pools of plasma. They are used in haemophilia and von Willebrand's disease.

Washed red cell concentrates are useful in patients who have severe recurrent urticarial or anaphylactic reactions.

Platelet concentrates can be stored for upto 5 days at 22°C. They are used to treat bleeding in patients with severe thrombocytopenia.

Albumin. 4.5% and 20% solutions are available. They are inappropriate fluids for acute volume replacement or in shock. They are indicated in acute severe hypoalbuminaemia, the 20% solution being particularly useful in patients with nephrotic syndrome or liver disease who are fluid overloaded and resistant to diuretics.

Immunoglobulins are used in hypogammaglobulinaemia to prevent infections.

Recycled blood. Because of the fear of AIDS as well as hepatitis, cardiac surgeons have started using 'recycled' blood. During an operation where a considerable quantity of blood is inevitably lost, a suction machine sucks up the blood from the cavity the surgeon is working in. The blood is passed through a highly efficient filter and allowed to flow right back into a vein. The system is quite safe. At the same time, because it is fresh, recycled blood has superior oxygen carrying and clotting qualities than banked blood once the heparin has been neutralized. Another advantage of recycling is that one can use an indefinite amount of blood. The same technique can be usefully employed in other branches of surgery.

PLASMA AND BLOOD SUBSTITUTES

Plasma substitutes. If massive bleeding has occurred or is taking place, the lost blood must be replaced promptly. If blood is not available immediately, at least the normal blood volume must be re-established immediately. Volume replacement can be carried out using one of a number of plasma substitutes available:

1. *Dextrans* are polysaccharides of different molecular weight. In the concentrations used, their osmotic pressure is the same as that of plasma. They induce rouleaux formation of the red blood cells and therefore interfere with blood grouping and cross-matching, so the blood sample for these tests must be taken before dextran is infused.

Low molecular weight dextran (40,000) restores blood volume promptly, but its action is of brief duration because the kidney rapidly excretes the small molecules. It prevents sludging of red cells in small vessels. In the kidney this action prevents the renal shutdown which can occur in cases of severe hypotension.

High molecular weight dextrans (110,000 and 70,000) are retained in the circulation for a longer time, so their action is more prolonged. However, they are associated with a higher incidence of allergic reactions.

2. *Gelatin* (molecular weight 30,000) is used as a 4% solution, and upto a liter can be infused.

Blood substitutes. *The future.* Natural haemoglobin when outside the red blood corpuscles breaks up into its two subunits. These are small molecules, which leak into the urine and damage the kidneys. Free haemoglobin therefore cannot be used for transfusion into patients. Recently, researchers have been able to grow large quantities of subunits a and b of human haemoglobin in the gut bacteria Escherichia coli. The subunits are next linked together to produce haemoglobin. These workers have been able to join the subunits in such a manner that they cannot split from each other when free in the blood, and therefore this haemoglobin can be administered to the patient without fear of haemoglobinuria. As haemoglobin can be manufactured on a large scale by E. coli, it appears that such haemoglobin will be available commercially in the near future, and will for the first time provide an oxygen-carrying blood substitute in abundant quantities to be used during wars and natural calamities. This preparation will have the advantage of being completely free of all infectious agents like the AIDS and hepatitis viruses. Besides, this kind of haemoglobin-based artificial blood requires no typing or cross-matching. It will therefore be a very great advance in the subject of blood transfusion.

COMPLICATIONS OF BLOOD TRANSFUSIONS

Although the availability of blood transfusions has greatly advanced the frontiers of surgery, it must be remembered that a number of serious complications can follow after blood transfusions, including the following:

1. Incompatibility. The ABO blood groups are of very basic importance in every case of blood transfusion. Let us see how a transfusion reaction develops. The ABO antigens are two, A and B. Each person carries in his red cells either one (A or B), or both (AB), or none (O). If he carries the antigen A, his blood does not have any anti-A antibodies. Now, many plants have both A and B antigens, and every human being gets exposed to them. So this person who belongs to group A develops anti-B antibodies at an early age. These antibodies are powerful haemolysins. Therefore, if he now receives blood of the B or AB groups, severe intravascular haemolysis is produced, which often results in disseminated intravascular coagulation and renal failure. Upto 10% of these cases end up in a mortality. At the same time, if a very large quantity of plasma containing anti-A or anti-B antibodies is infused into a recipient whose red cells contain A or B, haemolysis will occur, but usually will be less severe.

Misidentification the commonest cause of transfusion reactions. Although ABO incompatibility can and does occur from time to time, the irony of the situation lies in the fact that the majority of transfusion reactions occur from simple *misidentification;* either the patient or the blood is incorrectly identified, or the blood sample sent for cross-matching is wrongly labelled. The unnecessary deaths from some of these wrongly labelled units of blood can be prevented by being careful, and by strict adherence to a routine for proper identification.

The Rh antigens. A person either carries the Rh antigen in his red blood cells and is therefore Rh +ve, or he does not carry such antigen, and is Rh –ve. If a patient is receiving blood for the first time, no untoward reaction takes place even if the recipient is Rh –ve and the donor Rh +ve. However, with repeated transfusions of Rh +ve blood into an Rh -ve person, anti-Rh antibodies develop in the plasma of the recipient, and can cause a reaction. Thus Rh antigens are important only in Rh –ve persons, and then only if they have either been transfused previously with Rh +ve blood, or have been pregnant with an Rh +ve foetus.

O-negative blood. If blood is required in a dire emergency which allows no time for grouping and matching, group O Rh –ve blood can be used. Such blood is also very useful if there are mass casualties, where not only is there no time for grouping and cross-matching, but also the risk of a mix-up is greater.

Before O Rh –ve blood can arrive, the patient's blood volume can be restored by normal saline, Ringer's lactate, gelatin (e.g. Haemaccel), dextran or 4.5% human albumin. *If hypovolaemia is severe, it is the speed of infusion rather than the actual composition of the fluid that is important.*

Non-fatal haemolytic reactions occur once for every 6000 units of blood transfused, while the incidence of fatal reactions is about 1 per 100000 units administered. ABO and Rh incompatibility reactions occur because of labelling mistakes and technical errors in the laboratory. Intravascular destruction of red cells results in haemoglobinaemia and haemoglobinuria. The renal lesions consist of tubular necrosis and precipitation of haemoglobin in the tubules.

Clinical features. There is pain in the lumbar region and constricting pain in the chest with chills, fever, dyspnoea, hypotension and tachycardia. In patients under anaesthesia, abnormal bleeding and hypotension despite adequate volume replacement are seen. If a full unit of incompatible blood has been given, the mortality and morbidity rate is high. In about 20% of patients an acute haemorrhagic diathesis is seen with a fall in platelet count, increase in fibrinolytic activity, and consumption of coagulation factors due to disseminated intravascular coagulation.

Laboratory findings include haemoglobinuria with a free haemoglobin level of over 5 mg/dl, and evidence of antigen incompatibility of donor and recipient blood. A bladder catheter shows the dark colour and low volume of urine. A positive Coomb's test shows transfused cells coated with patient autoantibody.

Treatment. The transfusion is stopped, a sample of the recipient's blood is taken and sent to the blood bank with the suspected unit of blood. The serum bilirubin is determined. A Foley catheter is passed and the hourly urine output recorded. Mannitol or furosemide plus sodium bicarbonate are given intravenously. Dialysis is sometimes required. During recovery, losses of sodium and potassium due to the diuresis may require replacement.

2. Other transfusion reactions. i. *Pyrexial reactions.* The patient develops fever with rigors. The most common cause of these reactions is the presence of impurities in the donor apparatus. These reactions were very common in the past when red rubber tubings were repeatedly used in transfusion sets. Their incidence was greatly reduced by the introduction of plastic disposable transfusion sets.

ii. *Allergic reactions.* The patient develops an urticarial rash and tachycardia; rarely, acute anaphylaxis may occur. This is the result of an allergic reaction to plasma products in the donor blood. The transfusion should be stopped and an antihistaminic drug administered, e.g. chlorpheniramine, 10 mg.

3. Infections. Three common types of infection can occur in the recipient:

i. *Bacterial infection.* This usually occurs if the donor blood is left in a warm room for some hours before being transfused, as any bacteria in the blood can multiply their numbers. Septicaemia and even death can result.

ii. *Hepatitis.* A common and serious complication of blood transfusion is the transmission of the virus of serum hepatitis. Severe hepatitis arises about three months after the transfusion. The common type of hepatitis thus transmitted is not from the recognized types, and is called non-A, non-B hepatitis. It is not as lethal as hepatitis B, but can cause chronic active cirrhosis. The causative organism is the hepatitis B or hepatitis C virus (HBV or HCV). The advanced countries have a low incidence of HBV, which is widespread in the developing countries. HCV was identified as recently as 1988, and in countries where blood is tested for HBV markers, was responsible for the great majority of cases of post-transfusion hepatitis. However, since the introduction of screening for HCV in donor blood, this incidence has fallen to only 4%. All donors should be asked if they have suffered from jaundice in the past, and should be tested for hepatitis B antigen. However, the test is not sensitive enough to eliminate all possibility of the disease.

iii. *Thrombophlebitis* may occur in a vein into which the transfusion has been given, and usually *results from a lack of observation of aseptic precautions.* If suppuration develops, wide incision and drainage, or even excision of the vein, must be carried out for prompt relief from the infection.

4. Congestive cardiac failure. Congestive cardiac failure can occur if blood is transfused too rapidly specially in the elderly, or when there is cardiovascular insufficiency. If blood has to be transfused in a case of anaemia, it is better to give packed red cells; at the same time the transfusion should be given slowly, over a period of many hours.

5. Air embolism. Air may be sucked into an open vein at the end of the transfusion. If a drip chamber is used which contains a plastic float that plugs the exit when the fluid falls to a low level, this complication is prevented. Collapsible bags for blood and intravenous fluids are also relatively safe, unless they have been punctured by a needle for adding some drug to the infusate.

6. Coagulation defects. These may arise as follows:

i. *Stored blood* is low in platelets, factor V and factors VIII. Therefore, if large volumes of stored blood are used these factors may get diluted and haemorrhage can occur.

ii. *Disseminated intravascular coagulation (DIC).* This commonly follows ABO incompatibility. When coagulation takes place in the blood vessels the various coagulation factors namely fibrinogen, factor II, V, VIII and platelets, get used up, so that haemorrhage results. For the treatment of DIC these factors have to be replaced.

7 Fluid and electrolyte management

If the cells of the body are to function efficiently, their internal environment, i.e. composition of the extracellular and intracellular fluids, must remain constant. For this, it is necessary that water and different electrolytes used up in the various metabolic processes be replaced in like amounts. In the normal healthy person this takes place by ingestion of appropriate quantities of water and food as dictated by thirst and appetite, both of which are extremely elegant mechanisms for regulation of the internal environment; we are not sufficiently cognizant of their accuracy because we take them for granted.

Where oral intake is not possible for one reason or the other, the same must be provided by an alternative route, commonly intravenously. For this purpose one must know the normal amounts of fluids and salts ingested and excreted every day. At the same time in many surgical illnesses, as well as after operations, excessive quantities of water and salts are lost. In such situations we must know how to assess the amounts lost, in order to replace them accurately. It will thus be seen that fluid and electrolyte management is a very important part of the care of surgical patients.

NORMAL EXCHANGE OF FLUIDS AND ELECTROLYTES

The healthy 70 kg adult consumes on an average about 2,500 ml of water per day. About 1,500 ml of this is water taken as such by mouth. The rest is water extracted from solid food or gained as water of oxidation. The salt (sodium chloride) intake of this average adult is about 5 gm per day.

How to replace the water and salt? Before we discuss abnormal losses and their management, let us see how the above-noted basal amounts of water and salt can be replaced intravenously, if it is so desired.

If one was to replace all the 2,500 ml as plain water, one would require to make it isotonic, because if plain water was given intravenously in such a quantity it would cause intense haemolysis, being severely hypotonic, and would kill the recipient. In clinical practice water is made isotonic by adding 5% glucose to it, this being the amount of glucose which makes it exactly isotonic with plasma. An added bonus in using glucose is the fact that glucose is quickly metabolized, providing some ready energy, leaving behind just water. Thus, electrolytically speaking a 5% aqueous solution of glucose is simply water. In other words if one gives 2,500 ml of 5% glucose in water, one is really giving 2,500 ml of plain water.

Now, how does one add 5 gm of sodium chloride to this 2,500 ml of water? In clinical practice the most common method by which this is done is by replacing 500 ml of 5% glucose by the same volume of normal saline. This gives $500 \times 0.9/100 = 4.5$ gm of salt, which is fairly close to the 5 gm of salt required.

To sum up, then, the normal basal requirement of water and salt is made good by administering 2,000 ml of 5% glucose and 500 ml of normal saline. This is also called the *maintenance requirement.* Another method of giving the same quantities of water and salt is to administer 2,500 ml of 1/5th normal saline. This maintenance requirement never varies, i.e. in a 70 kg adult it is 2,500 ml of water, with 5 gm of salt.

Method of calculation in a patient. When calculating the fluid needs of any particular patient, this maintenance requirement is first noted down. To this are added any losses due to operation or fever. Finally, any losses from the gastrointestinal tract, due to vomiting, nasogastric aspiration, diarrhoea or discharge from an intestinal fistula, are recorded and added to the total. We shall see in detail, in due course, how the abnormal losses are assessed in different situations. However, the concept of maintenance requirement has been introduced at this stage for the sake of clarity, so that the full requirements can later be built up on this basic value.

Incidentally, every clinician should have a sip or two of 5% glucose, and of normal saline, to see how they taste. In fact if he tasted some of the other intravenously administered fluids as well, it would do him no harm!

CLASSIFICATION OF BODY FLUID CHANGES

Disorders of fluid balance may be of three types, namely disturbances of volume, concentration and composition. For ease of understanding, the three types are discussed in turn. However, it should be noted that in any patient more than one type of change is commonly present.

VOLUME CHANGES

The most common fluid disorder in the surgical patient is reduction in the volume of the extracellular fluid. Remember that the fluid lost is not water alone. Both water and electrolytes are lost, *in approximately the same proportion as that in which they exist in the extracellular fluid.*

Volume deficit. Volume deficit may be produced by two different kinds of processes:

1. Fluid is actually lost from the body; in surgical practice this commonly occurs when *gastrointestinal fluid* is lost due to:

   i. Vomiting.

   ii. Gastroduodenal suction, after operation or in cases of intestinal obstruction.

   iii. Diarrhoea.

   iv. Drainage from a fistula, usually intestinal.

2. No fluid is actually lost from the body. *However, fluid is lost from the blood vessels and is 'sequestrated' into the tissue spaces or body cavities.* Examples of such losses of fluids include the following conditions:

i. *Soft tissue injuries and infections*, fluid being lost into the injured tissues.

ii. *Peritonitis*, fluid being lost into the peritoneal cavity.

iii. *Intestinal obstruction*, large volumes of fluid collecting in the lumen of the intestine.

iv. *Burns*, where great quantities of fluid are trapped in the oedematous burn wound.

Clinical features. The symptoms and signs of volume deficit are manifested by the different organ systems as follows:

CNS. Sleepiness, apathy, anorexia.

Cardiovascular. Tachycardia, collapsing pulse, collapsed veins, hypotension.

Tissue signs. Decreased skin turgor.

Metabolism. Reduction in body temperature.

Volume excess. In surgical practice this happens commonly when too much fluid is given intravenously. At the same time, volume overload can take place in renal failure, due to the inability of the kidneys to excrete a normal volume of water. The signs are those of circulatory overload, e.g. distended neck veins, crepitations at the lung bases, and oedema of the feet. In the elderly patient congestive cardiac failure with pulmonary oedema may develop rather quickly even with a moderate volume excess. Our forensic colleagues tell us how frequently, at postmortem examinations, they find lungs overloaded with fluid in patients dying after stab or bullet wounds. We should therefore be careful not to overinfuse our patients.

CONCENTRATION CHANGES

If the serum sodium level becomes very low or very high, it can be diagnosed by clinical examination. However, one should not allow the situation to reach that stage. Serum electrolyte determinations should be carried out repeatedly, so that minor deviations from the normal are detected and corrected promptly. Disorders of sodium concentration include hyponatraemia and hypernatraemia.

Hyponatraemia. When the serum sodium level is low the osmolality of the extracellular fluid falls. This causes water to move into the cells to restore osmolality. In the brain increased intracellular water causes raised intracranial pressure, with muscle twitchings or even convulsions.

Hypernatraemia. In this condition CNS signs occur in the form of restlessness and weakness. In severe cases the patient is delirious and behaves like a maniac.

POTASSIUM ABNORMALITIES

Potassium is the major cation of intracellular water, 98% of the potassium in the body being located within the cells at a concentration of approximately 150 meq/liter. Disorders of potassium concentration include hypokalaemia and hyperkalaemia.

Hypokalaemia. The more common problem in surgical patients is hypokalaemia which may occur due to one or more of the following causes:

1. Loss of gastrointestinal fluids by diarrhoea, intestinal fistula, etc.
2. Prolonged administration of potassium-free parenteral fluids (because in the meantime obligatory renal loss of potassium continues).
3. Parenteral hyperalimentation with inadequate potassium replacement.
4. Excessive renal excretion of potassium.

Potassium plays an important role in the regulation of the acid-base balance. The physical signs of potassium deficit are produced by the failure of contractility of skeletal, smooth and cardiac muscle. There is weakness, progressing to flaccid paralysis. Abdominal distension occurs due to paralytic ileus. The ECG shows flattening of T waves and depression of ST segments.

Treatment. Treatment of hypokalaemia firstly involves prevention. While replacing gastrointestinal losses, potassium should also be replaced. It should be remembered that while treating hypokalaemia, *potassium should not be given into a vein*, as the sudden rise of potassium concentration in the blood can cause cardiac arrest. Instead, potassium is added to the intravenous fluids and given as a drip. No more than 40 meq should be added to a liter of intravenous fluid, and the rate of administration should not exceed 40 meq per hour.

Hyperkalaemia. The most common cause of hyperkalaemia is chronic renal failure. After severe injury or surgical operation, and also in a catabolic state from any cause, a large number of cells are broken down and a significant amount of intracellular potassium released into the extracellular space. Similarly, potassium also moves out of the cells in acidosis. *However, the serum potassium level rises markedly only if the kidneys fail to excrete the excess potassium*, in oliguric or anuric renal failure.

The *clinical signs* of hyperkalaemia are manifested in the cardiovascular and gastrointestinal (GI) systems. The GI symptoms include nausea, vomiting, intestinal colic and diarrhoea. The cardiovascular signs are first seen on the ECG: peaked T waves, widened QRS complexes, and depressed ST segments. At higher levels of potassium the T waves disappear, and heart block and diastolic cardiac arrest develop.

Treatment. Treatment of hyperkalaemia includes the following measures:

1. Exogenously administered potassium is withheld.
2. The following measures are taken to reduce the potassium level in the blood:

i. 50 ml of 50% glucose solution is given intravenously along with insulin. The glucose stimulates the synthesis of glycogen, resulting in an uptake of potassium and reducing its level in the serum.

ii. 50–150 meq of sodium lactate or bicarbonate are given intravenously. This raises the pH and shifts potassium into the cells.

iii. 10% calcium gluconate is given in a dose of 10-30 ml in a liter of intravenous fluid as an infusion. It helps counteract the effects of hyperkalaemia on the myocardium.

3. The underlying cause of hyperkalaemia is corrected if possible.

MIXED VOLUME AND CONCENTRATION CHANGES

The most common example is seen in a patient who is losing large volumes of gastrointestinal fluids but continues to drink plain water. The result is an extracellular deficit with hyponatraemia. This can also occur if, after operation, gastrointestinal losses are replaced by only 5% glucose in water. On the other hand, if a patient with oliguric renal failure is given an excess of water, the result is raised extracellular volume and hyponatraemia.

The importance of kidney function. Normally functioning kidneys minimize these changes. The result is that some of our mistakes in fluid administration are compensated and masked. However, when a patient is in oliguric renal failure, he is specially prone to develop these fluid disorders. In these patients, therefore, fluid management must be extremely precise.

'Functional' renal failure. It should be remembered that when a patient has a significant deficit of volume, even if he has normal kidneys his glomerular filtration rate (GFR) is reduced. Thus the patient is in a state of 'functional' renal failure, because with a low GFR the kidneys' ability of maintaining fluid haemostasis is lost. Fortunately, these changes are reversible with early correction of the extracellular fluid volume deficit.

COMPOSITION CHANGES

The most common change of composition involves an excess or deficit of hydrogen ions, i.e. acidosis or alkalosis. The other important changes of composition include excess or deficit of potassium, calcium and magnesium.

ACID-BASE BALANCE

In different disease states either acidosis or alkalosis may occur. Either of these may be due to a disorder of respiration or metabolism.

Respiratory acidosis. This condition occurs when alveolar ventilation is decreased, so that CO_2 is retained. Examples of these conditions include the following:

1. Airway obstruction.
2. Atelectasis.
3. Pneumonia.
4. Pleural effusion.
5. Hypoventilation due to the pain of upper abdominal incisions.
6. Abdominal distension from paralytic ileus limiting diaphragmatic movements.

These factors may operate singly or in combination. The problem can be particularly serious in the patient with chronic lung disease, because in such a patient pre-existing respiratory acidosis may be made worse in the postoperative period. After operation restlessness, hypertension and tachycardia are commonly due to pain. However, it must be remembered that *they can also be due to inadequate ventilation with a raised* Pa_{CO_2} which can be dangerous if it remains undetected and uncorrected.

Prevention. Strict attention to tracheo-bronchial hygiene during the postoperative period is an important preventive measure, specially in patients with chronic lung disease:

1. Deep breathing and coughing are taught before, and supervised after, operation.
2. Humidified air is inhaled to prevent hardening of secretions.
3. Oversedation is avoided, as it depresses respiration.

Management. Whenever possible the underlying defect should be corrected. At the same time, steps must be taken to ensure adequate ventilation. Occasionally, an endotracheal tube may have to be passed and the patient placed on a ventilator.

Respiratory alkalosis. After operation the patient may hyperventilate. The most common factors leading to such hyperventilation include apprehension and pain. Occasionally the cause may be hypoxia, and rarely nervous system injury.

Complications of respiratory alkalosis. Severe respiratory alkalosis can produce the following complications:

1. *Hypokalaemia*, producing ventricular arrhythmia and fibrillation.
2. Shift of the oxyhaemoglobin dissociation curve to the left. Thus haemoglobin cannot easily unload oxygen at the tissue level, and hypoxia may result.
3. The level of ionized *calcium* may be significantly depressed, and tetany and convulsions may result.

Treatment is directed towards preventing the condition by the proper use of mechanical ventilators and by correcting pre-existing potassium deficits.

Metabolic acidosis. This condition results when:

1. Fixed acids are either produced in excess or retained in the body. Some examples follow:
   i. In diabetic acidosis (due to excess production).
   ii. In lactic acidosis (due to excess production).
   iii. In azotaemia (due to retention).
2. Bicarbonate base is lost from the body, e.g. in:
   i. Diarrhoea.
   ii. Small bowel fistula.
   iii. Renal insufficiency, with inability to reabsorb bicarbonate.

Compensation initially occurs by an increase in the rate and depth of ventilation, which washes out CO_2.

Common causes of metabolic acidosis. The conditions commonly resulting in metabolic acidosis include the following:

1. One of the very important functions of the kidney is the regulation of pH, by the excretion of nitrogenous waste products and acid metabolites, and the resorption of bicarbonate. If *renal damage* occurs and these regulatory functions are lost, metabolic acidosis develops rapidly and may be difficult to control.
2. However, metabolic acidosis can occur even in a patient with normal kidneys. This happens when more chloride is given than the kidneys can handle. *The typical patient is one who has suffered excessive losses of alkaline gastrointestinal fluids* (biliary, pancreatic, small bowel secretions). He has been on intravenous fluids for many days, having been given mostly isotonic sodium chloride solution. Because these solutions have only chloride and no bicarbonate they will not correct the pH change. The use of a balanced salt solution, such as lactated Ringer's solution, is required.

Anion gap. Routine electrolyte estimations determine the levels of the cations sodium and potassium, and the anions chloride and bicarbonate. The total of the former exceeds that of the latter. This is due to the presence of organic anions which are not normally measured. The difference is called the anion gap.

Anion gap is a useful tool in the management of acid-base disorders. The value is found by subtracting the sum of the chloride and bicarbonate from the serum sodium concentration. The unmeasured anions that account for the 'gap' are sulphate, phosphate, lactate, and other organic anions.

If the acidosis is due to loss of bicarbonate (e.g. diarrhoea) or gain of chloride (e.g. administration of ammonium chloride), the anion gap will be normal. On the other hand if the acidosis is due to increased production of an organic acid (e.g. lactic acid in circulatory shock) or the retention of sulphuric or phosphoric acid (e.g. in renal failure), the concentration of these *unmeasured* anions (i.e. the anion gap) will be increased. The most common cause of an elevated anion gap is shock or inadequate tissue perfusion from any cause, resulting in accumulation of large quantities of lactic acid. Diabetic ketosis and starvation cause elevation of the anion gap by formation of ketoacids; renal failure produces the same effect by the retention of sulphuric or phosphoric acids.

3. A common cause of severe metabolic acidosis in surgical patients is *acute circulatory failure*. In this condition inadequate perfusion of the tissues results in tissue hypoxia. Due to the inadequate supply of oxygen, carbohydrates cannot be broken down to CO_2 and H_2O. Anaerobic glycolysis leads to formation of lactic acid.

4. *Acute haemorrhagic shock also* produces a profound drop in pH due to lactic acidosis. Attempts to raise the blood pressure with vasopressors simply worsen the situation. Similarly, efforts to correct the acidosis by infusing large quantities of sodium bicarbonate, without restoring the blood flow, are futile. The indiscriminate use of sodium bicarbonate during resuscitation of patients in hypovolaemic shock should be discouraged because:

i. A mild metabolic alkalosis is common following resuscitation, partly due to the alkalinizing effect of blood transfusions and the administration of lactated Ringer's solution.

ii. After restoration of hepatic blood flow the lactate in lactated Ringer's solution and the citrate in the transfused blood are metabolized and bicarbonate is formed.

iii. The lactic acid that accumulated during the shock episode is rapidly cleared once adequate tissue perfusion is restored.

If excessive quantities of sodium bicarbonate are administered at the same time, severe metabolic alkalosis can result. An alkaline pH is highly undesirable, because it shifts the oxyhaemoglobin dissociation curve to the left. Haemoglobin does not readily give up its oxygen, and oxygen unloading at the tissue level suffers.

On the other hand if volume replacement is carried out promptly, adequate tissue perfusion and therefore oxygenation is restored. The lactic acid is quickly metabolized and the pH returns to normal. This volume replacement should not be carried out using blood alone, but blood and lactated Ringer's solution should be used together. In this way the pH returns to normal more promptly. In fact the recent tendency is to use more Ringer's lactate than blood.

Metabolic alkalosis. Metabolic alkalosis results from loss of fixed acid, e.g. during the vomiting of pyloric stenosis, or due to gain of base bicarbonate. It is aggravated by any pre-existing potassium depletion. Compensation is primarily by renal mechanisms, because respiratory compensation is generally of a minor degree.

Most patients with metabolic alkalosis have some hypokalaemia. When cellular potassium is depleted sodium and hydrogen enter the cell. This produces an intracellular acidosis and extracellular alkalosis. The dangers of metabolic alkalosis are the same as those described under respiratory alkalosis, namely hypoxia, hypokalaemia and tetany.

In *pyloric stenosis* persistent vomiting or gastric suction produces a hypochloraemic, hypokalaemic metabolic alkalosis. Proper management requires replacement of the extracellular fluid volume deficit with isotonic sodium chloride solution, along with replacement of potassium. Volume restitution should be started first and a good urine output obtained before potassium is administered, otherwise dangerous hyperkalaemia could result. Temporary control of the alkalosis with this method is usually successful, but control of the underlying cause should be achieved as soon as possible.

CALCIUM ABNORMALITIES

The total amount of calcium in the body is about 1,000 gm in the average adult, most of which is found in the bones. The normal daily intake of calcium is 1 to 3 gm. Most of this is excreted via the gastrointestinal tract, and about 200 mg is excreted in the urine per day. The normal serum calcium level is 8.5 to 10.5 mg/dl (2.2–2.6 mmol/l). About half of this is non-ionized, and bound to protein and other substances in the plasma. The other half is ionized, and is responsible for neuromuscular stability. Disturbances of calcium metabolism are not a problem in the uncomplicated postoperative patient, and therefore administration of calcium is not required in such cases.

Hypocalcaemia. The common causes of hypocalcaemia include acute pancreatitis, chronic renal failure, hypoparathyroidism, and massive soft tissue infections (necrotizing fasciitis). The symptoms of hypocalcaemia (serum level less than 8 mg/dl i.e. 2 mmol/l) are numbness and tingling of the circumoral region, fingers and toes. The signs are muscle cramps, tetany with carpopedal spasm, convulsions, and prolongation of the Q-T interval on ECG.

Treatment consists of correction of the underlying cause alongwith repletion of the deficit. Acute symptoms can be relieved by intravenous calcium gluconate. Patients requiring prolonged replacement may be given calcium lactate by mouth. Routine administration of calcium during massive blood transfusions is probably not required. Only those patients who are receiving blood as rapidly as 100 ml per minute require calcium administration; in other cases dangerous levels of hypercalcaemia can result.

Hypercalcaemia. The two main causes of hypercalcaemia are cancer with bony metastases, and hyperparathyroidism. The former is most common in a patient with metastatic breast cancer who is receiving oestrogen therapy.

Treatment is urgent. Measures to lower the serum calcium level are instituted immediately. The extracellular fluid volume is depleted in these cases; the deficit is rapidly made good, and this immediately lowers the serum calcium level by dilution. The treatment of hypercalcaemia in the patient with metastatic cancer is that of prevention. If the serum calcium level is raised the patient is placed on a low-calcium diet, and measures are taken to ensure adequate hydration.

MAGNESIUM ABNORMALITIES

Magnesium deficiency occurs infrequently. Plasma magnesium concentration ranges between 1.5 and 2.5 meq/l (0.7–1.1 mmol/l). Most of the magnesium is excreted in the faeces, and the remainder in the urine.

Magnesium deficiency. Magnesium deficiency occurs in starvation, in the malabsorption syndrome, after very long-continued losses of gastro-intestinal fluids, and following the use of intravenous fluids with magnesium-free solutions. Other causes are acute pancreatitis, diabetic acidosis and the late stages of a major burn. The magnesium ion is essential for the proper functioning of most enzyme systems. Thus depletion is characterized by *neuromuscular* and *central nervous system hyperactivity*. The symptoms are similar to those of calcium deficiency, including muscle tremors and tetany, progressing to delirium and convulsions in severe cases.

The diagnosis of magnesium deficiency cannot be made without awareness of the syndrome. *In the surgical patient who exhibits disturbed neuromuscular or cerebral activity in the postoperative period, magnesium deficiency must be kept in mind.* This is specially so if he has had long-continued dysfunction of the gastrointestinal tract and has been maintained on magnesium-free intravenous fluids. Cases of small gut fistulas of many weeks' duration provide most of the examples.

Treatment is by parenteral administration of magnesium sulphate or chloride. If renal function is normal 80 meq of magnesium sulphate are given over 6–8 hours. The pulse, blood pressure, respiration and ECG are monitored for signs of magnesium toxicity, which can cause cardiac arrest. Calcium chloride or gluconate should be available to counteract any adverse effects of a rapidly rising magnesium level.

Magnesium excess. Magnesium excess is seen in massive trauma because large numbers of body cells are damaged, and the magnesium contained inside them is liberated into the extracellular fluid. However, *the most common cause of hypermagnesaemia (as of hyperkalaemia) is severe renal insufficiency*, when the magnesium which is liberated during the normal processes of metabolism cannot be excreted. Magnesium also moves out of the cells in acidosis.

Acute symptoms may be controlled by the slow intravenous administration of 5 to 10 meq of calcium chloride or gluconate. If elevated levels persist, peritoneal dialysis or haemodialysis is required.

NATURE AND QUANTITIES OF I.V. FLUIDS

Fluid requirements for metabolism. As stated before, an average adult consumes about 2,500 ml of water daily. About 1,500 ml water is taken by mouth, the rest being either extracted from solid food or gained as water of oxidation. The daily water losses include 800 to 1,500 ml as urine, 600 to 900 as insensible loss, and 250 ml in stools.

Even if a person is deprived of access to water he must still excrete a minimum of 500 to 800 ml of urine per day in order to excrete the products of catabolism, in addition to the mandatory insensible loss through the skin and lungs. This insensible loss is increased by hypermetabolism, hyperventilation and fever. The loss due to fever amounts to about 250 ml per degree centigrade of fever per day.

Nature of fluids lost during illness. Losses of extracellular fluid into the area of the operation or wound are isotonic. Gastrointestinal losses are usually isotonic or slightly hypotonic. Replacement of both these type of losses should be by isotonic salt solutions. The solution most suitable for this purpose is *lactated Ringer's solution.* Its composition is very similar to that of extracellular fluid. It contains 130 meq sodium balanced by 109 meq chloride and 28 meq lactate. This fluid has minimum effects on body fluid composition and pH even when infused in large quantities. Normal saline contains too much chloride for routine use. In Ringer's lactate this excess chloride is replaced by lactate, which has a very useful buffering action.

Constituents of available i.v. fluids. In the advanced countries the clinician describes the patient's clinical parameters as well as serum electrolyte values to the pharmacist, who prepares an appropriate mixture of fluids and electrolytes and sends it to the ward to be administered to the patient. Elsewhere in the world, however, the clinician has to fend for himself. Before we discuss the replacement of the fluids lost due to illness, we should be conversant with the composition of the different fluids which are commercially available (Table 1):

5% glucose in water. This solution contains no electrolytes, and therefore electrolytically speaking, this is plain water. As explained before, the purpose of the 5% glucose is to render the fluid exactly isotonic with plasma, so that there is no haemolysis on its administration. At the same time, the glucose provides instantly available energy. This fluid is used where plain water is required.

Table 1 Electrolyte content of parenteral fluids in meq/l.

SOLUTION	CATIONS					ANIONS	
	Na	K	Ca	Mg	NH_4	Cl	HCO_3
Extracellular fluid	142	4	5	3	0.3	103	27
Lactated Ringer's	130	4	3			109	28*
0.9% Sodium Chloride	154					154	
M/6 Sodium Lactate	167						167*

* Present as lactate, which is converted into bicarbonate.

Lactated Ringer's solution (Hartmann's solution). As can be seen in Table 1, this fluid closely approximates the composition of tissue fluid. Therefore when tissue fluid is lost during operations, whether on the surface or into the 'third space', Hartmann's solution constitutes the appropriate replacement. At the same time this is a more physiological solution than normal saline, which contains much more chloride than tissue fluid. In Ringer's lactate, some of this chloride is replaced by lactate, which acts as a useful buffer to neutralize the excess acid produced in infections, trauma etc.

0.9% saline ('Normal' saline). If excessive vomiting has taken place with resultant loss of chloride, this is a more suitable fluid than Ringer's lactate.

1/6th molar and molar lactate. These solutions are used to buffer excess acid produced in cases of metabolic acidosis, e.g. in diabetes, extensive trauma and fulminant infections. If the acidosis is severe, full-strength i.e. molar lactate is used; if more moderate, 1/6th molar lactate.

Which fluid to use? *Isotonic sodium chloride* contains 154 meq of sodium and 154 meq of chloride per liter. The high concentration of chloride is a load on the kidneys that cannot be rapidly excreted. Thus dilutional acidosis may result. However, this solution is ideal where there is a deficit of extracellular fluid volume with hyponatraemia, hypochloraemia and metabolic alkalosis, as in pyloric stenosis. On the other hand if volume deficit is present with metabolic acidosis, as in diabetes, *M/6 sodium lactate* may be given. The lactate is converted into bicarbonate and helps correct the acidosis.

If hyponatraemia is so *severe* as to produce symptoms, the choice of fluid would again depend upon the accompanying acid-base derangement. If acidosis is present *molar sodium lactate* is used. In the case of alkalosis *3% sodium chloride* may be employed. When the pH has returned to normal the remainder of the volume deficit can be corrected by a balanced salt solution like *Ringer's lactate.*

PREOPERATIVE FLUID THERAPY

Correction of volume changes. The most frequent abnormalities noted in the surgical patient are changes in the volume of extracellular fluid, specially depletion. This may result from external losses or internal redistribution. As explained in detail earlier, internal redistribution is also called loss into a '*third space*.' Examples are seen in extensive burns, crush injuries, generalized peritonitis and inflammation or strangulation of the bowel. Many liters of fluid may be lost into the tissues or the peritoneal cavity. Swelling of the bowel wall and secretion of fluid into the lumen of obstructed bowel causes even greater losses. Similar deficits occur with massive infections of the subcutaneous tissues.

Estimation of deficit. Exact measurement of these losses is impossible and unnecessary. An estimate of the deficit can be made from the severity of the clinical signs. A mild deficit represents a loss of approximately 4%, moderate loss about 7% and a severe loss about 10% of body weight. In a 70 kg man this would amount to 3, 5 and 7 liters respectively. It should be remembered that when such a loss of extracellular fluid volume occurs rapidly, cardiovascular signs e.g. tachycardia and hypotension predominate, with minimal or absent tissue signs.

Fluid replacement should be started, and changed according to the response of the patient noted on frequent clinical observation. Successful resuscitation is indicated by reversal of the signs of volume deficit, with stabilization of the pulse and blood pressure, and a urine volume of 30 to 50 ml per hour. It should be noted that in certain situations a high urinary output may be misleading. For example:

1. The excessive administration of glucose may produce an osmotic diuresis.

2. Similarly, an osmotic agent like mannitol produces urine at the expense of vascular volume.

3. Acute renal damage from shock and injury may impair the ability of the tubules to concentrate the urine, so that a large volume of dilute urine is produced.

When pure extracellular fluid volume loss has taken place, the use of a balanced salt solution such as lactated Ringer's is indicated.

Correction of concentration changes. The nature of the fluid required depends upon the type of disorder:

1. *For severe symptomatic hyponatraemia* 5% sodium chloride solution or molar sodium lactate is used, depending on the patient's acid-base status: chloride in cases with alkalosis, lactate for acidosis. The sodium deficit can be estimated as follows:

First estimate the deficit per liter by deducting the patient's serum sodium level from the normal sodium level. Then estimate the quantity of total body water in liters. Finally multiply the deficit per liter by the number of liters to obtain the total deficit.

Example. If a young adult female weighing 60 kg has a serum sodium of 125 meq/l, the total deficit is calculated as follows:

In females, body water constitutes 50% of body weight.
Thus total body water = $60 \times 0.5 = 30$ liters.
Now the deficit per liter = $140 - 125 = 15$ meq.
So the total deficit = $30 \times 15 = 450$ meq.

Half this calculated deficit is administered by intravenous infusion. Further correction is facilitated when renal function is restored by correcting the volume deficit.

2. For *mild hyponatraemia* isotonic sodium chloride is used in the presence of metabolic alkalosis, whereas M/6 sodium lactate is employed to correct acidosis. When the pH change has been corrected the remainder of the volume deficit can be repaired with lactated Ringer's solution.

3. *Hyponatraemia with volume excess* is treated simply by restriction of water. As the excess water is excreted the serum sodium level rises to normal.

4. In *severe hypernatraemia with a volume deficit* 5% glucose in water may be infused slowly until symptoms are relieved; as it is infused the volume deficit is made good, and at the same time the raised serum sodium level drops to normal due to dilution.

Correction of composition changes. Correction of a potassium deficit should be started only after an adequate urine output is obtained. Potassium chloride is available in 20 meq and 40 meq ampoules for addition to intravenous fluids. More than 40 meq should not be added to a liter of intravenous fluid.

Calcium and magnesium are rarely needed during preoperative preparation, except in acute pancreatitis, chronic starvation and massive subcutaneous infections.

Prolonged periods of fluid restriction, and the use of laxatives and enemas for preparation of bowel, may cause an acute loss of extracellular fluid. *Such losses should be recognized and corrected* to prevent complications during the operation.

INTRAOPERATIVE MANAGEMENT OF FLUIDS

If preoperative replacement of extracellular fluid volume has been incomplete, hypotension may develop during induction of anaesthesia. This should be prevented by replacing abnormal losses of fluids and electrolytes before operation.

At the beginning of this century it was discovered that after surgical operations changes occurred in urine output, blood volume and fluid and electrolyte composition. In the following 25 years saline solutions were given to patients undergoing operation, often in excessive amounts. Investigations carried out in the 1930s seemed to indicate that after surgical operations water and saline should be withheld, because most of the administered fluid is retained. More recent work has shown that proper management lies somewhere between the above two extremes. Some useful guidelines regarding fluid replacement during operations are as follows:

1. Blood should be replaced as it is lost.
2. Replacement of extracellular fluid should begin during the operative procedure.
3. Balanced salt solution should be given during operation at the rate of 0.5 to 1 liter per hour. The maximum should not exceed 2 to 3 liters during a 4 hour major abdominal procedure.

POSTOPERATIVE FLUIDS

The first day. Immediately after operation extracellular fluid may continue to be lost into the site of injury or operation. Several liters of extracellular fluid may be slowly deposited in such areas within a day or so after injury. This may produce circulatory instability. Postoperative hypotension and tachycardia require prompt investigation and proper therapy. The following parameters must be monitored carefully:

1. Pulse rate and volume.
2. Blood pressure.
3. Skin warmth and colour, and body temperature.
4. Hourly urine output.

Circulatory instability is most often caused by underestimated losses of fluids. Careful monitoring will show oliguria in addition to the rapid pulse and low blood pressure. An additional 500–1,000 ml of isotonic salt solution often resolves the problem. No potassium should be given during the first 24 hours unless a definite potassium deficit exists.

Later postoperative period. The problem is simply one of accurate measurement and replacement of all losses. This means the replacement of both the measurable losses which are mostly gastrointestinal, and the insensible losses. The insensible loss is usually relatively constant, between 600 and 900 ml daily. This may be increased by hypermetabolism, hyperventilation and fever to a maximum of about 1,500 ml daily. It is replaced by 5% glucose in water.

In the febrile patient, sweating seldom exceeds 250 ml per degree centigrade of fever per day, and should be replaced by 1/4 normal saline. Gastrointestinal losses are isotonic or slightly hypotonic, and are replaced by an isotonic salt solution. The amount of potassium required for replacement is 40 meq. daily for renal excretion of potassium, in addition to about 20 meq per liter for replacement of gastrointestinal losses if present.

FLUID NEEDS IN NEWBORNS AND INFANTS

Before going into the details of fluid needs in the newborn, the following background must be kept in mind. In nature, whenever a female mammal gives birth, not only is the mother exhausted but the infant animal is also unable to look after itself properly. Therefore nature stuffs extra fluid and salt in the neonate to last it a few days. Similar is the case with the human being. When a baby is born it looks bloated due to extra salt and water. During the first few days the baby loses weight, and it should be remembered that most of this weight loss occurs due to excretion of the surplus salt and water. The stable position is arrived at in about a week's time.

As the infant grows older, through the months and years, his weight increases at a greater rate than his surface area. Fluid requirements depend greatly on the area of the surface from which fluid losses take place. As the surface area becomes relatively less with growth, the fluid requirements *per kilogram* gradually get reduced.

With this background it is easy to understand the water and salt requirements during infancy, if these have to be given intravenously.

Water requirements. On the day of birth the baby requires only about 60 ml per kg per 24 hours. In 2 days time this figure rises to 80 ml and it peaks at the age of one week at 100 ml/kg/24 hours. After this the fluid needs gradually decline during childhood, as follows:

Below a weight of 10 kg the requirement remains at 100 ml/kg/day.

Table 2 Fluid requirements of an infant (in ml/kg/24 hours).

Age			Body weight	
0–2 days	3–7 days	7–days onwards (less than 10 kg)	10–20 kg	Greater than 20 kg
60	80	100	80	60

Note: The formula is somewhat over-simplified, consisting of average figures, but what it loses in accuracy it more than gains in the ease with which it can be committed to memory.

Between 10 and 20 kg body weight, it is reduced to about 80 ml/kg/day.

Above 20 kg body weight the need is further reduced to about 60 ml/kg/day.

All the above information can be expressed in an easy-to-remember formula (Table 2).

Salt requirements. How much *salt* should be added to this water? During the first one week the baby's body contains so much excess salt that he needs no more salt. Therefore, 5% glucose in water may be given. But the liver is immature and needs more glucose. So in fact 10% glucose in water is ordered. After one week the baby should be given the same proportion of salt as the older infant or adult, i.e. 1/5th normal saline.

To sum up, the basal fluid requirements of a baby work out to the following:

Age 0–2 days	60 ml of 10% glucose in water
Age 3–7 days	80 ml of 10% glucose in water
Age 7 days onwards (but less than 10 kg body weight)	100 ml of 1/5 normal saline
10–20 kg body weight	80 ml of 1/5 normal saline
>20 kg body weight	60 ml of 1/5 normal saline

ASSESSING FLUID LOSS AT OPERATIONS

The composition of the fluid. The fluid lost at operation is tissue fluid. This is closely mimicked by Ringer's lactate solution. Therefore, apart from any blood given for blood loss, the entire fluid lost at operation is commonly replaced by Ringer's lactate solution.

The amount to be replaced. A simple guideline for estimating third-space replacements after major abdominal surgery is as follows:

For each quadrant of the abdomen either affected by the disease process or involved in surgical dissection, one-fourth of the maintenance volume of fluid will be required as additional increment for volume replacement of third-space shifts. As mentioned above, the fluid will not be hypotonic solution but Ringer's lactate, preferably with 5% glucose. For example, if the maintenance volume was 2,000 ml, for a one-quadrant dissection 500 ml Ringer's lactate will be added.

Examples in a 10 kg infant

1. Procedure: *Appendicectomy* (1/4 quadrant).

Maintenance fluid: 10 × 100 = 1,000 ml of 1/4 normal saline.

Operation losses: 1/4 × 1,000 = 250 ml of Ringer's lactate solution.

2. Procedure: *Right hemicolectomy* for intussusception (2 quadrants).

Maintenance fluid: 10 × 100 = 1,000 ml of 1/4 normal saline.

Operation losses: 2 × 1/4 × 1,000 = 500 ml of Ringer's lactate solution.

3. Procedure: *Malrotation* (4 quadrants)

Maintenance fluid: 10 × 100 = 1,000 ml of 1/4 normal saline.

Operation losses: 4 × 1/4 × 1,000 = 1,000 ml of Ringer's lactate solution.

When calculating for an operation on an area other than the abdomen, the procedure should be assessed as equivalent to an abdominal operation affecting one, two, or more quadrants, and the fluid needs determined accordingly.

CALCULATING AN ACTUAL PATIENT'S REQUIREMENTS

A useful method of calculating the fluid needs of a patient over a 24 hour period is to prepare a proforma as in Table 3.

The various losses which commonly require replacement include maintenance requirements, operation losses (into the 'third space'), gastrointestinal losses (e.g. vomiting, diarrhoea or losses from fistulae), losses due to fever, and last but not least, summer losses in tropical countries:

1. The basal *maintenance* requirements never vary, and as explained at the beginning of this chapter, in the case of a 70 kg man amount to about 2,500 ml of 1/5th normal saline.

2. *Operation losses* depend upon the severity of the operation. As explained above, a simple guideline for assessing third-space losses after major surgery is as follows:

For each quadrant of the abdomen either affected by the acute illness or involved in surgical dissection, a quarter of the maintenance volume of fluid will be required as an additional increment for volume replacement of third-space shifts. This fluid is preferably Ringer's lactate, as it closely resembles the extra-cellular fluid which is lost.

3. *Gastrointestinal losses* also approximate Ringer's lactate in composition, except that during vomiting more

Table 3 Proforma for calculating a patient's requirements

	Glucose 5% in 1/5th normal saline	Ringer's lactate solution	Other e.g. blood, molar lactate etc. (where indicated)
Maintenance volume			
Operation losses			
G.I. losses			
Losses due to fever			
Summer losses			
Totals			

acid is lost, and during diarrhoea there is a greater loss of potassium.

4. As mentioned above, in a 70 kg man each degree centigrade of *fever* increases the water loss by about 250 ml per day. This fluid is probably about one fifth normal saline.

5. Similarly, due to acclimatization and salt conservation, *summer losses* are also probably about one fifth normal saline.

Example. Let us take the example of a 70 kg man who undergoes appendicectomy in a tropical country during the month of May. He is running a temperature of 39°C. The requirements can be worked out as follows:

Maintenance needs:	2500 ml G 5% in 1/5th normal saline.
Operation losses: (as 1 quadrant is dissected in appendicectomy)	2500 × 1/4 = 625 ml (Hartmann's).
GI losses:	Nil.
Fever losses (2 × 250 ml)	500 ml (1/4 N saline).
Summer losses (approx)	1000 ml (1/4 N saline).

In the author's practice, entering these data in a chart like the above is a useful method of ensuring that all the different types of losses are not only considered, but also their volumes are calculated and added to make up the total volume of fluid to be infused.

INTRAVENOUS ALIMENTATION

If fluids have to be administered intravenously for a prolonged period of time, water and electrolytes are not sufficient. Nutrients must also be given, otherwise the body's own tissues are burnt, and the patient starts losing weight rapidly. Each of the major types of nutrients must be given for optimal effect. Carbohydrates are utilized for ready energy, and proteins as replacement for wear and tear of cells and for synthesizing enzymes and hormones. Fats are given not only to serve as energy stores, but also for providing the essential fatty acids.

The nutrient fluids commonly available include the following:

1. *Glucose*, 10% and 25% solutions.
2. *Amino acid solutions.* Usually these contain a 5% solution of the different essential amino acids in 10% sucrose.
3. *Fat emulsions.* These come in two concentrations, 10% and 20%.

When nutrients are given parenterally, there is an optimal ratio between their quantities which is desirable. This is necessary in order to ensure the correct number of protein and non-protein calories, as well as enough fats for essential fatty acids. A suitable proportion of these for most cases requiring parenteral nutrition is as follows:

10% glucose solution	4 parts.
Amino acid solution	3 parts.
Fat emulsion	1 part.

It may be mentioned that such a solution is likely to contain insufficient quantities of the different electrolytes, namely sodium, potassium, and chloride, and these have to be topped up appropriately. All the above-mentioned solutions can be given through the peripheral veins, which is very convenient. However, if 25% glucose solution or 20% fat emulsion have to be employed, the infusion has to be given through one of the central veins.

CENTRAL VENOUS LINES

When fluids have to be given intravenously, they are normally administered through one of the peripheral veins, commonly in an arm or a leg. However, in two types of situations it is preferable to use one of the central veins, commonly either the subclavian or the internal jugular veins:

1. *Intravenous alimentation.* The hyperalimentation fluids, e.g. 25% glucose, are markedly hyperosmolar, and can cause thrombophlebitis if given into a peripheral vein. In the great veins the rapid flow of blood quickly dilutes the fluid, so that it cannot damage the intima of the vein. Therefore these concentrated fluids are best given into the great veins, i.e. the venae cavae.

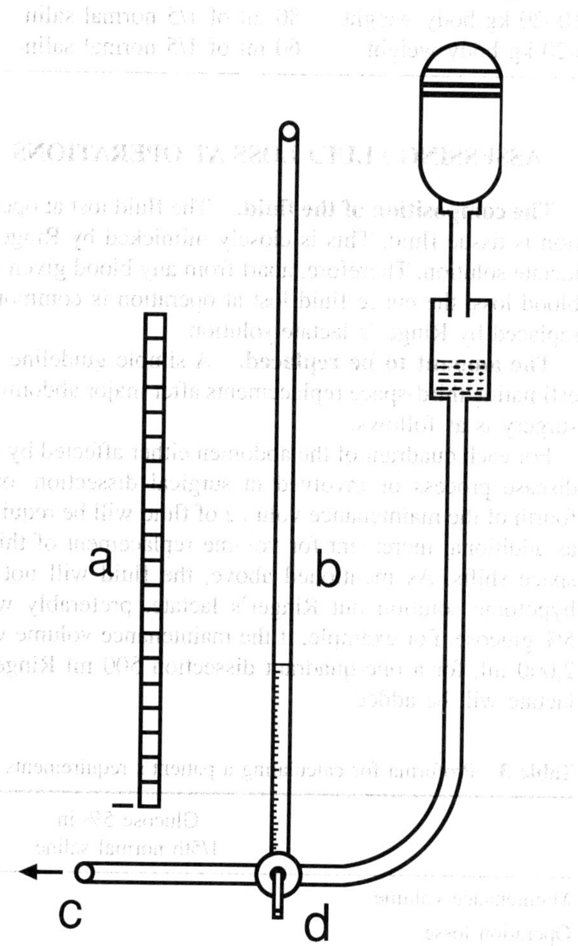

Fig. 1 Water manometer for measuring central venous pressure: (a) ruler, (b) water column, (c) tubing leading to patient, (d) 3-way stopcock.

2. *Conditions of haemodynamic instability.* If the patient is not haemodynamically stable, as in hypovolaemia or hypervolaemia, it is important to know the level of pressure in the central veins (*central venous pressure*) so that the correct volume of fluids can be infused. For this purpose a water manometer is constructed as follows:

A needle is passed into the subclavian or internal jugular vein, and through the needle a catheter is passed into the vein and advanced so that its tip lies in the superior vena cava. The catheter is now connected to the intravenous drip tubing through a 3-way stopcock. To the side-arm of the stopcock is attached a tubing which is fixed in a vertical position, with a measuring tape fixed along its side (Fig. 1). The intravenous fluid is allowed to flow into the vertically fixed tubing, and to fill it up. The zero level of the measuring tape is kept at the level of the manubrium sterni. When the lever of the stopcock is rotated so that the central veins are in communication with the vertically fixed tubing, the height of the fluid column in the tubing indicates the central venous pressure. The normal level of central venous pressure recorded at the sternal angle varies between 1 and 7 cm of water. If the pressure is low, the venous return should be supplemented by intravenous infusion; if excessively high, intravenous diuretics may be required. Electronic transducers can now be connected to the central venous tubing, and give more accurate and continuous readings.

8 Preoperative assessment and preparation

A surgical operation should ideally be carried out on a person who is in good health apart from the surgical condition from which he seeks relief. If he is suffering from one or more systemic illnesses, for every additional illness the risk of the operation is increased. It is therefore extremely important that the patient should be carefully interrogated and examined for the presence of any concomitant illness. If none is found, well and good; if a medical disorder is detected it should be corrected as far as possible. However, if it cannot be fully corrected, and the operation has to be carried out, the patient should be assessed as belonging to a higher risk category than the normal individual. This fact should be brought to the notice of the patient and his close relatives and the situation discussed with them. At the same time, the anaesthetist should be informed about the situation well in advance, so that he can examine and assess the patient and give his views in the matter. He would thus also be able to take any relevant precautions if the operation is finally decided upon.

It follows from the above that *examination of the patient from head to toe is more important for a surgeon than for a physician.* If a physician is treating a patient for dysentery, and he overlooks the fact that the patient is also suffering from a degree of heart failure, it does not matter that much, perhaps. After he has treated the dysentery he can attend to the heart failure. On the other hand if a surgeon is about to operate on a patient for a hernia and he misses the heart failure which is also present, he might not get a chance to treat the heart failure after the operation, because there may be no patient. The point which needs to be remembered is this: everyone should examine their patients thoroughly.

PREOPERATIVE ASSESSMENT

All the important organ systems should be systematically examined. Ideally, they should all be working perfectly; *if not, they should be put right as far as possible.*

Cardiorespiratory system. There should be an efficient mechanism for transport of oxygen to the cells:

1. *Lungs.* These should be in good working order; no asthma, no chronic bronchitis, no bronchiectasis etc., no cyanosis from any cause.
2. *Blood.* The haemoglobin level should be above 10 gm/dl for an elective operation. It may be mentioned that although this is desirable, recently the figure of 10 gm% as a *mandatory* requirement has been challenged.
3. *Heart.* The pulse should be regular with a good volume; there should be no cardiac murmurs; the blood pressure should be within normal limits. The ECG should be carried out before major operations, specially in patients over the age of 50, and should be normal.

The high-risk cardiac patient. ***Ischaemic heart disease.*** In patients with ischaemic heart disease who require surgery there is a critical balance between myocardial oxygen supply and demand. When this balance is unfavourable a myocardial infarction may result.

Drugs. Systemic hypertension should be appropriately treated. Antiarrhythmics should be used if indicated, and the patient's response to vasodilators for the treatment of angina assessed. Digitalis and diuretics are indicated in patients who have incipient or overt heart failure.

Angina. Filling of the coronary arteries takes place during diastole, as the myocardium compresses the coronaries during systole. With increasing heart rate diastole is shortened and coronary supply diminished. At the same time, if the blood pressure rises the heart has to pump blood against a higher pressure gradient and therefore has to work harder. Under these conditions if the patient has coronary disease, angina can occur. The presence or absence of angina should be noted. The more extensive the coronary disease, the lower the heart rate and blood pressure at which angina occurs, so much so that if the patient has very extensive disease, angina may occur at rest or may be initiated by minimal exercise.

The importance of the rate-pressure product. The product of the heart rate and blood pressure at which angina occurs is called the rate-pressure product. Above a rate-pressure product of 24000, even a healthy young adult can suffer coronary ischaemia. In patients with coronary artery disease the product should be kept below 15000, and preferably 12000. The beta-blocking agent propranolol lowers the heart rate and blood pressure. Both these effects reduce the oxygen requirements of the myocardium. Propranolol therefore allows the completion of longer periods of exercise before the rate-pressure product, which precipitates angina, is reached. In this way beta-blockage has greatly reduced morbidity in patients with ischaemic heart disease who undergo anaesthesia and surgery. High-risk cardiac patients are more stable when receiving propranolol. They are given 20 to 40 mg q.i.d. for at least three days before surgery. Finally, 5,000 units of heparin are given before surgery to reduce the chances of thrombosis. Postoperatively heparin is best used in an infusion, giving about 10000 units in 24 hours. The administration should be guided by repeated PTT and APTT measurements. These should be kept at around twice the normal values. The rate-pressure product should be determined in all high-risk patients before surgery, so that this figure can be used for management during surgery and in the postoperative period.

In patients with clinical or ECG evidence of previous myocardial infarction, the risk of reinfarction is increased by the combined effects of anaesthesia and surgery in the early post-infarct period. However, in about six months the risk falls to that seen in similar patients not undergoing surgery. Therefore, elective surgery should be postponed for this period of time.

Abrupt discontinuation of drugs may worsen pre-existing angina. Therefore β-adrenergic blocking drugs, calcium channel blockers, nitrates or diuretics should be continued upto the time that premedication is administered. Patients with angina at rest may require, in addition, perioperative medication, including transdermal or intravenous nitrates. After abdominal surgery the absorption of orally administered drugs may be interfered with, and medication must be provided by intravenous or sublingual routes.

Hypertension. Antihypertensive drugs may have to be withheld if the patient exhibits orthostatic hypotension, or if there is inadequate time available for optimization of drug therapy. The WHO recognizes four groups of patients:

1. Diastolic pressure between 95 and 110 mm Hg. There is no increase in the risk of surgery. A β-blocker may be utilized for premedication.
2. Diastolic pressure between 110 and 120 mm Hg on at least 3 occasions. The patient should be carefully monitored before, during and after surgery.
3. Diastolic pressure above 120 on at least 3 occasions.
4. Diastolic pressure normal, systolic between 200 and 250 respectively.

In groups 3 and 4, elective surgery should be postponed for 4 to 6 weeks and the blood pressure controlled with appropriate measures.

In the postoperative period, uncontrolled hypertension and tachycardia require aggressive treatment, as both these conditions cause an imbalance between coronary supply and demand, with the development of myocardial ischaemia.

Congestive cardiac failure. Both general and regional anaesthesia are contraindicated in the presence of acute heart failure, because cardiac muscle depression and hypokinesia may result. Intraoperative inotropic support with dopamine or dobutamine may be required. Evidence of left ventricular failure is associated with a poor prognosis.

Arrhythmias. Atrial flutter should be controlled to about 100 beats/min or less. It should be treated with digoxin or cardioversion before surgery. Multifocal ventricular tachycardias, and ectopics occurring more frequently than 1 in 5 beats, should be treated before operation. In patients with any kind of heart block the need for preoperative insertion of a temporary or permanent pacing wire should be considered.

Here it is pertinent to point out that tenderness in the right hypochondrium, which appears to be due to cholecystitis, could in fact be due to a congested liver due to right heart failure! One must be on one's guard in this, and in similar other potentially misleading situations.

Metabolism. Various metabolic parameters should be within normal limits:

Carbohydrate. There should be no sugar in a specimen of urine.

Protein. There should be no evidence of hypoproteinaemia, e.g. oedema. In certain countries undernutrition due to poverty is very widespread. This is aggravated by the massive loss of very valuable first-class proteins in the exudate of dysenteries which the population suffers from, due to poor social hygiene. Hypoproteinaemia is therefore quite common in these regions. On the other hand, in the affluent sections of society in any country, malnutrition is due to illnesses such as colitis and short bowel syndrome. In the presence of malnutrition not only is the risk of operation increased, but the wound also may take longer to heal, with a higher incidence of infection developing in it.

Weight. The weight should be reasonable. If the weight is more than twice the ideal body weight (200 to 225% to be exact) for the patient, he is defined as *morbidly obese*. If his weight is more than 225% of the patient's ideal body weight, he is classified as *superobese*. Obesity increases the risk of operation. Dissection is more tedious, so the operation takes a longer time to complete. Wound sepsis is more common, specially in the abundant subcutaneous fat, because fat has a poor blood supply. Obesity is also associated with a higher incidence of diabetes, hypertension, and heart disease, and these increase the operative risk. The increased amount of fat in the abdomen reduces the vital capacity i.e. causes pulmonary insufficiency. After major upper abdominal operations this results in retention of secretions in the basal areas of the lungs and increases the incidence of postoperative pulmonary complications. If weight is reduced, these complications of obesity are reversed and life expectancy improved.

Thyroid. The thyroid function should be normal, or should be brought back to normal before operation. Both hyperfunction and hypofunction of the thyroid are associated with a higher operative morbidity and mortality.

Body fluids. The patient should not be dehydrated or suffering from salt depletion.

Temperature. The patient's temperature should be normal. If it is raised, it may indicate an infectious fever or a septic focus.

GI tract. The appetite and bowel function should be normal. As a response of the body to any trauma the appetite becomes poor. So at least one should start from a normal baseline.

Urinary system. The kidney function should be good, as indicated by the urine volume and specific gravity. A routine laboratory examination of the urine should be normal. If in doubt the serum creatinine level should be determined.

CNS. The patient should be intelligent and cooperative. He should be able to move about. If he is bedridden the chances of hypostatic pneumonia, bedsores and pulmonary embolism are all greatly increased.

Skin. There should be no septic focus on the skin.

The above list is not all-inclusive, but does indicate the major areas which should be of concern to the surgeon before an operation, and the thoroughness required during the general examination.

ASSESSING THE OPERATIVE RISK

Age, obesity, specific organ failure, chronic illness and infection are all well-known causes of increased operative risk. *Cardiac arrest associated with complicated surgical problems is best treated by prevention.* In many cases cardiac arrest in the surgical patient can be avoided if careful attention is paid to the nine parameters outlined in Table 2, Chapter 5, and the patient's status corrected accordingly.

The ASA Scale. The American Society of Anaesthesiologists (ASA) has provided a very useful graded scale into which each patient is placed before anaesthesia. This scale, known as the ASA Scale, represents the significance of the patient's illness before anaesthesia:

ASA-I. Healthy person with *no systemic disease,* undergoing elective surgery. Patient not at extremes of age.

ASA-II. Patient with one-system, well-controlled disease which *does not affect daily activities.* (Other risk factors, e.g. mild obesity, alcoholism and smoking fall into this category).

ASA-III. Patient with multiple system disease, or well-controlled major system disease. Disease status *limits daily activity.*

ASA-IV. Patient with *severe, incapacitating disease.* Danger of death due to organ failure is present.

ASA-V. Patient in *imminent danger of death.* Operation a last resort attempt to save life. Patient not expected to live through next 24 hours.

The scale has great predictive value. The mortality rate in patients in ASA-I is a fraction of 1%, whereas in ASA-IV it is upwards of 10%!

PREOPERATIVE PREPARATION

The most important aspect of preparation is that the patient should be in good health, and if he is not, the specific abnormality of his health should be corrected before he is operated upon. Further, before any operation, everything about the operative procedure should be properly *explained* to the patient, and his *informed* and *written consent* obtained. This is specially important from a medico-legal point of view, to save the clinician from a charge of having operated without the patient's permission.

1. For *minor* operations under local anaesthesia no specific preparation is required. However, an oral sedative, e.g. 2 tablets of diazepam 5 mg taken about one hour before the operation, is useful. The patient has a considerable fear of the operation theatre, of the bright lights and the surgical appliances and equipment. The tranquilizer does not put him to sleep, it merely calms him down.

2. For operations under general anaesthesia the patient should have an *empty stomach.* This is necessary because during anaesthesia he may vomit. As his cough reflex is abolished under anaesthesia he may inhale the vomitus. If he does so, he may suffocate to death if the quantity of the vomitus is large; if not, he may develop a pneumonia or lung abscess. Thus ideally every operation should be carried out in the morning, when the patient is in any case normally fasting overnight. If operation has to be carried out at any other time, then 5 hours, or at the very least 4 hours, should have elapsed since his last meal.

3. It is an advantage if the patient has emptied his *bowel* on the morning of the operation, but this is not essential. In the past enemas were given routinely to all patients before major operations. They were quite unnecessary and caused dehydration, and the practice has been discontinued. However, before operations on the colon and rectum the large bowel is emptied of its contents by enemas, rectal washouts etc. This is discussed in detail elsewhere.

4. The part to be operated upon should be *shaved* with a good razor, avoiding skin cuts, as these may become infected. Before this shaving is carried out, the patient should have a bath and change of clothes on the evening before the operation, because nothing helps a wound heal cleanly more than all-round cleanliness. Some surgeons are not in favour of shaving; they point to the possibility of infection from the minor skin cuts, as mentioned above. However, when operating on hairy areas there is no escape from shaving, except by the use of hair-removing creams. After shaving, or without shaving, the area should be painted with alcohol (or methylated spirit) or with povidone-iodine, and bandaged over sterilized gauze. In the operation theatre this dressing is removed, usually after the patient has been anaesthetized, and the area again painted with methylated spirit or other antiseptic agent. In preparing the skin before operation, the utility of both the bath soap and the alcohol lies in their detergent action, by which they dissolve sweat, dirt and sebaceous matter from the skin. Alcohol, in addition, has a bactericidal effect on the micro-organisms present on the skin.

5. Finally, the whole body should be covered with *sterile drapes,* except the part to be operated upon.

If available a sterile, transparent, adhesive plastic drape may now be applied to the skin, and the incision made through it. This ensures that the skin is excluded from contact with the incised tissues, so that the skin bacteria have very little chance of getting into the wound. However, recent work has shown an *increase* in the incidence of infections after its use, presumably due to the warm, moist environment under the plastic drape encouraging the growth of bacteria!

9 Anaesthesia

For any operation to be carried out comfortably it is essential that the sensation of pain be abolished. This can be achieved either by general or regional anaesthesia. Each anaesthetic, even the simplest, creates a physiological disorder with a certain degree of risk. This risk may vary from slight to severe, but can never be eliminated. Studies on large series of patients have shown that of approximately 1,600 patients who are given an anaesthetic, one patient dies primarily as a result of having received the anaesthetic. With the extremely large number of anaesthetics administered the total resultant mortality is considerable. In the case of some of the more simple operations anaesthetic risk exceeds surgical risk. True patient safety can be achieved only by adhering to sound physiologic and pharmacologic principles.

PREMEDICATION

Premedication forms part of the anaesthetic technique. The objectives of premedication include anxiolysis, sedation and amnesia, as well as vagolysis to reduce salivary secretions. At the same time, drugs may be employed for prophylaxis against postoperative nausea and vomiting.

Most patients are afraid and anxious before operation, and sympathetic discussion of all the issues of concern to them allays most of their apprehensions. The most common *anxiolytics* employed include the benzodiazepines e.g. diazepam, and opioids e.g. morphine and pethidine. They also provide sedation and some amnesia. *Vagolytics* have the important side-effect of an unpleasant dry mouth, so are usually reserved for infants. Hyoscine is the most potent antisialagogue, and has the additional advantage of producing amnesia and sedation. *Antiemetics* include antihistaminics like promethazine which reduce the emetic effects of the anaesthetic agents employed; and drugs that aid gastric emptying such as metoclopramide. In the case of local anaesthesia these agents are best given by mouth an hour or two before the operation. With general anaesthesia parenteral administration is more appropriate. This is best carried out in the patient's bed, half to one hour before shifting him to the operation theatre. In this way he is spared the tension of the journey to the theatre, and the fright from the bright lights and the elaborate equipment in the operating room.

GENERAL ANAESTHESIA

General anaesthesia is administered when anaesthetics are either directly injected into the blood via the intravenous route or absorbed into the blood from the alveoli following inhalation. Safe general anaesthesia requires:

1. The administration and maintenance of an adequate anaesthetic dose without the development of adverse side-effects.

2. The monitoring of the depth of anaesthesia by clinical signs, e.g. heart rate, blood pressure and autonomic responses; or by an indicator of brain activity, such as EEG or evoked potentials.

3. The prompt recovery of normal brain activity by employing anaesthetic agents that undergo rapid elimination and leave no residual depressive effects in the central nervous system or other systems.

The airway. The cough reflex is abolished under general anaesthesia, and the airway has to be protected from aspiration of saliva or vomitus. A *laryngeal mask airway* is a curved tube with an inflatable cuff stuck at its end. The cuff lies in the laryngoparynx, against the upper opening of the larynx. However, if the muscles have to be paralysed and ventilation carried out under positive pressure, a *cuffed endotracheal tube* has to be used.

RISK FACTORS IN GENERAL ANAESTHESIA

The risks associated with both techniques of general anaesthesia are due to the same two factors, namely overdosage and inadequate ventilation. Almost all cases of cardiac arrest due to anaesthesia result from one or both of these two factors.

Overdosage. Avoidance of overdosage may be quite difficult, and there are two reasons for it. Firstly, individual variation of the patient's response to general anaesthesia is great. Therefore these drugs cannot be given in a predetermined dosage based on milligrams of anaesthetic agent per kilogram body weight, without risk of serious overdosage in some patients and inadequate anaesthesia in others. Secondly, evaluation of depth of anaesthesia is not precise. Many anaesthetics are such potent respiratory depressants, even in barely anaesthetic concentrations, that respirations become an inadequate guide to depth of anaesthesia. *In actual practice overdosage is said to be present when arterial hypotension or cardiac arrhythmias are produced by the general anaesthetic.* It is best avoided by repeated measurements of blood pressure and heart rate, and by continuous electrocardiographic monitoring.

Inadequate ventilation. The main causes of inadequate ventilation are obstruction of the airway and pharmacologic interference with respiratory mechanisms:

Airway obstruction. Obstruction to the airway may occur due to one of the following:

1. The tongue falling back into the pharynx.
2. Laryngospasm.
3. Bronchospasm.
4. Aspiration of blood, gastric contents or foreign bodies.

If left untreated, airway obstruction results in asphyxia, which may kill the patient; therefore action must be immediate:

1. If *blood or gastric contents* are present in the pharynx, these must be removed by one of the following methods:

i. By electric suction.

ii. By the use of a bulb sucker, specially in infants. This consists of a red rubber bulb with a nozzle. The bulb is squeezed to empty it of air. The nozzle is next placed in the pharynx and the pressure on the bulb released, allowing it to reinflate. As this is done, the secretions are sucked into the bulb and can be removed.

iii. If nothing else is immediately available, a gauze piece on the tip of an artery forceps may be employed to mop up the secretions.

2. If the *tongue has fallen back*, elevation of the mandible may open up the airway, by pulling the tongue forwards. A pharyngeal airway or endotracheal tube may now be placed in position in order to prevent the tongue falling back again.

Pharmacological causes of underventilation. These include interference with neural or muscular mechanisms of respiration. It should be emphasized that the signs of hypoxia and carbon dioxide retention are unreliable during anaesthesia. Respiratory rate, tidal volume, blood pressure, pulse rate and colour of skin are all inaccurate indices of dangerous degrees of hypoxia and hypercapnia.

The methods by which abnormal levels of oxygen or carbon dioxide can be reliably verified are two:

1. Measurement of the tensions of these gases in the arterial blood.

2. Pulse oximetry.

If these facilities are not available, it should be remembered that the *dangers of inadequate ventilation are very real,* while the risks of overventilation are only minor and rather hypothetical. Therefore it is better to overventilate patients artificially during anaesthesia rather than to permit underventilation to occur, because underventilation leads to hypoxia, which is dangerous.

Hyperventilation is readily accomplished by intermittent manual compression of the anaesthetic reservoir bag. Mechanical ventilators are not required. Also, an endotracheal tube is not required every time, but should always be handy in case of an emergency.

INHALATION ANAESTHESIA

The most important advantage of inhalation anaesthetics is *controlled reversibility.* In the case of modern inhalation anaesthetics, as soon as the supply of the anaesthetic is turned off the effect is reversed. Such is not the situation with conventional intravenous anaesthetics or muscle relaxants, because they have to be biotransformed or excreted before their effect can be terminated. Even their antagonists cannot always reliably reverse their action, because the antagonist often has a shorter duration of action than the drug itself, so that the patient may get reanaesthetized or recurarized after leaving the operating room. The inhalation anaesthetics in common use are nitrous oxide, halothane, enflurane and isoflurane. Others less commonly used are cyclopropane and ether.

Nitrous oxide (N_2O). Nitrous oxide is an inhalation analgesic, and is the most widely used drug in surgical anaesthesia. The reasons for its popularity are the following:

1. Unlike the narcotics it does not produce any marked respiratory or circulatory side effects.

2. Again, unlike narcotics its effects are immediately reversible.

3. It is non-explosive.

4. It is odourless.

However, nitrous oxide also has an important limitation. It cannot alone suppress the somatic, autonomic or haemodynamic responses to noxious stimuli. Therefore, it is rarely used alone. Instead, it is employed alongwith other more powerful agents, e.g. halothane, to decrease their required amounts, and thus to minimize their adverse side effects. In fact it is also used during intravenous anaesthesia; when nitrous oxide is used, smaller quantities of barbiturates are required.

Nitrous oxide should be avoided in the following situations:

1. During bronchoscopy and upper airway surgery; in these procedures high inspired oxygen concentrations are required, which are not possible in the presence of nitrous oxide.

2. During the first 4 weeks of pregnancy because of its effect on organogenesis.

3. In situations where it can diffuse into air-filled spaces, increasing their volume or pressure; this occurs in the presence of a pneumothorax, after pneumoencephalography, after tympanoplasty, and in patients with grossly dilated bowel due to intestinal obstruction.

Halothane. Halothane is a highly potent inhalation anaesthetic. Surgical levels of anaesthesia can usually be obtained with alveolar concentrations of about 0.7 vols % when used alone, and 0.4 vols % when used with nitrous oxide. Its advantages are that it is non-explosive, not unpleasant to breathe, and both onset and termination of effect are rapid. As it is such a potent drug it should be administered only by experienced persons using calibrated vaporizers.

The important disadvantage of halothane lies in the narrow margin of safety between its anaesthetic effects and cardiovascular properties. Surgical levels of halothane anaesthesia often produce cardiovascular depression, causing hypotension and decreased cardiac output, specially in persons who are aged or hypovolaemic, and in those with myocardial ischaemia or valvular heart disease. Halothane also increases the sensitivity of the ventricular pacemakers to irritant stimuli, predisposing the patient to the development of arrhythmias. The cardiovascular depression produced by halothane is dose-dependant. Halothane is therefore usually used alongwith nitrous oxide, which is beneficial. Nitrous oxide reduces the concentration of halothane required for anaesthesia, and therefore minimizes the chances of arrhythmias and cardiovascular depression resulting from its use. Its required dose can also be reduced by obtaining relaxation through the use of myoneural blocking agents.

Halothane dilates blood vessels, including cerebral vessels, leading to some increase in intracranial pressure. It is metabolized by hepatic microsomal enzymes. Occasional cases of hepatic damage following halothane anaesthesia have been reported, with development of 'halothane hepatitis' and jaundice.

Enflurane and isoflurane. Both these drugs belong to the family of ethers. Hepatotoxicity has been described with enflurane; it can also rarely produce mild epileptiform movements. Isoflurane exhibits all the properties of the other two volatile agents, combined with a faster intake and elimination and minimal biotransformation, so that it is less toxic to the kidney and liver.

Malignant hyperpyrexia can be triggered by all the three above-mentioned drugs.

Other inhalation anaesthetics. *Cyclopropane and diethyl ether* are both inflammable. In the advanced countries electrocautery is now used in virtually every surgical operation; therefore these anaesthetics have become quite obsolete. However, in the peripheral hospitals of the poorer countries *ether* continues to be used because of its cheapness and its relatively wider margin of safety, when used without sophisticated equipment, compared to more modern anaesthetics. Recovery after the use of either anaesthetic is very slow, therefore the patient needs to be watched very carefully in the early postoperative period. Also, ether irritates the respiratory passages, and the incidence of postoperative pulmonary complications is quite high after its use.

INTRAVENOUS ANAESTHESIA

General anaesthesia can also be produced by the intravenous injection of one or more drugs. An important *advantage* of intravenous anaesthesia is that it is agreeable for the patient. The rapid onset of unconsciousness without exposure to gases with different smells, and without the somewhat terrifying sensation of a mask over the face makes it popular with the patient. It is also convenient for the anaesthetist because anaesthesia is induced rapidly, without the longer and more exacting induction of inhalation anaesthesia.

However, the *disadvantages* of intravenous anaesthesia are also significant. The most important among these is the fact that although immediate and profound depression is produced, true anaesthesia i.e. absence of response to painful stimuli, may not be obtained. This can be dangerous, because although the patient's jaw and tongue can fall back into the pharynx due to the CNS depression and can obstruct his airway, yet he is not anaesthetized deeply enough to allow passage of an airway or endotracheal tube to relieve the obstruction. This problem can be solved by paralyzing the patient with a muscle relaxant and immediately placing an endotracheal tube in place for artificial ventilation. However, if the endotracheal tube cannot be passed immediately the situation can be dangerous.

Other disadvantages of intravenous anaesthesia are as follows:

1. It is difficult to maintain constant and predictable levels of anaesthesia with intravenous anaesthetics.
2. Because many drugs are used together, complex drug interactions may take place and complicate the situation.

It should therefore be remembered that *although it appears to be a simple technique, intravenous anaesthesia requires even more skill than inhalation anaesthesia if it is to be equally safe.*

Barbiturates. The most commonly used intravenous anaesthetics are the ultrashort-acting barbiturates, specially thiopentone. Their popularity is due to the fact that their action is rapid in onset and short in duration. This is due to their high solubility in lipids, which helps them cross the blood-brain barrier very quickly.

Thiopentone provides rapid, effective and safe onset of anaesthesia. The disadvantage of thiopentone is that it causes more cardiovascular and respiratory depression than inhalation anaesthetics when used in equianaesthetic doses. At the same time, in large doses its depressant effects last longer than those observed with inhalation anaesthetics. Because of these limitations thiopentone *is used mainly to induce general anaesthesia* prior to the administration of the more potent inhalation anaesthetics. It is also used to supplement other relatively weak anaesthetics such as nitrous oxide. As is the case with other general anaesthetics, thiopentone is contraindicated in the presence of a full stomach or in situations where the patency of the airway cannot be assured at all times.

Propofol (di-isopropyl phenol). This is one of a class of recently introduced intravenous anaesthetics which differ from the drugs used hithertofore in that their action is reversed almost instantaneously on discontinuing administration. If used with an infusion pump, they can be employed as complete substitutes for inhalation anaesthetics. Their advantage lies in their milder side effects. Propofol causes comparable cardiovascular and respiratory depression to thiopentone when used for induction of anaesthesia. It has a high clearance rate and can therefore be used for both induction and maintenance of anaesthesia, specially where prompt and complete recovery is important, as in day care surgery. The low incidence of nausea, vomiting and headache is appreciated by the ambulant patient.

Intravenous infusion anaesthesia. The use of intravenous infusions of anaesthetics has gained popularity due to the development of drugs with more rapid clearance and breakdown to inactive metabolites, such as propofol. Indications for the use of such techniques include day-care anaesthesia, military or 'field' anaesthesia, and as a supplement to regional anaesthesia.

Narcotics. Although they are not anaesthetics, narcotics are frequently used as adjuncts to anaesthesia. Firstly, they may be used for premedication, so that the patient is sedated before he is taken to the operation theatre. When used in such a manner these drugs are usually given intramuscularly or subcutaneously.

Secondly, narcotics may be used during general anaesthesia in combination with weak anaesthetics such as nitrous oxide to provide intense analgesia. Thirdly, they may be used during regional anaesthesia to provide relief of pain or discomfort. In such a situation they should be administered intravenously, otherwise absorption is slow and erratic.

The main disadvantage of narcotics as adjuvants to anaesthesia is that some degree of respiratory depression is always produced. The narcotics commonly employed include *morphine* (0.03–0.25 mg/kg) and *fentanyl.*

Ketamine differs from other narcotics in its action. It is the only hypnotic agent possessing analgesic activity. It produces profound analgesia with dissociation from the environment. It provides adequate anaesthesia for superficial operations not requiring muscle relaxation. As it does not cause relaxation of muscles, airway obstruction is uncommon. Its disadvantage lies in the unpleasant hallucinations it sometimes produces. Indications for its use include the following:

1. Poor-risk surgical patients, e.g. those with poor myocardial function or hypovolaemia.
2. Patients suffering from burns: for debridement, painful dressings and skin grafting.
3. Short diagnostic or surgical procedures, including cardiac catheterization.
4. Postoperative pain relief.

MUSCLE RELAXANTS

For gentle dissection of the deeper structures adequate relaxation of the muscles overlying them is essential. As the anaesthetic agent does not produce sufficient relaxation, a muscle relaxant is used. Such an agent produces profound relaxation of muscles without deep levels of anaesthesia, thus avoiding the adverse physiological effects of deep general anaesthesia. This benefit, however, is not obtained without any cost. Firstly, deep muscle relaxation greatly interferes with respiration, so that artificial ventilation has to be provided. Secondly, the effect of the muscle relaxant may last longer than the duration of the surgical operation, so that the patient is apnoeic after the operation has been completed. This can be extremely dangerous if the closeness of the patient's supervision is compromised even for a brief period.

Types of muscle relaxants. There are two types of muscle relaxants:

Firstly those, like *succinylcholine*, which interfere with myoneural transmission by producing *depolarization* at the motor end plate. These have a short duration of action, which is over in about 8 minutes.

Secondly those, like *curare*, which interfere with transmission at the myoneural junction by competing with acetylcholine *(non-depolarizing muscle relaxants).* They are longer-acting than the first type. For example, the effect of curare remains at a peak for about 20 minutes, and is terminated within 45 minutes.

Reversal of effects of muscle relaxants. If at the end of the operation the effect of a curare-type muscle relaxant is still continuing it can be safely reversed by intravenous administration of an anticholinesterase such as neostigmine. This drug must always be accompanied by atropine or a similar drug, to block the bradycardia produced by the anticholinesterases through stimulation of the vagi.

Malignant hyperpyrexia. Succinylcholine, in combination with halothane and other inhalation and local anaesthetics can produce, in certain rare individuals, malignant hyperpyrexia. This is a dangerous condition where the administration of succinylcholine is followed not by relaxation but by muscle rigidity. The body temperature rapidly rises upto 41.5°C (107°F) within minutes. It often proves fatal because of damage to the nervous and cardiovascular systems, and due to severe metabolic derangements.

The malignant hyperpyrexia syndrome probably results from an inherited susceptibility to succinylcholine and inhalation anaesthetics. It cannot be diagnosed in advance except after complex studies on muscle biopsies from patients at risk. A detailed family history of adverse reactions to anaesthetics can alert the clinician.

Routine monitoring of body temperature can help prompt recognition of the complication if it arises. Immediate aggressive measures to lower the body temperature, i.e. ice packs etc., may prove life-saving. Drug treatment consists of intravenous injection of dantrolene.

REGIONAL ANAESTHESIA

Apart from minor operations like those for sebaceous cyst or ingrowing toe-nail, more extensive procedures like herniorrhaphy and haemorrhoidectomy etc. can also be performed under regional anaesthesia. The advantage of the method lies in the fact that it produces maximal sensory anaesthesia without physiological side effects, provided the extent of the anaesthesia is limited. On the other hand if the region anaesthetized is extensive the physiological derangement may be greater than during properly conducted general anaesthesia.

Local anaesthetics produce a transient and completely reversible blockade of nerve function. They act by blocking sodium channels in the axon membrane and inhibiting nerve conduction. *Procaine* has low-grade potency and a short duration of action. *Lignocaine* is intermediate in its effects, while *bupivacaine* is highly potent and has a prolonged action.

Points in technique. When regional anaesthesia is being used the surgeon and his team must work quietly and unobtrusively to avoid upsetting the patient. Besides, the following steps should taken to make the procedure more smooth:

1. About one hour before operation a sedative and an analgesic should be given by mouth, e.g. diazepam 10 mg and paracetamol 500 mg.
2. The area of the operation should be screened away from the patient's view.
3. For the initial skin puncture a very fine needle, size 27, should be used to create a wheal in the skin, through which a longer needle can be introduced for infiltration.
4. The drug commonly used is xylocaine hydrochloride, available in a concentration of 2%. The drug should be diluted to a concentration of 1%, specially if the area of infiltration is extensive. If 1:100,000 adrenaline is added to the lignocaine, its vasoconstrictor effect decreases the absorption of lignocaine from the site of administration and prolongs its effect. Further, larger doses of lignocaine can be used due to the slower absorption.

The maximum volumes of 2% lignocaine allowable in an average adult are the following:

Plain lignocaine 2%:	15 ml.
Lignocaine 2% with adrenaline 1:100,000:	25 ml.

Before withdrawing the drug into the syringe the operator must always read the label on the ampoule to satisfy himself that he is administering the correct medicine.

Toxic effects. Most local anaesthetic agents cross the blood-brain barrier, initially causing excitation and later, at higher doses, central nervous system depression. At the same time they produce arterial dilatation and myocardial depression. At toxic concentrations peripheral vasodilatation, depressed myocardial contractility and depression of heart rate can produce circulatory collapse and cardiac arrest.

The ratio between the toxic and effective dose is low for bupivacaine. This has resulted in cardiovascular collapse following release of the tourniquet in patients given bupivacaine for intravenous regional anaesthesia, as well as after the use of bupivacaine in epidural anaesthesia in obstetric practice. Other toxic effects include methaemoglobinaemia, neurotixicity and malignant hyperpyrexia.

Systemic toxicity can be *prevented* by using appropriate doses, checking for accidental intravenous administration, employing vasoconstrictors where possible, and establishing venous access in all patients before instituting regional anaesthesia.

If systemic toxicity does occur, oxygen should be administered, cardiovascular effects monitored, and CNS excitation treated with diazepam. *Facilities for intubation and ventilation, as well as drugs for the support of the circulation should be available at all times.*

SPINAL ANAESTHESIA

In spinal anaesthesia a local anaesthetic is injected into the subarachnoid space, the needle usually passing between the laminae of the fourth and fifth lumbar vertebrae. This causes paralysis of the motor and sensory somatic fibres, producing both anaesthesia and muscle relaxation. However, besides these useful clinical effects, sympathetic paralysis and hypotension are also produced.

Sympathetic paralysis. The local anaesthetic agent causes blockade of the preganglionic sympathetic fibres. This sympathetic paralysis is responsible for all the profound physiological effects of spinal anaesthesia.

Certain anatomical characteristics of sympathetic nerve fibres have an important bearing on the extent of the paralysis produced. Firstly, sympathetic preganglionic fibres are smaller than either the somatic or sensory fibres, and are blocked by lower concentrations of the anaesthetic. Therefore sympathetic denervation usually extends about two spinal segments above the level made anaesthetic to pinprick, and the physiologic response is therefore greater.

Secondly, the highest preganglionic fibres leave the spinal cord at the level of T_1. Therefore if the sensory level of anaesthesia is at T_3 level, the physiological changes will be those seen after total sympathetic denervation.

Thirdly, each preganglionic fibre ascends and descends in the sympathetic chain, synapsing with a number of postganglionic fibres which are distributed to the periphery non-segmentally. Therefore, the sympathetic response to spinal anaesthesia may be more extensive than expected.

Hypotension. Sympathetic denervation produces arterial and arteriolar dilatation, which reduces the arterial pressure slightly. At the same time, and more importantly, it produces venodilatation. If the denervated vein is below the level of the heart gravity causes the blood to pool in it, reducing the blood pressure further.

The most common cause of impaired venous return during spinal anaesthesia is the head-up position. For this reason, after spinal anaesthesia the patient is nursed in a *head-down position* for a few hours. The other fairly common cause of hypotension after spinal anaesthesia is the use of this technique in a patient with reduced blood volume due to any cause. In such a case spinal anaesthesia should be avoided, or at least the deficit of blood volume should be made good first.

Respiratory function. Respiratory function during spinal anaesthesia remains normal even during high levels of sensory block. In high spinal anaesthesia the intercostal muscles are paralyzed, but this is compensated for by the diaphragm, specially as the abdominal muscles are relaxed. When respiratory arrest occurs during spinal anaesthesia it is commonly due to decreased cardiac output producing ischaemic paralysis of the brain-stem.

High spinal anaesthesia produces profound physiological derangements, whereas low spinal anaesthesia results in very little upset. Spinal anaesthesia is not normally used for operations above the level of the umbilicus, because the resulting total sympathetic denervation is too high a price to pay.

Complications. Apart from the hypotension mentioned above, the main complications of spinal anaesthesia are post-spinal headache, paralysis and meningitis. *Post-spinal headache* occurs fairly often after spinal anaesthesia. The cause is not known, but headache is more common after the use of larger-bore needles, which suggests that it is due to continued leakage of CSF from the puncture site in the dura. It is treated by analgesics and hydration. *Neurological complications* after spinal anaesthesia are commonly due to injury by the needle. Occasionally, they result from *incorrect identification* of ampoules, so that alcohol, phenol, etc. may be mistakenly injected, producing a chemical transverse myelitis which is irreversible. Therefore great care should be taken in this regard. The assistant should present the ampoule to the operator before breaking it, so that the latter can confirm that the correct drug is being used. He should present it again before the drug is actually injected, as a double-check. One cannot be too careful!

Meningitis. If a rigid aseptic technique is not employed while administering a spinal anaesthetic, meningitis can result. This should be avoided by strictly adhering to aseptic principles, e.g. autoclaving the needles or using disposable needles and syringes, thorough hand-washing, use of sterile gloves and sheets, and proper antiseptic sterilization of the skin.

EPIDURAL ANAESTHESIA

In this technique the local anaesthetic agent is injected into the epidural space. Its advantages are: firstly, a lower incidence of headache. Secondly, if it is desired to prolong the effect of the anaesthetic, the catheter can be left in place and the drug repeatedly injected in small doses.

Indications for epidural anaesthesia include: (a) For obstetric analgesia, to ensure painless labour; (b) For perineal operations; (c) For cervical analgesia for operations on the upper limbs, specially if bilateral; (d) For thoracic analgesia for crush injuries of the chest. Pain relief allows deep breathing, restoring ventilation to normal and preventing stagnation of secretions with its attendant complication of hypostatic pneumonia.

10 Critical care

When a patient is very ill and may die, his condition is referred to as critical. Such a patient has usually developed failure of one or more of the physiological systems. The assessment and management of the disturbed physiology in such a case is defined as critical care. The failure of each system is considered separately for ease of understanding. However, these failures often coexist. Patients dying in a critical care unit often develop what is called 'multiple organ dysfunction syndrome'. In the progression from single to multiple organ dysfunction syndrome, systemic or localized infection often plays a very important part and greatly decreases the chances of survival.

The critical (or 'intensive') care unit has become an integral part of a modern acute hospital, providing an environment for the observation and treatment of the severely ill patient. Many large hospitals are able to support separate medical, surgical, neurosurgical and respiratory units, while in smaller institutions a single multidisciplinary unit serves the needs of several specialties. The critical care clinician must be able to sustain the physiological equilibrium of the patient by pharmacological and mechanical means. This requires constant surveillance, anticipation of adverse events and aggressive and prompt intervention when necessary. The nurse occupies a key position in the provision of critical care, and a 'one to one' nurse to patient ratio is highly desirable. A major component of critical care is counselling and support for the relatives of the patient. This job should not be delegated to the junior medical or nursing staff but should be undertaken by the seniormost member of the surgical team.

MONITORING

Critical illness is normally severe. Many systems are affected, and changes in the different physiological variables take place rapidly. Traditional clinical evaluation cannot always be relied upon in critically ill patients, as major changes may occur which are not accompanied by obvious clinical findings. Therefore it is necessary to employ sensitive equipment to measure *('monitor')* these parameters continuously, or at least frequently. The different parameters repeatedly measured in the critical care unit relate to the hemodynamic, respiratory, renal, neurologic, metabolic and temperature regulating functions.

Haemodynamic monitoring. The haemodynamic state of the critically ill patient can be accurately assessed by measurement of the following parameters:

The ***ECG*** provides continuous information about heart rate and rhythm, and rapidly shows up any arrhythmias.

Arterial catheterization is indicated whenever there is a need for continuous monitoring of blood pressure and/or frequent sampling for blood gases.

States in which precise and continuous *blood pressure* data are necessary include shock from any cause, use of potent vasoactive drugs, high levels of respiratory support, high-risk patients undergoing extensive operations, and controlled hypotensive anaesthesia. The systolic, diastolic and mean arterial pressures can be continuously displayed.

Regularly repeated analysis of *blood gas* tensions and pH is necessary in any acute illness with cardiovascular or respiratory dysfunction. The *radial* artery is the commonly used site for arterial catheterization because of its superficial location and because of the dual blood supply to the hand. Problems associated with arterial catheterization include failure to cannulate, haematoma formation and disconnection from the monitoring system with bleeding. Infections at the catheter site are seen only if a catheter is left in place for longer than 4 days.

Central venous catheterization. The most common indications for central venous catheterization are: to secure access for fluid therapy, drug infusions or parenteral nutrition; and for central venous pressure monitoring.

Central venous pressure (CVP) is, by definition, the pressure in the right atrium. It is raised in the following conditions:

1. If the venous return is high.
2. If the venous tone is increased.
3. If the intrapericardial or intrathoracic pressure is high.
4. If the right ventricle is not functioning properly.

A low level of CVP may be the result of a hypovolaemia, a reduction of venous tone, or a combination of both of these. When monitoring CVP the catheter should be attached to a pressure transducer for electronic measurement rather than to a water manometer; the latter is less reliable as it cannot respond to the full range of pressure variations (transducer: a device that converts one form of energy into another, in this case pressure into an electrical signal).

Central venous cannulation. A radiopaque catheter is passed from a subclavian, internal jugular or antecubital vein into the right atrium. This should be done under full aseptic precautions. The head side of the table is lowered. This helps avoid air embolism. It also increases the venous return, which distends the veins and makes puncture of the vein easier. The actual method of insertion of the catheter differs according to the vein chosen for cannulation:

1. *Subclavian vein.* A 20-gauge needle on a syringe is inserted at a point below the midpoint of the clavicle and directed towards the tip of a finger in the suprasternal notch. When blood is aspirated freely the needle is used as a guide to insert the cannula through it into the subclavian vein. The needle is now removed, leaving the cannula in place.

2. *Internal jugular vein.* A line is drawn between the mastoid process and the sternoclavicular joint. The carotid artery is palpated on this line; the internal jugular vein lies immediately lateral to the artery at the mid-point of this line. A 7-cm needle on a syringe is inserted caudally at 45° to the vertical into the internal jugular vein. The syringe is

removed and the soft end of a Seldinger wire is passed through the needle into the vein. The needle is removed over the wire, and the catheter is passed into the vein over the wire. The wire is removed.

The catheter is sutured into position and covered with a transparent, sterile self-adherent dressing. Fluid should be infused only if blood can be easily withdrawn. The position of the catheter tip must be checked by a chest x-ray; it should be located at the lower border of the superior vena cava or the upper third of the right atrium. The CVP should be measured continuously using a pressure transducer. If such a facility is not available, a fluid manometer is used, when readings can be taken only intermittently. The midaxillary line in the fourth intercostal space is commonly used as the zero level, as it lies at the level of the right atrium. Alternatively, the sternal angle can be used for this purpose. Marked from the midaxillary line, the normal range of CVP is 3 to 7 mm Hg (0.4 to 1.0 kPa).

Complications of central venous cannulation include the following:

1. Damage to adjacent structures, e.g. pleura in the case of puncture of the subclavian vein, with resulting pneumothorax or haemothorax.
2. Occasional septicaemia due to introduction of infecting organisms through the catheter.
3. Air embolism: this is a constant threat, so infusion systems should be well sealed and examined frequently.

Pulmonary artery catheterization. In this method a balloon-tipped central venous catheter is advanced through the right atrium and ventricle into the pulmonary artery, and thence into one of the small branches of the artery. The balloon is now inflated to block the small artery. When this is done, the flow of blood in the distal segment of the pulmonary artery is interrupted. Now, a stagnant system in which no forward flow is present has the same pressure at its proximal as at its distal end, i.e. in this case the left atrium. Therefore the *pulmonary artery occlusion pressure (PAOP)* is a reliable index of the left atrial pressure. This in turn is roughly the same as left ventricular pressure at the end of diastole, and indicates the state of function of the left ventricle. Thus pulmonary artery occlusion pressure is a good indicator of the state of function of the heart. The pulmonary artery catheter is thus a very major advance in the methods of obtaining physiological information for the management of critically ill patients.

The *cardiac output* can be estimated using the *thermodilution* technique. A known volume of fluid at a known temperature (colder than the body) is injected through the proximal port of the pulmonary artery catheter. The fall in temperature is registered downstream by a thermistor located 4 cm from the catheter tip. The more generous the blood flow, i.e. cardiac output, the more the cold fluid is diluted and the less the fall in temperature. Applying an appropriate formula, the cardiac output can be calculated.

{Thermistor: a thermometer whose impedance varies with the ambient temperature, and which can measure extremely small changes in temperature}.

Complications of pulmonary artery catheterization include dysrrhythmias, apart from coiling, looping or knotting of the catheter in the right ventricle.

Low levels of PAOP are found in hypovolaemia. High levels are seen in hypervolaemia or with a failing left ventricle. However, it must be remembered that if mitral stenosis is present, blood is dammed in the left atrium and the PAOP may be raised even in the absence of either hypervolaemia or heart failure.

Respiratory monitoring. The critically ill patient may be unable to maintain a level of ventilation sufficient for adequate gas exchange. In such a situation ventilation may have to be carried out artificially by a ventilator. Monitoring ventilation and gas exchange is then of particular importance in deciding if ventilation is required, assessing response to therapy, making optimum use of the ventilator, and deciding if a weaning trial is indicated.

Tidal volume is the volume of air moved in or out of the lungs in any single breath. If the tidal volume is depressed the patient may have difficulty in both oxygenation and ventilation. In weaning patients from a ventilator rapid shallow breathing indicates that weaning is likely to fail. Tidal volume can be measured at the bedside using a hand-held spirometer (Wright respirometer).

Blood gases and *pH.* Arterial blood samples are assayed for partial pressures of oxygen and carbon dioxide (Po_2 and Pco_2), pH, base deficit, etc. At the same time, arterial oxygen saturation can now be measured percutaneously through a sensor applied as a clip onto a digit. The device measures the absorbance of light transmitted through well-perfused tissue, such as the finger or ear. However, it should be remembered that if the blood supply to the skin is reduced, the sensitivity of this device is impaired.

Renal monitoring. The reasons for monitoring renal function are three: firstly, the kidney serves as a monitor of the adequacy of tissue perfusion. Secondly, if acute parenchymal renal failure threatens, monitoring of the renal function helps guide therapy. Thirdly, if renal function is impaired, the doses of certain drugs have to be reduced proportionately to the degree of renal failure to avoid nephrotoxicity, and renal function monitoring helps indicate the degree of reduction required.

Blood *urea* nitrogen (BUN) has often been used to estimate renal function. However, BUN is affected by glomerular filtration rate and urea production. The latter may vary considerably from time to time. Therefore, BUN is an unreliable monitor of renal function. The value of plasma *creatinine* far exceeds that of BUN. In contrast to BUN concentration, plasma creatinine levels are not influenced by protein metabolism or rate of fluid flow through the renal tubules. If glomerular filtration rate is reduced by 50%, the plasma creatinine will double, assuming that creatinine production remains constant.

Neurological monitoring. Several methods have been used to evaluate brain function and the effects of therapy; these include the Glasgow coma scale, intracranial pressure monitoring and electrophysiological monitoring.

Glasgow coma scale (score). This scale was initially developed to help predict outcome after head injury. It is now also commonly used as an objective means of measuring the level of consciousness (Table 1, Chapter 44).

Intracranial pressure monitoring. This is important, because it allows calculation of *cerebral perfusion pres-*

sure, which is defined as the difference between the mean arterial pressure and the intracranial pressure (ICP). ICP values above 40 mm Hg represent dangerous and life-threatening levels of intracranial hypertension. The most common indication for ICP monitoring is head injury, in which monitoring is indicated if the Glasgow coma score after resuscitation is 7 or below. ICP monitoring is also recommended in cases of subarachnoid haemorrhage and hydrocephalus, and after craniotomy. The ICP may be monitored by the use of one of the following types of equipment:

1. A catheter passed into a ventricle and connected to a transducer.

(Transducer: a device for converting power into another form (in the present case hydrostatic pressure into electrical energy), which is displayed on a measuring scale).

2. A 'subarachnoid bolt' which is screwed through the skull and into the subarachnoid space.

3. Fiber-optic catheters carrying transducers at their tips, which can be placed into the subarachnoid space, cerebral parenchyma or ventricles.

The major risk of ICP monitoring is infection. The catheter or bolt should be removed as early as possible, because if monitoring is employed for less than 3 days, the infection rate is virtually zero.

Electrophysiological monitoring. The electroencephalogram (EEG) reflects electrical activity recorded on the surface of the scalp. Intraoperative EEG recording has been used for monitoring the adequacy of cerebral perfusion during carotid endarterectomy, cerebrovascular surgery, open heart surgery, and induced hypotension for a variety of surgical procedures.

Metabolic monitoring. During recovery from surgery and trauma if artificial feeding has to be carried out, the simple everyday function of ingestion of food becomes complicated, involving metabolic balance studies and mathematics, with the potential for serious side effects. The stress of illness, fever, etc. can increase the expenditure of energy, for example by 25% in multiple trauma patients and 50% in cases of extensive burns. However, even an increase of 50% results in a need for less than 3000 kcal in a patient weighing 70 kg. It should be kept in mind that excessive calorie administration is harmful. Carbohydrates given in excess are turned into fat. The liver may develop fatty infiltration resulting in hepatic dysfunction.

Indirect calorimetry. Oxygen consumption and carbon dioxide production by the patient are measured, and requirements of calories are derived from these figures. Methods of determination of oxygen consumption include the following:

1. The Fick equation, which calculates oxygen consumption from the product of the cardiac output and the arterial venous oxygen content difference.
2. Douglas bag collection of expired gases.
3. Commercially available computerized indirect calorimeters.

The benefits of metabolic monitoring include the following:

1. The increased calorie requirements resulting from the illness, with its accelerated metabolism, can be estimated.
2. Patients with hypometabolism or hypermetabolic states can be identified.
3. As the caloric requirements vary widely, metabolic monitoring is more desirable than administering quantities by rote or formula.

Commercially available indirect calorimeters can now measure oxygen consumption and carbon dioxide production, and can help more precise prescription of nutritional therapy.

C-reactive protein. During the acute phase of different inflammatory conditions a number of proteins are produced. The most clinically important of these 'acute phase proteins' is the C-reactive protein. It is synthesized exclusively in the liver and its value rises within 6 hours of an acute event. Its level in the plasma increases with temperature (being triggered by IL-1), in inflammatory conditions and after trauma. It follows the clinical state of the patient much more rapidly than the ESR and is not affected by the level of haemoglobin. It is easily and quickly measured using an automated immunoassay. It is being increasingly used in place of the ESR, which has traditionally been used to monitor the progress of inflammatory and degenerative conditions. However, determination of C-reactive protein requires more sophisticated equipment and is more expensive.

Temperature monitoring. Temperature is normally taken in the mouth, rectum or axilla. The temperature in these peripheral parts of the body is often influenced by such factors as mouth breathing, temperature of the environment, etc. Therefore it is recommended that core temperatures be taken in the critically ill patient. Core temperature is measured by a thermistor wire directly against the tympanic membrane, or a thermistor probe into the oesophagus or deep into the rectum.

(Thermistor: a thermometer whose impedance varies with the ambient temperature, and which can measure extremely small changes in temperature).

Three devices are now commercially available for measuring bedside core temperature in ICU patients: pulmonary artery thermistor catheters, urinary bladder thermistor probes and auditory canal probes. At the same time, pulmonary artery blood temperature is increasingly being used as a reliable indicator of core temperature, although the need for a catheter is an obvious disadvantage of this method. Urinary bladder catheters have the advantage of giving both exact measurements of urine output and continuous readings of core temperature.

CARDIOPULMONARY RESUSCITATION (CPR)

From the standpoint of the general duty doctor, the most important part of this chapter is this section, dealing with resuscitation of the patient from cardio-respiratory arrest. Cardiac arrest can take place at any time and any place. Therefore every member of the medical and nursing staff should be thoroughly trained in the procedure of resuscitation. At the same time the necessary instruments for dealing with this emergency should be available in all hospital departments and emergency services.

Causes of cardiac arrest. The common causes leading to cardiac arrest include hypoxia, drugs, a diseased myocardium and trauma.

Hypoxia. The most common and important precipitating cause of cardiac arrest is hypoxia of the myocardium. This in turn can be produced by serious haemorrhage, sudden severe hypotension, coronary air embolism or respiratory obstruction.

Drugs. Most anaesthetic agents can induce arrhythmias and hypotension, specially if anoxia is present at the same time. Inotropic drugs like isoprenaline, adrenaline and dopamine, if carelessly used, can cause arrhythmias leading to ventricular fibrillation. Beta-blockers, vasodilators, calcium antagonists, and hyperkalaemia, specially if in combination, can produce asystole.

Diseased myocardium. A healthy myocardium can withstand moderate hypoxia without ill effect, but a diseased heart has less reserve and relatively minor disturbances may cause failure.

Trauma. Trauma can cause ventricular fibrillation and cardiac arrest, either directly or through vasovagal inhibition.

Types of cardiac arrest. Absence of a circulation may be produced by:

1. *Circulatory obstruction.* A massive pulmonary embolism or air embolism may block the path of the circulating blood. It should be remembered that as little as 50 ml of air carelessly introduced at venesection can kill a patient.
2. *Asystole.* Absence of systole indicates severe depression of the myocardium. The heart beat first becomes slow and feeble and finally stops. The myocardium is dilated, toneless and cyanosed.
3. *Ventricular fibrillation.* This usually occurs when the heart is irritable, either from trauma or manipulation during operation, or due to drugs. A fibrillating heart is less depressed and more likely to recover than a heart where asystole has set in.

TREATMENT OF CARDIAC ARREST

Prevention. It is better to prevent cardiac arrest than to treat it. For a start *every surgical operation should be carried out under an ECG and blood pressure monitor and a pulse oximeter.* It is far better to detect any disorder at the stage of a simple arrhythmia than to allow it to develop into fibrillation or asystole due to lack of monitoring. All patients under intensive care are normally constantly monitored. Surely no patient needs intensive care, and therefore cardiac monitoring, more than one who is undergoing an operative procedure with all its surgical and anaesthetic hazards.

Secondly, *great care should be exercised while administering different drugs intravenously.* The sudden influx of almost any drug into the circulation can produce a severe arrhythmia; therefore intravenous injections should be given very slowly and after being diluted. Some agents, for example potassium ions, cannot safely be given through a syringe or into the drip tubing. These should be added to the contents of the drip bottle, for slow infusion.

Management. If cardiac arrest takes place and the circulation is not restored within three or four minutes irreversible damage to the brain may result. In any case, if the circulation remains suspended for more than ten minutes, death is the nearly certain consequence, and recovery highly unlikely.

Recognition. Because only a few minutes are available in which to reverse the situation, it is essential that cardiac arrest be recognized immediately. Diagnosis is based on three signs:

1. Absent major pulses.
2. Absent or gasping respiration.
3. Dilated pupils.

The first is the most important sign. If the carotid pulse cannot be felt, cardiac arrest must be assumed and immediate corrective action taken. It must be emphasized that *the ECG alone is of no value for the diagnosis of cardiac arrest* because electrical activity can continue on the ECG for some minutes after effective cardiac contractions have ceased. The main value of the ECG lies in its ability to detect ventricular or other arrhythmias or fibrillations, in which case defibrillation may be required. Ventilation is best carried out in such a situation by mouth-to-mouth insufflation of lungs initially, and then by an Ambu bag and endotracheal tube.

Treatment. Treatment can be divided into three phases:

1. *Immediate measures. The person immediately available should start mouth-to-mouth ventilation and closed cardiac massage at once.* It should be remembered that it is futile to start cardiac massage without ventilating the lungs, although under the pressure of the critical situation this obvious fact may be overlooked. The person providing first-aid should give one breath, then carry out ten chest compressions; and he should keep on repeating this cycle. An i.v. line should be immediately established. If two persons are available the situation is much better. On of them should give mouth-to-mouth respiration and the other should carry out cardiac massage. These manoeuvres should be carried out continuously until heart beats or spontaneous respirations return, or until appropriate equipment becomes available.
2. *Definitive management.* As soon as the equipment becomes available an *endotracheal tube* should be passed and positive pressure ventilation started with an *Ambu bag* or a ventilator using pure oxygen. If an endotracheal tube is available from the beginning there is no need for more than a breath or two of mouth-to-mouth ventilation, and the tube should be passed immediately.

Electrocardiographic monitoring should be started as soon as possible. It immediately allows us to identify the type of cardiac arrest, i.e. asystole or ventricular fibrillation. At the same time, any signs of recovery appear first on the ECG.

Further action now depends upon the type of rhythm shown by the ECG:

1. If *ventricular fibrillation* is present the *cardiac defibrillator* is used and external defibrillation is attempted. If this does not help, 100 mg of lignocaine may be given intravenously and defibrillation attempted after a few minutes, in the meantime continuing cardiac massage. If

even this is unsuccessful, the chest should be opened and open cardiac massage carried out.

2. If *asystole* is present, 10 ml of 1:10,000 adrenaline or 0.01 mg isoprenaline is injected intravenously to induce ventricular fibrillation. If fibrillation develops, it is dealt with as described above, i.e. by using a defibrillator. However, if there is no response the chest is opened and massage carried out, with further injections of adrenaline or isoprenaline.

3. *Open cardiac massage.* The chest is opened through the fifth left intercostal space. The wound does not bleed because there is no circulation. If a rib-spreader is available both hands can be passed into the chest, the pericardium widely opened, and cardiac massage carried out very efficiently between the two hands. Without a rib spreader only one hand can be introduced into the chest and massage is less effective. Massage should be carried out with the flat of the hand so as not to damage the myocardium. The rate should be 50 to 60 compressions per minute. The purpose of the massage is to improve the tone of the heart muscle, to increase the coronary flow, and to ensure a supply of oxygenated blood to the brain. The arrested heart is toneless, distended and blue. After massage it should become smaller and more firm and pink. After the tone has returned, an effort should be made to get it to beat normally. A toneless heart has a tendency to distend with blood returning from the body. This should be prevented by effective massage, otherwise irreversible damage can occur.

During cardiac arrest the normal aerobic metabolism of the tissues is replaced by anaerobic metabolism, resulting in the production of lactic acid, i.e. a metabolic acidosis results. This may prevent full resuscitation, and may be corrected by sodium bicarbonate (1 meq per ml) given intravenously. However, this should be given only after 10 minutes during which if possible the pH of the blood should be determined. Sodium bicarbonate should be given only if the pH is below 7.2. The dose should be calculated according to the base deficit.

4. *Later treatment.* When normal rhythm and blood pressure are restored the patient is still watched very closely, because another episode of cardiac arrest can occur. Any metabolic acidosis should be corrected. Unfortunately, the brain may have been damaged during the period of circulatory arrest. If return of consciousness is delayed, cerebral dehydration is carried out by the use of mannitol etc., and by reducing the intake of crystalloids. Total body hypothermia down to 32°C may help reduce the extent of cerebral damage.

Summary. In order to put the whole subject of cardiorespiratory resuscitation in a nutshell and to commit it to memory, the student need only remember the first five letters in the alphabet as follows:

A for Airway.
B for Breathing.
C for Cardiac massage.
D for Drugs.
E for Electrical monitoring and stimulation.

Thus the first priority is to ensure that the airway is fully patent; the second to see if the patient is breathing and if not, to start artificial ventilation. Next, cardiac massage is commenced. Finally, if necessary, drugs may be used as indicated by the results of electrical monitoring.

INFECTION IN THE CRITICAL CARE UNIT (CCU)

Nosocomial infection in the CCU. Nosocomial infection is that which develops at least 48 hours after admission to hospital (Gr. *nosocomium* a hospital). It affects 15 to 40% of critical care unit (CCU) patients and contributes to approximately 70% of late deaths in such units.

Definitions. Colonization is the presence of a pathogenic organism on two or more occasions. Infection is the presence of many pathogenic organisms, with leucocytes and the clinical signs of inflammation. Sepsis is a syndrome comprising inflammation (fever and leucocytosis) and organ system failure; a micro-organism may or may not be identified.

Predisposing factors. The incidence of nosocomial infection depends upon the length of stay in the CCU, the number of invasive procedures, the nature of the underlying illness and the mode of presentation. After 24 hours about 10% of patients are infected, while more than 90% can be infected after 2 weeks. These factors are to some extent interdependent; the longer a patient stays in the unit the more procedures are likely to be performed.

Endotracheal intubation and mechanical ventilation carries a 20 to 60 % incidence of pneumonia, while upto 30% of patients with urinary catheters develop urinary tract infections. Upto 15% of infections occur in vascular lines, and rules regarding the insertion and management of arterial and venous lines need to be strictly enforced. Factors associated with an increased incidence of vascular catheter infections include the infusion of hypertonic solutions, frequent disconnection of infusion lines and the length of time the catheter remains in place. Except for tunnelled feeding lines and those required for haemodialysis, no vascular lines should remain in position for more than 5 days.

Control of infection requires strict adoption of preventive measures, early recognition of infection, and application of disciplined antibiotic policies. Insistence on hand washing, disinfection, isolation procedures, and strict control of antibiotic prophylaxis and therapy pay dividends. The usual sites sampled in the microbiological survey of an infected patient include wounds and discharge sites, lungs and airways, blood, urine, the tips of invasive line tubes, CSF, and other needles and aspirates.

Nosocomial pneumonia. Overall, nosocomial pneumonia occurs in about 1% of hospital patients, but in critical care units the incidence may reach 5 to 25%. Such pneumonias may be responsible for upto a quarter of critical care deaths. The factors which predispose towards nosocomial pneumonia in critical care patients are the following:

Advanced age
Obesity
Cigarette smoking
Diabetes mellitus
Chronic heart, lung or kidney disease
Malignant disease

Low Glasgow coma score
Endotracheal intubation
Oropharyngeal colonization with Gram-negative organisms
Gastric colonization in ileus and reduced gastric acidity

For *diagnosis,* the purely clinical criteria of fever, leucocytosis, purulent sputum and new or progressive infiltrates on chest x-rays are not specific enough to use in the critically ill. Fever and leucocytosis may be due to a variety of infectious or even non-infectious conditions. A better diagnostic criterion consists of quantitative cultures of material obtained by a protected specimen brush and bronchoalveolar lavage. Significant infection is indicated by the presence of more than 10^3 colony forming units in 1 ml of lavage fluid. The number of infections increases from 10% at 10 days to over 25% at 30 days. Bronchoalveolar lavage offers the advantage that Gram staining of a centrifuged deposit of the fluid obtained may provide an immediate indication of pneumonia: if more than 25% of white cells in the deposit contain intracellular organisms it is highly likely that the patient has pneumonia. At the same time, blind bronchial lavage with an undirected catheter is almost as sensitive and specific as fibreoptically guided bronchoalveolar lavage.

Prevention. Measures to this end include:

1. Sheathed suction catheters which allow a single catheter to be used for 24 hours without repeated disconnection of the circuit.
2. Humidification using heat/moisture exchangers that also serve as microbiological filters.
3. Prevention of stress ulcer with the use of a cytoprotective agent like sucralfate, rather than antacids and H_2-blockers; the latter increase the gastric pH and may encourage bacterial colonization of the gastric secretions.
4. Change of posture every few hours to discourage the development of dependent lung collapse.

Management. All ventilated critical care patients who are considered to have nosocomial pneumonia should undergo fibreoptic bronchoscopy for bronchial lavage. Alternatively, lavage should be carried out through a non-directed catheter passed as far into a lobar bronchus as possible. If on cytological examination more than 25% of white cells contain organisms, empirical therapy should be commenced, based on the results of Gram staining. The most popular antibiotic regimen for nosocomial pneumonia consists of an aminoglycoside and an antipseudomonal β-lactam.

Infection in the immunocompromised patient. The most common causes of immunocompromise are malignancy, chemotherapy, corticosteroid treatment, splenectomy, and immunosuppression after transplantation and acquired immune deficiency syndrome (AIDS). Immunocompromise can take the form of failure of phagocytosis, defective cell-mediated immunity, and defective antibody-mediated immunity.

Treatment. Attempts to reduce infection using isolation procedures have failed. As the risk of infection is related to the number of interventions, invasive procedures should be limited to essential diagnostic interventions. The oropharynx and sinuses should be checked daily. The appearance of new infiltrates on chest x-rays indicates an opportunistic pneumonia until proved otherwise. Unfortunately, prophylactic antibiotics are very often associated with the development of bacterial resistance. Confirmed infection requires immediate and effective treatment. A combination of a third generation cephalosporin with an aminoglycoside (gentamycin or netilmicin) and a penicillinase-resistant penicillin (nafcillin or oxacillin) eliminates most of the likely organisms. Finally, persistent fever in the face of adequate antibiotic therapy should raise the suspicion of fungal infection.

CYTOKINES IN SEPSIS

A major breakthrough in the understanding of sepsis has occurred in the last decade with advances in molecular biology. The substances which are produced in severe inflammation and cause host autoinjury and death have been identified, and are called cytokines (cyto = cell; kinesis = motion). A cytokine is a soluble molecule produced by a cell to induce a biological effect elsewhere. It acts as a messenger at its destination. The effect varies according to the cytokine and the cell, but typically these molecules signal certain cells to activate, divide, or home in on a particular site in the body. The most important cytokines in the mediation of lethal sepsis are tumour necrosis factor and interleukin-1, the others being interleukins-6 and 8. They are synthesized not only by monocytes/macrophages, but by other cells including neutrophils, lymphocytes and endothelial cells.

Tumour necrosis factor (TNF) plays a key role in critical illness:

1. Administration of TNF to laboratory animals induces all the host alterations associated with severe infection.
2. In patients with overwhelming infection there is a close relationship between circulating TNF levels and death.
3. In animals given a lethal dose of live Gram-negative organisms, if monoclonal antibodies effective against TNF are administered, a fatal outcome is prevented. This shows that in lethal Gram-negative infection it is *substances produced by the host* (in this case TNF), and not bacterial poisons by themselves, that cause death.

Interleukin-1 (IL-1) exists in a and b forms, the latter being the more important. Administration of interleukin-1b to animals and human beings results in all the responses seen in acute infection. Stimuli for IL-1 release include all inflammatory, infectious and immunological processes. IL-1 acts on the CNS, inducing fever by stimulating local release of prostaglandins in the anterior hypothalamus, and inducing anorexia by direct action on the satiety center. It also multiplies the effects of TNF a hundredfold. The lethality of acute infection is due to TNF and IL-1b acting synergistically and causing hypotension, tissue injury and death in animals subjected to experimental sepsis.

Synergy between cytokines — the 'cytokine cascade.' (cascade = a series of waterfalls constituting a large waterfall; a series of stages of a process which, once initiated continues to the final stage, each stage being triggered by the previous one, with cumulative effect).

During health, the synthesis of TNF is strongly repressed. It is only when cells are triggered by endotoxins and other stimuli that they elaborate TNF. The result depends upon the amounts of TNF produced:

1. *Low* levels of endotoxaemia trigger TNF production. Fever occurs but without lethal responses like hypotension or coagulopathy.

2. If the levels of TNF are *high* enough for secondary synthesis of interleukin-1b, lethal responses can take place and result in death. The induction of a cytokine cascade represents an inappropriately severe response to an inflammatory stimulus, and leads to death through hypothermia, coagulopathy, visceral hypoperfusion and reperfusion injury, lactic acidosis, myocardial depression, peripheral vasodilatation, or the capillary leak syndrome. All of these alterations may be induced by TNF or interleukin-1b.

Blocking the cytokine cascade. The mortality in severe surgical sepsis is constant at 50 to 70%. It is not likely that better antibiotics or haemodynamic support will reduce it. However, modification of the cytokine cascade could reduce the death rate. This great advance could come, in future, through one of the following mechanisms:

1. If the endotoxin-induced generation of cytokines could be inhibited: an antibody against lipid A (the toxic part of the molecule common to all Gram-negative strains) has been developed and shown to reduce mortality from Gram-negative bacteraemia by 39%.

2. If effective monoclonal antibodies against cytokines could be developed (TNF and interleukin-1b): this is a promising approach, as these antibodies may be more applicable in severe inflammatory states rather than just those initiated by endotoxin. Experimentally they have been found to be most effective when given prophylactically.

3. If cytokine receptors could be inhibited.

After severe inflammatory or infective episodes the host releases not only large amounts of potentially lethal cytokines but also antidotes to these cytokines. Lethal effects of cytokines are seen when the antidotes are exhausted, leading to unopposed cytokine activity. Blocking the activity of either TNF or interleukin-1 prevents the full consequences of the disease.

Acute inflammation in a localized focus of infection is a 'friend' of the organism. On the other hand, intravascular activation of the same mechanism behaves as a 'foe', causing the entire body to behave like a massive wound, with intravascular mediator activation, capillary leak and often lethal consequences.

ADULT RESPIRATORY DISTRESS SYNDROME

Disordered exchange of gases in the lungs often follows shock and trauma, and is the most common cause of respiratory failure. In 1967 Ashbaugh described acute respiratory distress in twelve patients without underlying lung disease. This 'adult respiratory distress syndrome' (ARDS) may develop in a variety of clinical situations, of which severe sepsis is the most important. Apart from this, ARDS can occur as a non-specific reaction to a wide variety of insults including shock (specially septic shock), trauma, burns, fat embolism, cardiopulmonary bypass, amniotic fluid embolism and aspiration pneumonia.

Pathogenesis. In patients with trauma and sepsis, *endotoxaemia activates complement and other components of the immune-inflammatory cascade;* this causes leucocytes to be sequestered in pulmonary capillaries. The sequestered leucocytes release proteases, cytokines, and toxic superoxide radicals, which injure endothelial cells.

Pathophysiology. ARDS is the earliest manifestation of a generalized inflammatory response and is often followed by the development of multiple organ dysfunction syndrome. Severe infection or large areas of devitalized tissue can trigger a massive inflammatory response. Although beneficial when directed against local areas of infection or necrotic tissue, dissemination of this response can produce widespread tissue damage. The pulmonary epithelium is damaged, reducing surfactant production and lowering the threshold for alveolar flooding, thus leading ultimately to non-cardiac pulmonary oedema which is a cardinal feature of ARDS. The pathological changes result in reduced functional residual capacity, increased venous admixture (shunt), reduced lung compliance, and hypoxaemia which is refractory to treatment.

Obstruction of the pulmonary circulation results from:

1. Vascular compression by interstitial oedema as well as oedema of the vessel wall.

2. Constriction of the pulmonary vessels by:

i. Increased autonomic nervous activity.

ii. Circulating substances such as catecholamines, 5-hydroxytryptamine, thromboxane, fibrinogen degradation products (FDPs), complement and activated leucocytes.

Presentation. The recognition of adult respiratory distress syndrome is not difficult. The patient has acute respiratory distress, requires an increasing concentration of oxygen in the inspired air (greater than 0.5) to maintain a partial pressure of arterial oxygen (Pao_2) of more than 50 mm Hg, and chest x-rays show extensive lung infiltrates. With mechanical ventilation the lungs are stiff and require high inflation pressures. Cardiogenic pulmonary oedema should be excluded by measuring pulmonary artery wedge pressure.

Management. There is no specific treatment forARDS except to remove or suppress the injurious agent, and to support the patient until lung function returns. The clinician should anticipate its development by remaining aware of the precipitating causes. An aggressive approach to the management of these underlying disease processes may help prevent progression to respiratory failure.

The aim of *respiratory support* is to achieve adequate oxygen supply without impeding cardiac output. To ensure delivery of sufficient oxygen the haemoglobin concentration should be maintained at 11 g/100 ml of blood. Oxygen, intermittent positive pressure ventilation and positive end-expiratory pressure (PEEP) form the basis of respiratory support in this condition. 'Optimal' positive end-expiratory pressure opens up alveoli to restore the reduced residual functional capacity to normal. However, excessive positive end-expiratory pressure results in damage to the alveoli (barotrauma). The clinician should be alert to the signs of tissue hypoxia, such as metabolic acidosis, mental obtundation, and cardiac arrhythmias. If such signs are not present it is reasonable to assume that oxygen delivery is adequate.

Indications for *mechanical ventilation* fall into two categories:

1. Inadequate alveolar *ventilation* with increasing Pco_2.
2. Inadequate *gas exchange* with increasing alveolar-arterial oxygen gradient and arterial hypoxaemia: the clinician should anticipate problems before they arise.

Because the patient is often nursed for prolonged periods in the supine position, extensive collapse of the dependent parts of the lungs is common. Sitting the patient as upright as possible, or rolling him from side to side once every few hours, helps greatly in improving oxygenation.

Circulatory support. Fluid administration should be regulated to ensure adequate cardiac output without aggravating the pulmonary oedema. Measurement of pulmonary capillary wedge pressure provides a more reliable assessment of the filling status of the patient than determination of central venous pressure.

Prognosis. If multiple organ support is maintained, the chances of recovery are improved. Even after positive pressure ventilation for over 3 months a good functional recovery is possible. The mortality rate used to be as high as 50%. However, recent reports have shown a fall in mortality to about 20%.

11 Surgery and diabetes

Diabetes mellitus is a very common condition, affecting upto 10% of the population. It is of considerable importance for the surgeon for the following reasons:

1. Diabetes is a major metabolic defect of carbohydrate, protein and fat metabolism, and special management is required during a surgical procedure.
2. It can cause infection, vascular disease and neuropathy. If any of these conditions already exists, diabetes can aggravate it.
3. Surgical infection aggravates the diabetic state, so that the requirements of insulin are increased.
4. The perioperative mortality rate in diabetics is much higher than in the general population, being around 8%; most deaths occur due to diseases associated with diabetes, including atherosclerosis, nephropathy, hypertension, ischaemic heart disease and infection (63% of diabetics have cardiovascular disease, 44% have peripheral vascular disease, and 24% suffer from cerebrovascular disease). Also, many patients suffer from autonomic and peripheral neuropathies, which may lead to postural hypotension or cardiac arrest.
5. Hypoglycaemia must be considered as a possible cause whenever an unconscious patient is brought for treatment.

The *diagnosis of diabetes* is made on the basis of a fasting venous blood level above 140 mg/dl (7.8 mmol/l) and an abnormal glucose tolerance test, i.e. blood glucose above 200 mg/dl (11.0 mmol/l) two hours after ingestion of 75 g of glucose.

SURGICAL COMPLICATIONS OF DIABETES

The complications of diabetes which are of special concern to the surgeon include neuropathy, infection, and angiopathy; and specially in the case of the foot they lead to the clinical conditions of *ulcer* and *gangrene*.

Peripheral neuropathy. Peripheral neuropathy leads to the development of ulcers on the sole of the foot, as follows:

1. Loss of *sensory* nerve supply leads to anaesthesia, so that repeated minor trauma remains undetected and uncared for, predisposing to the development of an ulcer.
2. Loss of *motor* nerve supply results in muscle atrophy leading to the development of foot deformities. The pressure distribution on the sole of the foot becomes abnormal, with increased weight-bearing on the metatarsal heads. This leads first to the degeneration of the fat pads underlying the metatarsal heads, and later to the development of an actual ulcer.

Infection. Infection predisposes the part to the development of gangrene. It does so by producing hypoxia of the tissues, by increasing the demand for oxygen while reducing its supply:

1. The *increased demand* for oxygen results from the raised metabolic rate in the tissues due to the infection.
2. The *reduced supply* of oxygen results from vascular insufficiency, which itself is produced as follows:

i. Inflammatory oedema increases tissue tension and compresses the blood vessels.

ii. If gas-producing organisms are responsible for the infection, the pressure of the gas adds greatly to the tissue tension.

iii. Bacterial toxins produce thrombosis, which leads to occlusion of small vessels.

Angiopathy. 1. In patients suffering from diabetes, *arteriosclerosis* develops at a much earlier age than in the general population.

2. At the same time a *microangiopathy* occurs in the small blood vessels of diabetics; thickening of the basement membrane reduces the lumen of these vessels so that the flow of blood through them is diminished.

Ulcer and gangrene. In the development of an ulcer on the sole of the foot the major role is played by neuropathy, although infection and angiopathy probably also contribute their share. On the other hand, in the development of gangrene all three of the above-named factors make significant contributions.

THE DIABETIC FOOT

The foot, being farthest away from the heart, has a modest blood supply at the best of times. In old age arteriosclerosis further reduces the circulation to the foot. If diabetes supervenes, microangiopathy and neuropathy greatly increase the chances of onset of gangrene, as explained above. The widespread belief that diabetic arterial disease is primarily localized to the small vessels is erroneous. Although diabetics develop a microangiopathy, the primary pathology is that of typical large-vessel atherosclerosis.

Investigations. *Doppler pressure* determination in the toes accurately determines arterial insufficiency. Arterial disease is unlikely when the ratio between the pressure in the toe and in the brachial artery (toe-brachial pressure ratio) exceeds 0.70. *Arteriography* is frequently required to exclude the possibility of reconstructible arterial disease of the infrapopliteal or tibial vessels.

Management. 1. In every diabetic patient the peripheral pulses, the condition of the skin of the foot, and sensations in the foot should be carefully tested. If the circulation is *normal* and there is no neuropathy, the patient should be instructed in the meticulous care of his feet, and the feet checked periodically for the early onset of ischaemic changes.

2. If the circulation is even slightly *impaired* as indicated by the pulses, the sensations, or by the trophic changes, *urgent measures* should be undertaken to prevent damage to the skin which might lead to ulceration and gangrene. The most important precaution is the wearing of well-fitting shoes. The feet are protected from damage done by

tight fitting shoes, and corns and callosities can be prevented from developing. In countries with a warm climate where open sandals can be worn, specially in summer, this is not such a problem.

Instructions to the patient. The surgeon should explain to the patient that even minor ulcerations could get complicated, and lead to possible loss of the whole limb. However, it is no use just telling the patient to take good care of his feet, because he will not know what to do. A detailed set of written instructions should be given to him, on the following lines:

1. Inspect feet daily for blisters and cuts, specially between the toes.
2. Wash feet daily, dry carefully.
3. If feet are cold at night, wear socks; do not use hot water bottles.
4. Use properly fitted shoes, avoid pointed shoes, start wearing new shoes gradually.
5. Don't walk barefooted.
6. Cut nails straight across.
7. Don't cut corns yourself; get professional help.
8. See your doctor regularly and have your feet examined.

One of the reasons for including the above list of instructions in this book is to serve as a model. Whenever a patient is suffering from a condition where some of the medical care has to be entrusted to him at home, *an appropriate set of written instructions should be given to him.* The clinician will find that the patient's compliance with the instructions will improve greatly by the use of this simple device, to his great benefit.

3. If *ulcers or gangrenous spots* have already developed, a serious state exists. The part should be kept at rest. The ulcerated area is gently washed daily with lukewarm water and mild soap, and a dressing applied. The dressing should be kept in place by a bandage, adhesive plaster being avoided. Cultures of the area should be taken. Organisms will often be grown, but antibiotics should only be started if the ulcer is inflamed or there are systemic signs of infection. In most cases the ulcer can be managed by local cleansing and dressing.

4. If *rest pain* occurs the patient should sleep with the foot side of the bed a little lowered in order to increase the arterial supply. If this fails to give relief from pain, analgesics and even narcotics should be used.

5. If *ischaemia* is present, indicated by intermittent claudication or ulceration, and the pulses are diminished, arteriography should be carried out to see if reconstructive surgery is feasible and if so, operation should be performed.

INFECTION IN A DIABETIC

If infection develops in a diabetic it must be treated energetically, because it can have serious consequences for the patient. If ischaemia due to vascular disease is present, what might only be surface contamination in the normal patient can become invasive infection in the diabetic, because diabetes interferes with the ability of polymorphonuclear cells to kill bacteria. When infection occurs the insulin requirement of the diabetic increases, and if not provided for, can rapidly lead to ketoacidosis. Therefore, firstly every effort should be made to prevent infection; and secondly, if infection does take place, very effective medical and surgical treatment should be given to prevent ketosis.

If *elective surgery* is to be undertaken on a diabetic, every effort should be made to clear up any existing infection unless it is the reason for the operation. At the same time remote infections should be carefully searched for and eliminated before operation. If the infection cannot be eliminated, antibiotics should be started and continued for 3 to 4 days postoperatively.

Prophylactic antibiotics should be used only in contaminated and clean-contaminated cases. They must be started before operation, usually at the time of induction of anaesthesia, and continued for only a few hours, or at the most a day or two. Lengthy courses of antibiotics do not confer any added benefit. At the same time, antibiotics started after the operation are useless for prophylaxis.

Future developments in control of diabetes. Whatever the mode of administration of insulin, the glucose level in the blood fluctuates considerably. Damage to the blood vessels, nerves, and various other tissues occurs during the periods of hyperglycaemia. In order to stabilize the glucose metabolism *implantable insulin pumps* are being developed. The most sophisticated of these pumps can constantly monitor the blood glucose and keep on releasing insulin according to need. Such pumps, when perfected, will be a major advance in the control of diabetes, and will help prevent many of the complications of imperfectly controlled diabetes.

The only treatment of type 1 diabetes that establishes an insulin-independent euglycaemic state consists of *pancreatic transplantation.* However, the price which has to be paid for achieving such a state is the need for immunosuppression. If the patient is uraemic from nephropathy, he is already on immunosuppression. In that case pancreatic transplantation should definitely be carried out.

PREPARING THE DIABETIC FOR SURGERY

Preoperative management. The signs and symptoms of diabetes and any associated pathology should be assessed. Laboratory tests should include a full electrolyte, urea and creatinine screen, blood count with white cell differential, chest x-ray and ECG. If the patient is receiving treatment for other conditions, e.g. alpha-blockers, calcium channel inhibitors, other antihypertensives, digitalis, etc., it should be optimized before surgery.

Plasma potassium levels may be decreased in uncontrolled diabetes, and may need to be supplemented. A cardiac autonomic neuropathy is present in about one-third of all diabetics, and is associated with a poor prognosis. Its earliest manifestation consists of a lack of variation of the heart rate, with higher than average resting heart rates. Other features include postural hypotension and intraoperative episodes of bradycardia and hypotension.

Perioperative management. The major hazard in diabetes is hypoglycaemia. However, acute hyperglycaemia during surgery may result in altered host defence mechanisms, extracellular dehydration and electrolyte imbalance, intracellular dehydration and impaired wound healing. The blood glucose level is best maintained in the range 75 to 145 mg/dl (4 to 8 mmol/l).

Elective surgery. *Non-insulin-dependent diabetics* commonly secrete enough insulin to carry them through minor surgery (i.e. with no penetration of a body cavity or transection of a major limb bone), and do not need insulin provided glucose-containing solutions are avoided. In all patients oral hypoglycaemic agents should be discontinued before surgery and recommenced the next day whenever possible.

Insulin-dependent patients. Various regimens have been recommended for these patients. These include:

1. A 'split-normal-dose' regimen, a quarter or half the usual morning dose of insulin, plus 5% dextrose solution at a rate between 100 and 200 ml/hour.
2. Regular administration of low-dose i.v. insulin.
3. An infusion of insulin with the simultaneous infusion of 5% dextrose (with adjustment of the rates of infusion of the insulin or glucose based on frequent blood glucose estimates).

When monitoring these methods of diabetic control, blood glucose determinations are preferable to urine glucose analysis, because anaesthesia and surgery change the renal threshold to glucose excretion. The ready availability of glucose meters has made it simple.

Fluid replacement should be given as normal saline solution. Higher blood glucose levels (and hence higher insulin requirements) are seen in patients receiving either 5% dextrose or Ringer's lactate (the lactate being a precursor of glucose, specially in starved or catabolic patients).

Postoperative management. Neither sliding scale doses of insulin given every 4 to 6 hours, nor continuous infusions of insulin at a fixed rate are entirely satisfactory. A good method is the following: 5% glucose in water, with 16 units of insulin in each liter bottle, is given at the rate of 125 ml/hour. The blood sugar levels are determined 6 hourly and additional doses of insulin given as required. With this regimen hypoglycaemia is virtually insured against.

Emergency surgery. Sometimes a patient is admitted in severe diabetic acidosis or coma secondary to an urgent surgical problem, e.g. a perforated appendix. The diabetes may get out of control before the patient realizes it; his cerebral function may be impaired and he may be admitted as an emergency.

Apart from urine analysis, the patient's blood sugar, serum acetone and electrolytes must be immediately determined. Normal saline with regular insulin should be started through the intravenous line immediately. 50 to 300 units of insulin may be required; half the dose is given intravenously and the other half subcutaneously. If the patient is in shock the entire dose of insulin should be given intravenously, because of the poor absorption of drugs in shock. The blood glucose is measured every hour, and the state of fluid replenishment repeatedly assessed, with a central venous catheter and an indwelling urinary catheter. When the serum electrolyte levels are known the fluid may be changed to Ringer's lactate; the lactated buffer in the solution helps in correcting the acidosis.

As soon as an adequate urinary output has been achieved, potassium which has been lost due to the osmotic diuresis should be added to the intravenous solution. Further, as soon as acidosis is corrected and dehydration reversed, the patient may undergo the emergency operation.

12 Ulcers, sinuses and fistulae

Ulcers

An ulcer is a break in the continuity of an epithelial surface, usually produced by the sloughing of necrotic inflammatory tissue. There is progressive destruction of the tissue cell by cell. On the other hand in gangrene there is death of macroscopic portions of tissue. Ulcers may be non-specific, specific or malignant. Specific and malignant ulcers are discussed in the appropriate chapters.

Types of ulcers. The common types of ulcers include the following:

1. Traumatic ulcers, following incorrect treatment of wounds.
2. Pressure sores.
3. Venous ulcers.
4. Ischaemic ulcers.
5. Ulcers in skin diseases.
6. Neuropathic ulcers in diabetes and disseminated sclerosis, due to repeated trauma to an insensitive area of skin.
7. Infective ulcers:
   i. Specific infections:
   (a) Tuberculous, fungal and syphilitic ulcers.
   (b) Herpes simplex (seen in surgical practice in critical illness, chest infection, or in the immunocompromised patient).
   ii. Secondary infections following drainage of abscesses, and infection in operation wounds.
8. Aphthous ulcers: recurrent, painful ulcers in the floor of the mouth.
9. Ulcers artefacta, being inflicted by the patient himself.
10. Malignant ulcers of the skin and gastrointestinal tract.
11. Peptic ulcers.

The life-history of an ulcer. This consists of 3 phases: extension, transition, and finally either repair or chronicity.

Extension. In the stage of extension the floor of the ulcer is covered with exudate and sloughs. The base is hard from active inflammation, the edge is sharply defined, the discharge is purulent or blood-stained, and the surrounding skin is red and inflamed.

Transition. At this stage the floor of the ulcer is clear, the sloughs separate, the base is less hard, and the discharge is serous. Small areas of granulations appear and extend all over.

Repair or chronicity. Finally the ulcer may either undergo healing i.e. repair, or become a chronic ulcer.

1. *Repair.* The granulation tissue changes to fibrous tissue which contracts to form a scar. The skin edge grows over at the rate of 1 mm per day. The healing edge consists of three zones: the outer is white epithelium; the middle is blue, where granulation tissue is covered by a few layers of epithelium; the inner zone is red granulation tissue with a covering of a single layer of epithelial cells.

2. *Chronicity.* If conditions are not favourable for healing, the ulcer becomes chronic. The granulations are pale and the base, edge and surrounding areas are hard. The formation of weak granulation tissue may be due to a systemic disorder e.g. myxoedema, malnutrition, long-term therapy with steroids, local ischaemia or specific infections. Zinc-containing lotions e.g. red lotion and scarlet red, which stimulate granulation tissue formation, are useful in such situations.

CLINICAL EXAMINATION OF AN ULCER

During the clinical examination of an ulcer the following points must be noted:

Site. Most rodent ulcers occur on the upper part of the face. Carcinoma of the lip commonly arises on the lower lip.

Size and duration. A rodent ulcer grows extremely slowly, a carcinoma somewhat slowly, and an inflammatory ulcer rapidly.

Shape. A rodent ulcer is usually round, a syphilitic ulcer is irregular in shape.

Edge. A healing non-specific ulcer has a sloping edge, a tuberculous ulcer an undermined edge, a rodent ulcer a rolled edge, and an epithelioma a raised and everted edge.

Floor. In tuberculosis the floor is covered by gelatinous granulations, so also in amoebiasis.

Base. The base of the ulcer is hard in carcinoma, and fixed to the deep structures in a varicose ulcer.

Discharge. In acute infection the discharge is purulent, in *Pseudomonas pyocyaneus* infection it is bluish green, and in tuberculosis it is often watery.

Pain. Non-specific ulcers in the stage of extension are painful. Tuberculous ulcers are painless except when they occur on the tongue.

Lymph nodes. In rodent ulcer the lymph nodes are not enlarged, except from secondary infection. In carcinoma they may be enlarged, hard, and fixed.

General examination. During the general examination the clinician must look for evidence of anaemia, diabetes, tuberculosis, etc.

Pathology. Any discharge should be examined bacteriologically. If the diagnosis is not clear, a biopsy from the edge of the ulcer should be taken, including a part of the normal skin adjacent to the margin of the ulcer.

TREATMENT OF ULCERS

General treatment. In order to treat an ulcer successfully, it is essential to know its exact aetiology. Clinical findings often provide essential clues to the underlying disease. For example, the distal part of a limb the seat of arteriosclerosis may be cold, while a limb affected by the neuropathy of diabetes shows loss of sensation. If doubt still remains as to its exact nature, a *biopsy* of the edge should be carried out. Once the cause is found, it is eliminated as far as possible. At the same time any anaemia is corrected.

Local treatment. In the case of ulcers due to specific causes, the treatment varies according to the cause of the ulcer. However, in the case of non-specific ulcers the following applications have been found to be useful in dealing with different situations:

1. If granulations are excessive and oedematous, they can be made firm and pink by the application of *magnesium sulphate glycerine paste.* This paste is markedly hypertonic, and therefore withdraws fluid from the ulcer due to osmosis, making it less water-logged. It should not be applied over a fresh wound, as the effect of the salt on the raw nerve endings produces unbearable pain. When the endings get covered by a layer of granulation tissue this paste may be used; the patient still gets a twinge of pain but it soon passes away, as the paste gets diluted by the tissue fluid.

2. If the excessive granulations occupy a small area, they can be discouraged by the caustic effect of a 10 to 15% solution of *silver nitrate,* or by direct application of a crystal of silver nitrate. If a crystal is used, care should be taken to touch only the raw area with it. If silver nitrate powder is used by mistake, and this spills out over the surrounding skin, a severe burn with unbearable pain is the result.

3. If there is an excessive quantity of sloughs in the floor of the ulcer, gauze soaked in a solution of *Eusol* is a very useful dressing. Eusol is a clear watery solution of hypochlorite, with an odour like that of slaked lime. It clears up sloughs rapidly, and makes the ulcer look clean.

4. If the ulcer is chronic and non-healing, *infra-red radiation* is helpful. The healing agent is the heat produced by the infra-red rays, which causes hyperaemia. This brings in many times more blood to the part, which not only delivers more oxygen and nutrients but also carries away the waste products of metabolism more promptly. *Unfortunately, since the advent of antibiotics the healing properties of heat applied to an inflamed part have been forgotten, and this method of treatment is grossly underutilized.* The healing effects of heat are complementary to those of antibiotics; both can therefore be used together with advantage.

5. *Antibiotics.* In general, antibiotics are not required in granulating wounds, because healthy granulation tissue forms a very effective natural barrier against bacterial invasion, and is virtually impermeable to both topical and systemic antibiotics. Antibiotics are required only if the ulcer is infected with surrounding cellulitis, and in the case of ulcers of specific bacterial origin, e.g. syphilis or tuberculosis.

Decubitus ulcer (pressure sore). These ulcers occur over the sacral area, the heels and the back. Such an ulcer is one of the most common complications in the chronic invalid or critically ill patient, most occurring in patients who are old, and have impaired mobility and neurological disease, often along with incontinence of urine and faeces due to sphincter disturbances. Localized constant pressure over a contact area causes ischaemia, with eventual necrosis first of the subcutaneous fat and later of the skin. The gangrenous skin eventually separates, leaving necrotic subcutaneous tissue and fat, which overlies the developing granulation tissue. The ulcer may deepen to involve tendon and bone.

Prevention is much better than the long drawn-out healing process of the ulcer once it has formed:

1. Normally, a person in bed keeps changing his side periodically. Patients who are unable to move themselves *must be turned in bed every 2 hours,* as uninterrupted pressure due to the body weight results in ischaemia of the skin and the development of bedsores.

2. Twice a day, meticulous skin cleansing should be carried out using methylated spirit or cetavlon solution, followed by gentle massage and application of talcum powder.

3. *Ripple air beds* are available, in which alternate air cells are inflated and deflated by a motor every few minutes, and help to distribute pressure on the back.

4. Anaemia, uraemia, diabetes and hypothyroidism delay the formation of granulation tissue and should be corrected.

If an ulcer still develops, the above measures are continued. Slough and dead tissue are removed until capillary bleeding is just encountered. A silicone foam cushion is created as follows: the solution for producing the foam is poured into the ulcer. It 'rises' to create the foam cushion which is the exact size and shape of the defect, and distributes the pressure of the bandage evenly. The cushion can be removed, washed thoroughly and replaced in the ulcer. In most cases such treatment leads to healing of the ulcer, which gets accelerated as soon as the patient starts moving about. In a bedridden patient the ulcer is very resistant to treatment. Rotational flaps of skin and fat may need to be brought over from the buttocks.

Ischaemic ulcer. The ischaemic ulcer is usually initiated by minor trauma to a limb with impaired blood supply. The anterior tibial region just above the ankle is the most common site for these ulcers. Intermittent claudication or rest pain, and previous trouble with healing of skin, should lead one to suspect the condition. The clinical findings are due to the reduced blood supply. The skin is atrophic. The granulation tissue is pale. The limb feels cold and is hairless with deformed nails, often with a nail-fold infection. The pulses are weak or absent. The Doppler test and thermography show reduced blood flow. The cardiovascular and respiratory systems should be examined.

Arteriography demonstrates the presence or absence of a surgically correctable arterial lesion. Correction of a major vessel block may dramatically improve leg perfusion and lead to ulcer healing. Balloon angioplasty is not suitable due to the diffuse nature of the lesion. Lumbar sympathectomy increases blood flow to the skin in 60% of patients by opening arteriovenous anastomoses. Sympathectomy is usually considered if arteriography shows that direct arterial surgery is not feasible.

Sinuses and fistulae

Sinuses. A sinus is a discharging blind-ended tract which opens onto an epithelial surface and often leads to an abscess cavity. The key to the correct treatment of a sinus is the detection of any associated deep abscess cavity or complex deep extensions of the sinus tract. Failure to do so will result in recurrence of the sinus in the same or an adjacent location.

The discharge from a sinus should always be submitted for bacteriological examination. Most of the pathogens isolated will be skin organisms or gut commensals. However, occasionally specific infections such as tuberculosis, actinomycosis or fungus may be found. The sinus opening should be gently probed to assess the depth, direction and multiplicity of the tracts. If the opening is small, a fine tube may be introduced and a radiopaque dye injected for a 'sinogram' x-ray.

Fistulae. A fistula is an abnormal communication between two epithelial or endothelial surfaces. Commonly, this communication is between two internal organs, or between an internal organ and the skin. The fistula usually derives its name from the organs which it joins together. Thus a fistula between the rectum and vagina is called a rectovaginal fistula, one between the bronchus and pleura is a bronchopleural fistula, and so on.

Causes of sinuses and fistulae. Sinuses and fistulae may be congenital or acquired.

Congenital. Examples of congenital sinuses and fistulae include preauricular sinus, tracheo-oesophageal fistula, branchial fistula, etc. Most of these arise due to imperfect fusion of skin, or incomplete separation of hollow tubes from one another. Thus a preauricular sinus develops due to imperfect fusion between the auditory tubercles, and a tracheo-oesophageal fistula due to incomplete separation of the trachea from the oesophagus.

Acquired. These sinuses often result from inadequate drainage of an abscess, e.g. a perianal abscess may burst on the surface and lead to a sinus.

Causes of persistence of sinuses and fistulae. ***Congenital*** fistulae are lined by epithelium, and will persist indefinitely unless surgically closed, with excision of the epithelial lining.

Acquired sinuses and fistulae may persist due to one of many reasons:

1. A *foreign* body may be present in the sinus. For example a piece of unabsorbable suture may be responsible. Again, a piece of dead bone, i.e. a sequestrum, may lead to the persistence of an osteomyelitic sinus.
2. Inefficient drainage may prevent the healing of a sinus. Thus when a drain is introduced it should be placed in the most *dependent* part of a cavity, as otherwise some of the fluid remains undrained and stagnates in the cavity, resulting in persistence of the sinus.
3. Irritating *discharges*, e.g. urine or stool, may prevent healing.
4. Unrelieved *obstruction* of a hollow tube distal to a fistula can be the cause of non-healing of an intestinal fistula.
5. If dense *fibrous tissue* is present and prevents contraction of the cavity, the sinus or fistula will not heal.
6. *Specific infections*, like tuberculosis or actinomycosis, may prevent healing.
7. If the track is lined by *epithelium* the question of healing of a fistula does not arise unless and until the epithelium is excised at operation.
8. If a fistula between two organs has developed due to extension of a *malignant ulcer* in one of the organs, it will not heal unless the ulcer is excised along with some healthy tissue around it. In fact, in such cases even more radical operations are sometimes required.

Treatment. In the treatment of a sinus or fistula, its cause must be removed. As far as the local operation is concerned: while treating any sinus, after proper evaluation the sinus is laid open or excised and a piece of tissue from the wall of the sinus sent for biopsy. In most cases this will be seen to be ordinary granulation tissue, but occasionally a metastatic deposit or a specific inflammatory disease will be revealed, which would be missed if routine biopsy was not being practiced.

In the case of a fistula, if the track is lined by granulation tissue, laying it open with thorough curettage will often suffice. However, if the track is epithelialized, excision of the epithelial track is essential for healing.

Abscesses

An abscess is a localized collection of pus, which consists of a semiliquid debris of necrotic leucocytes and tissue cells. An acute abscess commonly starts as follows: a large inoculum of bacteria enters the tissues. Neutrophils are attracted to the area by chemotaxis; they surround the bacteria and liquefaction necrosis results. The lining of the abscess, which leads to the formation of more pus, consists of an inner layer of leucocytes surrounded by an outer zone of granulation tissue (*pyogenic membrane*). More neutrophils and macrophages are drawn into the cavity. At the same time the large protein molecules constituting the bodies of the bacteria and pus cells are broken down into smaller molecules which are more numerous and hence exert more osmotic pressure. Thus, both the size of the cavity and the pressure inside it continue to increase.

Antibiotics are not very effective in dealing with an abscess. The reasons for this are three:

1. The granulation tissue prevents adequate levels of antibiotics penetrating the cavity.
2. Most antibiotics are inactivated by different factors in the pus.
3. The bacteria in the pus are in a resting phase. This reduces the uptake of the antibiotics by the bacteria.

All the above factors render the antibiotic ineffective against the pus in the abscess. Now, antibiotics being relatively useless, *drainage is the only proper method of dealing with most abscesses,* and it is for this reason that such a great deal of stress is placed upon proper and adequate drainage.

Abscesses at different sites. Abscesses may form anywhere in the body, and the nature of the infecting organism varies with the site. Abscesses in the subcutaneous tissues are most often caused by *Staphylococcus aureus*. With penetrating wounds as in stabs, gunshot wounds, car accidents and crush injuries, dirt and bacteria get inoculated into the tissues. In these cases the risk of infection with clostridial organisms is high, specially in the presence of dead or crushed tissue. These wounds therefore always require prompt surgical excision and toilet.

Intra-abdominal abscesses are usually caused by perforations in the gastrointestinal tract, as in cases of appendicitis, diverticulitis, peptic ulcer and malignant ulcer of the colon. In other cases a leaking surgical anastomosis may be responsible. Usually many organisms are present, commonly from the enteric group: coliforms, *Streptococcus faecalis*, clostridia and bacteroides.

Factors increasing the risk of infection. In cases of perforation of the colon and oesophagus the risk of development of intra-abdominal abscesses is very high. The risk is less with perforation of the stomach and small bowel, as the normal resident count of bacteria in these organs is low. However, when the small intestine is obstructed or acid secretion is reduced in the stomach, bacterial overgrowth occurs. Other factors increasing the risk of sepsis include:

1. Advancing age of the patient.
2. Obesity.
3. Malnutrition.
4. Shock.
5. Decreased immunocompetence.

Following surgical treatment of intra-abdominal abscesses in such cases the mortality rate is high, upto 20%.

Clinical features. There is usually a systemic reaction with toxicity and intermittent fever. Pain and tenderness are present. The pain may become severe and throbbing if the pus is under tension. If an abscess is deep-seated and not under pressure, it may be silent even though large. However, the patient develops signs of toxicity and a hypercatabolic state, which may even progress to *multiple organ system failure*. At the same time, the risk of rupture of an abscess into the bloodstream and *septicaemia* is always present. Rupture of an intra-abdominal abscess results in widespread peritonitis.

Natural history. 1. An abscess may resolve after prompt and appropriate antibiotic therapy. The contents become liquefied by proteolytic digestion and the watery debris is gradually reabsorbed. The residual cavity occasionally calcifies.

2. If the abscess is near an external or internal surface, it may drain spontaneously and resolve.

3. The pressure effect of an expanding abscess may cause vascular thrombosis and cell death around it. The abscess may now track along fascial layers.

When an abscess gets drained, not only does this lead to evacuation of the pus and reduction of the bacterial load, but also it releases the pressure in the abscess and allows the penetration of antibiotics into the abscess cavity. The bacteria also start multiplying again and thus become more sensitive to antibiotics.

Treatment. The proper treatment of most abscesses consists of adequate drainage of the pus. In the past this meant open drainage. However, since the advent of ultrasound and computerized tomography, percutaneous drainage of the pus under ultrasound or CT control has become quite popular. The guidance provided by these imaging methods obviates the need for open operation. The catheter is left inside the cavity, and soon the drainage fluid from the abscess becomes more liquid. The rate of shrinkage of the abscess cavity can be monitored by x-rays taken after injection of a contrast medium. There may be more than one abscess, and if clinical improvement does not take place after adequate drainage of the abscess, the ultrasound examination should be repeated. An abscess may be secondary to a serious underlying disease; in that case appropriate treatment of the underlying condition should be carried out as soon as the abscess has been drained.

The onset of shock, rigors, a rising pulse rate and fever indicate septicaemia. Blood cultures should be taken, fluids replaced and antibiotic therapy commenced. Evacuation of pus should not be delayed. A biopsy of the wall of the abscess should be sent in all cases if a malignancy is not to be missed. A large quantity of pus should be sent for culture. A swab is less effective in obtaining an accurate culture unless sent in a transport medium.

13 Surgical infections

Infections are of great importance to the surgeon. If, after a major operation, the wound heals cleanly, the patient goes home in a few days. On the other hand if the wound becomes infected the patient may be in the hospital for many weeks. If the infection remains localized to the area of the wound it will delay wound healing and at the same time lead to a broad ugly scar. If it spreads through the blood-stream it could even kill him by causing septicaemia.

Historically, a surgical operation was a dreaded event, because almost all operation wounds became septic, and nearly half of all patients who had a major operation died as a result of invasive infection, so that compound fractures were treated by amputation! It was only after Lister and others, from the 1860s onwards, introduced the concept first of antisepsis and later of strict aseptic precautions in surgery that infection rates fell to the present low levels. Sterilization of instruments, first by chemicals and later by steam, was introduced during the 1880s, followed shortly by hand washing and wearing of gowns, gloves, caps and masks. Before this time surgeons used to wash their hands after, not before, operations! Antibiotics were first used in the treatment of infections in the 1940s, starting with penicillin and followed by streptomycin and others. Since then, an increasing number of antibiotics has become available, so that infections which in days gone by regularly resulted in mortality are treated successfully in the great majority of cases.

Surgical infections include those infections that either require, or result from, operative treatment:

1. Infections *requiring* operative treatment include the following:

   i. Body cavity infections, e.g. peritonitis, pericarditis, empyema.

   ii. Confined infections, e.g. abscesses, suppurative arthritis.

   iii. Soft tissue infections resulting in necrosis.

   iv. Infections associated with prosthetic devices.

2. Infections *resulting from* operative treatment include wound infections, postoperative abscesses and peritonitis, and hospital-acquired infections, e.g. pneumonias and infections resulting from catheters. If a surgical patient is immunocompromised, viral or fungal infections can overwhelm him.

FACTORS IN THE DEVELOPMENT OF INFECTION

Soon after birth a variety of micro-organisms colonize both the external and internal surfaces of the body. They do no harm and in fact may be beneficial. For example the normal intestinal flora act as a barrier against infections with pathogens such as Salmonella and Shigella species. Even in the case of pathogenic bacteria contamination becomes invasive infection only if either the micro-organism is excessively virulent or the resistance of the patient is reduced. The development of infection depends upon several factors:

MICROBIAL VIRULENCE

Whether infection develops or not depends upon the balance between microbial virulence and host defences. Microbes that cannot cause infection in a normal host can result in serious infection in an individual with immunocompromised defences.

Some bacteria have surface components which increase their pathogenicity by inhibiting phagocytosis, e.g. the capsule of Klebsiella. Other bacteria have surface components which are toxic, e.g. the enterobacteria. Still others, like clostridia and some strains of streptococci, produce exotoxins.

In clean wounds the common organisms found are skin bacteria like *Staphylococcus epidermidis*. In traumatic wounds the most common organisms are *Staphylococcus aureus* and *Streptococcus pyogenes*. When a body viscus is entered the natural or abnormal resident flora become the expected pathogens.

Number of bacteria required to produce infection. Bacterial contamination with greater than 10^5 organisms commonly leads to infection, whereas contamination with less than this number usually does not. In traumatic wounds foreign bodies and devitalized tissues are often found; in their presence fewer organisms are required to produce infection than in normal tissues. This is the reason why foreign materials and dead tissues are disliked so much by surgeons, and every effort is made to get rid of them.

Bacterial toxins. Bacterial infection causes damage to the host cells and tissues at the site of invasion. At the same time bacterial toxins are transported by the blood and lymph to cause cytotoxic effects at distant sites. Different micro-organisms vary in their ability to cause local and systemic damage. *Staphylococcus aureus* produces local damage but has little tendency to spread. *Streptococcus pyogenes* is both invasive and toxigenic. *Clostridium tetani* is almost solely toxigenic.

Types of toxins. Toxins are of two types. *Exotoxins* are specific proteins produced by certain bacteria. When they are denatured they lose their toxicity but retain their antigenicity. Such modified exotoxins are called *toxoids*. Those produced from *Clostridium tetani* are used to induce active immunity in man. *Endotoxins* are produced by gram-negative species. They are lipopolysaccharides of the bacterial cell wall, and are released only on dissolution of the bacterial cell. They do not form toxoids, so vaccines against them cannot readily be prepared.

HOST DEFENCES

Local host defences. Epithelia surround the tissues of the body and protect them from invasion by microbes. The skin as well as the epithelia around body orifices, e.g. pharynx, oesophagus and urinary tract, are multilayered for more effective protection. Mucous membranes are less resistant, but even here bacterial entry does not usually take place unless a small break occurs.

Phagocytes. For effective function by phagocytes, firstly they have to be delivered at the site of infection, and secondly they have to ingest the infecting bacteria.

Delivery of phagocytes. Any condition which reduces the delivery of phagocytes to an area of bacterial contamination promotes the development of infection. Examples include the following:

1. Reduced blood flow, e.g. in vascular occlusive states, in hypovolaemic shock, or after the use of vasopressors.
2. The presence of devitalized tissues, foreign bodies, haematomas and seromas.
3. Decreased vascular reactivity, e.g. in old age, in uraemia, and after the use of steroids.
4. Decreased production of phagocytes, e.g. after irradiation or cytotoxic chemotherapy, and in granulocytopenia from drugs or other cause.

Ingestion by phagocytes. In certain disease states the ingestive phase of leucocyte function is defective. Examples include the following conditions:

1. Uraemia.
2. Ketosis.
3. Hyperglycaemia.
4. Prematurity.
5. Certain malignancies.
6. Some immunologic deficiency diseases.
7. Malnutrition.

In extensive burns and wounds, as well as in severe sepsis, a hypermetabolic state exists, which may lead rapidly to protein malnutrition. When this occurs, phagocytic function is impaired, leading to bacteraemia and even septicaemia.

Many hospital-acquired infections result from therapeutic procedures which involve a *breach* in the skin or another epithelial surface. Prolonged use of indwelling urinary or vascular catheters, tracheostomies and ventilators are responsible for most iatrogenic infections.

Each site also provides a local environment that is not conducive to the growth of microbes. These local factors include the flushing action of tears and urine, the action of the cilia in the respiratory tract, the low pH and mucus in the stomach, etc.

Local environmental factors. If trauma has resulted in devitalization of tissue or if foreign bodies have become deposited in the wound, the likelihood of infection is greatly increased. Fluid collections inhibit phagocytosis and increase the likelihood of infection. Peripheral vascular disease as well as shock reduce the delivery of blood, and the systemic host defence factors it contains, to the infected part, and is accompanied by a greater incidence of infection.

Surgical technique. Last, but not least, surgical technique has a significant bearing on the incidence of postoperative infection. Gentle handling of tissues, removal of devitalized tissue, avoidance of excess use of cautery, ensuring adequate blood supply to bowel ends before anastomosis, etc., decrease the chances of infection.

Systemic host defences. These consist of phagocytes; the immune system; and molecular cascades, such as the complement system, the coagulation system and the kinins. The phagocytes include polymorphonuclear leucocytes (PMNs) and macrophages. As a result of interaction with complement and other activators, PMNs adhere to vessel endothelium, migrate across the endothelium, and move towards the microbe. They attach to and phagocytose the microbes. Finally lysosomes empty their enzymes into the phagosome and the microbe is digested. Macrophages not only phagocytose microbes but also initiate the immune response and can elaborate cytokines, tumour necrosis factor, interferons, etc.

Host defences are *impaired* in the very young and the very old, in malnutrition, after major trauma and burns, after extensive operations, in advanced malignant disease and after chemotherapy for the same, after immunosuppression to prevent rejection of organ transplants, and in patients on steroids.

Superinfections with viruses and fungi usually occur when the resistance of the host is diminished. Apart from immunologically deficient patients, they occur *mostly during a course of antibiotic therapy!*

The cytokine cascade. Cytokines are factors released by activated cells that act as messengers in cellular communication, at times spilling over into the circulation to function as hormones in response to haemorrhage, sepsis, inflammation and other forms of injury. They are proteins that are stimulated by the host defence system, and have autocrine effects (in the cells), paracrine effects (adjacent to the cells), and endocrine effects (at a distance).

The two most important cytokines are interleukin-1 and tumour necrosis factor.

Interleukin-1 (IL-1). Stimulants to the release of interleukin-1 include nearly all inflammatory, infectious and immunological processes. IL-1 acts on the central nervous system. It induces fever by stimulating release of prostaglandins in the anterior hypothalamus, produces anorexia by direct action on the satiety center, and lessens pain perception by increasing beta-endorphan release. IL-1 promotes skeletal muscle proteolysis. The amino acids thus released are used by the liver for energy as well as for synthesis of new proteins.

Tumour necrosis factor (TNF). This is a cytokine protein which acts synergistically with interleukin-1 to induce hypotension, tissue injury and death in animals subjected to experimental sepsis. TNF probably mediates the early hypotension of sepsis, and IL-1 participates in the later phases of sepsis-induced shock.

DIAGNOSIS

The signs and symptoms of acute infection are due to inflammation: redness and heat due to intense hyperaemia, pain and swelling due to the oedema. There is loss of function due to reflex and voluntary immobilization. Fever and chills indicate septicaemia, while a raised pulse rate is a sign of a toxic state.

Leucocytosis. Leucocytosis accompanies an acute bacterial infection; the more severe the infection the greater the leucocytosis. In most surgical infections the count is only slightly or moderately raised. A high leucocyte count (upto 35,000/mm^3) occurs in suppuration. A *reliable* total and differential leucocyte count is of great help to a surgeon in the diagnosis of the not-so-obvious infection. However in the elderly, in the severely ill patient, and during therapy with antibiotics, some anticancer and immuno-suppressive drugs, white cell counts may be normal or even low. In overwhelming sepsis there may be leucopenia, due to depression of the bone marrow and exhaustion of the supply of leucocytes. In some cases the total number of leucocytes is normal. However, there is a larger proportion of immature cells ('shift to the left'), which indicates an accelerated rate of production of white cells and points to the presence of an infection.

Pitfalls in diagnosis. It must be remembered that the only evidence of a chronic infection may be fatigue, low-grade fever and anaemia. At the same time, massive pyogenic abscesses may occur without leucocytosis, fever or tenderness. So the clinician should be on his guard in patients presenting with vague symptoms.

Appearance of pus. The pus should be examined for colour, odour and consistency. Bluish-green pus indicates infection with *Ps. pyocyaneus.* Foul-smelling pus usually means infection with anaerobes. Thin pus often indicates spreading infection, while thick pus definitely means that the infection has been confined (the 'laudable pus' of the past).

Gram staining. Micro-organisms causing a surgical infection may often be seen under the microscope on a gram-stained smear. This is a simple, rapid and inexpensive method which *provides very valuable information* for the surgeon. It should be used more often. Pus from abscesses may be obtained by incision-drainage or, in the case of deep-seated abscesses, by needle aspiration. Antibiotics should be started only after the pus has been collected. When the culture report is received from the laboratory, the drug may have to be changed.

Biopsy. In granulomatous lesions biopsy is useful in establishing the diagnosis, e.g. in tuberculosis, syphilis and the mycoses.

Blood cultures. Blood cultures can help in identifying the micro-organisms responsible for the infection. However, even a specimen taken at the height of a chill and fever may be negative, because phagocytes rapidly remove bacteria, while chills and fever occur about an hour later. This means that blood cultures, to be positive, have to be repeated frequently.

PRINCIPLES OF TREATMENT OF INFECTIONS

In the case of acute *spreading* infections, e.g., cellulitis and septicaemia, antibiotics are the primary treatment, and should result in clinical improvement in 24 to 48 hours; when the blood culture report is received, a change to a more effective antibiotic may be indicated. As far as *localized* infections are concerned, antibiotics cannot penetrate inside abscess cavities, and therefore incision and drainage must be carried out. At the same time, *necrotic* tissues or foreign bodies prevent the proper functioning of host defences, and have to be removed. *Perforations* of the gastrointestinal tract provide a continuing source of bacteria that overwhelm the defences. Operation is required to eradicate this constant source by closing the perforation, or by 'exteriorizing' it as in a colostomy.

Supportive measures to be taken for surgical infections include the following:

1. Bed rest.
2. Immobilization of the infected region to provide rest.
3. Elevation of a limb to promote venous and lymphatic drainage.
4. Relief of pain.

TYPES OF SURGICAL INFECTIONS

SOFT TISSUE INFECTIONS

Cellulitis is a nonsuppurative inflammation of the subcutaneous tissues and intercellular spaces. There is swelling, redness and pain without definite localization. The central area may undergo necrosis and suppuration. In severe forms, blebs and bullae form on the skin. The most common causative agent is the haemolytic streptococcus, but other aerobic and anaerobic bacteria may also be responsible. Treatment consists of antibiotic therapy and rest. For the streptococcus, penicillin G is the drug of choice. If after 72 hours there is no response this suggests that an abscess has developed and incision and drainage is needed.

Lymphangitis. Lymphangitis is an inflammation of lymphatic pathways, and is usually visible as red streaks under the skin. Again the most common aetiological agent is the haemolytic streptococcus. Lymphangitis and the associated lymphadenitis are a normal defence reaction against bacterial invasion, and are often seen on the forearm of a patient with infection of the hand or fingers. Most cases will respond to antibiotic therapy and rest.

Erysipelas. Erysipelas is an acute spreading cellulitis and lymphangitis, again usually caused by haemolytic streptococci which gain entrance through a break in the skin. There is a severe systemic as well as local reaction with fever, chills and marked weakness. The skin is red, swollen and tender, with a distinct line of demarcation. Recurrent erysipelas in a limb may lead to chronic lymphoedema by damaging the lymphatics. Antibiotic therapy halts the spread of the infection, but the erythema disappears more slowly.

Abscess. An abscess is a localized collection of pus surrounded by an area of inflamed tissue in which there is marked hyperaemia and infiltration by leucocytes. A *boil* or *furuncle* is an abscess in a sweat gland or hair-follicle. The course of a boil may be self-limited and may require no treatment. However, large boils and abscesses should be incised and drained and the patient treated with antibiotics.

The area of the face bounded by the bridge of the nose and the angles of the mouth is called the 'dangerous area'. This is because the veins of this area communicate with the cavernous sinus, and infection in their drainage area can produce septic cavernous sinus thrombosis, with serious consequences for the patient.

Carbuncle. A carbuncle is a multilocular suppurative extension of a boil into the subcutaneous tissues. The back of the lower part of the neck and the upper part of the chest are common sites. The carbuncle consists of a honeycomb of hundreds of tiny abscess cavities. When they rupture onto the skin, numerous sinuses develop. The most common organism concerned is *Staphylococcus aureus,* but streptococci and gram-negative bacilli may also be found. Incision of all the hundreds of cavities is impossible; therefore the only proper treatment of a carbuncle is to excise it completely. The wound contracts to a small scar, and a skin graft is usually not required. Carbuncles are almost always seen in patients suffering from diabetes mellitus; the diabetes should be brought under as effective control as possible before operation on the carbuncle.

Necrotizing soft tissue infections. Soft tissue infections that result in tissue necrosis are less common than other forms of infection but more serious because of extensive destruction of tissues and a higher mortality rate. Most are caused by mixed aerobic and anaerobic gram-negative and gram-positive bacteria. *Clostridium* species are common and cause the most severe infections, to which the term gas gangrene has been applied. These infections must be recognized early and treated aggressively. If the overlying skin is normal, diagnosis may be difficult. Early mental confusion, toxicity and failure to respond to nonoperative therapy may be the earliest clues to the presence of a necrotizing infection. Gas gangrene is described in detail later in this chapter.

BODY CAVITY INFECTIONS

These include peritonitis, intra-abdominal abscess, and empyema. They are described in the appropriate chapters.

PROSTHETIC DEVICE-ASSOCIATED INFECTIONS

These are seen in cases with prosthetic cardiac valves, vascular grafts and artificial joints. They are accompanied by failure of the operation besides great morbidity, and even death of the patient. Although the prosthetic devices have occasionally been salvaged by antibiotic irrigation, usually infected devices require removal.

HOSPITAL-ACQUIRED (NOSOCOMIAL) INFECTIONS

These are infections acquired during stay in a hospital. They lead to an increased hospital stay and a great deal of loss of time from work. They include infections of the urinary and respiratory tracts, vascular catheter-related infections, and wound infections.

Urinary tract infections account for 40% of hospital-acquired infections, the majority of patients having had operations on the lower urinary tract, instrumentation of the bladder, or catheterization. *The risk of bacteriuria in patients with indwelling catheters increases by 5 to 10 percent for each day the catheter is in place.* Therefore catheters should be placed only when necessary and should be removed as early as possible. If prolonged catheterization is required, suprapubic or condom catheters should be used to reduce the risk of infection. If catheters are inserted after careful cleansing of the urethral meatus and looked after properly, the risk of infection is reduced.

Lower respiratory tract infections. These constitute the third largest group of hospital-acquired infections. The common factors responsible include the following:

1. Abolition of cough reflex by anaesthesia permits aspiration of contaminated material.
2. Pain from thoracic or upper abdominal operations interferes with coughing and deep breathing and allows retention of sputum in the tracheobronchial tree and atelectasis which predisposes to infection.
3. Pulmonary oedema or adult respiratory distress syndrome arising due to overinfusion, cardiac failure, trauma, sepsis, etc. predisposes to pulmonary infection.
4. In intubated patients in critical care units, even low levels of aspiration may lead to pneumonia.

Vascular catheter-related infections. These are quite common, involving micro-organisms at the exit site of the catheter. Any evidence of phlebitis or cellulitis, or suspicion of septic complication due to an intravenous cannula, should be dealt with by immediate removal of the cannula.

WOUND INFECTIONS

Local factors in wound infection have been discussed above as well as in the chapter on wounds.

Systemic factors in wound infections. Many systemic conditions have an influence on the healing of wounds:

1. The *resistance* of the patient is deficient in a number of systemic conditions and diseases. These include old age, prematurity, advanced malignancy, burn or traumatic injury, leukaemia, diabetes mellitus, uraemia and inherited immunodeficiency diseases. In these conditions extraordinary precautions should be taken to prevent the development of wound infections, including correction of the underlying defect whenever possible.
2. *Malnutrition,* even when subclinical, can greatly impair host defences. The surgeon must correct any malnutrition before surgery, or as soon thereafter as possible by either oral or intravenous hyperalimentation. Malnutrition is widely prevalent in underdeveloped countries. There are two main causes: firstly, undernutrition due to poverty; secondly, the loss of valuable proteins in the diarrhoea of repeated episodes of dysentery due to poor food hygiene and impure water supply. Surgeons in these countries should be aware of this. The cause of malnutrition should be identified and corrected *before* elective surgery, rather than having to deal with a non-healing wound in an undernourished patient, which is a much more difficult undertaking.
3. If steroids, anticancer agents or antimetabolites are used there is an increased incidence of septic complications. Unnecessary use of these drugs in the surgical patient should therefore be avoided.

The above list of factors predisposing to infection in wounds shows how important it is *to take a meticulous and detailed history about the general health* of any patient who is about to undergo a surgical operation.

PREVENTION OF WOUND INFECTION

Prevention of infection is far more practical than treating it once it has become established. Fortunately, strict adherence to the principles of wound care can prevent the vast majority of infectious complications in surgical practice.

In the hospital. *Meticulous attention to every aspect of hygiene in every ward and operation theatre is important.* Severely infected cases should be *isolated* and barrier nursed. Surgical *audit* should be instituted to keep the infection rate under surveillance, so that adequate steps can be taken whenever necessary. If there is an *outbreak* of staphylococcal sepsis, elective operations should be stopped. Nasal swabs should be obtained from patients and staff to detect carriers, who should be treated and not allowed to return to work until the organism has been eliminated. Patients with sepsis should be isolated and discharged as soon as possible.

Preparation of the patient. *The longer a patient's preoperative stay in hospital, the higher is the incidence of infection* even in his otherwise clean wound, due to microorganisms accumulated by the patient during his hospital stay. Therefore, as far as possible each patient should be operated upon *soon* after admission to hospital. If a *remote* infection is present, the rate of wound infection is tripled; therefore elective operations should be delayed until the infection has been eliminated. A *preoperative shower*, preferably with an antiseptic soap, such as chlorhexidine or povidone-iodine, reduces the resident skin bacteria.

In the operation theatre. The theatre should be supplied with properly filtered *air*, using filters with a pore size of 2 mm. If clean air is introduced into the operating room close to the ceiling, and allowed to exit near the floor, it helps in limiting airborne contamination to very low levels. The air should be brought in at positive pressure, so that the flow of air is from the theatre outwards and not vice versa. The air in the theatre should be changed 5 times every minute; this is referred to as 300 changes of air per hour. The *number* of people in the operating theatre, their *movement*, as well as *conversation*, should be kept at a minimum.

The *instruments* should be sterilized by autoclave, antiseptics or ethylene dioxide, and the adequacy of sterilization checked regularly.

Gowns should be properly designed and *caps and masks* should be properly fitting. Recent studies have shown that when surgeons did not wear masks, wound infection rates did not increase. However, the above-named barriers should still be used, if only to prevent the patient's blood coming in contact with the operation room staff.

Hands should be washed for 5 minutes, using chlorhexidine or povidone-iodine. During operation a fair number of gloves get punctured; they should be immediately changed to avoid bacterial contamination of the wound.

The *patient's skin* around the operation area should be prepared with a soap, followed by painting with a bactericidal solution, e.g. 0.5% chlorhexidine in 70% alcohol or 1% povidone-iodine. The whole body apart from the operation area should be covered with cloth *towels* held in place by towel clips. An alternative is to apply a sterile, transparent, adhesive sheet to the operation area, with the incision made through the plastic sheet. This measure has gained popularity of late, although some very recent work has shown the use of this method to have increased the incidence of infection due to the warmth and moisture under the impermeable sheet!

During the operation. *Dissection* should be gentle, without bruising or forceful retraction of the tissues. *Haemostasis* should be adequate, as a haematoma acts as a foreign body. The surgeon should not spend an *unduly long* time over the operation, as the tissues are traumatized while the wound is open. If *non-absorbable* sutures have to be left in the wound, as far as possible they should be monofilament materials. *Open drains* should be avoided as far as possible; if used, they should be removed as soon as possible. If the gastrointestinal, respiratory or urinary tract has to be transected:

1. Before a hollow viscus is entered, the operative area should be carefully isolated by towels from the rest of the operative field.
2. A different set of instruments should be used for that part of the operation until the hollow viscus is closed.
3. All instruments, towels and sponges that may have come into contact with the contaminating bacteria should now be discarded.
4. The gowns and gloves of the surgical team should be changed before proceeding with closure of the wound.

Wound care. Wounds should be taken care of meticulously, specially if there is an impairment of host defence:

1. Gentle care of the tissues is important, as it minimizes local damage.
2. Devitalized tissues and foreign bodies should be removed.
3. If complete debridement is not possible the wound should not be closed; if such a wound is left open a much larger number of bacteria is required to produce invasive infection.
4. In contaminated wounds monofilament suture materials, e.g. polypropylene, are preferable to multifilament sutures like silk. This is because bacteria can get lodged in the interstices of multifilament sutures, where they are safe from the action of macrophages and antibiotics. If infection does take place in the presence of a multifilament suture it will not subside until the offending suture is removed. Monofilament sutures, having no interstices, are not associated with this complication.
5. The presence of haematomas, seromas or dead spaces favors bacterial localization and growth. If a large potential dead space results after an operation it is best to provide a system of closed suction drainage.
6. In heavily contaminated wounds the use of delayed primary closure will greatly reduce the chances of serious infection. The skin and subcutaneous tissues are left unsutured and packed loosely with gauze. The number of phagocytes at the wound edges increases to reach a peak in about five days. At the same time there is intense capillary budding. The exudate diminishes in quantity and becomes clear, and closure can usually be safely carried out at this time.

Prophylactic chemotherapy. When used for the correct indications, antibiotics help reduce the incidence of post-operative infections. However, blind and indiscriminate use of antibiotics does more harm than good by developing resistant strains of bacteria in hospitals. As far as the likelihood of development of infections is concerned, wounds can be divided into three categories.

Clean surgical wounds are those which are non-traumatic, where there is no break in aseptic technique, and where the respiratory or alimentary tracts have not been entered. In such wounds the incidence of infections is less than 1% when careful, gentle, meticulous aseptic technique is practised. Therefore there is no need to use prophylactic antibiotics in these cases. If infection occurs it is due to poor surgical technique or errors in aseptic routine.

Clean-contaminated cases are those in which the gastrointestinal or respiratory tracts are entered without significant spillage; or pharynx, vagina or non-infected genitourinary or biliary tract are entered; or there is a minor break in aseptic technique.

Contaminated cases are those which are either traumatic cases, or there has been a major break in aseptic technique or gross spillage from the alimentary tract, or the genitourinary or biliary tracts have been entered in the presence of infected urine or bile.

The acceptable infection rates for clean, clean-contaminated and contaminated cases are less than 1%, 3%, and 5% respectively. *If higher rates of infection are encountered, the matter should be investigated.*

Prophylactic antibiotics. In clean cases the use of prophylactic systemic antibiotics is clearly unjustified. However, in clean-contaminated and contaminated cases they are usually of benefit. The only proper exceptions to this rule are cases where any infection would mean disaster, as in vascular procedures like grafts, where secondary haemorrhage would be very dangerous, or even fatal. *When used prophylactically antibiotics should be started before the operation.* The idea is that if contamination with bacteria takes place during operation, the antibiotic should already be in position in the bloodstream and the tissues, so that it can destroy the small numbers of organisms before they get a chance to multiply to very large numbers. Antibiotics started even just 1 or 2 hours after operation are much less effective, and those started after 3 hours are quite useless. The usual practice is to give the first dose of prophylactic antibiotic intravenously just before induction of anaesthesia. Some surgeons give only this one dose; others follow it up with one more dose after 6 hours. Longer courses offer no added benefit. If heavy contamination has occurred antibiotics may be placed locally in the wound at the same time. It may be mentioned that topical applications of iodine preparations are highly effective. The reduced infection rates are comparable with those obtained with antibiotics. *It should again be stressed that prophylactic antibiotic therapy is no substitute for careful surgical technique and aseptic surgical principles,* and its indiscriminate or general use is not in the best interest of the patient.

MICRO-ORGANISMS IN THE BLOOD-STREAM

Bacteraemia. Bacteraemia is defined as the transient presence of bacteria in the blood with no toxaemia or other clinical signs, as a result of local infection or penetrating injury. It usually lasts only a few moments, as the macrophage phagocyte system destroys these organisms under normal conditions. The normal person probably experiences bacteraemia many times every year, e.g. after dental procedures, wounds etc. It is probable that infections in internal organs, e.g. osteomyelitis and subacute bacterial endocarditis, develop through this kind of bacteraemia.

Septicaemia. Septicaemia is a diffuse infection in which infectious bacteria or fungi are actually multiplying in the bloodstream, usually with the production of severe systemic symptoms such as fever and hypotension. It is commonly secondary to a focus of infection in the body. The majority of bacteria that produce suppurative lesions can give rise to secondary septicaemia, specially if the pus is not drained promptly.

Pyaemia. Pyaemia describes the serious situation when in a septicaemia organisms and neutrophil polymorphs embolize to many sites in the body producing abscesses, notably in the lungs, liver and brain. Just as the development of an abscess in any part of the body signifies a reduced level of resistance in that part, similarly the simultaneous appearance of abscesses in many different organs or parts indicates a generalized lowering of resistance. Thus *pyaemic abscesses point to a state of immunosuppression.* Therefore it is necessary not only to drain the abscesses but also to take steps to increase the patient's resistance to infection. Before the advent of antibiotics pyaemia was uniformly fatal; the mortality rate is still high.

The term *primary septicaemia* describes a situation where the focus of infection is not apparent. Such patients are generally elderly, undernourished or suffering from chronic disease, particularly alcoholic cirrhosis and diabetes. In the case of *secondary septicaemia,* the condition arises in a previously healthy person.

Toxaemia. In toxaemia toxins are circulating in the blood, but the micro-organisms producing the toxins need not be. In fact *Botulinum* toxin may be ingested directly and cause profound toxaemia without true infection.

SCORING THE SEVERITY OF INFECTION

Many scoring systems have been used to assess the severity of infections. The Apache II system has achieved the greatest measure of popularity. It judges the severity of the acute illness through an acute physiology score, while in the background it also assesses the general health of the patient utilizing chronic health evaluation points (**A**cute **P**hysiology **A**nd **C**hronic **H**ealth **E**valuation, **APACHE**). This point system is as follows:

Acute physiology score parameters include temperature, blood pressure, heart and respiratory rates; arterial oxygen and pH; serum sodium, potassium and creatinine; haematocrit and white cell count.

Every step-wise increase in the departure from the norm for each parameter adds a point to the score.

Neurology. Glasgow coma scale points are added.

Age. Every 10-year increase beyond 44 years adds 1 or 2 points.

Chronic health. Hepatic, cardiac, pulmonary, renal or immune dysfuntion each adds a point.

For patients with intra-abdominal infection a score of 21 indicates a mortality risk of 50 percent.

CLASSIFICATION OF SURGICAL INFECTIONS

The location of a lesion often provides a clue to the identity of the causative organism. For example, most wound infections are caused by *Staph. aureus* or a mixed flora. Abdominal infections with perforation of the gastrointestinal tract are always mixed, with aerobic and anaerobic gram-negative enteric bacteria, as well as gram-positive anaerobic bacteria. Infections in the genitourinary tract are mostly from gram-negative aerobes, specially *Escherichia coli.* A spreading cellulitis is usually due to *Streptococcus pyogenes.*

Staphylococcal infections. Most infections in surgical wounds are caused by *Staph. aureus.* They are localized with thick creamy pus, which is odourless and yellow or cream-coloured. Hospital-acquired infections are usually caused by antibiotic-resistant bacteria of increased virulence. Their treatment is surgical drainage with rest and elevation of the part. If such an infection occurs in the incision after an operation, the wound should be opened widely to facilitate free drainage of pus. Antibiotics should be started before the operation for drainage.

Streptococcal infection. Of all streptócocci, *Strep. pyogenes* is the one which is most commonly encountered in surgical practice. The lesions it produces are usually invasive, with a rapid course. There is cellulitis, lymphangitis, lymphadenitis and extension of the inflammation along fascial planes. The pus is thin and watery, abscess formation being rare. Thrombosis of small vessels may lead to gangrene of the tissues. Bacteraemia is common, with chills, high fever, thready pulse and signs of toxaemia.

Streptococcal gangrene is a spreading subcutaneous infection in which thrombosis of nutrient vessels results in sloughing of skin and fasciae. Treatment is wide surgical drainage along with antibiotics.

The microaerophilic streptococcus causes infections that develop slowly. Chronic burrowing ulcer and chronic cutaneous gangrene are good examples. Radical drainage is necessary for cure, antibiotics alone being useless.

It should be remembered that *where the correct treatment is surgical drainage, all the antibiotics in the world will not produce a cure without drainage.*

Infections by gram-negative bacilli. A variety of gram-negative bacilli are indigenous to the gastrointestinal and genitourinary tracts. Most wound infections by these organisms result from operative contamination of spilled gastrointestinal contents, and are due to careless operative technique. In other wound infections, and in many systemic invasive infections, these organisms act as opportunistic invaders. This is specially the case when host defence is impaired, or when incompletely removed devitalized tissues are present, e.g. in extensive burns and wounds. These infections are usually mixed, with both aerobic and anaerobic organisms. However, they are often not recognized as such, because anaerobic cultures are not routinely carried out in many hospitals. *If foul-smelling pus is found and anaerobic cultures are not available, the presence of anaerobic organisms should be presumed* and drugs effective against them, e.g. metronidazole or clindamycin, added to the regimen.

CLOSTRIDIAL INFECTIONS

Infections due to anaerobic clostridia cause three diseases important in surgical practice: clostridial cellulitis, gas gangrene and tetanus.

Clostridial cellulitis is a serious septic process of areolar tissues caused usually by *Clostridium welchii.* The cellulitis spreads along fascial planes. On palpation crepitus is felt due to the gas produced by the anaerobes. There is sloughing of skin and fasciae due to thrombosis of blood vessels. Pain is present, along with a greyish white discharge. Treatment should include surgical decompression with elevation of skin flaps superficial to the fascia. At the same time, systemic antibiotics are administered in large doses, usually penicillin and one of the tetracyclines.

GAS GANGRENE

Unlike clostridial cellulitis, gas gangrene is a clostridial *myositis*. The common organisms responsible are *C. welchi* and *C. septicum.* It primarily involves muscles, and is characterized by spreading gangrene and profound toxaemia, which is rapidly fatal if untreated. The toxaemia is due to the circulating exotoxins. In severe cases it may result in shock, haemolytic anaemia, renal failure and jaundice, and may contribute to the death of the patient.

Clostridial spores are very widespread in nature, yet gas gangrene is extremely rare in civilian practice. This is because the condition develops only in the presence of reduced oxygen tension. This in turn may result from severe contusion and laceration with necrotic tissue, devitalization of a wound by compression, or from an impaired blood supply. Most cases arise from contamination of large wounds as in agricultural tractor injuries, severe comminuted compound fractures sustained in road traffic accidents, and battle casualties. In the advanced countries gas gangrene is most commonly seen after criminal abortion and infections following intestinal surgery.

Gas forms in muscles, which exhibit crepitation. The infected muscles are soft, swollen and dark red. The overlying skin goes through a series of changes, from inflammatory erythema with ecchymosis to the formation of bullae and frank greenish black gangrene. There is a foul-smelling brown watery exudate with bubbles of gas, which contains many gram-positive rods when examined microscopically, thus giving an immediate definitive diagnosis. The patient is listless, sweats profusely, and is pale due to marked anaemia. Stupor and delirium develop near the end. *CT scan* is a sensitive method of detecting soft tissue gas and indicates accurately the extent of the tissue necrosis.

Treatment. *Surgical treatment* should be prompt, with extensive decompression of all involved muscle compartments by incision and fasciotomy. The aggressive excision of all dead and infected tissue at the first operation is crucial to the survival of the patient. If irreversible gangrenous changes have taken place in the extremity, amputation must be carried out. If amputation is the only way to save the patient's life from the severe toxaemia, no hesitation should be shown in proceeding with the operation.

The toxaemia in gas gangrene is due to exotoxins, but *antitoxin* therapy is relatively ineffective. *Antibiotics* cannot prevent or cure gas gangrene, but are useful as an adjunctive measure to surgery. Crystalline penicillin (1 to 2 mega units 6 hourly) is the drug of choice. If the patient is allergic to penicillin, metronidazole or clindamycin may be used instead. Hyperbaric oxygen can also be a useful adjunct to surgical treatment.

Hyperbaric oxygen. If oxygen is inhaled at two or three times the normal atmospheric pressure, the oxygen tension in plasma, lymph and tissue fluids is increased about 20 times. This greatly increases the effectiveness of surgical and antibiotic therapy in anaerobic infection, e.g. in clostridial myonecrosis, and dramatic clinical improvement may be seen within 24 hours. Large hyperbaric pressure chambers are available at only a few medical centres in the world, but much less expensive single-patient chambers are now available and can be used. The regimen consists of repeated treatments of 2 hours each at a pressure of 2.5 atmospheres.

TETANUS

This dangerous and sometimes fatal infection of wounds has been virtually eliminated from the advanced countries due to the universal practice of tetanus immunization in the neonatal period. However, in the remote and backward parts of the underdeveloped countries it is unfortunately still quite common. In such communities, hospitals contain special wards devoted to the treatment of patients suffering from tetanus.

The causative organism is *Clostridium tetani,* which is a Gram-positive spore-bearing bacillus. The spores require reduced oxygen tension for them to germinate. Thus, although the wound responsible for the development of tetanus is usually a minor one, it is nearly always *deep,* so that anaerobic conditions are produced in its depth. *Commonly the wound is located in the lower limb.*

Other causes of tetanus include the following:

1. Cases of septic abortion.
2. Septic umbilical stumps, where stump hygiene is less than perfect.
3. Imperfectly sterilized non-disposable syringes.
4. Unhygienic piercing of ear-lobes.
5. Burns.
6. Surgical operations on the gastrointestinal tract.

The important exotoxin of tetanus is a neurotoxin called tetanospasmin. It reaches the central nervous system along the axons of motor nerve trunks, and blocks the inhibitory impulses at the motor synapses. Two types of contractions of striated muscles are produced by the toxin: tonic (spasms) which are a feature of early disease, and clonic (convulsions) which indicate severe established disease.

Tetanus is a serious illness, the overall mortality even in leading centres being as high as 10 to 15%. The mortality rate is higher if the patient is either very young or very old, if the incubation period is short, and if the illness is severe.

Clinical features. *Neonatal tetanus.* In the underdeveloped countries neonatal tetanus constitutes the majority of the total number of cases. It usually results because of the unfamiliarity of untrained traditional birth attendants (TBAs) with elementary principles of asepsis and hygiene. It has often been stressed at conferences that so long as TBAs are going to manage a significant number of births in these countries, they should at least be exposed to short courses where they could be taught the essentials of aseptic techniques. However, unfortunately not much progress has been made in this important field so far.

The clinical picture usually becomes manifest on about the eighth day of life. In fact as early as the 3rd day the infant fails to suckle. Shortly thereafter, spasm of the facial muscles develops (*risus sardonicus*). At the same time the masseter muscles go into spasm (*lock jaw*). Generalized clonic spasms finally commence.

Children and adults. The vast majority of patients who develop tetanus have not previously been immunized. The incubation period ranges from 5 to 10 days; the shorter the interval the more severe the disease. Muscle pains, headaches, irritability and restlessness are followed by risus sardonicus, lock jaw and dysphagia (the last being due to spasm of the muscles of deglutition). Finally, generalized clonic convulsions come on, which are triggered by mild external stimuli (sound, movement of personnel, etc.). As the extensor muscles are more powerful than the flexors, the whole body, i.e. the back and the lower limbs, assumes a posture of hyperextension (*episthotonus*). The muscles do not relax between convulsive attacks; this distinguishes the convulsions of tetanus from those due to strychnine poisoning.

Tetanus is nowadays *classified* into the following degrees of severity:

1. *Mild,* if there is no dysphagia and no respiratory distress.
2. *Moderate,* if dysphagia and respiratory distress are present.
3. *Severe,* if gross spasticity and major spasms are seen.

Management. ***Prevention.*** 1. *Immunization.* The best method of prevention from tetanus is by active immunization with tetanus toxoid (a formolized preparation of the exotoxin adsorbed onto aluminium hydroxide), 0.5 ml being the usual dose. Three injections are administered, the second and third being given 6 weeks and 6 months respectively after the first. Booster doses should be given every 10 years.

At the time a wound is sustained, if more than five years have elapsed since the last booster, a fresh booster dose should be given, otherwise not. If more than 10 years have elapsed since the last booster, not only should a fresh booster dose be given, but passive immunization with human tetanus immunoglobulin (TIG) in a dose of 250 u intramuscularly is also indicated. This helps to cover the early 4-week period before the active immunity conferred by the booster comes into play. Horse serum should no longer be used because of its questionable value and the risk of serum sickness and anaphylactic reactions.

2. *Care of wounds.* Apart from active and passive immunization, prevention of tetanus requires that wounds should be looked after properly. In grossly contaminated wounds great care should be taken to remove all dirt, grit and foreign matter, after which the whole wound should be left open to be closed later by delayed primary suture.

Treatment. *Specific measures.* If a wound is present it should be excised and left open, being packed with antibiotic and hydrogen peroxide (the latter for creating aerobic conditions). One megaunit of benzylpenicillin should be administered every 4 hours for a week. Human tetanus immunoglobulin should be given in a dose of 4,000 i.u. intramuscularly. Recently, metronidazole (500 mg orally 6 hourly) has been found to be effective, but these studies require further confirmation. In neonatal tetanus intrathecal tetanus immunoglobulin (TIG) and prednisolone have given good results.

General measures. For *mild* tetanus sedation with diazepam is sufficient. In patients with *moderate* tetanus tracheostomy is usually required in addition to sedation. In *severe* disease the muscle spasms have to be abolished by curarization and the patient kept on intermittent positive-pressure ventilation. In *very severe* disease, sympathetic overactivity results in cardiac arrhythmias; these patients require adrenergic blockade. The severe muscle spasms need to be abolished by the use of anaesthesia and muscle relaxants; therefore the patient has to be placed on a ventilator for many days, until the effect of the toxins on the muscles is terminated.

OTHER INFECTIONS OF SURGICAL IMPORTANCE

Mixed bacterial infections. Many surgical infections are polymicrobial. The wound from a *human bite* contains oral spirochaetes as well as aerobic and anaerobic mouth bacteria, and produces a synergistic and locally destructive lesion. There is thick foul-smelling pus and necrosis of fasciae. Surgical decompression, antibiotics effective against both anaerobes and aerobes, and splinting are important in treatment.

Non-clostridial crepitant cellulitis. This usually occurs as a complication of wounds contaminated by gastrointestinal or genitourinary discharges. The common organisms are the residents of the GIT and GU tracts, namely anaerobic bacteroides, streptococci and the coliforms. There is necrosis of skin and fasciae due to thrombosis of vessels. Wide surgical decompression and intensive antibiotic therapy is required.

Synergistic gangrene. First described by Meleney, this condition is caused by synergism between an aerobic haemolytic *Staphylococcus aureus* and a microaerophilic nonhaemolytic streptococcus. One or two weeks after operation a pale red cellulitis develops around the wound, with a blue or purple central area which becomes gangrenous and ulcerates. The ulcer enlarges as its purple and painful margin extends outwards. *Treatment* requires radical excision of the lesion, systemic penicillin or erythromycin, and delayed skin grafting. Local bacitracin application is helpful. Prompt operation should be carried out to prevent increasing and sometimes fatal septicaemia.

Peritonitis. Infections that follow perforations of the gastrointestinal or genitourinary tract or contamination by their contents are always polymicrobial, both aerobic and anaerobic bacteria being present. Unfortunately, anaerobes are usually not detected, because they are difficult to culture. A good combination of antibiotics for infection by bowel bacteria consists of gentamycin and clindamycin.

The mycoses. *Actinomycosis bovis.* This infection occurs rarely, producing a granuloma. The area becomes swollen and indurated, with multiple sinus tracts. The pus shows sulphur granules. The areas affected are cervicofacial, thoracic and abdominal. In the neck the lower jaw is commonly affected, in the thorax the apex of the lung. In the abdomen the infection enters through the caecum, and sinuses form in the right iliac fossa. Treatment consists of incision and drainage of abscesses and prolonged therapy with penicillin or other antibiotic.

Moniliasis. Fungus infection occurs occasionally in the mouth, and suggests that the patient's immune mechanisms are depressed. A few drops of the anti-fungal remedy Nilstat are dropped on the tongue thrice daily, and help clear up the infection.

VIRAL INFECTIONS

Hepatitis. Hepatitis virus infections are a threat to patients receiving blood transfusion as well as to their surgeons. After open-heart operations upto 10% patients develop evidence of viral hepatitis, usually non-A-non-B, and 30% of these progress to chronic active hepatitis. At the same time a fair number of surgeons in practice develop evidence of hepatitis infection. An effective vaccine for prophylaxis is now available.

AIDS *(Acquired immunodeficiency syndrome).* The acquired immunodeficiency syndrome consists of a spectrum of illnesses which are caused by infection with the human immunodeficiency virus (HIV) and which lead, over a number of years, to serious disease and death. At present 13 million adults are estimated to be infected worldwide, and many more are likely to be infected with the passage of time. The virus is transmitted mainly via semen, cervical secretions and blood. Transmission takes place via the following routes:

1. *Sexual intercourse* (vaginal and anal). Heterosexual intercourse accounts for the vast majority of infections, followed by intravenous drug abuse.

2. *Mother to child.* As more women become infected, more babies are likely to acquire HIV from them *in utero, during childbirth or via breast milk.*

3. *Contaminated blood and blood products.* Transfusion of blood or clotting factors (e.g. in haemophilia) can be followed by HIV infection. In the advanced countries blood and its products are now screened and clotting factors are heat-treated, so that the risk of transfusion-related HIV infection is minimal. However, where such screening is not possible, the risk remains significant.

4. *Contaminated needles.* Intravenous drug users sharing common syringes and needles are a major route of spread of HIV infection. Doctors and nurses have an approximately 0.3% risk following a single needlestick injury with known HIV-infected blood.

5. *Surgeons* run additional risks of infection due to the possibility of a needle-prick during the placement of sutures, or a spurt of blood from a divided artery directly into the conjunctival sac. Therefore, they need to take extra precautions, including the wearing of goggles.

There is no evidence that HIV is spread by social or household contact.

Immunology. The cellular receptor for HIV is the CD4 molecule, which defines the cells that are susceptible to infection. Many cells within the immune system bear this molecule, and include $CD4^+$ lymphocytes (which are most affected). There is a progressive and severe depletion of CD4 'helper' lymphocytes, and it is this that leads to the clinical manifestations of HIV infection.

Clinical features. The spectrum of illness associated with HIV infection is broad. The Centres for Disease Control (CDC) classify patients into the following four groups:

Acute primary infection (CDC Group I). Most cases with a serum positive for HIV are asymptomatic. In a few cases a brief illness occurs 4 to 8 weeks after exposure, with fever, myalgia, arthralgia, lethargy, lymphadenopathy, sore throat, and a maculopapular rash. Neurological symptoms, e.g. headache, photophopbia, neuropathy and rarely encephalopathy occur commonly. The illness lasts upto 3 weeks and recovery is usually complete. Laboratory abnormalities include lymphopenia with atypical reactive lymphocytes, thrombocytopenia, and raised liver transaminases. CD4 lymphocytes are markedly depleted. Patients with a severe illness progress more quickly to AIDS.

Asymptomatic infection (CDC Group II). Most people with HIV infection are asymptomatic, but the virus continues to replicate and the person remains infectious. This state may last for as long as 10 to 12 years. The following laboratory markers are used to monitor asymptomatic patients:

1. Depletion of CD4 lymphocyte counts.
2. Raised CD8 lymphocyte counts, and reversed CD4: CD8 ratios.
3. Raised serum β_2-microglobulin.

Persistent generalized lymhadenopathy (CDC Group III). The lymph nodes are generally symmetrical, firm, mobile and non-tender, with hyperplasia of follicles and proliferation of capillary endothelium. The spleen may also be enlarged.

Symptomatic HIV infection (CDC Group IV). Progression of HIV infection is manifested by a variety of symptoms and signs. At the same time, CD4 lymphocyte counts decrease. The patient becomes more susceptible to both conventional and opportunistic pathogens as immunosuppression becomes more profound, so that multiple infections may be present at the same time. It should be remembered that due to lack of inflammatory response, typical signs and symptoms of infection may be missing. Therefore, body fluid or tissue is required for direct identification of infecting organisms.

Encapsulated bacteria such as *Strep. pneumoniae* and *H. influenzae,* as well as non-typhoidal *Salmonella* spp., show an increased incidence in HIV infection. The response to antibiotic therapy is good, but recurrent infection is common and long-term suppressive therapy is usually necessary. Similarly, the incidence of tuberculosis (TB) in HIV patients is quite high. TB can cause disease when there is only minimal immunosuppression, and thus often appears early in the course of HIV infection. At the same time, many cases of HIV-related tuberculosis represent reactivation of latent TB.

Constitutional symptoms include lassitude, weight loss, night sweats, and diarrhoea. Skin and mucous membranes are often the sites of bacterial, fungal and viral infections, in the form of seborrhoeic dermatitis and folliculitis, stomatitis, aphthous ulcers, and oral and vaginal candidiasis.

Neurological disease (CDC Group IV B) manifests itself through a sensory neuropathy, a progressive myelopathy, loss of memory and poor concentration, sometimes accompanied by depressive or psychiatric features. Gastrointestinal manifestations include weight loss, diarrhoea and malabsorption. Anorexia, nausea and vomiting often complicate acute episodes of opportunistic infection and their therapy. Haematological complications include anaemia, neutropenia and thrombocytopenia.

Specified secondary cancers (CDC Group IV D). These include Kaposi's sarcoma, non-Hodgkin's lymphoma and primary cerebral lymphoma.

Diagnosis. The most commonly used marker of HIV infection consists of the detection of IgG antibody to envelope components. The routine tests are based on ELISA techniques. Other tests include the detection of Viral p24 antigen, and IgG antibody to p24.

Treatment. The aims of management are to maintain health, avoid transmission of HIV and provide palliative support. Confidentiality must be strictly adhered to, and psychiatric support provided to the patient as well as his family.

Zidovudine (AZT) is an analogue of thymidine and inhibits reverse transcriptase. It is now widely used in the advanced countries in symptomatic HIV disease. Survival is improved and opportunistic infections reduced in intensity and frequency. Any benefits of this drug in asymptomatic patients have still to be proved. The most common toxic effect is bone marrow suppression. Dosage varies from 500 to 1000 mg daily in divided doses.

Attempts are being made to develop an effective vaccine against HIV, but such an agent in unlikely to become available in the near future. Education programmes should provide factual information and strategies to avoid infection, including the use of condoms and access to clean needles and syringes among drug users.

ANTIMICROBIAL AGENTS

A number of different antibiotics and other antimicrobials are employed in the treatment of surgical infections.

Selection of antibiotics. Ideally, the identity and sensitivity of the organism should be known before an antibiotic is started. However it is quite proper, and in fact the usual practice, to send the pus for culture and immediately start an antibiotic which is likely to be effective. On receipt of the culture report, the drug may have to be changed. Normally the culture and sensitivity report takes two or three days to arrive. However, in urgent situations information may be obtained much more quickly. Firstly, *immediate gram staining* of the purulent exudate will often show the organism. Secondly, *direct sensitivity testing* may be carried out by plating the pus directly on a blood agar plate and simultaneously testing with sensitivity discs. Preliminary information can thus usually be obtained within 12 hours. *In critically ill patients this early receipt of information can make the difference between life and death* by guiding the clinician in the choice of the correct antibiotic. Unfortunately this is a grossly underutilized method, because many clinicians are not aware of it.

Resistant strains. These emerge most often when contamination from external sources continues, as in open wounds, leg ulcers and burns.

Penicillins. Penicillins, as well as cephalosporins, have a beta-lactam ring fused to a thiazolidine ring. Penicillins block the cross-linking between alanine and glycine which is an important step in the final stages of formation of the cell wall. Benzylpenicillin can be given only parenterally, and is the drug of choice for serious infections including pneumonia, streptococcal and gonococcal infections, clostridial infections (tetanus, gas gangrene), actinomycosis, anthrax and spirochaetal infections e.g. syphilis.

Flucoxacillin is insensitive to bacterial penicillinase, and is therefore used in infections caused by penicillinase-producing staphylococci. Ampicillin is sensitive to penicillinase, but its activity includes Gram-negative organisms such as Salmonella, Shigella, *E. coli, H. influenzae* and Proteus. It is useful in the treatment of urinary tract and upper respiratory infections. Amoxycillin has a similar activity to ampicillin, but is better absorbed if given by mouth. Carbenicillin and ticarcillin are active against Pseudomonas infection. Generally, the penicillins are very safe drugs. However, hypersensitivity (skin rash, urticaria, anaphylaxis), encephalopathy and tubulo-interstitial nephritis can occur.

Cephalosporins. Like the penicillins, the cephalosporins inhibit bacterial cell-wall synthesis. Cephalexin and cephradine can be taken by mouth. At the same time, highly potent parenteral preparations are available, in the form of cefuroxime, cefotaxime and ceftazidime. They are resistant to staphylococcal penicillinase and are active against both Gram-negative and Gram-positive organisms. They are inactive against enterococci and *Pyocyaneus aeruginosa* (except ceftazidime). The cephalosporins are useful for the treatment of serious systemic infections. They are commonly used for serious postoperative sepsis and in immunocompromised patients.

Monobactams. The only member of this class in current use is aztreonam. Its spectrum of activity is limited to aerobic Gram-negative bacilli, thus resembling aminoglycosides. It is commonly used in combination with metronidazole (for anaerobes) and penicillin or erythromycin (for Gram-positive cocci).

Aminoglycosides. These antibiotics are derived from *Streptomyces* spp. They interrupt bacterial protein synthesis by inhibiting ribosomal function. Streptomycin is not often used in the advanced countries. However, in the poorer communities it still has a place because of its low cost. Neomycin is only used for the topical treatment of eye and skin infections and orally for preoperative 'sterilization' of the bowel.

Gentamycin and tobramycin are given parenterally. They are highly effective against many Gram-negative infections including *Pseudomonas.* The newer antibiotics, amikin and netilmycin, have a similar activity. Their use should be restricted to gentamycin-resistant organisms. Aminoglycosides are nephrotoxic and ototoxic, specially in the elderly, therefore their blood levels should be checked.

Tetracyclines. These are bacteriostatic drugs. They inhibit bacterial protein synthesis by interrupting ribosomal function. They are effective against Gram-positive and Gram-negative bacteria, but their use is now limited, specially in surgical conditions.

Erythromycin. This drug belongs to the group of macrolides, which also inhibit protein synthesis by interrupting ribosomal function. It has a similar antibacterial spectrum to penicillin, and can be used both orally and parenterally. It is included in the treatment regimens of all pneumonias as many are due to Mycoplasma. Prolonged treatment with erythromycin can be followed by cholestatic jaundice. The newer macrolides, *azithromycin and clarithromycin* are active against Gram-negative organisms as well. At the same time they have enhanced tissue and intracellular penetration, and a longer half-life that allows once or twice daily dosage.

Chloramphenicol. Chloramphenicol contains nitrobenzene, which is probably responsible both for its activity against bacteria as well as its toxicity. It competes with messenger RNA for ribosomal binding. Despite its toxicity, it is indicated for the treatment of severe infection due to *Salmonella typhi* and *S. paratyphi* (enteric fevers), and meningitis due to *H. influenzae.* It is also useful in plague and purulent conjunctivitis. It should be remembered that it enhances the activity of anticoagulants, phenytoin and oral antihyperglycaemic agents. *Severe irreversible* bone marrow suppression can occur with the use of this drug. Therefore its use should be restricted to the above indications. Again, it should not be used in neonates or premature infants, as they cannot conjugate and excrete this drug, and high blood levels lead to circulatory collapse.

Fusidic acid. The structure of fusidic acid resembles that of bile salts. It is used mainly for penicillinase-producing *Staph. aureus* infections such as osteomyelitis and endocarditis, and for other staphylococcal infections associated with septicaemia. The drug is well absorbed orally, and is concentrated in bone. Resistance occurs rapidly; therefore it is used in combination with another antibiotic. It may occasionally be hepatotoxic, but is generally safe and can be given in pregnancy.

Sulphonamides. Sulphonamides block the synthesis of thymidine and purine. Trimethoprim also inhibits folic acid synthesis. Sulphamethoxazole is used mainly in combination with trimethoprim (as co-trimoxazole) for *P. carinii* infection. Trimethoprim alone is now used for urinary infections and bronchitis. Sulphapyridine in combination with 5-aminosalicylic acid (i.e. sulphasalazine) is used in inflammatory bowel disease. Bacteria may become resistant to sulphonamides by altering bacterial cell permeability to these agents. Sulphonamides potentiate oral anticoagulants and hypoglycaemic agents. They also cause thrombocytopenia, folate deficiency and haemolysis in individuals with glucose-6-phosphate dehydrogenase deficiency, and therefore should not be used in such persons. At the same time, co-trimoxazole should be avoided in the elderly.

Quinolones. Ciprofloxacin, norfloxacin and ofloxacin are useful oral broad-spectrum antibiotics related structurally to nalidixic acid. The latter achieves only low serum levels, and therefore its use is restricted to the urinary tract where it is concentrated. Quinolones inhibit bacterial DNA synthesis by inhibiting DNA gyrase. They should be reserved for infections resistant to other drugs. The extended spectrum quinolones such as ciprofloxacin are active against Gram-negative and some Gram-positive bacteria, and are useful in Gram-negative septicaemia, skin and bone infections, gastrointestinal, urinary and respiratory infections, gonorrhoea and infection with *Chlamydia trachomatis.* The newer quinolones are the only oral anti-pseudomonas antibiotics available. Toxic effects include gastrointestinal disturbances, photosensitive rashes and occasional neurotoxicity.

Nitroimidazoles. Metronidazole is the most important member of this group of drugs. Minor modifications in its structure have produced tinidazole and nimorazole. They act by breaking down the strands of DNA in the microbes. Metronidazole is important in the treatment of anaerobic bacterial infection, particularly that due to *Bacteroides.* It is also widely used prophylactically in colonic surgery. Apart from this, it is the treatment of choice for amoebiasis, giardiasis and *Trichomonas vaginalis.* It can be used both orally and intravenously. Nitroimidazoles result in a metallic taste, and produce peripheral neuropathy with prolonged use. They should be avoided in pregnancy.

Vancomycin. Vancomycin is a complex glycopeptide produced by *Streptomyces orientalis.* It exerts bactericidal activity against Gram-positive bacteria by inhibiting cell-wall synthesis. It is not a drug meant to be used routinely. It is given orally for pseudomembranous enterocolitis produced by *Clostridium difficile,* and intravenously for methicillin-resistant *Staph aureus.* It is also employed in Gram-positive infections in patients allergic to penicillins.

Antifungal drugs. *Amphotericin B* is used intravenously in severe fungal infections. The drug is nephrotoxic, so that renal function must be taken into account. *Nystatin* is not absorbed through mucous membranes and is therefore useful in the treatment of candidiasis affecting the mouth, intestines and vagina. It can be given orally or as pessaries. *Griseofulvin* is concentrated in keratin, and is therefore a useful remedy for chronic fungal infection of nails, as well as for ringworm.

Antiviral drugs. *Zidovudine (AZT)* is a thymidine analogue. It inhibits HIV reverse transcriptase and thereby impairs replication of the virus. It is recommended for HIV patients with symptomatic infection, particularly those with opportunistic infections and neurological disease. Serious bone marrow toxicity occurs commonly, while polymyositis and an encephalitis-like syndrome can also be encountered.

Ganciclovir is a guanine analogue. It is used for cytomegalovirus retinitis and gastrointestinal disease in patients with HIV infection. The major complication is neutropenia. *Interferon* is a naturally occurring substance produced by T lymphocytes during virus infection. It is produced in response to infection by many different viruses, and production stimulated by one virus may confer protection against a second viral invader. It is used in hepatitis B and C, as well as in certain malignancies.

Other antiviral agents. Unexplained fever, postoperative atypical pneumonia and herpes may occur in the surgical patient due to virus infections, the incidence of which is underestimated. In the case of the more common infections, e.g. herpes, cytomegalic, and influenza viruses, diagnosis can be arrived at by finding a rising titre of antibodies against the virus. At the same time, more and more drugs are becoming available against virus infections, like amantadine against influenza and acyclovir against herpes.

14 Neoplasia

A neoplasm is a group of cells which have become unresponsive to control mechanisms, and which show excessive, useless proliferation. *Benign* neoplasms contain normal-appearing cells that do not invade locally and do not metastasize. *Malignant* neoplasms or cancers show uncontrolled proliferation of cells, invasion of surrounding tissues and metastatic spread to distant sites. Cancers of various organs differ a great deal in their biological behaviour. However, taken as a whole cancer is a frequent cause of serious illness and death. The sites most commonly causing death in males are lung, large gut, prostate and pancreas. In females these sites include breast, large bowel, lung, ovary and uterus.

Geographical distribution. Environmental variation is probably the major cause of the disparate geographic distribution of different tumours. Thus in southern India chewing a mixture of betel, tobacco and lime results in a high incidence of oropharyngeal tumours. The common occurrence of gastric cancer in Japan is considered to be due to ingestion of smoked and highly salted foods. Hepatocellular carcinoma is common in parts of Africa with a high incidence of hepatitis B infection. Caucasians living in subtropical zones are at increased risk of skin cancer.

BIOLOGY

When cells become malignant they revert to more primitive cell types, i.e. they de-differentiate:

1. The normal orderly cell patterns are lost and are replaced by the random piling up of malignant cells without a definite pattern.
2. Other histological changes which take place include cellular pleomorphism, a high rate of mitosis and hyperchromatism in the nucleus and nucleoli.
3. Invasion of adjacent normal structures also may be seen microscopically.

These morphological changes are the basis of the histological and cytological diagnosis of cancer, and usually allow very accurate diagnosis of neoplastic disease. That is why a tumour is declared as malignant only after the histopathology report has been received.

Similarly, the cellular biochemistry sometimes reverts to that of the embryonal cells, so that *such substances are produced which are normally manufactured only by embryonal structures.* The presence of these *abnormal* materials in adult cells can be used to diagnose cancer. Examples of this type include:

1. *Carcinoembryonic antigen* found in gastrointestinal cancers.
2. *Alpha-fetoglobulin* associated with hepatomas and embryonal cancers.

Hormones. Tumours may produce different types of hormones:

1. Malignant cells may produce hormones that are *normally produced* by the cells from which the tumour originated, and may cause symptoms due to the same. For example, hyperparathyroidism may be produced by parathyroid carcinomas.
2. Other neoplasms may produce hormones that are *not normally produced* by the cells of origin of the tumour. For example some bronchogenic carcinomas may produce ACTH, antidiuretic hormone, etc.

The mechanism of the production of such abnormal hormones is quite interesting and can best be explained as follows:

– All cells in a human being contain the same genes.
– However, only about 10% of these genes are expressed in any one adult cell type, the remainder being repressed.
– Cancer cells are primitive cells.
– When normal cells de-differentiate into the more primitive cancer cells they develop the ability to express these previously repressed genes.
– When these new genes express themselves, a new specific messenger RNA is produced, and new (abnormal) hormones are manufactured.

Gompertzian progression. Biologic growth, whether of normal tissues or of neoplasms, follows a particular pattern. In the beginning growth is very rapid. It then continues to become steadily and progressively slower. The specific equation describing this relationship was derived by the eighteenth century mathematician Gompertz, hence the term Gompertzian growth.

Carcinogenesis. In experimental tumours if the dose of the carcinogen is large the tumours are induced in a shorter period of time. In humans many tumours arise slowly, suggesting that they are the result of prolonged exposure to low doses of carcinogens. Tumorigenesis takes a long time to have its effect; this is why tumours are common in middle and old age.

Physical carcinogenesis. Tumour induction by physical agents occurs by essentially two mechanisms: firstly, induction of cell proliferation over a period of time, which increases the opportunity for events leading to transformation; and secondly, exposure to physical agents that induce changes in DNA replication. A *foreign body* rarely induces a tumour itself. However, the irritation induced by the foreign body promotes cellular proliferation, thereby increasing the chances for errors in DNA replication that may lead to neoplastic transformation. A similar role is played by chronic inflammatory conditions such as inflammatory bowel disease.

Ionizing radiation. In experimental animals alpha, gamma, and x-radiation, as well as ultraviolet light, induce tumours. X-rays commonly result in the induction of leukaemias, lymphomas and thymomas. Ultraviolet light induces skin tumours. The mechanism usually involves chromosomal changes, mutations, and activation of oncogenes. In the presence of oncogenic viruses radiation may accelerate tumour induction. In addition to its direct effects, radiation is also a potent immunosuppressive, decreasing the effectiveness of an important mechanism of inhibition of tumour formation. Both gamma and x-rays affect the function of lymphocytes.

Chemical carcinogenesis. For thousands of years colours created by nature, as well as foods designed by her for consumption by animals and humans, have come into contact with or passed through animal and human bodies without inducing allergies or tumours. Chemicals created by man are not equally sophisticated; they are much more often followed by harmful effects. The list of chemical carcinogens is a long one, and includes heavy metal residues from fossil fuel combustion and industrial processes.

Immunodeficiency. Immunodeficient individuals and immunosuppressed recipients of organ transplants are at a greater risk for neoplastic disease, mostly of the lymphoreticular system. In the normal host several types of lymphoid cells including T, B, and NK lymphocytes participate in the destruction of aberrant cells and prevention of neoplasia.

Development of neoplasia. The progression of the cell to frank malignancy passes through different stages. *Hyperplasia* is an increase in the number of cells. Following injury the local growth rate increases over the baseline in the normal process of wound healing. As wound closure is achieved, the rate of cell division returns to that of the adjacent tissue. Hyperplasia increases the chances of development of malignancy, but to a very slight extent. In the breast marked hyperplasia is associated with just a 2-fold increased risk of carcinoma. On the other hand hyperplastic polyps are common in the colon, and are potential precancers in the evolution of colonic malignancy.

Metaplasia is reversible transformation of one mature cell type to another, the replacing cell type being present in an area where it is not normally found. For example, in gastro-oesophageal reflux the normal distal oesophageal squamous epithelium exhibits metaplasia to a 'gastric-type' columnar epithelium.

In *dysplasia* the cell size, shape and organization is altered. The cells show polymorphism and hyperchromatism, often with complete loss of cellular and epithelial polarity. Mitoses are frequent. There is no penetration of abnormal cells through the epithelial basement membrane. Carcinoma in situ shows all of these changes. Not all dysplastic tissue progresses to carcinoma. However, close clinical, endoscopic and x-ray surveillance should be maintained, with consideration of prophylactic resection of all tissue at risk.

Final induction of neoplasia. Normal cell multiplication takes place only when the cell is stimulated by a growth factor. If a growth factor receptor in the cell undergoes a mutation and becomes 'constitutively active' (i.e. active itself, without need of being stimulated), it sends uncontrolled mitogenic signals to the cell nucleus, and unrestrained multiplication results. The cell ceases to respond to the growth factor regulatory networks within the tissue system. Its requirement for growth factors diminishes, and it may begin to synthesize its own growth factors.

Inheritance. In all cancers changes take place in the normal cellular genes:

1. In the vast majority of cancers (especially in older people) these genetic changes occur in the somatic tissues of the individual and do not enter the germ-line, so even close relatives of the patient do not run an increased risk.
2. In a few cancers close relatives may have an increased susceptibility to neoplastic change, but the cancer is not caused by a single gene defect; rather, multiple factors are responsible.
3. Finally, in some very rare cancers the changes can be inherited as a single gene defect.

Cancer tissues are clonal and a cancer arises from changes in only one cell which then proliferates in the body.

The genes that are damaged by the genetic changes which lead to cancer fall into two categories:

1. *Oncogenes.* These lead to the formation of proteins that regulate normal cellular proliferation. Therefore, alteration in the structure of these genes can lead to abnormal cell proliferation. When genetic damage to an oncogene gives rise to a signal for uncontrolled growth, the gene is said to be 'activated'. Oncogenes can be activated by:

   i. *Mutation.* For example, carcinogens such as those found in cigarette smoke can cause point mutations in DNA. By chance some of these mutations occur in regions of the oncogene that lead to activation of that gene.

   ii. *Chromosomal translocation.* During cell division an error occurs during which portions of two chromosomes exchange places with each other i.e. get 'translocated'. Sequences of one part of this abnormal gene are inappropriately expressed because they are under the control of the other part of the gene.

   iii. *Viral stimulation.* Some viruses, such as retroviruses, can cause cancerous changes by activating oncogenes when they infect a cell.

2. *Tumour suppressor genes.* These genes normally restrict undue cell proliferation, as opposed to oncogenes which enhance signals for cell growth. Therefore mutations in these genes also lead to uncontrolled cell growth.

CLASSIFICATION OF NEOPLASMS

The most useful classification is based upon the cell type of the tissue of origin of the tumour. When a benign tumour arises from any tissue, the suffix *-oma* is added after the name of the tissue, e.g. a benign tumour arising from fibrous tissue is called a fibroma, a tumour arising from a bony tissue is named an osteoma, and so on. Malignant tumours arising from connective tissues are called sarcomas; those originating from epithelia are named carcinomas.

Examples of tumours. *Connective tissue tumours.* Benign tumours arising from fibrous, fatty and vascular tissues are called fibroma, lipoma and angioma respectively. Malignant tumours arising from the same tissues are named fibrosarcoma, liposarcoma and angiosarcoma respectively.

Epithelial tumours. The different epithelia belong to two main types:

1. In the first type the cells line an external or internal surface without forming glandular structures, and are usually of ectodermal origin. The lining usually consists of

squamous epithelium. Examples are seen in the skin, and close to various orifices in the body, e.g. mouth, larynx, oesophagus and vagina, etc. Benign tumours arise on these epithelia as papules, and are called *squamous cell papillomas;* malignant tumours are called *squamous cell carcinomas.*

2. In the second type of epithelium the cells form acini. Examples are seen in the case of the breast, pancreas, liver, stomach and colon. Benign tumours are called *adenomas* and malignant tumours *adenocarcinomas.*

Teratoma. This is an unusual tumour. It is a neoplasm in which anaplastic, immature somatic cells comparable to blastoderm are usually dominant. It exhibits varying degrees of differentiation into mature cells of ectodermal, mesodermal and entodermal types. Teratomas occur in the testis, ovary and mediastinum.

GRADING OF MALIGNANCY

Broders has classified tumours into four grades, depending upon their degree of differentiation. The most differentiated tumours are classified as grade 1, the least differentiated as grade 4. In general, the lower grade tumours are less malignant and tend to metastasize less often than the higher grade, more anaplastic ones. *Although the grading of neoplasms is useful, growth rate and presence of metastases are usually more important in determining prognosis.*

Carcinoma *in situ*. Carcinoma *in situ* is a lesion with the cytological characteristics of a malignant tumor, but with no detectable infiltration into the surrounding or deeper tissues. Most probably these *in situ* lesions develop into invasive cancer after variable periods of time. In the case of the cervix the interval between detection of a carcinoma *in situ* and the development of invasive carcinoma may be as long as 10 to 15 years. Carcinoma in situ also occurs in the skin, bronchus, stomach and pharynx. If such a lesion is adequately treated, a complete cure is assured.

ROUTES OF SPREAD OF MALIGNANT TUMOURS

There are four main routes of spread of tumours. A great deal is known about these routes, but very little about the conditions which determine that spread. Some tumours have already metastasized by the time they are discovered, while others of the same type and in the same organ may remain localized for years. Metastases may dominate the clinical picture while the primary tumour remains latent and asymptomatic. For example, a metastasis to the brain from a silent cancer of the lung may be mistaken for a primary brain tumour.

A tumour may spread by direct extension, via lymphatics, by vascular invasion, or by implantation in serous cavities. However, many cancers spread by more than one route and an orderly course of metastases cannot be relied upon. For example a cancer of the breast may metastasize to the lungs or liver but not develop secondaries in the regional lymph nodes.

Direct extension. Cancer cells may spread directly by infiltrating the surrounding tissues. Invasion of surrounding tissues requires the active participation of hydrolytic enzymes. Many human malignant neoplasms possess higher levels of lytic enzyme activity than benign tumours or normal tissues. Some tumours, such as adenocarcinomas of the stomach or oesophagus, may extend upto 10 cm along tissue planes beyond the palpable tumour mass. Others, such as basal cell carcinomas of skin, rarely extend for more than a few millimeters beyond the visible margin.

Lymph spread. Tumour cells readily enter lymphatics and extend along these channels by permeation or embolism. *Permeation* is the growth of a colony of cells along the course of the lymph vessel. This occurs commonly in the skin lymphatics in carcinoma of the breast. Spread by *embolism* to the regional or distant lymph nodes is of much greater importance. When a lymph node containing tumour is more than 3 cm in diameter, this means that the tumour has already gone through the capsule into the surrounding fat. According to many oncologists *the presence of cancer cells in the lymph nodes indicates an unfavourable host-tumour relationship*, and the likelihood of distant metastases.

According to classic teaching epithelial tumours commonly spread through the lymph nodes, and mesenchymal tumours through the bloodstream. However, recent work suggests that this division may be artificial, and that tumour cells pass from one system to the other. Further, there is no clear evidence that lymph nodes serve as barriers to the spread of the neoplasia.

Vascular spread. Cancer cells may reach the blood stream either through the thoracic duct or by invasion of blood vessels. When the vascular endothelium is destroyed a thrombus is formed which is invaded by tumour. This combination of thrombus and tumour may get detached to form a tumour embolus. *Vascular invasion is commonly seen in both carcinomas and sarcomas, and indicates a poor prognosis.* Most tumour cells are destroyed within the bloodstream. However, the greater the number of cells released by a primary tumour, the greater the probability that a few will survive to form metastases.

Malignant tumours do not produce their own blood vessels; they induce the ingrowth of new capillaries from host tissue by releasing tumour angiogenesis factor. The penetration of these new vascular channels by the tumour cells is aided by their defective endothelium and increased permeability. In this way metastatic spread is rendered more likely.

Spread through serous cavities. Tumour cells sometimes gain entrance to serous cavities by direct growth of the tumour through the wall of an organ, and then spread widely throughout the cavity. Common examples include peritoneal seeding of gastrointestinal and ovarian tumours.

CLINICAL FEATURES OF CANCER

The clinical presentation of cancer varies from case to case. It may appear as a mass without any other symptoms, or the patient may complain of certain symptoms which are found on investigation to be due to an underlying malignancy. Finally, the cancer may be so small that it produces no symptoms or signs, but may be shown up by *routine screening*, e.g. by a mammogram.

Clinical features may be produced either directly by the mass, or by physiological derangements produced by it. By publicizing the key symptoms of cancer, earlier diagnosis may be achieved. The American Cancer Society has formulated the *Seven Danger Signals of Cancer* which are as follows:

- A lump in the breast or elsewhere.
- A sore that does not heal.
- Change in the bowel or bladder habit.
- Unusual bleeding or discharge.
- Indigestion or difficulty in swallowing.
- Obvious change in a wart or mole.
- Nagging cough or hoarseness.

This short list may be helpful in the effort to educate people and increase the frequency of *early* diagnosis for certain common cancers, and should be made widely known. *Screening* programmes should cover those who have an inherited susceptibility to cancer. These include individuals with a family history of breast cancer, colon cancer, and medullary thyroid cancer, as well as those with predisposing conditions such as polyposis of the colon.

Signs of expansion. These depend upon the site of the tumour. If it is near the surface, there is simply a mass. If it arises in a hollow tube, the signs may be those of obstruction of that tube. For example, a tumour in the gastrointestinal, biliary or urinary tract may produce vomiting, jaundice and urinary obstruction respectively. Expansion of the tumour may result in destruction of host tissues. Examples are seen when tumour cells replace bone and result in a pathological fracture. Similarly, malignant cells may replace the greater part of the liver parenchyma and result in hepatic insufficiency.

Other clinical features. With the passage of time clinical features may appear which show that the cancer is in an *advanced* stage:

1. When a tumour *infiltrates* nerves pain, numbness or paralysis may be produced. For example, a cancer of the rectum may infiltrate the sacral plexus, resulting in pain in the parts supplied by this plexus.
2. When a tumour becomes necrotic it may *ulcerate* and bleed. In carcinoma of the stomach or right colon ulceration may cause bleeding which results in anaemia. The patient presents with fatigue and weakness, and only by keeping a high index of suspicion and by carrying out the relevant investigations can the underlying cancer be detected.
3. If an ulcerated cancer becomes *infected* there may be pain, tenderness and fever. In this way a cancer of the caecum may be mistaken for appendicitis.
4. The primary tumour may remain undetected while *metastases* present clinically, e.g. in supraclavicular nodes, lungs, liver, bones and brain.
5. Finally, the *cachexia* of carcinomatosis may result from competition between the tumour and the host for basic components of the same metabolic pool.

DIAGNOSIS

Diagnosis of cancer should be pursued in an orderly fashion: very careful history, thorough physical examination, appropriate laboratory tests, x-rays, ultrasound examination, CT and radioisotope scans and biopsy, as indicated by the clinical findings.

BIOPSY

It is essential that microscopic proof of malignancy be obtained before treatment is started for any cancer, because significant morbidity and mortality may result from all forms of cancer therapy. At the same time, the specific type of antitumour therapy will depend upon the histological type of the tumour which can only be determined by biopsy. The common methods of biopsy include needle biopsy and open biopsy. Finally, exfoliative cytology can be considered a form of biopsy.

Needle biopsy. This is the simplest method and may be used for subcutaneous masses, muscular masses and some internal organs, such as the liver and kidney. Its disadvantage lies in the fact that the specimen may be small and not representative.

A ***Tru-cut needle*** gives a fairly good-sized biopsy specimen. Local anaesthesia is used. The sheath of the Trucut needle is advanced to the tumour surface. The needle is next pushed into the tumour. The side of the needle carries a groove, and the tissues of the tumour bulge into this groove. The sheath is now advanced into the tumour, its forward cutting edge acting as a knife which cuts off the piece of the tumour in the groove. The whole instrument is now withdrawn, the tissue removed from the groove, and processed as usual. This biopsy needle usually provides tissue adequate for a histological rather than a cytological report. However, sampling errors are possible, and if the pathologist desires the whole tumour or lymph node, then this technique cannot be used. A negative report for malignancy should be followed by incisional biopsy if there is any doubt.

Fine-needle aspiration cytology, in which thin strands of cells are obtained for cytology, is being used increasingly. A 22-gauge needle on a 10 ml syringe is commonly used. The needle is introduced into the tumour and suction applied, when a small quantity of tumour tissue is obtained in the syringe. No anaesthesia is required and the procedure can be carried out in the outpatients department. The technique is extremely useful but requires considerable skill to interpret it, and should only be carried out by a pathologist trained in the method.

Open biopsy. This can take one of two forms: incision biopsy and excision biopsy.

Incision biopsy. This entails removal of a small piece of the tumour for pathological examination. If possible, a margin of normal tissue should be taken with it.

Excision biopsy. This means local removal of the whole tumour, and is suitable for small neoplasms 2 to 3 cm in diameter. It is ideally suited for small squamous or basal cell carcinomas and malignant melanomas. It is also used for polypoid lesions of the colon, for breast and thyroid nodules, and when the pathologist cannot make a definite diagnosis from an incision biopsy.

Lymph nodes which are to be biopsied should be carefully selected. *Cervical lymph nodes should not be biopsied until a careful search for a primary has been made,* e.g. by endoscopies of the upper respiratory tract, thyroid scans etc. Enlargement of upper cervical nodes is usually due to tumours from the larynx and pharynx. Supraclavicular nodes are more often enlarged from metastases arising from the abdomen or thorax.

Exfoliative cytology. Cancer cells are shed from the surfaces of some neoplasms arising in epithelial-lined body cavities and orifices, such as the vagina, bronchus and stomach. These cells can be collected, stained and recognized as malignant because of their morphological changes. This method can help in the early diagnosis of cancer of these organs. However, a pathologist trained in cytological diagnosis is required. The advent of fibreoptic endoscopy with the facility of direct biopsy has reduced the need for exfoliative cytology.

Examination of the biopsy specimen. The specimen may be examined either by frozen or paraffin section. For *frozen* section the specimen is immediately handed over to the pathologist, who gives the report within 15 to 20 minutes. For a *paraffin* section the specimen is placed in formal saline and requires 1 to 2 days of processing. Although in the case of a few tumours frozen section gives a reliable diagnosis, most pathologists prefer to make a definitive diagnosis on paraffin sections. Frozen section is used only when the diagnosis is required *during the surgical procedure,* so that the decision about the type of resection can be guided by it; otherwise a paraffin section is always preferable.

STAGING OF TUMOURS

The extent of spread of a tumour at a given time is called its *clinical stage.* Before treatment is started it is not only necessary to have a histological diagnosis of cancer, but the stage of the tumour should also be determined. A number of attempts have been made on an international level to stage tumours, none of which have been as yet universally accepted. However, stage I usually indicates a neoplasm confined to its primary site of origin, stage II indicates metastases to the regional lymph nodes, stage III indicates infiltration into surrounding tissues, and stage IV denotes distant metastases.

TNM system. The Union International for the Control of Cancer (UICC) has standardized a system of staging of cancer for world-wide use. It is called the *TNM system.* T stands for the extent of the primary tumour, N for the presence or absence of node involvement, and M for the presence or absence of distant metastases. T_1, T_2, T_3 and T_4 stand for primary tumours of increasing size. N_0 denotes absence of lymph nodes and N_1 their presence. Similarly M_0 and M_1 indicate absence and presence of distant metastases respectively. A small tumour without nodal or distant metastases is designated as $T_1N_0M_0$. A very large tumour with both nodal and distant metastases is identified as a $T_4N_1M_1$ lesion.

In spite of its relative complexity the TNM system *has become universally accepted* because it helps in staging the tumour precisely. The importance of accurate staging when designing a treatment programme for a patient with cancer cannot be overemphasized. Without this, the results of therapy in different centers cannot be properly compared, nor can new forms of therapy be correctly evaluated.

Unfortunately one of the great deficiencies of the present methods of staging is their *inability to detect subclinical microscopic metastatic lesions.* For example, about half the patients who undergo mastectomy for cancer of the breast have subclinical distant metastases at the time of the operation. If a test is developed which can show up these micrometastases it will be a major advance in the management of cancer.

THE TREATMENT OF CANCER

The methods available for the treatment of cancer include surgery, radiotherapy, chemotherapy and immunotherapy. So long as the tumour is localized to the primary site and the regional lymph nodes, surgery and radiotherapy are the most successful means of dealing with it. Once the disease has metastasized beyond the local region these methods cannot be considered curative, although they may be used for palliation.

On the other hand, chemotherapy and immunotherapy represent systemic forms of treatment effective against tumour cells which have already metastasized. These methods have a greater chance of curing patients with a minimum number of tumour cells than those with clinically evident disease. Thus, though surgery and radiotherapy cannot be curative unless the disease is confined locally or regionally, they can be used to decrease the patient's tumour burden so that chemotherapy or immunotherapy may become more effective. Treatment combining surgery, radiotherapy, chemotherapy and possibly immunotherapy significantly improves cure rates above those achieved with any single method of treatment. Therefore in the treatment of cancer *surgeons, medical oncologists, radiotherapists, pathologists, etc. should work in very close cooperation with each other.*

Once the diagnosis of malignant disease has been made, before aggressive therapy is started *it must be decided whether the disease is curable or not.* Patients are generally judged as incurable if they have distant metastases or extensive local infiltration. However, solitary pulmonary metastases may be curable by resection. Similarly, at operation it may be found that the local infiltration is not as extensive as it appeared on clinical examination, and that wide resection with a clear margin of normal tissue is possible.

SURGERY

Surgical treatment represents the most frequently used single method of cancer therapy. However, only about one third of cancer patients are cured by surgery alone, because surgical treatment is effective only when the disease is localized to the primary site and regional nodes.

Most malignancies, after starting from a single cell, have a relatively long latent period. Unfortunately, during this period they often shed cells into the blood vessels as they grow. Surgery is a means of local control of the disease, and obviously can have no effect on the cells which have been swept away into the blood stream and have produced metastases at distant sites. However, the decrease in tumour burden following local resection can alter the host-tumour balance to favour the patient with minimal metastases, so that it can become easier to deal with these micrometastases by chemotherapy.

Preoperative preparation. In advanced cancer the patient's condition may be relatively poor. Many cancers have a greater degree of toxic effect on the host than would be expected from their size. In cancers of the oesophagus and intestinal tract there may be malnutrition due to interference with normal alimentary function. Anaemia, vitamin deficiencies, defects in the coagulation mechanisms and hypoproteinaemia must be corrected before an operation can be safely performed.

The operation. *The operative procedure for a case of cancer must be very carefully planned, because the best, and often the only, opportunity for cure is at the time of the first operation.* If the tumour is incompletely excised at that time tissue planes, lymphatics and blood vessels are violated and tumour cells seeded throughout the wound. Therefore, enucleation of tumour masses is never the correct treatment for a cancer.

Prevention of dissemination during operation. During the operation cancer cells should not be transferred by inoculation into the surrounding tissues. If preliminary biopsy is done and the tissue sent for frozen section, the entire operative field should be prepared again after the biopsy incision is closed. The instruments and gloves, and even the saline used during the biopsy, are not used again, because they may have been contaminated. During the operation cancer cells can also be disseminated via the blood stream. To prevent this, manipulation of the tumour during the operation is avoided. At the same time, the vascular pedicle of the tumour is ligated early during the operation to prevent venous spread.

RADIOTHERAPY

Radiotherapy, like surgery, can cure only localized cancer. It can destroy neoplastic tissue with minimal damage to the surrounding tissues, and when successful provides good functional and cosmetic results. Often, radiation therapy and surgery are combined to increase the cure rates for certain neoplasms.

Mechanism of action. Radiation collides with the atoms in the irradiated tissue. This releases energy that causes ionization of water in the cells into hydroxyl and peroxide radicals. These radicals cause breaks in the DNA of the chromosomes in both tumour cells and normal cells. Within a few minutes of irradiation vacuoles appear in the cytoplasm of the cell, which becomes swollen. The nuclear chromatin forms clumps. The cell may die, or may be rendered incapable of division. *Because the mechanisms of repair are more adequate in normal cells, they suffer less damage than tumour cells.*

The *rad* is the unit of measurement of the radiation dose. The total dose to many tumours, usually given over a period of four to six weeks, ranges between 4,500 and 6,000 rads. In order to deliver larger doses of radiation to the tumour-bearing area than to the surrounding tissues, various techniques are used, such as multiple ports, rotational fields, lead shielding, etc.

The rad is gradually being replaced, as the unit of measurement of radiation dose, by the gray (Gy), which is equal to 100 rads.

There are three types of radiation: alpha particles, beta particles and electromagnetic rays, such as gamma rays and x-rays. *Alpha* particles penetrate only a few microns and are stopped by the epidermis. *Beta* particles penetrate only a few millimeters. *Gamma* rays can penetrate through several centimeters of metal. At the same time, the higher the voltage of the machine the greater the penetration. Supervoltage machines, producing 1,000 to 50,000 KV of energy, are now available. Such radiation penetrates to a greater depth and causes less skin damage than the 250 KV machines used in the past.

Planning the therapy. *Palliation or cure?* After evaluation of the patient, the objective of the treatment must first be defined. If the cancer is curable, a prolonged course of therapy and a moderate risk of serious morbidity are often accepted in an effort to eradicate life-threatening disease. On the other hand if the object is palliation of symptoms, treatment must be designed to minimize morbidity and maximize symptom relief.

Alone or in combination? Radiotherapy *alone* is curative in many clinical situations. Local or local plus regional treatment yields high cure rates in many cancers of the head and neck, anal canal and prostate, gynaecological malignancies, Hodgkin's disease, and other tumours. Most sarcomas are radiosensitive. As far as carcinomas are concerned, squamous cell carcinomas are radiosensitive. Adenocarcinomas have been generally considered as radioresistant. However, this was the position with conventional radiotherapy. With the higher voltages of the linear accelerator, even adenocarcinomas exhibit some response to radiotherapy.

In other cases radiation is used *in combination* with surgery or chemotherapy. The use of combined treatment may allow less morbid treatment than would be possible with either method alone. Such planned treatment is better than the use of one method to salvage the failure of the other, as in that case the effectiveness of the second method is greatly reduced.

Finally, *late sequelae* of radiotherapy may appear months or years after treatment, and should be discussed with the patient before deciding upon the mode of treatment.

Treatment planning is becoming increasingly sophisticated. The *target volume* is defined by synthesizing information from the history, physical examination, x-rays, operation findings, and pathology reports. Treatment is now designed to maximize tumour control and minimize side effects.

Delivery. The best method of delivery of radiation is selected from different options, including multiple beams of photons and electrons, sometimes aided by intracavitary or interstitial applications. Various types of beam shaping devices may be used. Computer-assisted programs allow accurate calculations of the different options. Marks on the patient's skin make it possible to reproduce the fields during the treatment. The patient may be immobilized to improve the reproducibility of the treatment, so that repeated delivery can be accurate to within a few millimeters.

The *location* of a tumour may make it more accessible to radiotherapy. For example, tumours of the cervix can be controlled locally with minimal risk, due to the opportunity to deliver high doses with *intracavitary* radiotherapy. On the other hand carcinomas in the upper abdomen cannot be controlled with radiotherapy alone because the surrounding organs such as liver, kidneys, bowel and spinal cord limit the doses of external beam radiotherapy that can be delivered safely. When such tumours are exposed during operation, they are accessible to direct irradiation. Investigations are therefore continuing into the possibility of *intraoperative* radiotherapy, to increase the dose of irradiation that can be delivered in such situations.

Radiosensitivity versus radiocurability. Radiosensitivity does not necessarily mean radiocurability. As an example, although Ewing's sarcoma responds very well to radiotherapy, very few patients are cured, because they develop metastases.

In general, tumour cells which are undifferentiated or in active mitosis are more sensitive to radiation. Furthermore, if the cell of origin of a tumour is radiosensitive the tumour also generally responds to radiation. Haemopoietic cells, epidermoid cells, lymphocytes and germ cells of the gonads are most sensitive to radiation, and tumours derived from these cells are also usually radiosensitive.

Complications of radiotherapy. Although radiation therapy is not usually associated with any immediate mortality, *the morbidity, complications and long-term effects of radiotherapy may be considerable.* The acute changes are caused by oedema and inflammation, the chronic changes by scarring, fibrosis and ischaemia. Megavoltage radiation has mostly eliminated the skin changes seen in the past with lower voltage radiation. Many patients undergoing radiotherapy develop malaise, nausea, vomiting, weakness and weight loss. These symptoms are directly related to dose, volume and rate of delivery. Antiemetic drugs help prevent and treat this *radiation sickness.*

Late *carcinogenic* effects may be seen from time to time. In the early days after the discovery of x-rays, before the malignant potential of radiation became known, radiologists used to take no precautions to protect themselves from x-rays. It was only when they started developing skin cancers on their hands, and leukaemias, that rigid protocols for the protection of the personnel of x-ray departments were instituted, and are now in routine use. Similarly, some decades ago radiotherapy was freely prescribed for benign conditions in the neck in childhood, specially in the USA. It was only when these children grew up, and a large number of them started developing thyroid cancers, that the practice was discontinued. With proper precautions, such problems are seen much less often nowadays.

Linear accelerator. Compared to the conventional radiotherapy machines, the linear accelerator produces a higher voltage, in the order of 4 to 50 MeV in clinical practice. This is accompanied by many benefits:

1. The rays penetrate deeper, thus delivering a higher dose to the tumour.
2. The skin dose is lower, so that there are fewer changes in the skin.
3. A smaller dose is absorbed in the bone, so that bone necrosis and pathological fractures are rare.
4. The beam is more sharp, so that the treatment area can be better defined.

Indications for radiotherapy. Radiotherapy may be used either for cure or palliation. *When it is used for cure, the doses and complications are much higher than those for palliative radiation. It is therefore essential that the stage of the tumour be established* in order to ensure that the disease is still localized and therefore curable by radiotherapy. A good example is Hodgkin's disease which is treated by aggressive, curative radiotherapy for stages I, II, and possibly III without organ involvement other than the spleen. If other organs are involved systemic chemotherapy is indicated. *Thus, the importance of careful clinical examination and staging cannot be over-emphasized.*

Radiotherapy can relieve symptoms such as pain, haemorrhage, dysphagia and spinal cord compression.

Combined radiotherapy and surgery. Radiotherapy is a local adjunct to surgery for treating many locally advanced neoplasms. *Preoperative radiotherapy* often improves cure rates in cancers of the larynx, oesophagus, bladder and uterus. It can sometimes convert an inoperable tumour into an operable one by decreasing both its size and its fixity to the surrounding structures. *Postoperative radiotherapy* confers benefit in lung carcinoma, seminoma and Wilms' tumour. When the margin of normal tissue is inadequate or it is felt that further surgery would be excessively mutilating, postoperative radiation therapy is indicated.

CHEMOTHERAPY

During the last few decades the chemotherapy of cancer has achieved considerable importance. In the case of some cancers, e.g. lymphomas, chemotherapy is used on its own as the method of treatment. In other tumours it is administered as an adjunct after surgery, and greatly improves the cure rates. In the beginning chemotherapy was used in an attempt to cure macrometastatic disease. However dramatic responses were rare. Attention is therefore now directed more towards pre- and postoperative chemotherapy for presumed micrometastatic disease.

The importance of recognition as foreign. In antimicrobial therapy for bacterial infections, after the antibiotics have killed the bacteria or arrested their proliferation, the host antibodies and immune cells eliminate the remaining viable bacteria. In this activity they are greatly helped by the fact that they recognize the bacteria as foreign. On the other hand, tumours arise from normal cells through mutations that usually do not alter the cell surface. Therefore, even after significant cell kill by cytotoxic chemotherapy, *the host does not recognize the remaining few viable tumour cells as foreign*, allowing the regrowth of tumours. This makes the chemotherapy of tumours much more difficult than the treatment of infections.

Most antineoplastic drugs affect either enzymes or substrates of enzymes systems. In most cases the effects relate to deoxyribonucleic acid *(DNA) synthesis:*

Table 1 Common chemotherapeutic agents.

Class	Type	Action	Example
Alkylating agents	Non-cell cycle-specific	Contribute unstable alkyl group to cross-link nucleic acids	Cyclophosphamide Cisplatin
Antibiotics	"	Interfere with synthesis of nucleic acids	Actinomycin D Doxorubicin
Plant alkaloids	Phase-specific	Bind microtubules and cause arrest in metaphase	Vincristine Vinblastine Etoposide
Antimetabolites	"	Interfere with DNA and RNA synthesis	Methotrexate 6-Mercaptopurine

1. Drugs which act by *inhibiting enzymes of nucleic acid synthesis* are called *antimetabolites,* e.g. methotrexate and 5-fluorouracil. They lead to the synthesis of abnormal DNA due to:

i. The inclusion of an abnormal building block in the DNA molecule, or

ii. The disruption of DNA synthesis due to the lack of an essential building block.

2. Drugs *acting on substrates* include the following:

i. *Alkylating agents* e.g. chlorambucil and cyclophosphamide. They substitute an alkyl group for the hydrogen atoms of DNA, thus interfering with DNA replication.

ii. A second group of drugs acting on substrates are certain *antibiotics*, e.g. actinomycin D and adriamycin. They form stable complexes with DNA, thereby inhibiting the synthesis of DNA and RNA.

Necessity of repeated courses of chemotherapy. Antitumour drugs cannot kill all cancer cells at any given exposure; they kill a variable fraction of cells, from a few upto 99.99%. Therefore, treatment must be repeated many times in order to achieve control. Thus every treatment regimen commonly consists of a number of 4-week courses, and not just one course.

The target of chemotherapeutic drugs is the tumour stem cell. Complete destruction of all tumour stem cells is essential to effect a cure. Drugs generally kill *nearly* all cells, but not all cells. A 1-cm tumour contains about 10^9 cells and even a 99.999 percent kill will leave behind 10^4 viable tumour cells and fail to cure the tumour. Therefore the larger the tumour the less easy it is to obtain cure. Thus the so-called complete clinical response, defined as the disappearance of all measurable disease, is often followed by recurrent disease, as millions of viable but undetectable and proliferating cells are still present.

Tumour growth rates are highest when the tumour mass is small. Therefore small volume disease is more responsive to drugs acting against proliferating cells, and provides the rational basis for adjuvant chemotherapy.

Timing of chemotherapy. Maximum cell kill is achieved by giving the highest tolerated dose over the shortest possible time. The interval between doses depends on the pattern of toxicity to normal tissues. For most drugs with bone marrow toxicity, leukopenia and thrombocytopenia become evident by about day 9 and are most marked by day 16. Recovery then commences and is nearly complete by day 28. This provides the rationale for the 28-day cycle of marrow suppressive agents.

Multidrug therapy. When a number of drugs are combined in the chemotherapy of cancer, the results are considerably improved. In such cases the cytotoxic effects of the different drug are summated, but the side effects are not. Treatment with as many as 5 drugs is used in the case of some cancers, with great benefit. Careful selection of drugs with complementary actions and non-overlapping toxicities is essential to avoid life-threatening injury to normal tissues.

Which drugs to combine? Some cytotoxic drugs affect particular phases of cell division, others act independently of the cell cycle. Drug combinations can benefit from the complementary effects of phase-specific agents on rapidly dividing cells, and non-cell cycle-specific drugs on all cells. Of the major classes of chemotherapeutic agents, alkylating agents and antibiotics are non-cell cycle-specific, while antimetabolites and plant alkaloids are phase-specific (Table 1).

Multidrug resistance. A tumour may be found to be resistant to several unrelated drugs. Sometimes this is due to the presence of a 'multidrug resistance gene' (*mdr* gene). The protein produced by this gene is P-glycoprotein. High levels of this protein are found in the lumina of the gastrointestinal tract, liver and kidney. The normal function of this substance is the ejection of environmental toxins from the body. This protein treats some cytotoxic drugs similarly. It ejects several drugs, including vincristine, actinomycin D and etoposide, from the target host cell.

If the action of this protein could be prevented, it would help greatly. It so happens that this protein can be blocked by calcium channel blockers like verapamil; these drugs are therefore currently being studied in this connection. At the same time, antibodies against P-glycoprotein have been prepared and are being investigated.

Applications of chemotherapy. Chemotherapy may be used independently, or before or after surgery or radiotherapy.

Induction chemotherapy. Here chemotherapy is used as the sole form of treatment, usually for multiple sites of metastatic disease, where local-regional treatment by surgery or radiation would not address the systemic illness. If the patient fails to respond, a change to another agent or modality may be considered.

Adjuvant chemotherapy. This describes the use of systemic or regional chemotherapy after local-regional tumour ablation by surgery or radiotherapy. *All adjuvant chemotherapy is the treatment of presumed micrometastases.* This kind of treatment is given only to patients considered to be at moderate-to-high risk of local or distant recurrence. A limited but intensive duration of therapy is usually employed, as any benefit against micrometastases is likely to occur during the first few courses.

Neoadjuvant (primary) chemotherapy. Here primary chemotherapy is used for different solid tumours before surgery. Examples include tumours of the breast, gastrointestinal and paediatric carcinomas, localized lymphomas and sarcomas. The method has obvious attractions:

1. Locally advanced tumours may be down-staged before operation.
2. Tumour responsiveness can be determined while gross tumour is still present, and can guide postoperative chemotherapy; if the response is poor, other methods can be used.
3. Possible micrometastases are treated immediately, instead of after several weeks' delay due to surgery or radiotherapy.

However, the method also has important drawbacks:

1. If chemotherapy produces its effect on the tissues, it may cause confusion in the pathological staging of resected tissues, complicating future treatment decisions and prognosis.
2. If there is no response, local-regional treatment of the tumour may be delayed.
3. If the tumour progresses despite chemotherapy, a safe resection may become impossible.

IMMUNOTHERAPY

The biochemical and subcellular constituents of both normal and cancer cells are similar. Hence any treatment, e.g. radiotherapy or chemotherapy, designed to inhibit the proliferation of cancer cells also inhibits the function of normal cells. If the attack could be directed against only those cells possessing tumour antigens while sparing normal cells, it would specifically kill more tumour cells than any other known method of treatment. Immunotherapy achieves precisely this goal. This is a recently introduced form of treatment which *depends upon the antigenic difference between neoplastic and normal cells* for its therapeutic effect.

Immunotherapy depends upon host defences. These can destroy small numbers of cancer cells, but are ineffective when the number of cells is large. Thus it is most useful for the treatment of *subclinical* microscopic metastases following surgery, radiotherapy or chemotherapy, as also for disease in the earlier stages, for the following reasons:

1. The immune response is specific, and thus it reaches small numbers of cancer cells like no other method can.
2. Patients with early disease have intact immune systems and are therefore more likely to respond.

When immunotherapy is used in clinical practice, either antitumour sera or lymphocytes from an immunized donor are employed. This method of treatment appears to have great potential, but as it is in its infancy, at present its value is limited and its use confined to a few centres.

Gene therapy. Work is proceeding on introducing genes capable of producing cytokines (e.g. tumour necrosis factor) into tumour-infiltrating lymphocytes. These lymphocytes would then ensure a high concentration of the cytokine at the tumour site to maximize tumour cell killing, while sparing the host tissues of the harmful effects of high-dose systemic cytokine.

COMBINED MODALITY THERAPY

When a number of methods of treatment of cancer are combined, the results are often superior to those obtained by the use of a single method. For example, if Wilms' tumour is treated by surgery alone, the cure rate is only about 35%; when radiation and chemotherapy are added to surgery, as many as 75% of patients are cured.

Management of distant metastases. *The lungs and pleura* are the most common sites of metastases. A standard chest x-ray is the best screening test, suspicious metastases being evaluated by CT scan or tomograms. Pulmonary metastases are generally asymptomatic, but sooner or later symptoms arise. Resection should be considered only if there are no metastases at other sites, if the primary tumour has been controlled, and if the potential for complete resection exists. Pleural effusions are usually associated with a short survival time. If symptomatic, they can be dealt with by aspiration.

Liver metastases are very common, again with few symptoms. They are shown up on ultrasound or CT scans. If they are multiple, biopsy is not required to confirm the diagnosis. In most cases surgical excision is not beneficial and chemotherapy is the treatment of choice. However, patients with isolated liver metastases from colorectal cancer may benefit from resection.

Bone metastases are common in advanced breast or prostate cancer. They lie in the medullary canal and destroy bone, with little new bone formation, except cases with prostate cancer. The best screening test is the radionuclide bone scan, but as the findings are non-specific, they should be correlated with x-rays to distinguish between benign and malignant causes. In non-weight-bearing bones, irradiation relieves the pain. In weight-bearing bones, if there is cortical destruction, prophylactic intramedullary nailing should be carried out, followed by radiotherapy.

In *brain* metastases headache and mental deficits are the common symptoms. CT scan shows up the metastases clearly, and MRI gives an even better picture. Steroids, specially dexamethasone, are the mainstay of treatment, by reducing oedema around the tumour and relieving symptoms. In the case of a solitary, surgically accessible metastasis, resection followed by cranial irradiation is the treatment of choice.

CANCER PAIN

Advanced, infiltrating cancer produces a great deal of pain and distress. A patient suffering thus needs all the support and sympathy the doctor can give him, apart from the analgesics and other drugs that are administered to him. In the terminal stages of cancer one should not be miserly in respect of the use of analgesics and narcotics.

Cancer pain. Oral codeine and morphine are the most practical, and should be available. Cancer pain is persistent, and often gets worse with the passage of time. It is felt more intensely if the patient is lonely and is a highly emotion-laden subject. The most common causes of cancer pain include bone metastases, nerve compression, and visceral distension.

Treatment includes the following measures:

1. Treat the disease: in this respect, radiotherapy is most effective.
2. Raise the pain threshold.
3. Distract the patient, e.g. by entertainment, prayer, etc.
4. Divide the nerve pathway, by dividing the coeliac plexus by an injection of alcohol, or by dividing the spino-thalamic tracts after laminectomy.

For the relief of pain due to cancer, increasingly strong *analgesic* agents can be tried, and the one selected which gives effective pain relief. In this respect, the concept of a 'ladder' is useful:

i. At the lowest rung of the ladder non-opioids are employed, e.g. aspirin and paracetamol.

ii. If pain persists in spite of these agents, weak opioids, e.g. codeine, may be used, either alone or in combination with non-opioids.

iii. If these agents also fail to control the pain, strong opioids, e.g. morphine, may be listed into service. For cancer pain, morphine is best administered orally. It is usual to start with a dose of 10 mg every 4 hours, and to increase it gradually until pain control is achieved.

The above drugs are often used along with 'adjuvants', e.g. antiemetics.

Rehabilitation. The clinician should be concerned not only with eradication of the disease but also with reconstruction of any loss of symmetry or contour of the body and full return of function.

Counselling. Most patients take an active part in decision-making about their illness; others need more guidance and support. Sympathetic listening and discussion reassures the patient. Sufficient time should be available to the clinician to discuss all aspects of the patient's illness and to advise him about the best course to be followed. This should be the practice not only in cases of cancer but in all major illnesses.

Should the patient suffering from cancer be told the truth? A great deal depends upon his personality and level of education. It is usually better to tell the patient, though in a gentle and optimistic manner. When a mutilating operation has to be carried out for the cancer, e.g. an amputation or a mastectomy, it is unreasonable to assume that the patient will agree to the operation unless he is told that he has cancer. Finally, the patient must never have the feeling that his medical attendants have deserted him. Moral as well as therapeutic support must be continued till the very end of any illness, whether due to cancer, or from any other cause.

Cancer prevention. Surgical removal of tissue may occasionally be justified for cancer prevention alone. For example, lobular carcinoma of the breast sometimes arises in the opposite breast also. If a patient with such a cancer also has a family history of breast cancer, she would be a fit candidate for prophylactic contralateral mastectomy.

Prognosis. Predicting the future course of a cancer is a difficult matter. However, a number of factors are important in determining prognosis. These include the site of origin, the stage of disease, the histology, the host immune factors, the age of the patient, and the centre where his treatment is carried out.

Soft tissue sarcomas

These tumours are discussed here as the chapters in Part II of the book are organ-specific, while these tumours are not confined to any one organ.

Soft tissue sarcomas can arise anywhere in the body and usually present as painless lumps. When they arise in the retroperitoneum or deep in the thigh they may be quite large before they are noticed. The larger and more rapidly growing the mass the more likely it is to be a sarcoma. This diagnosis should be considered for any mass that lies under the deep fascia. The misleading feature of soft tissue sarcomas is their 'benign' presentation that induces a false sense of security.

Diagnosis. Whenever a soft tissue sarcoma is suspected a biopsy specimen must be obtained. *Fine needle aspiration* indicates a malignancy but cannot help classify and grade it. Even with a core-needle biopsy the specimen consists of a thin core of tissue and this hinders an accurate diagnosis and grading. *Incision biopsy* is therefore the technique of choice. General anaesthesia is preferable as most of these tumours lie under the deep fascia.

Staging. Accurate TNM staging of these tumours requires careful physical examination followed by CT or MRI imaging. The risk of distant metastases increases with increasing size and more advanced grade of the tumour, from 0% for a grade 1 tumour of any size to 83% for a grade 2 or 3 tumour larger than 20 cm. The search for metastases is focussed on the lungs and requires a CT scan of the chest.

Types. *Rhabdomyosarcomas* are rare, although they are the most common soft tissue sarcomas in children under 15 years of age. If all tumour can be removed with minimal morbidity, resection followed by adjuvant chemotherapy gives excellent control, radiation being reserved for those cases where it has not been possible to resect the tumour with wide margins. *Liposarcomas* may be multicentric. They may be quite large, and commonly arise in the proximal part of an extremity or the retroperitoneum. They may regress quite rapidly following radiotherapy. Tumours that would have been classified in the past as fibrosarcomas or pleomorphic rhabdomyosarcomas are now grouped together as *malignant fibrous histiocytomas*. This diagnosis implies a high-grade sarcoma that lacks specific features of differentiation. *Leiomyosarcomas* can arise from the walls of blood vessels anywhere in the body, apart from their origin in the gastrointestinal and genitourinary tracts.

Neurofibrosarcomas often arise in patients with von Recklinghausen's disease, about 15% of whom develop sarcomas. *Angiosarcomas* are usually high-grade and behave aggressively. *Lymhangiosarcoma* arises in an oedematous extremity. It is often diffuse, and amputation is required for its control. *Kaposi's sarcoma* consists of multiple pigmented sarcoma nodules. This tumour occurs in nearly half of male homosexuals with AIDS. It is also seen in transplant patients who are receiving immunotherapy.

Treatment. ***Surgery.*** The goal of treatment is to eliminate the primary tumour as well as any metastatic disease. Local control of soft tissue sarcoma requires resection with a generous margin of apparently normal tissue. For low-grade tumours this may be as little as 1 cm of clear margin; for high-grade tumours 4 cm. Such margins cannot be provided in all tumours; in such cases amputation is required.

Radiation. This may be combined with surgery. Radiation is used to eliminate subclinical extensions of tumour into surrounding tissues; this is followed by resection of gross tumour, thus sparing adjacent major nerves and vessels.

Combined treatment. Chemotherapy followed by limited surgical resection and irradiation results in excellent local control while sparing the extremity.

15 Transplantation

Transplantation of entire organs is one of the most impressive advances in the field of surgery. However, before this stage could be reached, scientific progress spread over many fields and many decades was required. During the first few decades of this century sufficiently fine suture materials were produced, and techniques of anastomosis of arteries and veins were perfected. However, some very important problems remained to be solved before whole organs like the kidney or the heart could be transplanted.

Firstly, it was necessary that after removal from the cadaver and before being transplanted, the organ should not suffer such damage as would affect its function or its viability in the recipient's body. For this purpose methods were devised by which the organ could be *perfused* with a physiological solution e.g. plasma at low temperatures. The cooling greatly reduced its metabolic needs, while the plasma contained most of the nutrients, including fatty acids, required for its metabolic activity. If the plasma was passed through a membrane oxygenator, oxygen could also be supplied.

Secondly, it was necessary to ensure that once the organ was transplanted it was not rejected by the recipient's body through an antigen-antibody reaction. For this purpose such methods had to be devised which could suppress the immune response to the transplant (*immunosuppression*).

Thirdly, in the case of the heart it was essential that during the period between removal of the patient's diseased heart and its replacement by the new heart the circulation be carried out artificially. Therefore heart transplantation could only be attempted when *heart-lung machines* had not only been developed but their use had become commonplace.

ORGAN PRESERVATION

Graft damage must be minimized from the time the organ is removed from the donor to the time it is implanted into the recipient, i.e.:

1. While the graft is still within the donor in preparation for graft procurement.
2. During removal, storage and transport of the graft.
3. During the transplantation operation.

Many different measures help in organ preservation. Cooling from 37°C to 0°C, by reducing the metabolic rate, extends the storage time of most organs from 1 to 2 hours to about 12 hours. The large-molecule and impermeant sucrose provides osmotic force to oppose cellular oedema. Phosphate provides a buffer to counter intracellular acidosis. *Continuous cold perfusion* combines all these benefits: hypothermia, continuous buffering, continuous provision of oxygen and nutrients, and continuous washout of accumulating toxic metabolites.

If during storage the organ could be treated to deplete it of antigen presenting cells, this could dramatically improve results and would be a major advance in the future.

PREVENTION OF REJECTION

The most important problem in organ transplantation is not the surgical problem of removing the organ and joining the arteries, veins, and excretory ducts of the donor organ to the vessels of the recipient. The most difficult matter is to ensure that the foreign proteins introduced into the recipient's body in the form of the donor organ are not rejected. Before methods could be devised by which rejection of transplants could be prevented or suppressed, it was necessary to understand the process of rejection.

The ideal transplant is one where there is no antigenic difference between the donor and the recipient. If the tissues of the transplanted organ are 'foreign' to the recipient they will elicit an antigen-antibody response and the organ will be rejected. The strongest transplantation antigen is expressed in a single chromosomal region called the major histocompatibility complex (MHC), which in human beings is located on chromosome 6. Transplantation antigens were first investigated on leucocytes and were therefore named human leucocyte antigens (HLA).

The less antigenic the graft the less the host will react against it. When the donor and recipient are identical twins there is no antigenic difference and the tissues are accepted. If they are siblings or if a parent is the donor there is a greater likelihood of antigen-sharing between donor and recipient than when an unrelated donor is used.

Several methods have been developed for *demonstrating antigenic similarities* between donor and recipient, so that donor and recipient pairs which are relatively histocompatible may be selected. This lessens the need for large doses of immunosuppressive drugs and increases the likelihood of a successful outcome. The common methods are *leucocyte typing* and *mixed leucocyte culture*.

The role of the small lymphocyte. Mature lymphocytes lie in a state of immunological readiness. The small lymphocyte can recognize whether or not a molecule is foreign and can react to it. It does so by producing antibodies that can react with the antigen, and can recruit other mediators of the immune response. In addition, lymphocytes carry immunologic memory. The most striking feature of the immune response is its specificity. For each unique stimulus a distinctive population of antibodies or immune cells is elicited.

Graft destruction. The recognition of antigens by sensitized cells or antibodies marks the beginning of the active disposal of the foreign graft. However, the reaction of an antibody with a graft will not by itself destroy the graft. The recognition merely triggers the activation of several cascading enzyme systems, which include the complement pathway. The process of allograft rejection thus has two phases. In the first phase the foreign material is recognized as such. This process is immunologically specific, and is called the *recognition* phase. The second phase consists of the actual process of rejection, which is greatly enhanced or amplified in the presence of complement. This process is immunologically non-specific, and is called the *amplification* phase.

When an unsensitized patient is allografted, the first change is perivascular infiltration of round cells, followed by macrophages. Antibody and complement are deposited in the area of the capillaries, and the lymphocytes produce immunoglobulins. Thus both recognition molecules (antibodies) and sensitized cells (lymphocytes, etc.) are present. On recognizing the foreign tissue, sensitized cells release mediators of inflammation and cell damage. Complement is fixed, producing chemotactic factors and finally cellular damage. Capillary permeability is increased by anaphylotoxins and kinins. Damaged cells release additional compounds that attract polymorphonuclear leucocytes. These release vasoactive amines (histamine and serotonin) and other factors increasing vascular permeability. The small vessels become plugged with fibrin and platelets. The intima and media of vessels is thickened, and the lumen narrowed as a result. These changes reduce perfusion and prevent function.

The myocardial cell of the transplanted heart, the tubular cell of the kidney, and the acinar and islet cells of the pancreas are highly specialized structures which require an abundant supply of oxygen. If destroyed, they cannot be replaced by further cell division. Therefore, compromise of oxygen supply by endothelial and medial hypertrophy, intravascular platelet aggregation, and interstitial oedema result in their atrophy and death, with replacement by fibrous tissue.

IMMUNOSUPPRESSION

If an allograft is to be successful one must make sure that the rejection response described above will be suppressed. In theory many different methods can be employed towards this end. However, in practice the common methods depend upon destroying the immunocompetent cells and inhibiting their differentiation and proliferation. At the same time, to be most effective immunosuppression must be commenced *before* the time of transplantation, because once the immune response is under way it is more difficult to suppress it.

IMMUNOSUPPRESSIVE AGENTS

Immunosuppressive therapy plays a very important role in organ transplantation by preventing rejection of grafts. The important agents in use include antiproliferative agents, cyclosporin and corticosteroids.

Antiproliferative agents. Most of the commonly used immunosuppressive agents have been borrowed from cancer chemotherapy for their antiproliferative activity. They inhibit the full expression of the immune response by preventing the differentiation and division of the immunocompetent lymphocyte after it encounters the antigen.

Antiproliferative agents fall into two broad categories. The first type, the antimetabolites, structurally resemble needed metabolites; the second type, consisting of alkylating agents and toxic antibiotics, combine with certain cellular components, such as DNA, and thereby interfere with cell function.

Antimetabolites. These are structurally similar to the normal cell metabolites, e.g. purine, pyrimidine and folic acid. They get incorporated during synthesis to produce faulty molecules. The purine analogue *azathioprine* has been the most widely used immunosuppressive drug in organ transplantation. Its toxicity is due to bone marrow suppression leading to leucopenia. The folic acid antagonist *methotrexate* prevents the conversion of folic acid to tetrahydrofolic acid, a step which is necessary for the synthesis of DNA, RNA and certain coenzymes. It has been used in bone marrow transplantation but not much in kidney transplants.

Alkylating agents. The usefulness of alkylating agents like *nitrogen mustard* and *cyclophosphamide* is limited by their toxicity. Even so, cyclophosphamide has been used in kidney transplants when liver toxicity prohibited the use of azathioprine.

Antibiotics. The immunosuppressive antibiotics include *actinomycin D* and *mitomycin C*. However, none of these is clinically useful as an immunosuppressive agent for transplantation.

X-rays. Total body irradiation has not been used much in transplantation because the toxicity is too high. It is utilized only to reduce the immune reactivity of patients before bone marrow transplantation. The toxicity of total body irradiation is predictable. The rapidly multiplying cells of the skin and gastrointestinal tract are affected most and nausea, vomiting, diarrhoea and skin changes occur. Late problems also occur due to damage to the cellular genetic apparatus: growth retardation, sterility, cataracts and a higher incidence of cancer.

Cyclosporin. Cyclosporin represents an entirely different class of immunosuppressive agents. It selectively inhibits the activity of T lymphocytes, leading to inhibition of IL-2 production. It is not antiproliferative, and therefore it does not suppress the bone marrow. *This lack of myelosuppression is a major advance over other immunosuppressants.* It is therefore one of the most frequently used immunosuppressive agents, and its use made liver and heart transplantation feasible. In combination with modest doses of prednisolone and/or azathioprine, it provides effective control of graft rejection with fewer side effects. Stopping the drug permits rejection to proceed again, so that it does not lead to permanent tolerance.

Specially in liver transplants FK 506, a macrolide antibiotic, has given results as good or better than cyclosporin.

Corticosteroids. These are the immunosuppressants which have been most often used in clinical practice. Glucocorticoids have many anti-inflammatory actions, which make them potent immunosuppressants. Steroids cross the cell membrane and bind to specific receptors in the cytoplasm of most cells, including lymphocytes. The steroid-receptor complex then enters the nucleus and interacts with DNA. In lymphocytes the synthesis of DNA, RNA and proteins is inhibited, with degeneration and lysis of lymphocytes, specially of T cells. Within a few hours of administration of steroids a profound fall in the blood lymphocyte count occurs. Furthermore, the ability of macrophages to respond to lymphocyte-derived signals is blocked by steroids. Steroids alone cannot prevent allograft rejection, but along with other compounds, they help in preventing and reversing rejection reactions.

Side effects of steroid therapy include a cushingoid appearance, hypertension, weight gain, peptic ulcers and gastrointestinal bleeding, personality changes, cataract formation, diabetes, pancreatitis and osteoporosis. Transplantation will be greatly facilitated when more specific immunosuppressants are developed and the present steroid dosages can be reduced.

Monoclonal antibodies. The rapid development of monoclonal antibodies recognizing different cell markers on lymphocytes is making immunosuppression increasingly specific and precise. Already OKT3, a monoclonal antibody against T cells, is being used to treat steroid-resistant rejection.

The introduction of *multimodal therapy* using a combination of drugs which act synergistically allows maximum immunosuppression with a minimum of side effects, because lower doses of each drug are required.

Complications of immunosuppression. Immunosuppression is not obtained without paying a significant price in terms of side effects. Infection and malignancy are the most frequent complications encountered with the use of non-specific immunosuppressive agents.

Infection. Transplant recipients who receive immunosuppression encounter a greatly increased incidence of infection, which remains the most common cause of mortality. Most deaths used to be due to invasive infections. These have been controlled by antibiotics. Nowadays most infections are caused by opportunistic pathogens, including fungi, protozoa and viruses, the latter being specially common among kidney transplant patients.

Candida albicans and *Aspergillus* species are the most common *fungi* encountered in transplant patients. The latter produces upper lobe pulmonary cavities. The protozoan *Pneumocystis carinii* is also a frequent cause of pulmonary infection, producing an alveolar infiltrate with severe dyspnoea and cyanosis. However, it is seen less often since the use of prophylactic trimethoprim and sulfamethoxazole in transplant recipients.

Among the *viruses,* cytomegalovirus (CMV) and Epstein-Barr virus (EBV) commonly infect transplant patients. CMV is the most important virus infection seen in immunosuppressed transplant patients. The virus itself produces severe immunosuppression, rendering the patient susceptible to bacterial and fungal opportunists. The prophylactic use of acyclovir has caused a significant reduction in the incidence of viral infections.

Prevention of infection. The following measures help reduce the incidence of severe infections:

1. Sources of infection should be sought by routine preoperative cultures and eliminated.
2. Organs should be obtained from well-matched cadavers as far as possible.
3. If the white cell or platelet count drops, the dose of azathioprine should be reduced.

Isolation of the patient is probably ineffective and imposes much psychological stress; it is therefore not recommended.

Malignancy. Cancer is seen more often in transplant recipients than in the general population, but not so often as to contraindicate transplantation. Most cancers are either epithelial or lymphoid. The former, consisting of carcinomas of the cervix and lip and basal cell carcinomas, constitute about one half of these; B-cell lymphomas form the other half. Many lymphomas are not true cancers, as they are not monoclonal. They represent proliferation of B cells in response to EBV infection, and respond to treatment with acyclovir. The reasons for the high incidence of malignancies in immunosuppressed transplant patients probably include the following:

1. Surveillance by lymphocytes may be responsible for elimination of tumour cells as they arise; when lymphocyte function is suppressed, tumours arise.
2. Azathioprine may cause mutations in the cells of the patient.
3. Herpes virus, to which the immunosuppressed patient is susceptible, could induce these malignancies.

Other complications are mostly considered to be due to the use of steroids: Cushing's syndrome, cataracts, gastrointestinal bleeding, hypertension, pancreatitis, and avascular necrosis of the femoral heads.

TRANSPLANTATION OF INDIVIDUAL ORGANS

KIDNEY

Indications. All patients with end-stage renal failure are potential candidates for renal transplantation, there being no absolute contraindications. The patient should have a normal urinary outflow tract, and should not have active infection, severe malnutrition, disseminated malignancy or incapacitating systemic disease. As far as the actual cause of the irreversible renal failure is concerned:

1. Type I diabetes is the most common, accounting for 10 to 20 percent of all patients coming to transplantation.
2. *Chronic glomerulonephritis* and *chronic pyelonephritis* similarly provide many candidates for transplantation. Often patients do not present a classic history of either disease, and the kidney lesions are so far advanced by the time biopsy is performed that the pathogenesis is not definite. Rather than make a definitive diagnosis suggesting a cause it is best to regard such patients as having end-stage renal disease of unknown cause. Recently however, with the more widespread use of renal transplantation, patients are arriving at earlier stages of their illnesses.
3. A patient with a malignant *tumour* arising in a solitary kidney can be treated with nephrectomy followed by dialysis and later transplantation.
4. Among children, patients with *congenital obstructive disease* of the urinary tract with an advanced degree of renal damage are suitable candidates for renal transplantation.

The operation. A renal transplant has been a standard operation for many years now. Through an oblique incision in either iliac fossa, the muscles are divided in the line of the incision. The peritoneum is reflected upwards and medially to expose the iliac vessels. The renal vein is anastomosed end-to-side to the external iliac vein, and the renal

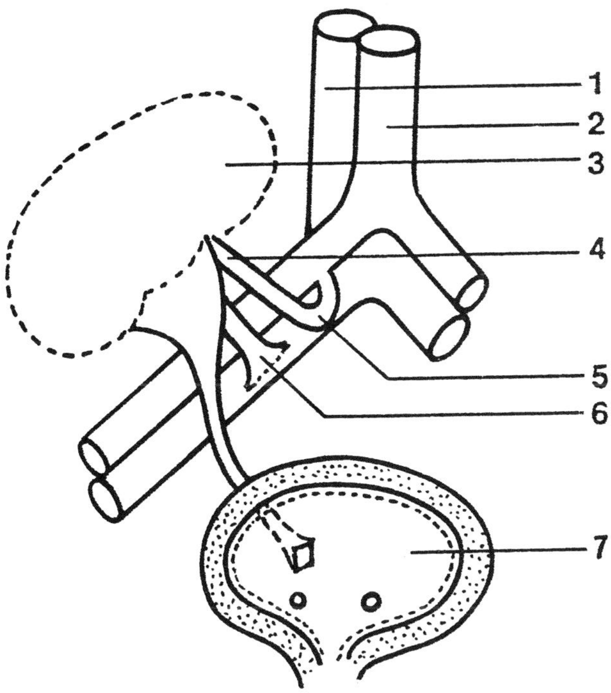

Fig. 1 Kidney transplant, recipient operation. 1. inferior vena cava, 2. aorta, 3. donor kidney, 4. renal artery, 5. internal iliac artery, 6. renal vein, 7. bladder.

artery end-to-end to the internal iliac artery. The ureter is implanted in the bladder through an anterior cystostomy with a submucosal tunnel (Fig. 1). The wound is usually closed without drainage, and an indwelling catheter left in the bladder for a few days.

A kidney from a living related donor always starts functioning immediately, that from a cadaver donor only about 70% of the time. During the first 24 hours the urine output varies from 5 to 25 liters, and requires careful replacement employing a central venous pressure line for 2 or 3 days.

Results. Most grafts carried out in the Western world are cadaveric, most of those in the underdeveloped countries are from living related donors. Around 80% of grafts are functioning at 1 year, and about 65% at 5 years. Patient survival rates are around 90% at 1 year and 80% at 5 years.

DIALYSIS

Besides renal transplantation, renal failure can also be managed by dialysis. Before we examine the relative indications of dialysis and transplant we shall briefly consider the essential principle underlying the process of dialysis.

In clinical practice dialysis is carried out by one of two methods, namely haemodialysis and peritoneal dialysis. The *principle* underlying these two different methods is basically similar. In both these procedures blood is circulated in such a way that only a semipermeable membrane separates it from a reservoir of fluid which has roughly the same composition as interstitial fluid. The blood of the anuric patient contains sodium, potassium, chloride and various waste products at concentrations higher than in normal extracellular fluid. Due to the osmotic gradient these substances move out to the reservoir, so that when equilibrium is attained the blood contains these electrolytes etc. at the same levels as the normal plasma or tissue fluid, i.e. it has got rid of the excess of waste products. As far as the actual set up is concerned, the two methods are very different from each other.

Haemodialysis. In haemodialysis blood is withdrawn through a cannula placed in an artery, e.g. the radial. It is pumped through coils of synthetic tubing which lie immersed in a reservoir of fluid with a composition resembling interstitial fluid. It is then returned to the body via a cannula passed into a vein, e.g. the basilic. The circulation of blood is continued for 2 or 3 hours, this period of time being sufficient for attaining a state of equilibrium. Such a session of dialysis is usually repeated every two or three days, either for the rest of the patient's life, or until a renal transplant is carried out. If haemodialysis is to be used for a prolonged period, the outer ends of the arterial and venous cannulae are joined together to form a small shunt, in order to avoid thrombosis in the cannulae. However, infections at the entrance sites of the cannulae cause problems from time to time.

Continuous haemofiltration. In *intermittent* haemodialysis, as described above, dialysis is carried out for a few hours every few days, the patient in between carrying on his normal social activities. With patients in critical care units such intermittent provision of haemofiltration is not necessary, and *continuous* haemofiltration can be carried out. Although haemodialysis removes certain solutes such as potassium more efficiently, haemofiltration causes less haemodynamic disturbance.

Peritoneal dialysis. In peritoneal dialysis a catheter with numerous holes in its distal half is mounted on a trocar and introduced into the peritoneal cavity through a small incision at the umbilicus. The trocar is removed and the catheter advanced so that its tip lies in the rectovesical or rectovaginal pouch. A couple of liters of dialysis fluid is now gravitated into the peritoneal cavity. It is left there for about an hour, after which it is siphoned out through the other limb of the Y-connection and discarded. The process is repeated over a period of 24 to 48 hours until the blood urea and creatinine levels fall to normal values. Unlike haemodialysis, the blood in peritoneal dialysis circulates not in synthetic tubing but in the vast capillary network lying under the visceral and parietal peritoneum. The semipermeable membrane is not the wall of the tubing but the vascular and peritoneal endothelia. And finally, the reservoir consists of the fluid which has been placed in the peritoneal cavity. But otherwise the principle underlying the two methods is the same.

Haemodialysis requires a very elaborate and expensive artificial kidney machine. On the other hand peritoneal dialysis requires only a catheter with trocar, some Y-tubing, and a number of bottles of dialysis fluid. Recently, catheters made of pure silicon are being left in more or less indefinitely, so that patients at home can have repeated peritoneal dialysis. The method is called *chronic ambulatory peritoneal dialysis.*

In the affluent communities peritoneal dialysis is gradually being replaced by haemofiltration.

Dialysis in reversible renal failure. Apart from their use in *end-stage* renal disease, both methods of dialysis are used in *reversible* renal failure. Some examples follow:

1. Acute anuria due to *simultaneous blockage of both ureters* by stones: in this condition dialysis is used for a few days to bring the serum creatinine level down to normal. When this has been achieved, the calculi are removed at operation. Once this has been carried out free drainage of urine is established, so that dialysis is no longer required.
2. A*cute tubular necrosis* due to drug toxicity, etc.: in this condition dialysis is continued for a few weeks in order to tide the patient over the time it takes for the kidney to recover from the effects of the tubular necrosis. Once the kidney has recovered, dialysis is no longer needed.
3. Acute renal failure in the *sepsis syndrome*, usually as a part of multiple organ system failure.

In the underdeveloped countries the use of peritoneal dialysis for the above two indications is eminently feasible, in view of the relatively modest cost of the equipment and bottles of fluid.

Indications for renal replacement therapy. The need for renal replacement therapy must be evaluated in each individual patient. Commonly, the following are considered threshold values: potassium > 6 mmol/l, blood urea > 40 mmol/l, and pH < 7.2. However, the overall clinical status needs to be considered. The aim of therapy is to remove uraemic toxins and maintain fluid, electrolyte and acid-base balance. In the patient with uncomplicated renal failure a plasma urea level below 30 mmol/l is generally considered acceptable. In the critically ill patient lower target values close to 20 mmol/l are preferred.

Transplant or dialysis? Renal transplantation is nowadays the treatment of choice for most patients with renal failure, haemodialysis and peritoneal dialysis serving as temporary substitutes. Even if renal transplantation is planned, usually the patient is kept on haemodialysis while the investigations and preparation for transplantation are proceeding. In the poorer communities kidney transplants sometimes cannot be used because of the exorbitant cost of the immunosuppressive agents, which are required thereafter for the rest of the patient's life.

When it is successful, transplantation provides a greater degree of rehabilitation to the uraemic patient than dialysis. The risk is also slightly greater because of the immunosuppression required indefinitely. Transplantation is superior to dialysis with respect both to quality of life and medical costs. In children growth is more active; similarly diabetics have fewer problems. Most patients who have had a transplant - even one that has failed - prefer life with a renal transplant to life on dialysis.

HEART

A few decades ago no one could have imagined that it will ever become possible to take out a living person's heart, replace it with another, and make it work. Because if Shylock had known it, he would not have insisted upon the heart as his chosen pound of flesh! Today, thousands of heart transplants are being done every year around the world, with 5 year survival rates of around 70%. At the same time, a high degree of rehabilitation is achieved in as many as 90% of the surviving patients in some centres.

Before a heart could be successfully transplanted, researchers had encountered and tackled the following technical problems:

1. They had developed a technique of resuscitation and preservation of the cadaver heart.
2. They had developed a surgical technique for the actual transplantation, consisting of anastomoses of the pulmonary artery, aorta and the atria.
3. They had demonstrated that the denervated heart would function adequately after operation.
4. They had devised methods of early detection and prevention of homograft rejection.

It was only after all the above hurdles had been overcome that the first heart transplants were attempted. The successes achieved upto date have been impressive.

Indications. A heart transplant is indicated only if the patient is suffering from terminal heart disease for which all alternative methods of treatment have been exhausted. Most patients have severe *coronary* disease with multiple infarctions and extensive loss of left ventricular myocardium. Another group includes patients with *cardiomyopathy* who do not respond satisfactorily to medical therapy. Valvular and congenital heart disease provide the remaining few patients.

Recipients are usually less than 60 years of age, although recently patients have been accepted for the operation upto the age of 70 years! The patient should not have irreversible systemic illness or active infection, and should be emotionally stable, so as to be able to comply with a rigid postoperative protocol of immunosuppressive drugs. The pulmonary vascular resistance should not be unduly elevated; if it is, a *heart-lung transplant* might be more suitable.

Recipient operation. After a median sternotomy the aorta and venae cavae are encircled and controlled. The patient is heparinized and cannulae placed into the superior and inferior venae cavae. The aorta is cannulated and cardiopulmonary bypass commenced. Systemic cooling to 26°C is initiated. An aortic cross clamp and snares are applied and the heart excised, dividing the aorta, pulmonary artery and the middle of the atria. The donor heart is placed in position and anastomoses carried out with running sutures successively of the left and then right atrium, aorta and finally pulmonary artery. The last-named is anastomosed with the heart beating, and is vented for about 20 minutes to allow reperfusion of the new heart, before weaning the patient from the cardiopulmonary bypass. The patient is resuscitated, with pressor support as necessary.

Complications. Rejection and infection are the most common complications, together accounting for about half the deaths in cardiac transplant recipients. After 1 year the incidence of both these complications decreases greatly. Rejection is managed by intravenous methylprednisolone and if necessary monoclonal antibodies; infection is controlled by the aggressive use of antibiotics. If rejection still persists, retransplantation should be considered.

Results. Cardiac transplantation is very effective in the treatment of end-stage cardiac failure, over 70% surviving at 5 years. The operation can no longer be considered experimental and should be offered to all appropriate candidates.

LIVER

Liver transplant has been successfully used in a large number of patients suffering from congenital and acquired disorders. The grafted liver may be placed in the normal anatomical position after total hepatectomy of the recipient (*orthotopic transplantation*). Alternatively, the donor organ is placed in an ectopic site *(heterotopic transplantation)*, usually with retention of the host's liver *(auxiliary transplantation)*. Most clinicians prefer orthotopic transplantation.

Indications. The indications for liver transplantation are the following:

In ***infants***, *biliary atresia* which is incorrectable surgically is the most common indication. If the initial Kasai portoenterostomy fails, the baby should be immediately considered for transplantation, as multiple attempts at revising biliary drainage compromise the likelihood of success of the transplant.

In ***later childhood***, inborn errors of metabolism, postnecrotic cirrhosis, and otherwise unresectable hepatic neoplasms provide the common indications. In children, the non-availability of suitable-sized donors has led to the development of *reduced-size liver transplants*, one lobe of the liver being used.

In ***adults***, the leading indication has been *postnecrotic cirrhosis*. Patients with high levels of hepatitis B antigens are at a higher risk of developing recurrence, and are often excluded from consideration for transplantation. On the other hand hepatic replacement for other conditions leading to end-stage cirrhosis, such as primary biliary cirrhosis, sclerosing cholangitis, and autoimmune hepatitis is highly successful. The recent trend is to carry out the operation early, instead of allowing the patient to deteriorate to the point of repeated gastrointestinal bleeding, malnutrition, sepsis and coma.

Patients with small-sized *primary carcinomas of the liver* with pre-existing cirrhosis, which precludes partial hepatic resection, should be offered hepatectomy and liver transplantation; 50% survive disease-free in the long term. *Acute liver failure* represents a difficult indication for liver transplantation. If stage III-IV encephalopathy has set in, the mortality rate will be forbiddingly high. To be successful, therefore, hepatic replacement should be carried out before stage IV coma is established.

Contraindications to liver transplantation include the following:

1. Widespread malignancy.
2. Concurrent disease seriously impairing survival.
3. Irreversible infection.
4. A high risk of recurrent disease in the organ to be transplanted.

At centres with considerable experience of liver transplantation, 5 year *survival* rates of over 60% are being obtained. Most deaths occur in the first 3 months after operation, due to early graft dysfunction or infection. Most of the surviving patients are adequately rehabilitated, 80% resuming their previous occupations. Some of the earlier patients have survived for over 20 years, and death in patients who survived over 5 years has occurred only rarely. This suggests that the prognosis of those expected to survive 5 years is excellent.

SMALL BOWEL

Improvements in total parenteral nutrition have significantly improved survival of patients with short-bowel or severe malabsorption syndromes. However, prospects remains poor for patients whose remaining bowel does not hypertrophy enough to allow at least partial enteral nutrition. The reasons are mainly two: recurrent infections at venous sites take their toll; and liver function progressively deteriorates from prolonged high-calorie intravenous feeding. The only viable alternative is replacement of the diseased or absent bowel by a functioning allograft.

Adult candidates include patients who have survived massive bowel resection for extensive Crohn's disease, vascular compromise or trauma. In children the short-gut syndrome commonly results from resection for extensive atresia, midgut volvulus or necrotizing enterocolitis. Three main problems make small bowel transplantation difficult: the allograft inevitably becomes colonized by microbes; huge numbers of immunocompetent donor lymphocytes are necessarily transplanted; and the incidence of thrombotic complications is high. A few transplants have succeeded in the short term. The procedure as yet is only to be considered in highly selected patients in whom all other options have been exhausted.

PANCREAS

In spite of the availability of insulin and oral hypoglycaemic agents, diabetics are 17 times more liable to kidney disease, 5 times to gangrene of the extremities, and twice as likely to develop heart disease, for the simple reason that the control of the blood sugar level is both inaccurate and intermittent. If control could be continuous as well as accurate, it would be a very great advance. Transplantation of whole pancreas or islets provides precisely that.

The major problem in pancreatic transplantation is difficulty in establishing drainage of the pancreatic duct. In the most popular technique the whole pancreas and the second part of the duodenum are taken from a cadaver. The superior mesenteric artery of the donor is anastomosed to the iliac artery of the patient, while the portal vein is joined to the recipient's inferior vena cava. The duodenum is anastomosed to the urinary bladder, so that the pancreatic juice is drained via the urinary tract (Fig. 2). One advantage of the technique lies in the ease with which urinary amylase levels can monitor the survival and function of the graft.

The immediate effect of successful pancreatic transplantation is dramatic. Within 24 hours the allograft provides a self-regulating source of insulin: the patient does not require any intra- or postoperative insulin. As far as long-term prospects are concerned, as many as 60% are still functioning at 3 years.

Pancreas and kidney transplants. Thousands of clinical pancreatic transplants have been performed, and an

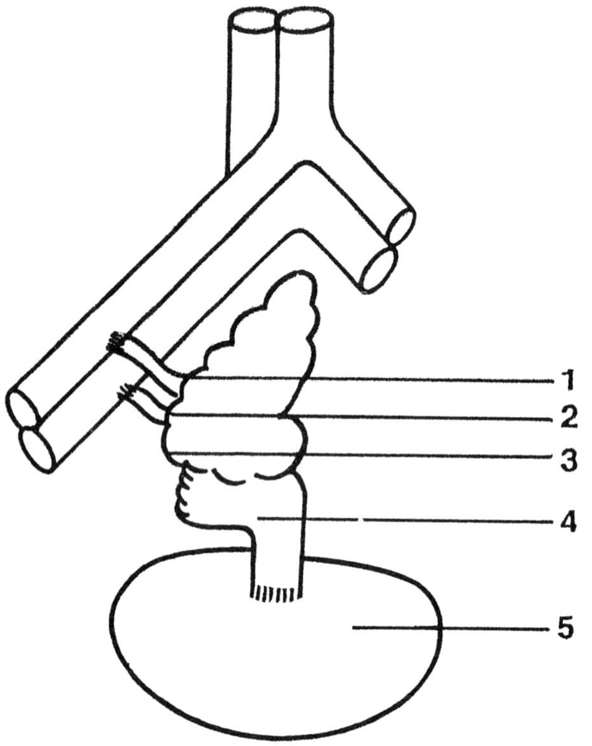

Fig. 2 Pancreas transplant, recipient operation. 1. arterial anastomosis, 2. venous anastomosis, 3. pancreas, 4. duodenum, 5. bladder.

International Human Transplant Registry is maintained, in order to pool together the experience gained world-wide. Most recipients have end-stage diabetic renal disease; therefore the kidney is also transplanted at the same operation. Combined pancreas and renal transplant should be carried out before renal function deteriorates to the stage of dependence on dialysis, because the restoration of normal glucose metabolism at this earlier stage of the disease will more effectively prevent microangiopathy. With the passage of time, pancreatic transplants are being carried out before advanced renal disease occurs.

Islet transplants. The results of transplantation of the vascularized pancreas now compare reasonably with those of other organ transplants. However:

1. To transplant an entire organ to cure a non-lethal condition when all that is required is a small fraction of the transplanted tissue does not sound proper.
2. Transplantation late in the disease does not reverse the complications of diabetes. And yet, a young diabetic cannot be expected to agree to transplantation with the necessary life-long immunosuppression.

It is therefore gratifying to note that it is not necessary to transplant the entire pancreas in order to cure diabetes; transplantation of pancreatic *islets* suffices. In this method the pancreas is mechanically disrupted and digested by enzymes, and the islets are separated. Isolated islets infused into the portal vein produce long-lasting control of diabetes in rats. This technique has been applied successfully to the autotransplantation of islets in patients who require total pancreatectomy for chronic painful pancreatitis, their own islets being used for the purpose. When it comes to transplantation from a human donor, rejection poses a problem. However, the evidence from animal experiments that islet tissue graft can prevent, halt, and even improve the vascular and neurological lesions of diabetes provides an incentive for research despite the difficulties.

CELLULAR TRANSPLANTATION

Cellular transplantation is a newly emerging specialty. Historically, bone marrow was the first successful cellular allograft. Grafting of pancreatic islets is now accepted as a clinical approach to the treatment of diabetes. Grafting of liver, muscle and nerve *cells* is the next likely field of research, with exciting possibilities in the treatment of hitherto incurable illnesses.

16 *Investigative procedures in surgery*

Upto the middle ages the only way a clinician could diagnose a patient's illness was by the use of his five senses, specially sight (inspection), touch (palpation and percussion), and hearing (auscultation). Compared to the medical worker of today he was at a very serious disadvantage. Great advances in the science of physics have changed all that during the last two centuries. These advances could not even be imagined in those days. In order to understand the rationale and concept of each advance it is best to see how each method evolved to its present state of refinement. To a greater degree than in the case of internal medicine, the surgeon depends upon endoscopic and imaging techniques rather than biochemical investigations. These techniques are therefore highlighted in the following pages.

ENDOSCOPIC TECHNIQUES

The electric bulb. Before the advent of electricity no reliable and accurate source of light was available for looking inside the various body cavities. The development of the electric bulb placed such a source at our disposal at the flick of a switch. Further, as smaller and smaller bulbs were crafted, these could be mounted on the tips of slim endoscopes, so that narrower and narrower body tubes could be illuminated and investigated. This led to the design first of *sigmoidoscopes,* and later of *oesophagoscopes* and *bronchoscopes,* of which the last-named have the narrowest lumen and require the smallest bulbs. However, these tiny bulbs frequently broke down, and this was a great nuisance.

Fibreoptics. The realization that fine, transparent synthetic fibres could transmit light though their substance led to great advances in endoscopic techniques. As these fibres were flexible, the endoscopes no longer needed to be rigid and could be passed more comfortably and for much longer distances. In fact the modern colonoscope can be passed all round the colon to the caecum. Secondly, as the light source could be kept outside, much larger and more powerful bulbs could be used. This not only led to greater intensity of illumination, but also made sure that the bulbs did not break down as frequently as in the past. As the endoscopes became finer, it became easy to swallow them for gastroduodenoscopy or bronchoscopy. Through the lumina of these endoscopes fine forceps could be passed for biopsy of lesions and for short procedures under diathermy. Catheters could also be passed up the bile duct and pancreatic duct for injection of radiopaque dyes for cholangiography and pancreatography respectively.

With these brilliantly lit endoscopes, the interior of the hollow viscus under investigation can be inspected by direct vision, leaving no doubt about the presence or absence of a suspected lesion. Similarly, the procedure of cystoscopy has benefited greatly from the introduction of fibreoptic cystoscopes.

Endoscopy. Modern endoscopes play an ever-increasing role in the diagnosis of surgical conditions. The common endoscopes used by surgeons include bronchoscopes, oesophagoscopes, gastroduodenoscopes, proctoscopes, sigmoidoscopes, colonoscopes, cystourethroscopes, and last but not least laparoscopes. The different types of endoscopic procedures are described in the appropriate chapters.

IMAGING TECHNIQUES

X-rays. Before the advent of x-rays the only way the human body could be examined was by inspecting or palpating it from outside, or by examining the blood or various excreta. The discovery of x-rays was one of the most important milestones in the history of medicine. It is difficult to imagine the thrill felt by Roentgen when he was able to take an x-ray picture of his own hand. What was concealed uptil now became revealed. Pathological processes in bones and joints could be elucidated without exposing them at operation. The lungs were now like an open book, and most pulmonary diseases could be diagnosed by a simple chest x-ray. Changes in the outline of the heart could indicate cardiac pathology. Urinary tract stones and opaque gallstones could be seen. The distribution of air bubbles in obstructed intestines could point to the site of obstruction. Soft tissue shadows of the kidney, etc. could provide valuable information. And so on and so forth.

Contrast media in radiography. Soon after the discovery of x-rays researchers thought of outlining the various body cavities by radiopaque media:

1. The first system to be explored was the *gastrointestinal tract,* and soon barium sulphate became accepted as the standard medium to outline it. Again it is not easy to imagine the excitement of those early workers when they found they could see the whole outline of the oesophagus (by a barium swallow), the stomach and intestines (by a barium meal follow-through), or the colon and rectum (by a barium enema). In any of these hollow tubes, a stricture, an ulcer, a tumour etc. could now be easily shown up.

2. Soon after this an opaque medium (a precursor of the modern day lipiodol) was prepared, suitable for introduction into the *bronchial tree.* Cases of bronchiectasis, tumours of bronchi, etc. could be investigated by this method.

3. Similarly, radiopaque dyes suitable for introduction into the *spinal theca* through a lumbar puncture (in myelography) were invented. The cause of compression of the spinal cord could now be detected with a fair degree of accuracy.

4. Next, such radiopaque dyes were prepared which could be safely injected *intravenously,* and which had the property of being excreted by the kidney into the urine (for intravenous urography) or by the liver into the bile (for intravenous cholangiography). The whole of the urinary

tract could now be outlined, showing up any stricture with dilatation above it, any diverticulum, the filling defect produced by any tumour or radiolucent stone, and any congenital anomaly of the urinary tract. Intravenous urography also indicated the function of each kidney.

5. Dyes suitable for injection into *arteries* (in arteriography) were next produced. Because a dye injected into an artery is quickly washed away, rapid-changing x-ray cassettes had to be produced before arteriography could be usefully employed.

Arteriography is used in two types of conditions:

1. In diseases of arteries, e.g. aneurysm, coarctation, atherosclerosis etc., to outline the artery itself.
2. Where a tumour is thought to be present which may be displacing the arteries to one side, or have a characteristic pattern of circulation in its mass. This application of arteriography is employed in many different parts of the body.

SECTIONAL IMAGES

Although x-rays provide good images, the x-ray tube is positioned on one side of the body while the film is on the other. In the x-ray picture the images of various structures lie on top of each other; the result is that the less opaque structures cannot be shown up.

If an image could be created where the structures in the body could be seen as if a section had been cut across the body, it would be a very major advance. The section of each structure would lie side by side with the other organs; there would be no overlap, and each viscus would be seen clearly.

In an attempt to obtain cross-sectional images, three different forms of energy have been used, namely:

1. Ultrasound waves (in ultrasonography).
2. X-rays (in computerized tomography i.e. CT scan).
3. Magnetic waves (in magnetic resonance imaging, i.e. MRI).

Ultrasonography. In this technique sound waves of a frequency higher than that which is suitable for hearing *(ultrasound* waves) are beamed at the selected part of the body. If they encounter an interface between two tissues of different density, some of the waves are reflected back in the form of *echoes,* which produce images on the screen.

If the waves come across a clear fluid, they pass right through it so that no echoes, and therefore no images, are produced and the area appears quite black on the screen. While passing through turbid fluids, and even more so when they encounter solids, some of the waves are reflected back and the area appears as a dark or light shade of grey, depending upon the number of echoes produced. If the waves come across a dense solid, such as a stone, they are all reflected back, so that a dark area appears on the screen on the far side of, i.e. behind, the stone. This area is called an *acoustic shadow,* and its presence confirms the presence of the stone (Fig. 1).

Air acts as a barrier to the passage of ultrasound waves. This has significance in at least two respects. Firstly, to avoid the layer of air between the probe and the patient's skin, a jelly-like material has to be smeared on the skin before the probe is moved over it. Secondly, the gas contained in the intestines usually prevents good visualization

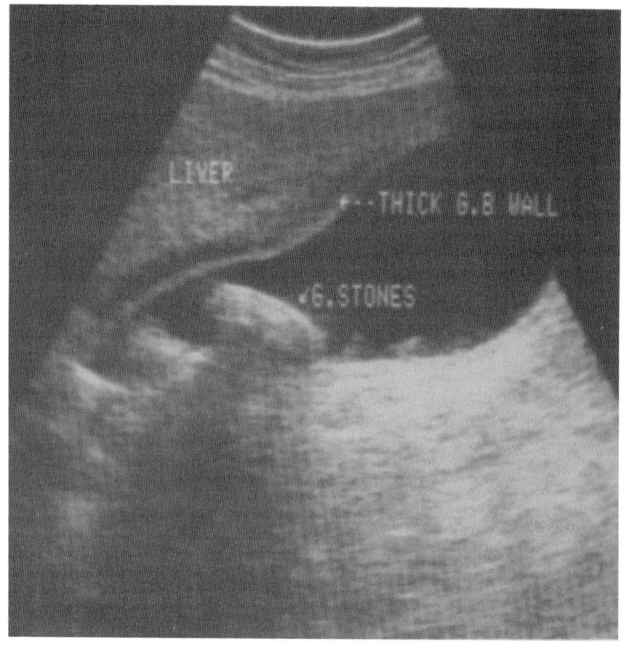

Fig. 1 Ultrasound picture of gallbladder showing gallstones, with acoustic shadows behind them. The thickness of the gallbladder wall can also be assessed.

of the pancreas and the lower end of the common bile duct, both of which lie behind the intestines.

Applications. The most common applications of ultrasound are to be seen in the gastrointestinal (GI) tract and the urinary tract. In the *GI tract,* conditions of the liver, gallbladder, spleen and pancreas lend themselves to elucidation by this technique. The intestines are not ideally suited to investigation by this method. However, dilated intestines and thickened walls of gut loops can be shown up, and can be interpreted in the light of the clinical findings.

In the case of the *urinary tract,* ultrasound examination has nearly replaced intravenous urography, except in respect of the following:

1. Ultrasonography cannot tell us anything about kidney function.
2. If a plastic repair on the renal pelvis i.e. a pyeloplasty is contemplated, intravenous pyelography gives a very clear picture of the anatomy of the pelvis and helps in planning the surgery.

Apart from the gastrointestinal and urinary tracts, cystic lesions in the thyroid and breast can be examined by the ultrasound probe. Similarly, in the newborn the open anterior fontanelle provides a window through which dilated ventricles can be visualized.

Ultrasound examination findings should be interpreted intelligently. This requires knowledge of basic anatomy, and of the changes produced by different diseases in the ultrasound pictures of the various organs. Recently the author came across an ultrasound report on a swelling of a testis. It stated that, as the swelling contained fluid, it was either a hydrocele or a meningocele! The finding of fluid in the swelling was correct; the interpretation was wide off the mark.

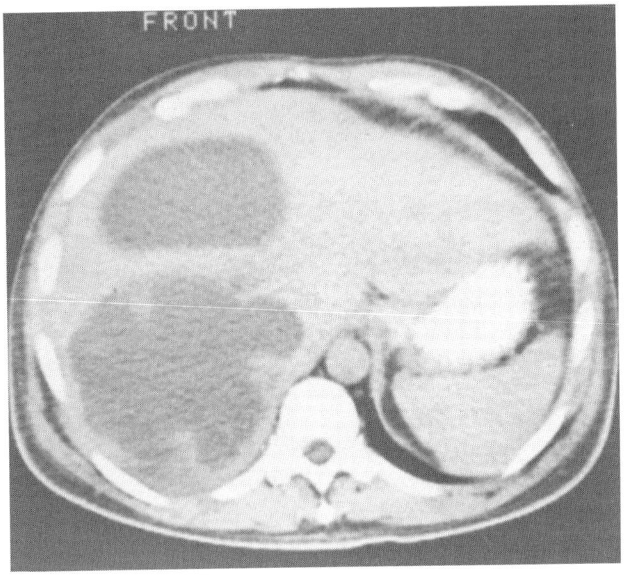

Fig. 2 CT scan through liver showing a large multilocular liver abscess. Note the transverse section of the vertebra, and the oblique sections of the ribs. In front of the vertebra lies the aorta, and behind it the mass of the erector spinae muscle. The spleen is seen at the back on the left side.

Computerized tomography (CT scan). Computerized tomography is a very major advance in the field of investigations. In this technique an x-ray tube rotates around the body in the transverse plane. During this process x-rays are beamed across the body from different angles and pictures taken. A computer synthesizes these different images to produce a single picture which makes it appear as if the body had been sectioned transversely and one was looking at the section from below (Fig. 2). A series of sections are taken at different thicknesses, such as 8 mm, 10 mm, and so on, according to the situation.

Applications. A CT scan can be used for most of the conditions for which ultrasonography is used. Further, it allows transverse sections to be taken at regular distances, allowing a standardized record of the lesion to be kept. Finally, whereas ultrasound waves cannot penetrate through the skull, the CT scan is one of the most useful methods of investigation of the cranial contents. However, it must be mentioned that CT scan is a very much more expensive method of investigation than ultrasonography. In other words the latter can be called the poor man's CT scan, and has great relevance in the poorer communities.

Magnetic resonance imaging (MRI). Magnetic resonance imaging is another new method of imaging in which 'sections' of the body can be obtained. The selected part of the body is placed in the field of a very powerful magnet. When the magnet is switched on, the protons in the body tissues get aligned according to the magnetic field. The magnet is now switched off. The protons return to their original positions and a signal is emitted, which results in the creation of the image.

MRI produces a picture with a sharper resolution than CT, specially in the case of the soft tissues. At the same time it allows 'sections' to be taken not only at right angles to the long axis of the body, but also in other planes, because there is no x-ray tube which has to rotate around the body. However, it is much more expensive than CT, which itself is a very costly method of investigation.

CT scan and MRI have completely revolutionized the process of imaging throughout the body. For example, before their advent carotid angiography, air encephalography, and myelography were the only imaging methods available for gaining information about the brain and spinal cord. All three were invasive and potentially dangerous investigations. CT and MRI have nearly replaced those techniques.

17 Modern surgical materials

Numerous advances in optics, metallurgy, plastics, etc., are continuing to make hospital equipment more and more efficient with each passing decade. Some illustrative examples follow.

Optics. The development of extremely fine transparent plastic fibres has made it possible to transmit light through bundles of these fibres. There are two benefits of this development. Firstly, one no longer requires a tiny and fragile light bulb to be mounted at the tip of an endoscope; the light source can take the form of a sturdy and powerful bulb, and its light can be conveyed along the fibres (*fibre-optics*). The intensity of light can thus be much greater than in the past. Secondly, as the fibres can be bent, we have flexible endoscopes. Not only can they be passed through tortuous tubes, like oesophagus and stomach, or colon, but their tips can be bent backwards through 180° to visualize every nook and corner of the viscus under investigation. This means that the lumina of the bronchi, the stomach and duodenum, as well as the whole colon, can be examined directly under excellent illumination, and with great clarity.

Metals. In the old days needle-holders could not hold the more delicate curved needles, as their crude jaws would crush them. Nowadays these jaws can be covered with a layer of tungsten carbide which is softer, and therefore more gentle than stainless steel; thus, the finer needles can be held more firmly yet delicately.

Plastics. A few decades ago only red rubber tubes were available. The rubber had a rough surface, and also caused a marked inflammatory reaction around it. Also, as the material was not very strong, the wall of the catheter had to be thick, so that the lumen was narrow and clogged easily. At the same time very fine tubes could not be made out of this rather brittle material.

Modern plastic materials have changed all that. The best materials are strong, so that fine tubes can be made from them. The wall can be thin, so that the bore can be made wider for a better flow of fluids. The surface can be very smooth, so that the lumen does not clog easily. The tube can be transparent, so that the flow of fluids through it can be monitored visually. Finally, when placed in the tissues the tubes induce very little reaction. Because of such properties these tubes can be used for much more refined procedures than in the past. These tubes made from man-made materials are making it possible to carry out more and more refined surgical procedures with their use. Similarly, sutures made from plastic materials are stronger, smoother, and less reaction-inducing than natural fibres.

SUTURES

Sutures are required to accurately appose the wound edges and to hold them together until the reunited tissue has acquired a sufficient degree of strength to support itself. However, as they are foreign bodies they irritate the tissues and increase the chances of development of infection. In this connection, the following characteristics of sutures are of special significance:

Thickness. About a century ago only crude suture materials were available. Three sizes of sutures were made, and were called sizes 1, 2 and 3. Later, when surgeons wanted to carry out more delicate suturing they started asking for finer materials. The thinner silk which was made was given the number zero. When even more fine sutures were produced they called them 2/0, 3/0 and so on until today some of the finest sutures are 10/0 or so. However, this numbering by zeroes was illogical and cumbersome, therefore recently the metric system of numbering has been introduced. Table 1 shows the equivalent numbers of the two systems. Students would be well advised to learn the metric system, as in the next many decades of their expected working life this system will be employed more commonly. The thicker the suture, the more foreign body is introduced into the tissues. Therefore, sutures should be selected at the finer end of the range. Modern synthetic sutures are generally stronger than the natural ones, so finer sizes can be used without sacrificing strength.

Number of filaments. Monofilament sutures cause less reaction than multifilament threads, because their smoother surface presents less of an area to the tissues. Monofilament sutures are also attractive because infection does not persist if it occurs; with multifilament sutures bacteria lodge in the recesses of the suture and are outside the reach of phagocytes and antibiotics, so that infection persists until the offending suture is removed, thus requiring another operation. However, monofilament sutures have two important disadvantages: firstly, they are difficult to knot, and

Table 1 Equivalence between old and new systems of numbering of suture sizes.

Old system	Metric system	
	Silk Polypropylene Polyglactin	Catgut
6/0	0.7	
5/0	1	
4/0	1.5	2
3/0	2	3
2/0	3	3.5
0	3.5	4
1	4	5

Table 2 Absorbable suture materials.

Type of suture	Absorbed in (weeks)	Strength	Knotting
Plain catgut	2	+ –	Loose
Chromic catgut	3	+	Reasonable
Polyglactin	6	+++	Good
PDS	8	++++	Good

Table 3 Non-absorbable suture materials.

Type of suture	Number of filaments	Strength	Knotting
Silk	Multiple	++	Good
Multifilament nylon	Multiple	+++	Good
Polypropylene	Single	+++	Slips

the knot can slip unless extra ties are thrown. Secondly, the larger-sized sutures are more stiff than multifilament sutures in equivalent sizes. This property is a drawback in two situations:

1. When used to close the muscular abdominal wall, the end of the stiff suture can sometimes erode through the skin and result in a sinus.
2. Removal of skin sutures can be painful due to the stiffness of the suture.

Absorbability. In the beginning surgery was limited in its scope to superficial operations. The commonly available threads namely linen and silk were employed. It was only when surgeons started proceeding deeper into the body that the need arose for sutures which would get absorbed spontaneously, rather than result in longstanding granulomas around them. Only then was catgut, consisting of collagen from the submucosa of sheep, employed. Having served its purpose of bringing tissues or walls of hollow tubes together for union, it got absorbed. It should be remembered that absorbable sutures generally cause more reaction than non-absorbable ones in equivalent sizes, because nature's vultures, the macrophages, collect in large numbers to devour them. Over a period of time a large number of both non-absorbable and absorbable sutures have been synthesized, the more commonly used sutures being listed in Tables 2 and 3.

DIFFERENT SUTURES

Non-absorbable sutures. ***Silk.*** Before the introduction of synthetic sutures, silk was the most commonly used non-absorbable suture. It had adequate tensile strength. Further, being flexible and having a matt surface, it was easy to knot and its knot did not slip. Finally, silk is a soft suture, and stitch removal was painless.

The main problem with silk as with other multifilament sutures arose from the fact that if infection developed, it was very difficult to eradicate it because of the bacteria lurking in the interstices of the suture. Because of this important drawback, multifilament sutures have mostly been supplanted by monofilament sutures.

Polypropylene. This is an extremely useful suture. Because it is monofilament, it has no interstices into which bacteria could lodge and hide away from the body's defences. It has great tensile strength, so that smaller sizes can be used. At the same time where extra strength is required as in the repair of tendons, it is a suitable suture. It also causes very little reaction in the tissues. For all these reasons the incidence of infection after its use in clean cases is very low. Because of these qualities it is one of the most popular non-absorbable suture materials today.

The smooth surface of polypropylene, however, creates problems. The knot slips, and therefore not only does the thread have to be pulled rather tight, many loops of the knot have to be thrown. When pulled tight, it can result in more pain, oedema and venous congestion, and a greater likelihood of infection. Further, polypropylene is stiff, specially in the larger sizes. When used to repair the muscular abdominal wall its ends can burrow through the overlying skin, specially in a lean person, and result in bothersome sinuses.

Multifilament nylon. This type of suture has most of the advantages and disadvantages of silk, and is similarly used less often than monofilament sutures.

Absorbable sutures. ***Catgut.*** Catgut is used in the deep structures when it is desired that the suture should get absorbed within a few weeks. Plain catgut lasts only two to three weeks, chromic catgut approximately twice that long. Plain catgut is best for use in the subcutaneous tissues, where fat has a poor blood supply and a suture is required which is easy to absorb. On the other hand chromic catgut is used to suture intestines, urinary bladder, bile duct etc. In the last-named two structures its early absorbability is attractive, as it ensures that there is no foreign body around which stones could form afresh. It is not a very strong suture, and is not suitable for bringing together tissues requiring strength, such as aponeuroses. Catgut is attractive in communities where the higher cost of polyglactin is significant.

Polyglactin is a synthetic suture. It is a great deal stronger than catgut, hence much finer sizes can be employed. It lasts in the tissues for many more weeks, and for this whole period lends its strength to the tissues it has joined. It is suitable not only for the gastrointestinal tract but also for joining together the muscular layers of the abdominal wall.

PDS is another synthetic suture which is even stronger than polyglactin, but more expensive.

18 Miscellaneous

In this chapter it is proposed to discuss the importance of clinical methods in surgical practice, a few basics of operative surgery, and the use of lasers in surgery.

Clinical methods

This is not a book on clinical methods, for which the reader is referred to the various excellent volumes on the subject. However, the author would impress upon the surgical trainee the over-riding *importance* of clinical methods in diagnosis. *It is also proposed to emphasize the significance of the most important clinical method in surgical illnesses, namely the examination of a swelling.* Unless a clinician is thoroughly conversant with the correct methods of examining a patient, he cannot elicit the different physical signs on which the diagnosis of the patient's illness is based. The *history* and the *physical signs* each have their importance.

THE HISTORY

It is axiomatic that about 80% of diagnoses are made on the basis of the history alone. The reason is this: physical examination tells us only about the state of affairs at the present moment. On the other hand the *history gives us information about all the events that have taken place since the onset of the illness*, which may be as far back as many years ago. If the patient has been having epigastric pain off and on, it has significance. If the pain has recently increased greatly in severity it has added importance. If he has, in addition, had haematemesis repeatedly, it has further significance. Now, it is self-evident that physical examination, however thorough, cannot tell us about these things; *it is only history which can.* Every medical teacher stresses upon the students the value of listening to the sick person patiently, methodically, in fact skilfully, because each sentence uttered by the patient narrating his story is likely to unfold one event in the development of the illness.

PHYSICAL SIGNS

A few centuries ago the only way in which a clinician could find out about a patient's physical condition was by the use of his five senses. Modern investigative methods have placed many very effective tools at his service. However, the value of the use of physical signs for diagnosis is still undiminished. At the same time, these signs are available to the clinician even where sophisticated investigations are not; for example, away from the hospital setting.

SWELLING AS A PHYSICAL SIGN

The importance of a swelling as a physical sign in surgery cannot be over-emphasized, for the simple reason that *the majority of surgical conditions result in the development of a swelling.* If a kidney is diseased a swelling appears; if the thyroid is abnormal it is swollen; if the testis is diseased a swelling is the result. And so on, and so forth. Therefore, it behoves the surgical trainee to thoroughly familiarize himself with the method of taking a proper history, as well as the conduct of a proper physical examination, of a swelling in any organ or part of the body. If he knows all the ins and outs of the examination of a swelling, it means he has mastered at least half of all clinical surgery. The student should thoroughly familiarize himself with all the important points to be remembered while taking the *history* of a case with a swelling. Next he should both understand and commit to memory all the dozen or so points of importance in both *inspection* and *palpation* of a swelling, and should constantly practice the methods of eliciting the relevant signs. Only thus will he be able to form a correct opinion about the nature of the swelling and the underlying illness. *Complete familiarity with the method of examination of a swelling will pay him rich dividends throughout his clinical career.*

Some basics of operative surgery

Being allowed the privilege of helping restore the function of a person's most precious possession, his body, every surgical operation should be carried out gently, to the best of one's ability, and with attention to detail. Only general guidelines are given below, while special situations may require special steps.

Sterilization. Attention to the details of sterilization pays rich dividends by ensuring the healing of wounds by first intention, and by preventing the development of life-threatening septicaemia. Sterilization can be achieved by the use of heat, chemicals, gamma-irradiation and ultraviolet light.

Heat. Boiling kills bacteria but not spores, therefore for effective sterilization temperatures have to be raised above the boiling point of water. This can be achieved either by the hot air oven or the autoclave.

The *hot air oven* can raise the temperature to 120°C and beyond. It is used for the sterilization of blunt instruments and glassware. However, fabrics get burnt in such an oven, therefore a different method of sterilization is required for linen.

In the *autoclave* steam is generated at similar high temperatures. This is suitable for linen, as the steam penetrates through all its layers. However, the linen should be packed loosely to allow this to happen. At the same time, heat sensitive chemicals on paper strips are placed in the deepest part of the linen. These change colour, and show the effectiveness of sterilization.

The sharp edges of cutting instruments are damaged by all kinds of heat. Therefore *chemical* methods have to be employed, and these instruments are kept dipped in appropriate solutions for varying periods of time. The time-honoured liquid is pure phenol (carbolic acid). Recently other solutions have come into use, like Cidex, which are milder in spite of having a rapid action on the micro-organisms.

Instruments can also be sterilized by *gamma-irradiation.*

Finally, the interior of the operation theatre can be exposed to *unltraviolet light* from a lamp overnight.

Position on the table. It is often not realized that a proper position on the table is of the utmost importance. One of the important reasons for the apparent difficulty of an operation is the unsuitability of the patient's position on the table for the particular procedure.

Lighting. Good theatre lights contain numerous bulbs for shadowless viewing. Further, they can be rotated through large arcs to provide light from almost every conceivable angle. Before the operation starts one should have the light fixed at the best angle. Working under imperfect illumination can have dangerous consequences.

Assistants. Most average-sized operations can be carried out with one assistant and one scrub nurse, apart from a runner. In the usual type of case it is more convenient for the assistant to stand across the table, so that both the nurse and himself can assist the surgeon more efficiently.

If an operation is proving to be unexpectedly difficult, the surgeon should check to see if the position of the patient on the table, position of the lights and of the assistants, even the method of draping, are all as they should be.

Shaving. Hair should be shaved off from the area of the operation. However, care should be taken that cuts are not produced in the skin, which could become infected.

Scrubbing. At the operation table the area to be operated upon should be scrubbed with a detergent to remove any grease etc. The time-honoured detergent is ordinary soap, which is perfectly adequate for the purpose. However, antiseptic detergents are available, like cetavlon, and should be employed. This should be followed by painting with methylated spirit, povidone iodine or other antiseptic.

Draping. Autoclaved linen sheets are used to drape the patient, leaving only the area of the operation exposed. An adhesive transparent plastic sheet may be fixed to this area to completely exclude bacteria from the wound; however, recent work has shown *higher* infection rates following its use.

Incisions. These are made keeping in view the requirements of exposure. As far as possible they should follow the lines of skin tension, as healing then takes place with the least conspicuous scars. The length of the incision should be quite sufficient for adequate exposure to enable the operation to proceed smoothly.

Diathermy. During the operation small blood vessels can be sealed off by this technique, obviating the need for individual ligature. Thus not only is time saved; the quantity of foreign matter left in the wound as ligature material is also minimized. A diathermy machine passes electric current through the body. One electrode, which is applied at an area away from the site of the operation, has a large surface. The second electrode is applied to the artery forceps which is holding the small vessel. This electrode is pinpoint; the large quantity of current converging on this point coagulates the tissue, resulting in arrest of bleeding. Only a minimum amount of tissue should be taken into the grip of the haemostat before applying the diathermy electrode to it, so as to minimize the amount of tissue coagulated.

A higher frequency of diathermy can also be employed. This cuts the tissue, acting in place of the 'cold' knife. Even the cutting current produces a haemostatic effect, so that there is minimal loss of blood. Whether using it for coagulation or for cutting, one should hold the active electrode like a pen, not like a sword.

Speed. Some surgeons can operate at a faster speed than others. In driving a car, if one proceeds at a pace slightly slower than one's comfortable speed, the journey proceeds most satisfactorily; the same is true during surgical operations. The temptation to rush the pace should be avoided. The utmost gentleness should be exhibited while handling and dissecting the tissues; it pays rich dividends in trouble-free healing and a relatively pain-free postoperative period.

Closure of wounds should be carried out meticulously. The edges of the skin should not be allowed to overlap each other, otherwise a granulating broad ugly scar results.

Drainage. If a large cavity is left behind after the operation, drainage of the wound should be employed. *Tube* drains are most commonly used. *Corrugated* drains function smoothly and rarely get blocked; however, they can allow introduction of infection from outside, specially if left in for long. *Suction* drains evacuate fluid before it can collect, allowing the walls of the wound to come together. They thus greatly expedite healing.

Lasers in surgery

If a photon (a particle of light) hits an atom, it can either get absorbed, or it can stimulate the emission of another photon from the atom. If the latter event takes place, this stimulated emission causes amplification of the light. The phenomenon is called 'Light Amplification by Stimulated Emission of Radiation' and the light thus emitted is called LASER light.

Unlike ordinary light, the light produced from lasers is coherent, the photons being in step with each other in both time and space. Therefore there is little divergence of the beam which can be focused onto a very small spot, producing enormous irradiance and localized power.

On striking a tissue if the light is reflected, transmitted through or scattered in a tissue, it produces no biological effect. It is only if the light is absorbed in the tissue that a biological effect is produced. The effect of absorption in a tissue depends on its constituents such as melanin, haemoglobin, myoglobin and water; lasers of different wavelength are preferentially absorbed by different tissues. For example carbon dioxide laser is particularly absorbed by water, argon laser by haemoglobin and other pigments.

The biological effect is dependent on the temperature attained in the tissue. Upto 45°C selective hyperthermic destruction of malignant tissues takes place; above this all cells are rapidly killed, and further heating causes contraction and coagulation of proteins. As the tissue shrinks, small vessels can be sealed, arresting haemorrhage; thrombosis of the vessel then follows. The Nd YAG laser is able to seal vessels upto 1 mm in diameter. If more energy is used tissue necrosis occurs, with vaporization and tissue ablation.

APPLICATIONS

Nd YAG laser is used for lithotripsy in the endoscopic fragmentation of *biliary calculi.* Laser beams are transmitted down flexible optical fibres, the ends of which are placed just touching the stone. The laser pulses produce a localized shock wave that can pulverize stones. Interstitial laser hyperthermia is being investigated for unresectable *liver and pancreatic cancers.* Multiple fibres are inserted into the tumour under ultrasound control. The progression of the damage to the tumour can be monitored by ultrasound or MRI, and the area of destruction can be matched to the size of the lesion.

In cases of *upper GI haemorrhage*, surgery can be avoided if the laser is used as an endoscopic haemostatic device to produce thermal contraction of the bleeding vessel. The bleeding vessel is identified, any clot washed off, and the lesion ringed with several pulses of laser energy. The tissue turns white when it is coagulated and the feeding vessel has been occluded. The method is associated with a 1 percent mortality compared with a 12 percent mortality in control patients.

Laser therapy is now widely used for the *palliation* of malignant dysphagia caused by oesophagogastric cancer and for the palliation of the symptoms produced by advanced, inoperable rectal cancer. Treatment is entirely local and is used at high power to coagulate and vaporize the tumour. In the *oesophagus* laser treatment is most useful for the treatment of totally obstructing tumours and for tumours which are unsuitable for endoscopic placement of prosthetic tubes. It is not suitable if a tracheo-oesophageal fistula is present; in that case intubation is to be preferred. A few *colorectal cancers* have advanced metastatic spread or severe concomitant disease that render them unfit for surgery. In such cases laser therapy aims to remove all of a cauliflower tumour, improving bleeding, discharge and obstructive symptoms.

The laser fibre is passed through the operating port of a ureteroscope. The small fibre size, accuracy and safety allow successful *ureteral stone fragmentation* with minimal invasiveness. The low energy pulse, the selective absorption of the particular wavelength by the stone, and its minimal absorption by the tissue, makes this a safe and effective method of stone fragmentation.

Laser prostatectomy is the method which probably holds the most promise for the future. The laser probe directly touches and vaporizes the prostatic tissue, the result being the immediate removal of obstructing tissue in a manner similar to transurethral prostatectomy. Improvement in the urinary stream is usually prompt. It is expected that reduced bleeding may lead to reduced requirement for transfusion and the possibility of avoiding catheterization. If this can materialize, selected patients could be treated in this way in a day surgery unit.

PART II

PRACTICE

Section 1

Gastrointestinal tract and abdominal wall

19 *Oesophagus*

OESOPHAGEAL ATRESIA

Atresia is defined as the congenital absence or closure of a normal body orifice or tubular organ. Oesophageal atresia is a serious illness of the newborn, and occurs in 1 in 4,000 births.

In the common type of this abnormality, which accounts for about 85% of the cases, the upper pouch ends blindly, while the lower communicates with the trachea (Fig. 1). Because of the upper blind pouch the infant cannot swallow his saliva. When the baby breathes and the air goes in and out through the pharynx, it mixes with the saliva to create a froth, and therefore the baby is seen to blow bubbles. He also gets repeated attacks of coughing, choking and cyanosis. Because the lower pouch communicates with the trachea, some of the air breathed in goes into the stomach and can cause abdominal distension. At the same time reflux of gastric juice can occur into the lungs, resulting in bronchitis and pneumonia.

If a baby presents in this manner oesophageal atresia should be suspected. The diagnosis can be confirmed by passing a stiff size 10 catheter through the mouth, when its passage will be arrested at 10 cm from the gums. 0.5 ml of meglumine diatrizoate can be injected down the catheter and an x-ray taken, which will outline the blind pouch. However, the contrast medium must be immediately and completely aspirated from the pouch, otherwise it can spill over into the lungs and cause pneumonia.

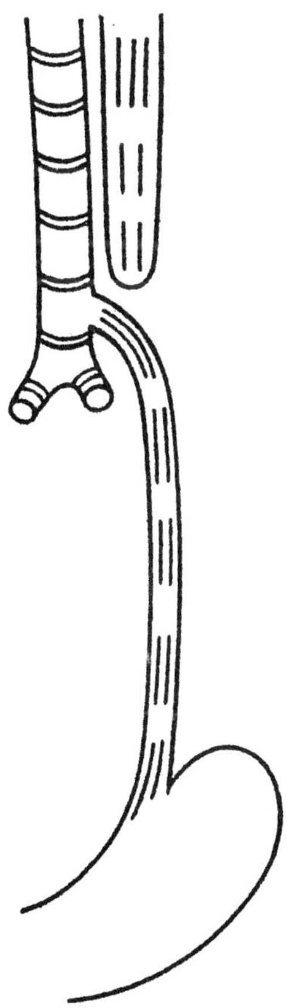

Fig. 1 Oesophageal atresia of the common type. The upper end is blind, the lower is communicating with the trachea.

In many cases of oesophageal atresia there is at the same time a congenital heart lesion, an anorectal anomaly or a duodenal atresia. In these cases the operative morbidity and mortality are higher. The prognosis is also made worse if the baby's birth weight is low or if pneumonia has already set in.

Treatment is by urgent operation. If the baby has been born in hospital and the diagnosis made within a few hours, operation should be carried out immediately. If pneumonia has already set in, 12 to 24 hours may be required to control the lung infection with intensive antibiotic therapy. During this waiting period the secretions from the upper pouch must be dealt with very carefully. A double-lumen (*Replogle* type) tube is ideal for this purpose. It is passed into the pouch and connected to a low pressure suction pump. The advantage of the second lumen lies in the fact that when suction is applied air can go down this lumen. Otherwise, with the usual single-lumen catheter the blind pouch collapses onto the catheter and no suction can take place. If a double-lumen tube is not available an ordinary catheter should be passed and aspiration ordered every 5 minutes.

Operation is performed through a right thoracotomy. The fistula is divided and the tracheal end closed. End-to-end anastomosis using fine silk sutures is carried out between the upper and lower pouches. If the oesophagus is approached extrapleurally the results are superior, because if any leakage occurs it does not lead to the development of an empyema. Most surgeons carry out a gastrostomy as a safety valve, as otherwise the air belched up through the oesophagus can disrupt the delicate anastomosis. After the operation oral feeds are withheld for 8 to 10 days. In a few cases a narrowing develops at the site of the anastomosis, which requires dilatation.

Awareness about this anomaly is important in order to diagnose and treat it in time. *All medical students and midwives should be taught to pass a size 10 catheter if the condition is suspected.*

Before concluding, two other uncommon forms of this anomaly may be mentioned:

1. Oesophageal atresia without fistula. Both ends are blind in this form. The abdomen is airless.

2. Tracheo-oesophageal fistula without atresia, i.e., an H-type fistula. Choking and coughing after feeds are almost always present, and respiratory infections are common.

Detailed discussion of these types is outside the scope of this book.

FOREIGN BODIES IN THE OESOPHAGUS

Coins, pins and dentures are the most common foreign bodies in the oesophagus. If the swallowed object is radiopaque, an x-ray confirms the position. If not, a barium swallow may outline it. It is removed by passing an oesophagoscope. Occasionally, a large denture may require cervical oesophagotomy for removal.

Oesophagoscopy. Two types of oesophagoscopes are available:

1. The classical instrument is straight and rigid and has a large lumen. It is more useful for removing foreign bodies.

2. The modern version employs fibreoptics and is flexible. It is used much more commonly because of the ease with which it is swallowed. The latest models have a smaller diameter than the earlier ones, which were quite difficult to swallow. The patient is sedated with a small dose of diazepam given intravenously immediately before the procedure. He is asked to lie down on his left side. The throat is sprayed with a local anaesthetic solution, and he is asked to swallow the scope, the instrument being advanced under vision. The only difficult point is the oesophageal sphincter; once it is passed the instrument moves quite easily onwards, and the whole of the lumen of the oesophagus can be visualized. Suction is employed as necessary to clear the saliva. The presence of a polyp, a diverticulum, a growth, a stricture, oesophagitis, etc. can be noted. Biopsy of a suspicious mass can be taken, and oesophageal varices injected if present.

DYSPHAGIA

Dysphagia is the sensation of swallowed material sticking on its journey from the mouth to the stomach. Odynophagia, or painful swallowing, is unusual but occurs if oesophagitis or diffuse spasm is present. The causes of dysphagia are many. They may lie in the lumen, in the wall, or outside the wall of the oesophagus:

1. In the lumen, foreign bodies or polyps may make swallowing difficult.

2. In the wall, oesophagitis may render swallowing not only difficult but also painful. Growths produce dysphagia by mechanical blockage, and achalasia by the failure of the cardia to relax. Neurological disorders produce dysphagia by the failure of the oesophagus to propel its contents forwards.

3. Outside the wall a goitre, an aortic aneurysm or a rolling hiatus hernia may produce dysphagia by compressing the oesophagus, while a bronchial carcinoma may produce the same effect by infiltrating it.

The ***history*** should be taken carefully. In general, the longer the duration of dysphagia, the greater the chances that it is caused by a benign condition. If dysphagia commenced for both solids and liquids together, a motor disorder is likely; if with solids alone then mechanical obstruction should be suspected. If an initial dysphagia for solids progresses to liquids, malignancy is suggested. If the dysphagia is intermittent, achalasia, diffuse spasm or impacted food above a stricture should be considered. Difficulty in starting the act of swallowing usually arises from neurological disorders. Finally, diffuse oesophageal spasm may simulate angina pectoris.

Investigations. A *barium swallow* is carried out first. *Cinefluoroscopy* allows visualization of any abnormality of swallowing at the hypopharynx or upper oesophagus. A *plain chest x-ray* can help, by showing a large mediastinal gas shadow in a case of achalasia or hiatus hernia. If a stricture is discovered, *oesophagoscopy* and *biopsy* should be carried out. Motility disorders should be evaluated by oesophageal *manometry*.

Treatment. Once the cause is determined, it must be treated. Carcinoma is best treated by resection, and benign stricture by dilatation or an anti-reflux procedure. Achalasia is best dealt with by myotomy, although some cases respond to pneumatic dilatation.

PERFORATION OF THE OESOPHAGUS

Causation. Perforation of the oesophagus may be seen in the following situations:

1. Perforation most commonly occurs from inexpert use of an oesophagoscope or gastroscope. Due to the very common use of fibreoptic *endoscopy,* perforations are seen more often than previously, occurring in about 1 in 1,000 endoscopies.

2. Oesophageal *dilatation* results in a number of perforations. The risk is increased:

i. When early dilatation is carried out after a caustic burn, because it is performed through friable tissues.

ii. When forceful hydrostatic or pneumatic dilatation is carried out for achalasia.

3. *Celestin plastic tubes* passed transorally through an unresectable carcinoma of the oesophagus as a palliative measure ocasionally end up in a perforation.

4. Forceful *endotracheal intubation* can perforate the oesophagus just below the cricopharyngeus muscle.

5. *Hiatal hernia* repair, *vagotomy* and *sclerotherapy* for variceal haemorrhage can occasionally result in perforation.

6. After prolonged vomiting from any cause, spontaneous perforation of the oesophagus may take place (*Boerhaave's syndrome*).

7. Foreign bodies, mostly bones, coins, and artificial dentures, can perforate the oesophagus.

The injury takes place just above the cricopharyngeus, or just above a stricture. It may go unnoticed. However, severe chest pain, fever, dysphagia, mediastinal and subcutaneous emphysema and ultimately dyspnoea and sepsis may occur. X-ray may show widening of the mediastinum along with surgical emphysema. Pleural effusion or hydropneumothorax may be seen, usually on the left side. If lipiodol is swallowed it may leak out and be seen on x-ray. A CT scan after contrast swallow may visualize a tiny perforation which has been missed by conventional x-ray studies.

If perforation has occurred urgent operation is required to repair it, through a cervical incision or a thoracotomy. It should be carried out under full antibiotic cover for aerobes and anaerobes. After the repair, a pleural pedicled flap may be wrapped round the oesophagus, suturing it firmly over the area of leakage. A gastrotomy may be performed at the same time for drainage, as well as a jejunostomy for feeding. Morbidity and mortality result from extensive mediastinal or pleural infection.

MALLORY-WEISS SYNDROME

If repeated vomiting or retching takes place due to any cause, a mucosal tear may occur at the gastroesophageal junction resulting in upper gastrointestinal (GI) bleeding. This condition is called the Mallory-Weiss syndrome, and is responsible for about 10% of severe upper GI bleeds. The diagnosis is confirmed by upper GI endoscopy, which should be delayed in shocked patients until resuscitation is achieved by blood transfusion. If bleeding is continuing, the tear may be electrocoagulated at the same time. The treatment is conservative with H_2 receptor blockers and antacids. Surgical treatment is required only if the haemorrhage continues or recurs after the above measures, the bleeding mucosal tear being suture-ligated through a generous gastrostomy. In poor risk patients such as cirrhotic individuals, percutaneous embolization of the left gastric artery may be carried out.

CORROSIVE OESOPHAGITIS

Ingestion of strong acids, alkalies, etc. produces extensive chemical burns with severe oesophagitis. Sloughing of the mucosa, inflammation of the submucosa, thrombosis of oesophageal vessels, perforation and mediastinitis may develop. In severe cases the patient looks toxic, with high fever, prostration and shock. Swelling of the lips, tongue and pharynx may produce respiratory distress and severe dysphagia.

Complications include perforation, mediastinitis and tracheoesophageal fistulas. Circular burns result in strictures.

Treatment. Emergency treatment consists of washing the oesophagus with large volumes of water. Dilute acid or alkali are used to neutralize the ingested fluid. Broad-spectrum antibiotics are started immediately to prevent bacterial invasion of the oesophageal wall. Corticosteroids are used to reduce fibrous tissue formation and stricture. If severe stricture develops, the oesophagus must be replaced by stomach, which is mobilized and brought up into the chest.

BENIGN STRICTURES

The most common cause of a benign stricture is corrosive oesophagitis. Other causes include gastroesophageal reflux, indwelling nasogastric tubes, radiation therapy, congenital oesophageal atresia, and postoperative (anastomotic) stricture. Corrosive strictures are usually multiple, the narrowest being at the level of the crossing of the left bronchus. The presenting symptom is increasing dysphagia. Diagnosis is established by barium swallow x-ray and oesophagoscopy.

Investigation. Barium swallow can help assess the length and diameter of the stricture as well as provide clues to other causes of dysphagia. If the stricture is longer than 20 mm and located in the upper or middle oesophagus, if it looks like an 'apple core' and reflux is absent, it raises the suspicion of neoplasia. *Endoscopic biopsy* and *cytological brushings* are essential to rule out malignancy. *Oesophageal pH studies,* and specially 24-hour continuous pH monitoring, help detect gatroesophageal reflux disease as a cause of oesophageal stricture.

Treatment. ***Conservative.*** *Medical.* In cases due to reflux, medical therapy includes elevation of the head of the bed, avoiding eating before bedtime, and antacids. *H_2 blockers* such as cimetidine and ranitidine are the mainstays of medical treatment. Omeprazole is a *proton pump inhibitor* that inhibits acid production in the stomach. It is very effective against gastroesophageal reflux disease, most cases of oesophagitis healing at a daily dose of 20 to 40 mg. *Metoclopramide* and *cisapride* increase the lower oesophageal sphincter pressure and improve gastric emptying, correcting two factors responsible for gastroesophageal reflux disease. These two agents may be used with H_2 blockers and omeprazole for maximal effect.

Dilatation. Dilatation plays an important part in stricture management. The aim is to break up the fibrous stricture and improve dysphagia and alimentation. Dilatation is also used to allow endoscopic inspection and biopsy. Objective results of dilatation are transient, lasting less than 12 weeks.

Surgical therapy is reserved for patients who fail to improve from conservative management or suffer complications from dilatations. The operations include the following:

1. Dilatation and fundoplication (Nissen), in which the fundus is wrapped around the lower oesophagus.
2. Gastroplasty and fundoplication.
3. Resection with replacement by stomach or interposition of jejunum (the colon is used less often nowadays). Jejunum has a better blood supply than the colon. At the same time it avoids the need for vagotomy and gastric drainage which is required if gastric pull-up is used for reconstruction.

HIATUS HERNIA AND REFLUX DISEASE

Physiology. The oesophagus passes through the oesophageal hiatus of the diaphragm into the abdomen and travels downwards and to the left for a distance of 3 to 4 cm before it enters the stomach at the cardia. Normally, reflux of gastric contents back into the oesophagus is prevented by the following factors:

1. The muscle fibres of the right crus exert a pinch-cock type of action.
2. The intra-abdominal segment of oesophagus is pressed upon and closed when the gastric fundus distends, and this prevents reflux.
3. The valvular action of the angle between the oesophagus and the fundus of the stomach has the same effect of closing the oesophagus when the gastric fundus distends.
4. The folds of mucosa at the cardia help further in closing it tightly.

Pathophysiology of reflux. Some reflux is normal, and therefore pathological reflux is defined as more reflux than

95% confidence limits for the population, (or simply stated, more reflux than occurs in 95% of the normal population). In actual figures, reflux is pathological if the lumen of the distal oesophagus is at a pH below 4 for more than 4% of the day, or if there are more than 10 reflux episodes (i.e. pH below 4) per 24 hours. Prolonged exposure of the oesophagus to acid is caused by:

1. Frequent episodes of reflux.
2. Large volume reflux.
3. Defective oesophageal clearance.
4. A combination of all three.

Anatomical changes at the hiatus such as a *sliding hernia* or *resection of the distal oesophagus* make reflux more likely. *Obesity* often accompanies sliding hernias and contributes to the development of reflux by raising the intra-abdominal pressure. *Age* is important, reflux being common at the extremes of life. In infancy the gastroesophageal mechanism is not fully developed. In old age not only does this mechanism become degenerate, peristalsis is also less efficient; further, a hiatus hernia is often present.

Reflux is both painful and damaging to the oesophagus. Gastric contents are corrosive and burn the oesophageal squamous epithelium. Gastric and duodenal juices together are more destructive than either alone, indicating that the damage is not purely pH dependent. Deep chronic ulcers or peptic strictures may be produced. The oesophagitis is graded macroscopically from 0 (normal) to grade 4, although there is poor correlation between severity of inflammation and symptoms.

There are two types of hiatus hernia, the sliding and the paraoesophageal (Fig. 2).

SLIDING HIATUS HERNIA

More than 90% of hiatus hernias are of this type. The upper stomach slides up into the thorax through the hiatus, so that the cardia lies in the chest (Fig. 2a).

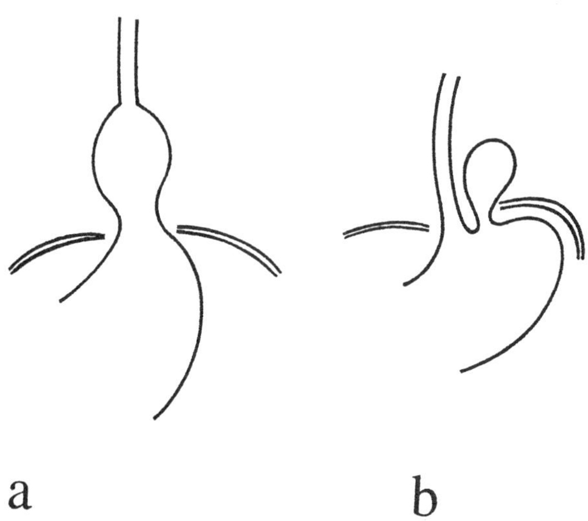

Fig. 2 Hiatus hernia. (a) sliding; the gastro-oesophageal junction (GEJ) is above the diaphragm. (b) paraoesophageal (rolling); the GEJ is below the diaphragm. The gastric fundus has rolled up into the chest by the side of the oesophagus.

Of the above-mentioned factors preventing reflux the first three are operative only so long as the cardia lies in the abdomen. When it slides up into the chest they are put out of action and reflux occurs. Reflux is increased by lying down, and by anything which raises the intra-abdominal pressure e.g. stooping, straining, overeating, late pregnancy and advanced obesity.

Clinical findings. Most patients are above the age of fifty, this being a disease of middle and old age. Half the cases have no symptoms. When symptoms do occur, they can be classified into three types:

1. *Typical symptoms.* Retrosternal and epigastric burning pain i.e. 'heartburn' often occurs after meals or while lying down. It is relieved by drinking water or by antacids.

2. *Atypical symptoms.* Nocturnal reflux with frequent aspiration may present in the elderly as recurrent respiratory tract infection. In rare cases reflux may be responsible for attacks of asthma in younger patients. Laryngitis from the refluxed acid may lead to hoarseness. The acid acting on the teeth may cause loss of enamel. Chest pain and night sweats may be seen from time to time.

3. *Complications.* Peptic strictures present in older patients with gradually progressive dysphagia, but little weight loss. In contrast, carcinoma of the oesophagus presents with marked weight loss despite the brief history.

Diagnosis. The *history* is important in diagnosis. Symptoms resembling those of sliding hiatus hernia can be produced by gallstones, peptic ulcer, achalasia and coronary artery disease. Confirmation of the diagnosis is obtained by *endoscopy*. This demonstrates the oesophagitis or the columnar transformation of the distal oesophageal mucosa. A hiatus hernia is often visible, with the squamocolumnar junction between stomach and oesophagus lying at a variable distance above the crura of the diaphragm. If history strongly suggests reflux but oesophagitis is absent, 24-hour oesophageal *pH measurement* may demonstrate pathological reflux. If the symptoms are atypical an *acid infusion test* (Bernstein test) may help. The test is positive if the patient complains of pain when 0.1M hydrochloric acid is infused into the oesophagus and the pain disappears when the infusate is changed to saline. Rarely oesophageal *manometry* helps in the diagnosis of diffuse oesophageal spasm due to reflux as a cause of non-cardiac chest pain in the presence of a normal ECG and exercise test. *Barium swallow* shows up a hiatus hernia. *Cineradiography* helps in the diagnosis of dysphagia caused by neurological or pharyngeal muscular disorders, some of which may be secondary to pathological reflux.

The main *complication* of sliding hiatus hernia is oesophagitis, which can lead to ulceration and stricture formation.

Treatment. ***Medical.*** Half the cases have no symptoms and require no treatment. Of the other half the great majority can be managed conservatively. In *moderate* cases the following general corrective measures alone are usually sufficient: weight reduction, avoidance of heavy meals just before retiring to bed, stopping smoking, avoiding anticholinergic drugs and excess alcohol, and taking antacid alginates. These latter agents give better relief than antacids alone, because they line the oesophageal epithelium and provide added protection from contact with acid.

More *severe* symptoms and oesophagitis require, in addition to the above, acid suppression with H_2 antagonists. If this proves insufficient, a proton pump inhibitor such as omeprazole is employed, as it provides more complete acid suppression. If symptoms still persist, a prokinetic drug such as metoclopramide may be used to enhance gastric emptying and oesophageal clearing. For maintenance therapy, 40 mg of omeprazole daily prevents recurrence over a period of 5 years in 80% of cases.

Surgical. Surgery is indicated in the few patients in whom:

1. Severe symptoms are present which cannot be controlled medically.
2. Complications arise, e.g. oesophagitis, haemorrhage, or stenosis.
3. Associated lesions are present, e.g. gallstones, peptic ulcer etc., which require operation in any case.

Operative treatment. The aim of surgical management is to prevent excessive reflux while allowing physiological reflux. Most operations are performed through the abdomen. The guiding principle of repair is to ensure a length of at least 4 cm of intra-abdominal oesophagus, and to prevent this segment from returning to the chest. The most popular operation is that by *Nissen* where the abdominal oesophagus is mobilized and the fundus of the stomach wrapped around it. It ensures an intra-abdominal segment of oesophagus and also re-constitutes the oesophagogastric angle. The Nissen fundoplication is a 360° fundal wrap. Modifications of the operation vary the amount of wrap to as little as 180° around the distal oesophagus. The more the wrap, the better is reflux prevented; however, the greater also are the risks of gas bloat and dysphagia. 90% of patients have a good result after operation; the remainder have persistent reflux.

PARA-OESOPHAGEAL ('ROLLING') HERNIA

Here the greater curvature or the whole stomach herniates into the thorax to the left of an undisplaced gastroesophageal junction (Fig. 2b). As the cardia lies undisturbed below the diaphragm, reflux of gastric contents does not occur. If left untreated, the intrathoracic stomach may undergo volvulus or acute dilatation, which are dangerous complications; therefore such a hernia should be repaired early.

Clinical features. Symptoms rarely appear until the hernia attains a large size, and are mostly due to pressure on adjacent organs by a recurrent gastric volvulus. There may be a good deal of belching. The patient may also complain of difficulty in swallowing. Palpitations may occur due to cardiac arrhythmias, and hiccough may result from irritation of the phrenic nerve which passes near the hernia before reaching the muscle of the diaphragm.

Treatment. Medical treatment is of no avail. Surgical correction is required if the patient is disabled by symptoms or is acutely ill. In the latter situation with a gastric volvulus, rapid fluid replacement, gastric decompression, oxygen therapy and intravenous antibiotics are important preoperative measures.

Operation. An *elective* operation in an old patient is best performed through an upper midline incision. The stomach is reduced into the abdomen, the hernia sac excised, and the crura approximated by non-absorbable sutures to close the hiatus around the oesophagus. An anterior gastropexy, fixing the lesser curve of the stomach to the anterior abdominal wall with three or four non-absorbable sutures, prevents recurrence. A posterior gastroenterostomy ensures adequate gastric drainage and also provides additional fixation for the stomach. In a very frail old patient gastroenterostomy alone may suffice.

In acute cases it is dangerous to attempt to draw the stomach down from the thorax through an abdominal incision because of the risk of gastric rupture. For these cases a left thoracotomy through the bed of the 7th rib is the best approach, and provides good access to decompress and mobilize the stomach. The left chest is opened, the hernia is reduced, the sac is excised and the hernial orifice repaired by overlapping sutures of a non-absorbable material. However, this operation is much more traumatic for elderly and frail patients and carries a greater risk of complications.

GASTROESOPHAGEAL REFLUX IN INFANTS

Besides middle age, gastroesophageal reflux occurs in newborns. There is effortless vomiting of small amounts, usually blood-tinged, soon after birth. The cause of this reflux is the absence of both an intra-abdominal segment of oesophagus and an acute angle between the oesophagus and the gastric fundus. The baby should be nursed in an upright position in a legless chair made of plaster of Paris or other material. In most infants all symptoms disappear when they start to walk; some others require the Nissen fundoplication procedure. In this operation the gastric fundus is wrapped around the lower oesophagus to prevent reflux.

PLUMMER-VINSON SYNDROME

This condition occurs nearly only in middle-aged women. The patients complain of dysphagia which can be shown on endoscopy and radiography to be due to a fibrous web partially obstructing the oesophageal lumen a few millimeters below the cricopharyngeus muscle. Severe retching spells may occur. On examination the tongue is smooth and pale, the corners of the mouth are cracked, the finger-nails are spoon-shaped and brittle. The spleen is enlarged and the bone-marrow is devoid of stainable iron stores. There is hypochromic anaemia and usually achlorhydria. The lesion is precancerous.

Treatment. The condition has been shown to be due to a dietary deficiency, and responds to oral iron and bougie dilatation of the web. Ferrous sulphate with vitamins is prescribed. Sometimes blood transfusion is required. Hyperalimentation through a nasogastric tube accelerates the regeneration of the desquamated epithelium of the oesophageal mucosa.

ACHALASIA

In this condition the cardioesophageal sphincter fails to relax in response to swallowing. Due to this functional obstruction the oesophagus dilates and hypertrophies, without organic stenosis. The dilatation terminates abruptly at the cardia. There is atrophy of ganglion cells in Auerbach's plexus. There is marked stasis and retention oesophagitis due to the presence of the foul-smelling stagnant fluid. The cause of the condition is not known.

Clinical features. Achalasia of the oesophagus occurs in middle age. There is progressive dysphagia of many years' duration. Although the patient says she vomits, in fact there is regurgitation of fluid several hours after the meal. The retention oesophagitis results in retrosternal discomfort. The retained food stagnates and putrefies, so that there is foul-smelling belching. Some of the fluid overspills into the bronchi, producing aspiration pneumonia. A 'rheumatoid' arthritis due to toxic absorption may occur. Due to malnutrition the patient remains in poor health. In infants respiratory problems due to overspill may be the first symptom to prompt evaluation and diagnosis.

Characteristic features on *x-ray* include widening of the mediastinum and a posterior mediastinal air-fluid level. Chronic aspiration may produce abnormalities of the lung fields. Barium swallow demonstrates dilatation and tortuosity of the oesophagus, a smooth pencil-shaped narrowing of the lower end of the oesophagus (bird's beak deformity), and lack of a gas bubble in the stomach. An oesophageal diameter of less than 4 cm qualifies as mild disease, 4 to 6 cm as moderate, and greater than 6 cm as severe disease ('mega-oesophagus').

The most reliable and accurate method of diagnosis consists of *oesophageal manometry*. In this method pressure-sensitive catheters (transducers) are used to measure the intra-oesophageal pressures and to detect and record the occurrence of peristaltic activity. If it is found that organized peristaltic activity is absent throughout the intrathoracic oesophagus, and that the lower oesophageal sphincter does not relax, the diagnosis of achalasia is confirmed. On *endoscopy* the oesophagus appears as a cave filled with dirty water.

Differential diagnosis. Achalasia may be confused with a benign stricture or carcinoma at the cardia. In these cases the huge dilatation of the oesophagus seen in achalasia does not occur. Also, in carcinoma the lower end of the barium column is irregular (rat-tail appearance).

Treatment. The aim of treatment is to relieve the functional obstruction at the cardia. This can be accomplished by disruption of the constricting fibres of the cardia, either from within by an inflatable bag, or from without by Heller's operation. Neither method restores coordinated peristalsis of the oesophageal body. However, disruption of the sphincter relieves the dysphagia and regurgitation. Forceful *dilatation* involves rapid pneumatic expansion of an inflatable bag placed at the oesophagogastric junction. Usually three or four dilatations are required. *Heller's* operation is best carried out through the left thorax, as exposure of the whole of the lower oesophagus is direct. At the same time the hiatus is not stretched, which could have been followed by reflux. The muscle coat of the lower end of the oesophagus is divided longitudinally, care being taken to divide all the muscle fibres, and to reach proximally to include all dilated oesophagus. Distally, the incision should extend less than 1 cm onto the stomach wall. Results are good to excellent in 90% of patients.

BENIGN TUMOURS

Benign tumours of the oesophagus are very rare. They produce dysphagia, and are discovered on barium swallow as indentations of the oesophageal lumen. Oesophagoscopy with biopsy confirms the diagnosis. A leiomyoma or lipoma may be removed transthoracically. A papilloma, as it is pedunculated, may be excised by diathermy through an oesophagoscope. A cavernous haemangioma may cause haematemesis. Injection of a sclerosing agent may help; if not, partial oesophagectomy is required.

CARCINOMA OF THE OESOPHAGUS

Incidence. Carcinoma of the oesophagus is more common in males, occurring most often between 50 and 60 years of age. The incidence varies considerably around the world, from 5 per 100000 in the United States to 100 per 100000 in parts of China.

Risk factors. The important risk factors include the following:

1. Heavy alcohol use.
2. Smoking, the risk being even greater when combined with excessive alcohol intake.
3. Malnutrition, specially:
   i. Plummer-Vinson syndrome, from iron and vitamin B deficiencies.
   ii. Coeliac disease, due to multiple deficiencies from malabsorption.
   iii. Molybdenum, zinc and magnesium deficiencies.
4. Chronic irritation: chronic corrosive strictures, achalasia, oesophageal diverticula.

Pathology. The vast majority of tumours are squamous cell carcinomas, from the squamous epithelium of the oesophagus. However, tumours arising at the cardia are usually adenocarcinomas, mostly of gastric origin. Three gross patterns of growth are commonly seen. The ulcerating type has a well-defined ulcer with a raised margin. The fungating type has a large intramural component with an irregular surface. The infiltrating type shows extensive circumferential intramural growth without ulceration. The tumour spreads by direct invasion into the surrounding structures, through the blood stream, and by lymphatic dissemination. Lesions of the lower oesophagus metastasize primarily to the coeliac lymph nodes. As far as blood-borne metastases are concerned, they develop mostly in the lungs, bones, liver and brain.

In a high-risk population in China, extensive *mass screening* was carried out by abrasive cytology using a swallowed balloon which is inflated and pulled back through the oesophagus, thus collecting a sample of epithelial cells. Dysplastic cells were almost always found in association with carcinoma. When patients were followed for 12 years, no patient with normal cytology progressed to carcinoma. On the other hand, 1% of patients with mild dysplasia, and as many as 15% with severe dysplasia developed cancer. Surgical treatment of early, cytologically diagnosed, asymptomatic cancers provided over 90% survival at 5 years, emphasizing the importance of early diagnosis.

TNM staging is given in Table 1.

Table 1 TNM staging of oesophageal carcinoma.

T0	No tumour
Tis	Carcinoma-*in-situ*
T1	Invades submucosa
T2	Invades muscularis propria
T3	Invades perioesophageal tissues
T4	Invades adjacent structures
N0	No node metastases
N1	Regional node metastases
M0	No distant metastases
M1	Distant metastases

Clinical features. Dysphagia is the most prominent symptom, causing marked weight loss. At first solid foods cause difficulty, later even liquids are difficult to swallow. This is a late symptom and usually indicates that two-thirds of the circumference is involved. There is weakness and anaemia. Steady deep chest pain usually indicates mediastinal invasion. Cough and hoarseness are common in upper oesophageal tumours from invasion of the airway or recurrent laryngeal nerve. Aspiration pneumonia may be present due to obstructive overspill, or from a malignant oesophageal-airway fistula.

Complications. Occult anaemia is frequent, though massive bleeding is rare. Invasion of superior vena cava, aorta, trachea or pericardium may occur, producing fatal haemorrhage, tracheal obstruction or cardiac arrhythmias respectively. A fistula with the trachea may produce aspiration pneumonitis and lung abscess.

Investigations. ***Radiology.*** *Barium meal x-ray.* This shows an irregular mass whose upper border is roughly horizontal like a 'shelf'. Annular lesions show a narrow lumen with an irregular mucosal outline. Angulation of the long axis of the oesophagus suggests mediastinal invasion and predicts unresectability. *Chest x-ray* may show an oesophageal air-fluid level, lung infiltrates suggesting aspiration, mediastinal widening from tumour or lymphadenopathy, and pulmonary nodules suggesting lung metastases. *CT scan* shows the oesophageal wall, mediastinal structures and metastatic sites clearly. However, it does not predict invasion accurately. Gross distortion of a mediastinal structure indicates invasion, while the presence of a fat plane between the tumour and the structure indicates the absence of invasion.

Endoscopy. *Oesophagoscopy* with biopsy confirms the diagnosis and helps measure the length of the lesion and the distance from the incisors for staging and treatment planning. *Bronchoscopy* is necessary in upper and middle third carcinomas to detect involvement of the trachea or bronchi. *Laparoscopy* allows biopsy of the liver, perigastric lymph nodes and peritoneum, if indicated by ultrasound or CT. *Thoracoscopy* can confirm invasion into local structures and sample lymph nodes for staging. The role of video-assisted thoracoscopy for oesophagectomy needs to be defined. *Endoscopic ultrasound* improves the ability to determine wall penetration and abnormal lymph nodes, thus improving preoperative staging.

Treatment. There are only two methods of treatment proved to benefit patients with carcinoma of the oesophagus: surgical resection and irradiation. Most patients present with advanced disease (Stage III) with full-thickness invasion of the oesophageal wall and lymph node metastases; this precludes cure, so that the aim is palliation.

Irradiation. Squamous cell carcinoma of the oesophagus is a radiosensitive and theoretically radiocurable tumour. Unfortunately, although the primary lesions may be controlled, failures result from the presence of tumour outside the irradiated fields, and few permanent cures are obtained. Radiotherapy for adenocarcinoma of the gastroesophageal junction is much less effective.

Radical radiotherapy (5,000 to 6,000 rads) is followed by only 5 to 10% 5 year survivals. At the same time, the complications of such radiotherapy are many: radiation pneumonitis, local recurrence, stricture, tracheoesophageal fistula, perforation, spinal cord injury and pericardial effusion. *Preoperative radiotherapy* (2,000 to 4,000 rads) followed by surgery improves the resectability rate slightly, but does not affect survival. *Palliative low-dose radiotherapy* (2,000 to 4,000 rads) relieves distressing symptoms such as pain, dysphagia, and bleeding, with minimal risk of morbidity.

Preoperative or *postoperative* radiotherapy is not recommended, as neither confers any benefit.

Surgery. Surgical treatment quite effectively controls local disease and restores normal swallowing. 5 year survival rates are also good: (Stage I, 85%; Stage II, 34%; Stage III 15%; overall 22%). Today, the most popular operation is resection of the oesophagus and its replacement by the mobilized stomach. Because of its thick and tough wall, its richer blood supply, and the absence of bacteria in its lumen, the stomach is better than colon for use as replacement for the oesophagus. Colon is used only when stomach is not available for some reason. The stomach is taken up either through the right chest, or through the posterior mediastinum i.e. the normal route of the oesophagus. It can be taken all the way to the neck, and can therefore be used in cases of carcinomas arising anywhere along the thoracic oesophagus.

The different *approaches* are as follows:

Left thoracoabdominal approach through the left sixth interspace, the diaphragm being divided circumferentially to avoid injury to the phrenic nerve; best for lower third lesions.

Laparotomy and right thoracotomy, best suited for middle or lower third lesions. Through an upper midline laparotomy the stomach is first mobilized on the right gastric and gastroepiploic arteries. The hiatus is enlarged and the lower oesphagus mobilized. The patient is now turned on his left side. Through a right thoracotomy the oesophagus can be mobilized right upto the apex of the right chest, resected, and anastomosed obliquely to the gastric fundus to prevent reflux.

Transhiatal oesophagectomy. The chest is not opened. Dissection is carried out downwards form the neck and upwards from the abdomen. The middle third of the oesophagus has to be dissected by the fingers. The advantage of the method consists of the avoidance of a thoracotomy. The disadvantage lies in the necessity of blind dissection of the middle third of the oesophagus, and the possibility of injury to thoracic duct, trachea, azygos vein and recurrent laryngeal nerve. The method can be used only for upper and lower third lesions.

In the case of cancers of the cervical oesophagus and hypopharynx, radiotherapy is superior to surgery, and has the added advantage of preserving the voice if the local tumour is controlled. However, if the tumour recurs, the surgeon has to carry out en bloc removal of the larynx, pharynx and oesophagus in an irradiated field, which is a difficult undertaking.

Chemotherapy alone has had very little effect in palliating patients with either squamous cell carcinoma or adenocarcinoma of the oesophagus. Because of the belief that this disease is often systemic at the time of diagnosis, combined modality treatment using chemotherapy, irradiation and resection has gained popularity. Initial reports are encouraging, but it is too early to make any long-term predictions. Preoperative adjuvant chemotherapy has shown promising results, partial and complete response rates upto 66% being reported.

Palliation of inoperable oesophageal cancer. *Transoral intubation.* In patients with far advanced malignancies, distant metastases, or recurrence after radiotherapy the aim is palliation, so that the patient can swallow. This has classically been achieved by placing a plastic tube in the lumen of the oesophagus and passing it down through the growth. Many different types of tubes are available, e.g. Celestin, Mousseau and Souttar, and go by the names of the workers who designed them. Unfortunately, transoral intubation has a high morbidity and mortality, due to perforation of the oesophagus, obstruction of the tube by food or tumour, and migration of the tube. The average survival after such palliation is about six months. This method is best suited to patients with a carcinoma of the oesophagus which has fistulated into the trachea, because the tube occludes the fistula and allows oral feeding for the remaining months of the patient's life.

Laser. Laser therapy is now widely used endoscopically for the palliation of malignant dysphagia caused by oesophagogastric cancer. The laser is used to coagulate and vaporize the tumour. It is most suitable for tumours which are unsuitable for endoscopic placement of prosthetic tubes. It is not suitable if a tracheoesophageal fistula is present; in that case intubation is to be preferred.

A *feeding gastrostomy* provides no palliation for oesophageal obstruction and should be employed only as a temporary measure for maintaining nutrition during outpatient radiotherapy or between stages of oesophageal reconstruction.

Causes of death. If the growth is not removed, death is caused by progressive cachexia and dehydration; pneumonia from perforation into the bronchial tree; mediastinitis; or erosion into the aorta.

20 Stomach and duodenum

INFANTILE HYPERTROPHIC PYLORIC STENOSIS

This condition results from hypertrophy of the muscle of the pylorus and distal antrum of the stomach. The cause is not known. However, there is a strong familial element, with a 5% incidence in children whose mothers suffered from the condition. Males predominate 4:1. The condition is seen in the newborn, and is more common in first-born infants.

Clinical features. The baby is usually full-term, and *feeds well for one or two weeks.* At that time occasional regurgitation of some feeds starts. In a few days the vomiting becomes more frequent, forceful, and projectile. However, in the weak premature infant there may be effortless regurgitation of stomach contents. The vomitus contains no bile. Shortly after the vomiting the infant wants to feed again. Because of the obstruction at the pylorus, constipation with hard faeces develops. Due to diminished absorption from the intestines, weight is lost. Gastric peristaltic waves can usually be seen moving across the epigastrium from left to right. In some cases the thickened pylorus can be palpated as a lump when the baby is relaxed by sedation or by feeding clear fluids.

X-rays. If the pyloric tumour cannot be palpated, an x-ray picture is taken after giving a small amount of meglumine diatrizoate. The pyloric canal may be outlined by a 'string sign' or a pyloric 'beak' may be seen where the pyloric entrance from the antrum occurs. X-rays taken two or three hours later show most of the dye still lying in the stomach.

Differential diagnosis. Repeated vomiting without bile in the newborn may also be due to feeding problems, intracranial lesions, an incompetent cardiac sphincter, pylorospasm, duodenal atresia, malrotation of the bowel or adrenal insufficiency. It is extremely important to remember that *the vomiting of infantile pyloric stenosis does not start at birth but one or two weeks later.* This fact helps distinguish this condition from duodenal atresia.

Complications. Repeated vomiting leads to loss of water and nutrients producing dehydration and starvation with weight loss. Chloride and potassium are lost in the vomitus, resulting in hypochloraemic hypokalaemic alkalosis. Aspiration of vomitus can produce pneumonia.

Treatment. Medical treatment is of no avail. The proper treatment is surgery. Before operation, the deficiency of water, potassium and chloride must be corrected; for this purpose the level of serum electrolytes is determined. The baby is resuscitated with 0.5N saline solution (0.45 percent NaCl) with 2g of potassium chloride per 500 ml bag initially to correct the hypokalaemia and alkalosis. When the bicarbonate falls below 30 mmol/l the baby is taken to the theatre. A nasogastric tube is placed in position before operation to empty and wash out the stomach. Operation is carried out through a right upper transverse incision. The pyloric tumour, which is an olive-shaped mass upto 2 cm in diameter, is delivered and a longitudinal incision made over it, from the pyloroduodenal junction at least 2 cm on to the antrum, dividing all the muscle fibres and exposing the mucous membrane, which bulges into the incision. Some air is squeezed from the stomach into the duodenum to demonstrate adequate division of the muscle. The cut in the muscle is left unsutured. The abdominal wall is repaired. This procedure, which is essentially a pyloromyotomy, is called *Rammstedt's operation.* Small feeds of 5 ml hourly are started next morning and rapidly increased over a period of one or two days. If diagnosed and treated promptly, the mortality rate in this condition approaches zero. However the greater the delay the worse the prognosis.

Peptic ulcer

Peptic ulcers result from the corrosive action of acid gastric juice on a vulnerable epithelium. They are commonly seen in the duodenum and stomach and occasionally in the oesophagus. They may also be encountered in the jejunum after a gastrojejunostomy, or in the ileum in a Meckel's diverticulum adjacent to ectopic gastric mucosa. Thus it will be seen that peptic ulcers normally arise at sites adjacent to acid-secreting epithelium. The common locations are the lesser curvature of the stomach and the first part of the duodenum. Realization of the central role of acid has led to therapy by antacids and H_2 ion antagonists, and to operations that reduce acid secretion. Peptic ulcer is a very common condition nearly all over the world. Men are affected 3 times as often as women. Duodenal ulcer is 10 times more common than gastric ulcer. Duodenal and gastric ulcer are fundamentally different diseases whose major common feature is acid-pepsin-dependent ulceration.

PATHOPHYSIOLOGY

Ulcers of the stomach and duodenum are caused chiefly by the effects of hydrochloric acid produced by the parietal cells of the stomach, and by lack of protection of the mucosa against this acid.

As far as *duodenal ulcer* is concerned, acid production is by far the most important factor. However it cannot be the only factor, because the severity of duodenal ulcers does not vary directly with the amount of gastric acid secreted. Firstly, the disease is more common in persons with blood group O. At the same time stress and anxiety, irregular and highly spiced meals, inadequate mastication, alcohol, caffeine and excessive smoking are all considered important in causation.

With *gastric ulcer,* additional factors are important. Gastric contents can be *retained* for much longer periods than duodenal contents, and are *not neutralized* as rapidly as by duodenal chyme. The gastric mucosa is protected from the damaging effect of the hydrochloric acid which it secretes by an adherent layer of mucus. Further, under the mucus lies a layer of bicarbonate which neutralizes any acid diffusing back through the mucus layer. The mucus layer also protects the mucosa from other noxious agents such as bile, alcohol and aspirin and other irritating drugs.

The causes of *gastric ulcers* vary with location of the ulcers. In this respect two categories of ulcers are seen:

1. To the first category belong (Johnson's) type 1 ulcers, i.e. ulcers which are located in the *body* of the stomach. In these cases gastric secretion levels as determined by secretory tests are low. Here *inadequate mucosal protection* and back-diffusion of hydrochloric acid through the mucus and bicarbonate layer into the gastric mucosa seems to be involved.

2. In the second category we find two types of ulcers: type 2 gastric ulcers are those combined with a duodenal ulcer, while type 3 describes ulcers arising in the prepyloric area. Both these types behave more like duodenal ulcers; here the effects of *acid production* are more important.

Ulcers that develop *after gastroenterostomy*, and those which recur *after various operations* for duodenal and gastric ulcers, are due to persistent secretion of hydrochloric acid. Finally, *extragastric* lesions can lead to increased levels of serum gastrin and consequent acid production. Thus in the Zollinger-Ellison syndrome a non-beta cell tumour secreting large quantities of gastrin occurs in the pancreas, and produces extremely intractable duodenal ulceration.

DUODENAL ULCER

Duodenal ulcer is most common in the young and the middle-aged (20–45 years), and occurs more often in men than women. 95% occur in the duodenal bulb i.e. the first 2 cm of the duodenum.

Clinical findings. Aching, burning or gnawing pain occurs in the epigastrium. Pain occurs one hour or more after breakfast. The pain is relieved by lunch, but recurs in the afternoon. It is most likely to occur at night, several hours after food. Food, milk or antacids give temporary relief. When the ulcer penetrates posteriorly into the head of the pancreas, the pain bores through to the back and may become more persistent. On examination there may be tenderness in the epigastrium to the right of the midline. The symptoms typically come and go, each relapse lasting for several weeks. This periodicity of pain is an important feature of duodenal ulcer. The diagnosis of a duodenal ulcer with only minimal symptoms is made on the basis of the typical pain and the response to food or drugs that reduce acid secretion or protect the mucosa. In such cases neither endoscopy nor barium contrast x-rays are necessary. Diagnosis in more severe cases is preferably made by endoscopy; repeated endoscopies to monitor healing are not required unless the patient responds poorly. Barium studies are helpful, particularly if an operation is contemplated, because the extent of the duodenal deformity can be delineated.

Laboratory findings. The *stool* should be examined for occult blood. If the Zollinger-Ellison syndrome is suspected a gastric analysis is indicated, along with an estimation of the serum gastrin level.

The standard *gastric analysis* measures acid output under basal fasting conditions, the basal acid output. It also measures acid production during stimulation by histamine, given in a dose which is maximal for this effect — the maximal acid output. The upper limits of normal are: basal, 5 meq/hour and maximal, 30 meq/hour. However, the overlap between the values found in either type of peptic ulcer and in normal individuals is so marked that gastric analysis is of little value in clinical practice.

Serum *gastrin* levels above 200 pg/ml are abnormal. These levels are raised in two different types of conditions. Firstly, serum gastrin is markedly increased in the Zollinger-Ellison syndrome; in this condition a gastrin-secreting islet cell tumour produces a greatly increased quantity of gastric acid and results in peptic ulceration. Secondly, serum gastrin levels are raised in atrophic gastritis and pernicious anaemia. In these conditions achlorhydria occurs, and the absence of acid in the stomach results in a loss of the normal inhibition for gastrin release.

X-ray findings. The first inch of normal duodenum shows up on the barium meal x-ray as a triangle with rounded sides and corners. This appearance is called the duodenal cap. A duodenal ulcer produces distortion of the duodenal cap due firstly to inflammatory swelling and later to scarring. At the same time, after the duodenum has emptied of barium, a speck of barium may be held up in the ulcer and show up on the x-ray.

Gastroduodenoscopy. Fibreoptic gastroduodenoscopy has nearly replaced barium meal x-ray for the diagnosis of peptic ulcer, as the whole interior of the stomach and proximal duodenum can now be clearly visualized. Endoscopy can also accurately localize the site of bleeding in haematemesis and assess the response to therapy. As the end of the gastroscope can be turned backward on itself through 180°, the area of the fundus can also be visualized.

Differential diagnosis. The most common diseases simulating duodenal ulcer are the following:

1. *Chronic cholecystitis.* In this condition pain is usually felt more to the right side i.e. in the right hypochondrium. Also, if pain radiates backwards it does not bore through to the back but spreads around the chest to the inferior angle of the scapula and often to the right shoulder. Ultrasound examination shows up the stones in most cases.
2. *Pancreatitis.* In severe forms of this illness shock is present to a degree out of proportion to the severity of pain, and serum amylase is raised to a very high level.
3. *Functional indigestion.* In this case x-ray and other tests are normal. So-called 'gastritis' may be included in this category, or may represent a precursor of peptic ulceration.
4. *Reflux oesophagitis.* In this condition the pain commonly radiates upwards retrosternally.

Complications. Besides the distress caused by pain, the common complications of duodenal ulcer are haemorrhage, perforation and duodenal obstruction. They are discussed later.

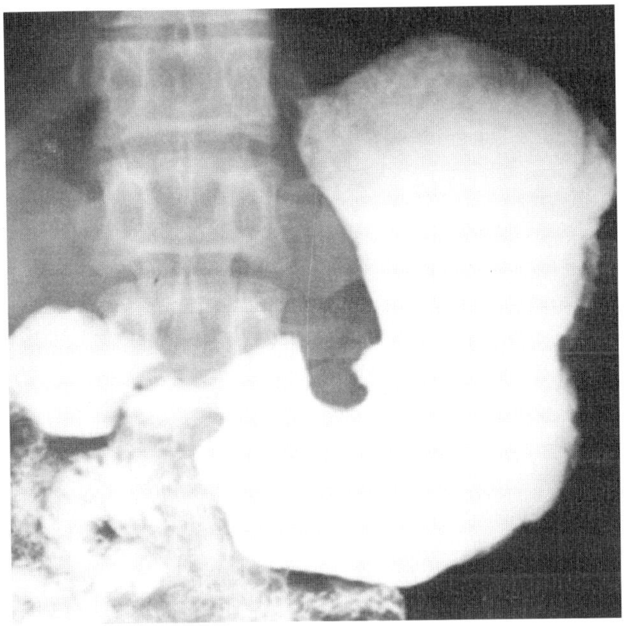

Fig. 1 Benign gastric ulcer, located at the typical site on the lesser curvature.

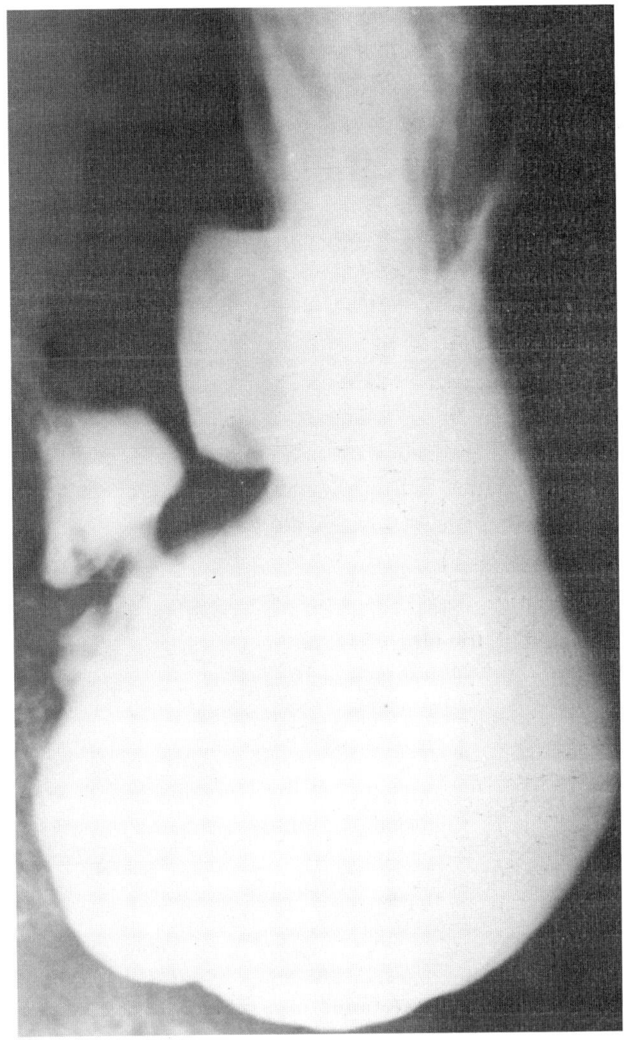

Fig. 2 Malignant gastric ulcer on lesser curvature; diameter greater than 2 cm.

GASTRIC ULCER

Gastric ulcer is most common between the ages of 40 and 60 years. 95% of the ulcers occur on the lesser curvature. A few gastric ulcers occur near the pylorus at the same time as a duodenal ulcer; their treatment should follow the guidelines for duodenal ulcers. Most gastric ulcers, however, occur by themselves, without a duodenal ulcer.

Clinical features. The main symptom of gastric ulcer is epigastric pain relieved by food or antacids, as in duodenal ulcer. Epigastric tenderness usually occurs. The pain tends to occur early after eating, within about 30 minutes. Vomiting, anorexia and aggravation of pain by food is more frequent than with duodenal ulcer. However, the two diseases cannot be distinguished on the basis of the history, and endoscopy is required.

Gastric analysis. Basal and maximal acid output are low or normal. But if a duodenal ulcer is also present they are high. In the absence of acid in the stomach no benign peptic ulcer can develop. Therefore, *if achlorhydria is present in a case of gastric ulcer, it must be a malignant lesion.*

Barium meal. On barium meal x-ray a gastric ulcer is usually located on the lesser curvature (Fig. 1).

If a tumour mass is not present, the following suggest that the ulcer is malignant:

1. Ulcer greater than 2 cm in diameter (Fig. 2).
2. The meniscus sign on barium meal x-ray, i.e. a dark ring around the ulcer caused by the raised edges of the tumour.

Gastroscopy. On gastroscopy the rolled-up margins of a malignant ulcer can be distinguished from the flat edges of a benign ulcer. Biopsies are taken from the edges of the ulcer in each quadrant (four-quadrant biospy).

Differential diagnosis. Hiatus hernia, atrophic gastritis, chronic cholecystitis, irritable colon syndrome and functional problems can mimic gastric ulcer. The clinical features of each of these conditions differ somewhat from those of gastric ulcer. Endoscopy and barium meal x-ray help distinguish the first two conditions, and gallstones are shown up on ultrasound examination.

Complications. The common complications of gastric ulcer are the same as those of duodenal ulcers, namely haemorrhage, perforation and stenosis. They are discussed in detail later.

MANAGEMENT OF PEPTIC ULCER

Prevention. Ulcerogenic drugs and other substances, e.g. caffeine, alcohol, nicotine and highly spiced foods, should be avoided in susceptible individuals. In this connection it should be remembered that nearly all non-steroidal anti-inflammatory drugs (NSAIDs) are ulcerogenic, and should be avoided. Elimination of unusually stressful environmental factors may also be helpful.

MEDICAL TREATMENT

Medical treatment is similar for gastric and duodenal ulcer and includes the use of specific medications and elimination of known gastric irritants. At the same time attempts are made to relieve social problems and irregular habits of eating, working and sleeping.

Gastric *irritants* include tobacco, alcohol, caffeine, aspirin, ibuprofen, indomethacin and salicylates, as well as most other non-steroidal anti-inflammatory drugs (NSAIDS). In the past *diet* was considered as closely related to ulcer disease; this is not true. Normal food taken at regular intervals is best. Food buffers gastric acid, so during acute episodes the patient should take frequent meals, or snacks between the three main meals. A drink of milk and a few biscuits are valuable at bedtime and also for rapid control of pain that appears in the middle of the night.

Specific *medications* to control ulcers include antacids, H_2 antagonists, mucosal coating agents, omeprazole and prostaglandins. Controlled studies have shown all except the last-named to be equally effective as far as pain relief is concerned. 80% of ulcers healed within one month, although gastric ulcers took longer to heal. The recurrence rate within 6 months was high.

Antacids should be prescribed to be taken 1 and 3 hours after each meal. Magnesium trisilicate plus aluminium hydroxide is the antacid of choice; the former is a mild laxative, the latter has the opposite effect, the two together balance each other out. The advent of *H_2 antagonists* has radically altered the prognosis and course of peptic ulceration. Cimetidine (300 mg four times a day) reduces acid secretion and is more effective than antacids in the treatment of duodenal and gastric ulcers. Treatment with cimetidine can be continued for very long periods, and the ulcer remains healed so long as this drug is being used. However, when the drug is stopped a recurrence may take place. The advent of long-term therapy by cimetidine has greatly reduced the incidence of operations for peptic ulcer, although this may also be attributed to a decreasing incidence of the disease. Recently, another H_2 ion antagonist, ranitidine (150 mg twice a day), has been introduced. Its action is similar to that of cimetidine, but it is more expensive.

The most effective *mucosal coating agent* is sucralfate (1g four times daily). Omeprazole inhibits the intracellular *proton pump* and can eliminate gastric acid production altogether. *Prostaglandins* increase the blood supply to the gastric mucosa and decrease the damaging effect of NSAIDS. The only prostaglandin approved by the FDA (Food and Drug Administration of USA) is misoprostol. Anticholinergic drugs have not been shown to confer any therapeutic benefit, and therefore should not be relied upon.

A *gastric ulcer* which is unhealed after a full course of medical treatment could either be simply an intractable ulcer, or it could be a malignant one. Four quadrant endoscopic biopsies should now be carried out. If the biopsy shows malignancy, operation is the only method of treatment which offers hope of cure, and should be carried out, unless contraindicated by evidence of widespread disease or very poor general condition of the patient. If the biopsy shows that the ulcer is benign the decision has to be made between continuing medical treatment or resort to surgery. Gastric ulcers are generally difficult to cure medically, recur frequently and cause more severe symptoms than duodenal ulcers. Therefore, surgery should be offered earlier than in the case of duodenal ulcers. However, in the elderly poor-risk patient medical treatment should be continued.

SURGICAL TREATMENT

If medical treatment has been properly carried out, an ulcer that fails to heal may be judged intractable, and surgical treatment is indicated. Each surgeon will have his own ideas about how many episodes of recurrence make operation mandatory. The patient and the surgeon should discuss this matter to arrive at a decision. Haemorrhage, perforation or obstruction are also manifestations of intractability in the wider sense.

Excision of the ulcer itself is not sufficient for either duodenal or gastric ulcer. Recurrence always take place following such a procedure. *Therefore all the different operations available for peptic ulcer aim at reducing the level of acidity in the stomach*

Methods of reducing acidity. The objective of reducing gastric acidity may be achieved in one of the following ways:

(a) Abolishing the nervous phase of gastric secretion.

(b) Draining the acid gastric contents into the duodenum or jejunum.

(c) Providing for reflux of alkaline duodenal or jejunal contents into the stomach to neutralize the acid.

(d) Removing the gastrin-secreting area i.e. the antrum.

(e) Removing the whole or a part of the acid-secreting area i.e. the parietal-cell bearing regions of the stomach.

Operations available. The operations available are the following:

Vagotomy. This abolishes the nervous phase of gastric acid secretion. There are three types of vagotomy:

1. *Truncal vagotomy.* (Fig. 3a) 1 to 2 cm of each vagal trunk is excised, just below the oesophageal hiatus. This procedure denervates the entire stomach and the gastrointestinal tract to the midcolon. Combined with other operations, it is highly effective in reducing the number of recurrent ulcers. However, it carries some deleterious side-effects; it reduces the ability of the stomach to empty, and is followed by other late motility disturbances, like diarrhoea and reflux alkaline gastritis. As it is followed by gastric stasis it cannot be used alone; it has to be combined with a drainage procedure.

2. *Selective vagotomy.* The vagi are divided below their hepatic branches. Although this operation is more time-consuming and difficult than truncal vagotomy it gives similar results, therefore it has attracted few supporters.

3. *Proximal gastric vagotomy.* The branches of both anterior and posterior vagi running from the main trunks to the lower 7 cm of oesophagus and the upper stomach down to 8 cm above the pylorus are divided, those supplying the antrum being spared. The main trunks are also left intact. Thus the antrum remains innervated, gastric emptying takes place normally, and this type of vagotomy does not have to be supplemented by a drainage procedure.

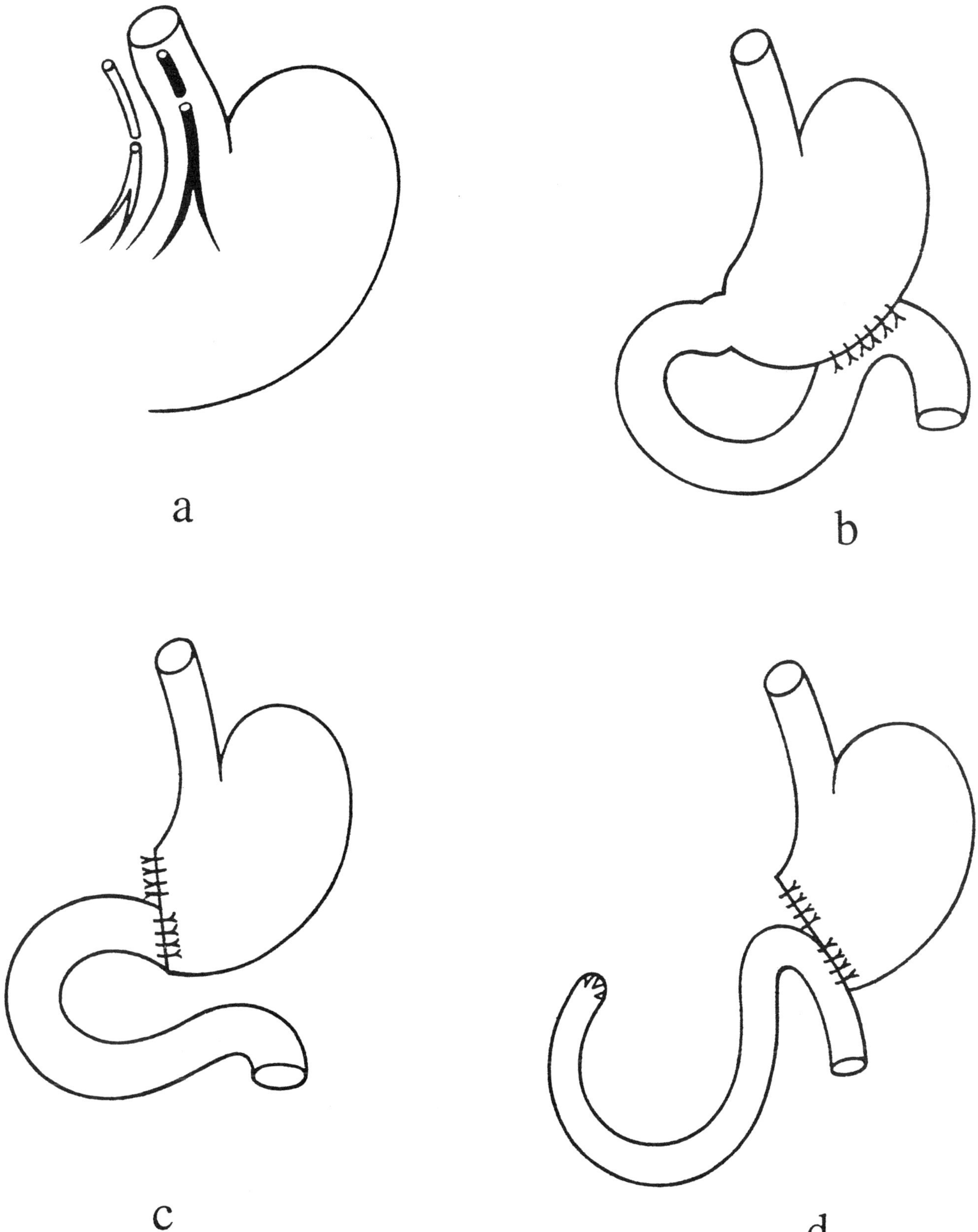

Fig. 3 Different operations for peptic ulcer:
a: Vagotomy, b: Gastrojejunostomy, c: Antrectomy (Billroth anastomosis), d: Partial gastrectomy (Polya anastomosis).

Table 1 Ways in which different operations on the stomach reduce acidity.

	Abolishes nervous phase (a)	Drains acid contents (b)	Allows alkaline reflux (c)	Removes gastrin secreting area (d)	Removes parietal cell area (e)
Vagotomy	+				
Gastrojejunostomy		+	+		
Vagotomy + gastrojejunostomy	+	+	+		
Antrectomy		+	+	+	
Vagotomy + antrectomy	+	+	+	+	
Total gastrectomy	+	+	+	+	+

Gastrojejunostomy. (Fig. 3b) An anastomosis is made between the posterior wall of the stomach and the most proximal loop of the jejunum.

Pyloroplasty. The pyloric sphincter is divided and rendered incompetent; the wall of the stomach and duodenum is then repaired.

Antrectomy. (Fig. 3c) The gastric antrum is removed. The stomach is anastomosed to the duodenum (Billroth I operation).

Partial gastrectomy. (Fig. 3d) The distal 2/3rd to 3/4th of the stomach is excised. The stomach is joined to a loop of proximal jejunum, the duodenal stump having been closed (Polya operation).

The ways in which these operations achieve the objective of reducing acidity are given in Table 1.

Operations carried out in actual practice. In actual practice vagotomy is almost never used alone, because it produces severe stasis in the stomach. Similarly, gastrojejunostomy is not used alone; it does not adequately reduce acidity, and so is quite often followed by an ulcer in the jejunum just distal to the anastomosis (anastomotic ulcer). But fortunately these two operations ideally complement each other. Vagotomy abolishes the nervous phase; gastrojejunostomy not only helps drainage of the stomach contents and allows regurgitation of the alkaline contents, but also remedies the main defect of vagotomy, namely stasis. Thus added together, the acidity-lowering effect of the two operations becomes sufficient to deal with the situation by combining a, b and c (Table 1). For similar reasons, antrectomy is not used alone but is combined with vagotomy (a, b, and d).

Total gastrectomy is used only for the extremely severe hyperacidity produced by the Zollinger-Ellison syndrome.

To sum up, the operations used commonly are:

1. Proximal gastric vagotomy.
2. Vagotomy and gastrojejunostomy (or pyloroplasty).
3. Partial gastrectomy (distal 3/4 stomach).
4. Vagotomy and antrectomy.

Choice of operation. ***Duodenal ulcer.*** Proximal gastric vagotomy causes the least physiological derangement, but is a difficult operation technically. For a healthy well nourished man vagotomy and antrectomy is best, because there is a low rate of recurrent ulcer with minimal early and late complications. But if the patient's general condition is suboptimal or technical difficulties are likely during gastric resection, vagotomy plus pyloroplasty minimizes the immediate morbidity and mortality rates. The long term results of this procedure are slightly poorer than vagotomy and antrectomy or partial gastrectomy, mainly because of a higher rate of recurrent ulcer. Finally, partial gastrectomy has mostly been replaced by vagotomy and antrectomy in the treatment of duodenal ulcer.

Gastric ulcer. For patients with gastric ulcer *without* duodenal ulcer, a 50% gastrectomy with Billroth I reconstruction is usually advised. The recurrence rate is low (2%) and the long-term results excellent. If the ulcer is high on the lesser curve the distal gastrectomy is combined with local excision of the ulcer.

In patients with a prepyloric ulcer *along with* a duodenal ulcer, the duodenal lesion should be regarded as the primary one, and the case should be dealt with as described under duodenal ulcer, i.e. by vagotomy plus drainage or vagotomy plus antrectomy. The recurrence rate after the former operation is a good deal higher than after the latter; therefore, it is used only in poor-risk patients.

Recording the results. Visick's criteria allow us to record the postoperative result objectively. They are as follows: Visick I, totally asymptomatic; II, minor symptoms; III, symptoms interfering with daily life; IV, totally incapacitated.

Prognosis after treatment. *Duodenal ulcer* patients who do less well with *medical* treatment are those with a high acid secretion. Bleeding occurs in 15% and perforation and obstruction each in about 5%. The onset of back pain is a bad prognostic sign. The results of *surgery* are good in 90% patients. The mortality rate following elective surgery is 1–2%.

With *gastric ulcers,* the recurrence rate in the first two years after *medical* therapy is as high as 40%. In ulcers that fail to heal, malignancy cannot be excluded. For these reasons, and because gastrectomy cures gastric ulcer so efficiently, *surgery* is advised in many of these patients.

COMPLICATIONS AFTER GASTRIC OPERATIONS

Apart from the usual pulmonary, cardiac and thrombotic complications which can follow any major upper abdominal operation, a variety of specific complications can occur after operations on the stomach and duodenum.

Duodenal fistula. The most serious early complication after an operation for a peptic ulcer is blow-out of a duodenal stump. This occurs after the Polya operation, in which the duodenal stump is closed. Many liters of duodenal contents pour out from the duodenum, producing severe dehydration and electrolyte depletion, as well as skin excoriation due to the digestive enzymes in the leaking fluid. Treatment consists of fluid and electrolyte replacement, intravenous alimentation, suction of the discharge to remove it from contact with the skin, and barrier creams like zinc oxide paste to protect the skin. If no drain was placed near the stump at the surgery, immediate operation should be carried out and drains inserted. If the condition is treated promptly and efficiently, healing usually takes place.

Recurrent ulcer. A recurrent ulcer usually occurs just distal to the anastomosis (anastomotic ulcer) and arises due to insufficient reduction in gastric acidity. There is severe persistent boring pain. If the stoma is adequate and acid hypersecretion is present, vagotomy will cure the ulcer. If an anastomotic ulcer remains untreated it may erode into the transverse colon and produce a gastrojejunocolic fistula. There is severe diarrhoea after every meal, with foul eructations. The fistula should be resected and the colon and jejunum repaired. At the same time, vagotomy or a high partial gastrectomy should be carried out.

A gastric ulcer in the body (type 1) does not produce much acid. If it is dealt with by gastric resection even without vagotomy, the operation is followed by a low rate of recurrence. On the other hand a gastric ulcer with a duodenal ulcer (type 2), or a pyloric or prepyloric ulcer (type 3), has a high acid output. If it is treated by proximal gastric vagotomy, the recurrence rate is high; these ulcers should therefore be treated by antrectomy plus bilateral truncal vagotomy.

The lowest recurrence rate is seen after gastric resection and bilateral truncal vagotomy, the highest after proximal gastric vagotomy. However, recurrent ulcers after proximal gastric vagotomy can be successfully treated by gastric resection.

Postgastrectomy syndromes. After partial gastrectomy the food passes rapidly into the small intestine. This may give rise to the *early dumping syndrome* (sweating, palpitations, abdominal cramps and diarrhoea) within half an hour after a meal; this is seen particularly after liquids with a high osmolality, such as milk shakes. The *late* dumping syndrome is also related to the intake of carbohydrates. About 2 hours after the meal, the hyperglycaemia induces an oversupply of insulin which then leads to a reactive hypoglycaemia with symptoms of sweating and extreme weakness. Moderation of carbohydrate intake usually controls the symptoms.

Reduced acidity in the proximal intestines impairs calcium absorption, leading to *osteoporotic* changes in bones. Other less specific symptoms have been included in this category, e.g. early satiety, regurgitation and reflux gastritis.

Steatorrhoea and anaemia. In the Polya type of gastrectomy the stomach is anastomosed directly to the jejunum, and the duodenum is bypassed. Here two additional problems arise. The poor mixing of food with bile and pancreatic juice may cause steatorrhoea. At the same time, bypassing the duodenum hinders iron absorption and results in anaemia.

Weight loss. The combined effect of all the above factors leads to diminished absorption, with weight loss.

COMPLICATIONS OF PEPTIC ULCERS

The three most important complications of peptic ulcer include haemorrhage, perforation and stenosis.

UPPER GASTROINTESTINAL HAEMORRHAGE

Upper gastrointestinal (GI) haemorrhage may be mild or severe, but *should always be taken seriously* and investigated thoroughly. Bleeding is the most common serious complication of peptic ulcer, portal hypertension and gastritis, and these conditions account for most episodes of upper GI bleeding.

Haematemesis. Vomiting of bright red or dark blood indicates that the source of bleeding is proximal to the duodenojejunal junction. Vomitus looking like ground coffee ('coffee-ground vomiting') indicates that blood has been in the stomach long enough for gastric acid to convert haemoglobin to methaemoglobin.

Melaena. Melaena can be produced by blood entering the bowel at any point from mouth to caecum, but most patients with melaena are bleeding from the upper gastrointestinal tract. The red cells in the blood disintegrate, and the released haemoglobin is broken down into haem and globin. Intestinal and bacterial enzymes now oxidize haem to haematin, which gives melaena stools their black colour. Bright red blood from the rectum is not called melaena.

Haematochezia. Haematochezia means the passage of bright red blood from the rectum; the blood comes from the anus, rectum or colon. But if very brisk bleeding is occurring in the upper intestine, bright red blood may be passed in the stool due to rapid transit.

Management of upper GI haemorrhage. If in a healthy looking patient melaena has continued for a week or more, it suggests slow bleeding. Such a case should be admitted to hospital and investigated.

On the other hand, haematemesis or sudden melaena should be regarded as a much more serious emergency, and urgent resuscitative measures should be taken as follows:

1. The circulatory status should be assessed. The pulse rate and blood pressure are recorded, and one should look for the presence of pallor, cold extremities and air hunger, which indicate loss of a large volume of blood.
2. The amount of blood lost and the rate of bleeding should be estimated, and the deficit made good by rapid blood transfusion.
3. Stomach lavage with ice-water should be started to slow down or stop bleeding.
4. Emergency endoscopy should be carried out to detect the site of bleeding, and if possible to arrest the haemorrhage, e.g. by sclerosing injection into oesophageal varices, or diathermy or laser coagulation of a bleeding artery in the base of a peptic ulcer.

The following findings indicate that surgical treatment will probably be required:

1. The presence of hypotension on admission.
2. The need for more than 4 units of blood to achieve circulatory stability.
3. High rates of bleeding.
4. Continued bleeding.
5. Recurrent bleeding.
6. Age above 60 years, because these patients tolerate continued blood loss less well.

Bleeding ulcers in the duodenum are usually located on the posterior wall. As the ulcer becomes deeper the gastroduodenal artery may get eroded, leading to very severe haemorrhage.

Treatment of bleeding peptic ulcer. Most patients with bleeding peptic ulcer can be managed medically, whereas about 25% require emergency surgery.

Early upper gastrointestinal endoscopy is the most valuable diagnostic procedure. However, profuse bleeding may make it useless. If a wide-bore nasogastric tube is passed into the stomach and irrigation continued until the bleeding slows down to a trickle, endoscopy can be carried out and the source can usually be determined. Even so, the diagnosis of the source of bleeding sometimes has to be made by laparotomy. If necessary, a wide gastrotomy incision that extends across the pylorus gives the best exposure to help find the source.

Medical measures for acute massive bleeding include irrigation of the stomach for removal of blood clots, elimination of oral intake, continuous nasogastric suction, intravenous replacement of blood, and injection of vasopressin into a peripheral vein. A careful chart of the vital signs and repeated assays of haematocrit are essential.

Patients over the age of 60 do not tolerate massive bleeding well; they respond much better to early operation. Under that age mortality is not increased by the delay imposed by attempts to control the bleeding by endoscopic techniques such as electrocoagulation or laser.

If *laser* is used as an endoscopic haemostatic device to produce thermal contraction of the bleeding vessel, surgery can be avoided. The bleeding vessel is identified, any clot washed off, and the lesion ringed with several pulses of laser energy. The tissue turns white when it is coagulated and the feeding vessel has been occluded. The method is associated with a 1 percent mortality compared with a 12 percent mortality in control patients.

Angiographic embolization of the gastroduodenal or left gastric arteries may be effective, but there are dangers involved. The foreign material injected into the left gastric artery may cause necrosis of the upper portion of the stomach; that in the gastroduodenal artery may slip into the hepatic artery and cause hepatic necrosis.

Early *operation* is indicated in patients bleeding from the gastroduodenal artery or a gastric ulcer. If the patient's general condition is good, a bleeding gastric ulcer is best treated by a partial gastrectomy, and a duodenal or prepyloric ulcer by a vagotomy and antrectomy.

PERFORATED PEPTIC ULCER

A perforated peptic ulcer is a very serious emergency. Most perforated ulcers are on the anterior surface of the duodenal bulb, much less often on the anterior surface of the stomach. In most cases there is a long history of peptic ulcer. In a few cases a 'silent' ulcer perforates, specially if the patient has been on cortisone.

Clinical findings. At the moment of the perforation either gastric acid, or (in the case of a duodenal ulcer) bile and pancreatic enzymes, suddenly pour into the peritoneal cavity. Due to the intense chemical peritonitis the patient cries out in agony. Peritoneal fluid is now secreted in liberal amounts. This dilutes the irritants and gives temporary relief. However in a few hours the stage of bacterial peritonitis sets in. The patient is in severe pain. The temperature may be subnormal. The abdomen is held still. The whole abdomen is tender and rigid like a board. The escaping gas may change the normal liver dullness to a tympanitic note. Peristaltic sounds are absent due to paralytic ileus.

It should be noted that in occasional cases the presentation may not be as dramatic, and diagnosis may be missed because the clinical manifestations are not sufficiently severe, specially in the elderly.

X-rays. Plain x-rays in the erect posture show free air under the diaphragm in the great majority of patients. If no air is seen, gastrografin is given by mouth and x-rays may show escape of contrast material from the lumen.

Differential diagnosis. The differential diagnosis of a perforated peptic ulcer includes acute cholecystitis, acute pancreatitis, strangulating intestinal obstruction, acute appendicitis and mesenteric thrombosis. In pancreatitis there is more shock than would be expected from the degree of pain. In cholecystitis pain often radiates to the inferior angle of the scapula and the right shoulder.

Treatment. The treatment of a perforated peptic ulcer is immediate operation. A right paramedian incision is commonly employed. All pus and food debris are removed. The perforation is closed by interrupted sutures of silk, taking care to avoid the sutures cutting through the oedematous and friable edges of the ulcer. A patch of greater omentum is sewn over the suture line to provide further protection from leakage. Drains are placed in both paracolic gutters. If the patient is young and in good condition and the operator is experienced, the definitive operation for the ulcer may be carried out instead of simple closure of the perforation. Of patients treated by simple suture, one-third remain free of symptoms. Of the other two-thirds, about half require a definitive operation.

Most perforated gastric ulcers are located in the prepyloric area. They behave as perforated duodenal ulcers and require similar treatment. However, perforation of an ulcer elsewhere in the stomach introduces the possibility of malignancy, and immediate definitive resection of the stomach is recommended. If the patient's condition is poor and simple closure is carried out, biopsy of the margin of the ulcer should be taken to rule out malignancy.

PYLORIC OBSTRUCTION DUE TO PEPTIC ULCER

Pyloric obstruction usually occurs from fibrosis around a duodenal ulcer. Most patients have a long history of dyspepsia. The ulcer pain gets worse, and there is anorexia and vomiting. The vomitus contains food taken many hours previously. There is no bile in the vomitus. Weight loss and dehydration are obvious. A succussion splash may be elicited from retained gastric contents in the dilated stomach. Occasionally, peristalsis in the distended stomach may be visible, passing from left to right in the epigastrium. Tetany may occur due to advanced alkalosis. Anaemia is common.

Metabolic disturbances. Prolonged vomiting causes dehydration and alkalosis. Vomiting depletes the patient of sodium, potassium and chloride. The loss of hydrochloric acid in the gastric juice causes the extracellular bicarbonate level to rise. The kidney excretes this excess bicarbonate, which takes large amounts of sodium with it as sodium bicarbonate. The loss of sodium activates aldosterone. In order to maintain the extracellular fluid volume, sodium is conserved and potassium and hydrogen are excreted instead. The glomerular filtration rate falls and produces prerenal azotaemia. A marked deficit of Na^+, Cl^-, K^+ and H_2O is the result. While replacing the fluid and electrolyte losses the usual practice is that water and NaCl are replaced first till a satisfactory urine flow starts. KCl replacement is then started. If potassium is given before a good flow of urine is obtained, dangerous hyperkalaemia may result.

Treatment. In the vast majority of cases of pyloric stenosis operation is required to relieve the obstruction and reduce acidity. The common operations carried out are: either vagotomy and gastroenterostomy, or partial gastrectomy. Elderly patients in poor condition who are considered to have burned-out ulcers can be treated by gastroenterostomy under local anaesthesia. Operation is carried out only after the electrolyte disturbances have been corrected.

ZOLLINGER-ELLISON SYNDROME

The Zollinger-Ellison syndrome consists of peptic ulcer disease caused by a gastrin-producing tumour (gastrinoma). These are mostly non-beta islet cell carcinomas or adenomas in the pancreas, or uncommonly in the duodenum. Rarely the condition is due to multiple endocrine neoplasms (MEN syndrome).

Clinical features. Symptoms result from the extremely severe hyperacidity. Abdominal pain occurs due to the peptic ulcer. Diarrhoea is common, and is due to hypersecretion of acid. The duodenum is flooded with acid. This destroys pancreatic lipase and produces steatorrhoea and also damages the small bowel mucosa. Symptoms often persist in spite of large quantities of antacids. Anastomotic ulcers appear even after surgical operations that would heal ordinary ulcers.

The *serum gastrin* level may be many times the normal upper limit of 200 pg/ml. On *x-ray* an ulcer may be seen in the duodenal bulb. Occasionally the ulcer may be in the distal duodenum or upper jejunum; an ulcer in that location is diagnostic of gastrinoma, as the 'normal' duodenal ulcers occur only in the first part of the duodenum.

Treatment. Total gastrectomy is effective treatment for the Zollinger-Ellison syndrome, and has been the standard treatment uptil now. Cimetidine controls the acid hypersecretion, and patients are now being managed on continuous cimetidine. Because the tumour is often multiple, its removal is successful in only 20% of patients. Laparotomy should be carried out after controlling the ulcer with cimetidine. Any pancreatic adenoma should be removed. Proximal gastric vagotomy should also be carried out, so that if removal of the adenoma is incomplete, management with cimetidine is made easier. If all else fails total gastrectomy is available.

After total gastrectomy most patients lead a relatively normal life. *Life-long iron e.g. ferrous sulphate 1 tablet b.d. and parenteral vitamin B12 are required.* Until recently most gastrinomas could not be found, therefore the best treatment was total gastrectomy. However these days gastric hypersecretion can be effectively controlled by H^+-K^+-ATPase inhibitors like omeprazole. At the same time, most gastrinomas can be localized by CT scan, digital subtraction angiography, ultrasonography and selective angiography. Exploratory laparotomy with duodenal illumination and duodenotomy finds many more gastrinomas. Therefore, the treatment of choice these days consists of excision of the tumour.

GASTRIC SURGERY FOR MORBID OBESITY

If the weight is more than twice the ideal body weight (200 to 225% to be exact) for the patient, the patient is defined as *morbidly obese*. If his weight is more than 225% of ideal body weight, he is classified as *superobese*. In such cases the complications related to obesity are severe; at the same time, long-term weight reduction cannot be achieved by conservative methods and surgery is required. In the past, short-circuiting of the small intestine used to be employed for this purpose. However, this was found to lead to extremely severe nutritional and metabolic deficiencies, and has been given up. The most successful method of dealing with morbid obesity and superobesity consists of restricting the surface area of the stomach available for contact with food (*gastric restrictive surgery*). Not only does this kind of surgery cure morbid obesity, it also helps in connection with the different obesity-related complications. For example, hypertension related to morbid obesity is cured in as many as two-thirds of the patients.

CARCINOMA OF THE STOMACH

Carcinoma of the stomach is an important cause of death. The highest incidence is between 45 and 65 years of age. Premalignant conditions are gastric polyps and pernicious anaemia. More than half the tumours arise in the pyloric region. Microscopically the tumours are nearly always adenocarcinomas. A few squamous cell tumours are seen at the cardia, but they actually arise from the oesophagus. Macroscopically there are five types:

1. A cauliflower-like growth.
2. An ulcer with irregular indurated edges.
3. Colloid carcinoma
4. Scirrhous carcinoma
5. Carcinoma secondary to gastric ulcer.

Aetiological factors. *Familial* and *racial* factors play a part in the causation of gastric carcinoma. 4 percent of the patients give a family history of the disease, which is slightly more common in patients with blood group A. In

Japan gastric cancer occurs in almost epidemic proportions, being responsible for nearly half the deaths from all malignancies. *Atrophic gastritis*, along with its resultant achlorhydria and high gastric pH, is associated with an increased incidence of the condition. Finally, *nitrates* as food preservatives have been incriminated. It may be mentioned that in the advanced countries, recently there has been a remarkable decrease in the number of cases of carcinoma of the body and antrum. While the reason for this dramatic decrease is still speculative, it could be due to better refrigeration and more rapid transport of commercial meat prior to ingestion.

Spread. Extension of carcinoma of the stomach occurs by spread in the wall, direct spread to adjacent organs, and lymphatic metastases. Transperitoneal implantation may occur. These cells gravitate to the pelvis and produce tumours there.

Clinical findings. The first symptom is gastric distension with inability to take a normal meal. Anorexia and weight loss develop. Epigastric pain is persistent. The patient is anaemic and weak, and gets tired easily. He may present with obstruction at the cardia (dysphagia), or at the pylorus (fullness, belching and vomiting). A lump in the epigastrium may be palpated incidentally without any symptoms. Carcinoma in the body of the stomach is usually silent, but may give rise to features in other organs e.g. obstructive jaundice (from secondary deposits in the liver), ascites (from carcinomatosis of peritoneum), etc.

Investigations. A thorough investigation should be undertaken in every case of persistent indigestion, specially in middle and old age. Anaemia is present in 40%, achlorhydria in 20% and occult blood in stools in 80% of cases of gastric carcinoma. The E.S.R. is raised in 70% cases.

X-rays. A skilled radiologist is required. A little barium is given first. It smears the mucosa of the stomach, and outlines lesions which would be obscured once the stomach is full of barium. After this, more barium is given and pictures taken from different angles.

Gastroscopy. All patients with a newly discovered gastric ulcer should undergo fibreoptic gastroscopy. Carcinoma is recognized by its nodularity, multicoloured base, and immobility. Multiple biopsies must always be taken. Usually, biopsy is taken from each quadrant of the mass or ulcer (four-quadrant biopsy). Fibreoptic gastroscopy has revolutionized the diagnosis of carcinoma as well as of other mucosal lesions of the stomach, and has nearly replaced barium meal x-rays.

Exfoliative cytology. Exfoliative cytology has become much less important since the introduction of excellent fibreoptic gastroscopes through which biopsies can be taken.

Treatment. Surgical resection is the only curative treatment for carcinoma of the stomach. Emaciated patients should be nutritionally resuscitated by a 2-week course of high-calorie parenteral nutrition before surgery (3,000–4,000 kcals/day). In the advanced countries 80% of patients are operable. At operation the lesions are resectable in 50% of cases. Of these one half are potentially curable, (i.e. there are no signs of spread beyond the limits of resection).

Pyloric tumours require distal 2/3rd gastrectomy with removal of omentum and nearby lymph nodes, all in one piece. Restoration of continuity may be achieved by the Billroth I or Polya procedures. In the Billroth I procedure the remnant of stomach is joined to the duodenum. In the Polya operation the duodenal stump is closed and the stomach remnant is anastomosed to the most proximal loop of jejunum.

Tumours of the proximal half of the stomach require total gastrectomy. After removal of the stomach a loop of jejunum is taken up to the hiatus and joined to the oesophagus. Tumours of the cardia require resection of the distal oesophagus and proximal stomach, with oesophagogastrostomy. For palliation of a pyloric tumour a limited resection utilizing a Polya resection is better than a diverting gastrojejunostomy. For advanced disease chemotherapy with a combination of methyl-CCNU and fluorouracil (5-FU) gives objective improvement in nearly half the cases.

Prognosis. In the developed countries the 5 year survival rate is 12%, although in the absence of lymph node involvement the figure is as high as 50%. Death may follow dissemination to other organs or be the result of progressive obstruction and malnutrition.

ACUTE GASTRITIS

This condition has been recognized with greater frequency since the use of fibreoptic gastroscopy in acute upper gastrointestinal bleeding. Ingestion of large amounts of alcohol or salicylates etc. is an important causative factor. There may be acute epigastric pain, or no symptoms. Tiny mucosal ulcers develop and occasionally cause massive haemorrhage. Diagnosis is made by gastroscopy and biopsy. Gastric lavage with cold solutions usually halts blood loss. If haemorrhage continues undiminished, operation may have to be performed. Vagotomy and drainage is usually carried out. If this fails, subtotal or rarely total gastrectomy might be necessary to save the patient's life.

VOLVULUS OF THE STOMACH

This is a serious though rare condition. The stomach usually rotates around the axis made by its two fixed points — cardia and pylorus. The greater curve with the colon moves up to lie under the diaphragm. A paraoesophageal hiatus hernia often occurs with it. Rotation around the transverse axis is rare. There is severe abdominal pain, vomiting, retching, epigastric distension and inability to pass a nasogastric tube. Immediate laparotomy is required to prevent death from acute gastric necrosis and shock.

DUODENAL ATRESIA

In duodenal atresia there is congenital occlusion of the second part of the duodenum, usually just distal to the ampulla of Vater. The baby starts vomiting right from birth, and the vomitus contains bile. This is in contradistinction to the situation in infantile pyloric stenosis, where vomiting starts one or two weeks after birth, and the vomitus contains no bile. The plain x-ray shows just two gas shadows: a large one in the stomach, and a small one in the duodenum (the double-bubble sign). Operation should be carried out urgently, through an upper right transverse incision. The most suitable procedure is a duodenojejunostomy, i.e. joining up the distended duodenal loop to a collapsed loop of the proximal jejunum.

DUODENAL DIVERTICULA

These are fairly commonly seen in autopsies and barium meal series. But only 1% of those detected by x-ray require surgery. Dyspepsia may occur and require antacids and anticholinergics. Complications are haemorrhage, perforation and biliary obstruction.

DUODENAL FISTULA

A duodenal fistula may occur:

1. Due to traumatic rupture of the duodenum.
2. As a complication of Polya gastrectomy: this used to be the most common cause. However, with the decrease in the number of gastrectomies carried out since the advent of cimetidine, it is taking second place.
3. Due to injury to the duodenum during nephrectomy or colectomy.

Both bile and pancreatic juice are discharged in large quantities through the fistula and produce excoriation of the skin. Dehydration, electrolyte depletion and hypoproteinaemia can quickly arise if the fistula is a large one.

Treatment. Treatment consists of protection of the skin with a barrier cream, drainage of the fistula, which may be aided by the patient lying on his right side, and total parenteral nutrition until the fistula heals. In common with other intestinal fistulae one must ensure that there is no distal obstruction if the fistula is to heal on conservative treatment.

21 *Liver*

INJURIES TO THE LIVER

Liver injuries may be penetrating or blunt.

The common *penetrating* injuries are stabs and bullet wounds. Stabs usually cause less damage; high velocity bullet wounds shatter the parenchyma over a wide area. More commonly, however, liver injuries are *blunt*. They are most often sustained during traffic accidents. They may produce bursting wounds with much damage. Problems are caused by haemorrhage, bile leakage, and devitalization i.e. infarction of liver tissue. Overlying ribs may be fractured.

Bleeding may be profuse and free into the peritoneal cavity producing collapse, or it may occur within the liver as a large haematoma. This may become infected to form an abscess, or may burst into the bile duct to give rise to haemobilia. *Bile leakage* can cause chemical biliary peritonitis with abscess formation. *Infarction* of the liver can also result in an abscess.

Clinical findings. If the liver is badly shattered, there may be hypovolaemic shock with hypotension, decreased urinary output, and low central venous pressure. Abdominal distension may be present. Haemoperitoneum may produce shifting dullness. If liver rupture is suspected on clinical grounds, peritoneal tap may be carried out to detect blood in the peritoneal cavity. If the tap is negative, peritoneal lavage may be carried out to look for blood-staining of the aspirate.

CT scans. Until recently nearly all liver injuries were treated by laparotomy. CT scans have revolutionized treatment; they have shown that in many of these injuries blood loss is less than 500 ml. For these stable and relatively minor injuries observation alone is satisfactory. If, in an injury to the right hypochondrium, a CT scan shows that the hepatic flexure of the colon and the right kidney are not damaged, the case can be treated conservatively. However, unstable patients do not benefit from the use of CT scans, because the time taken in the scan is too long for safety. Unstable patients need an urgent laparotomy.

Treatment. In severe abdominal injury the only safe course is laparotomy. *The morbidity caused by delay while waiting for diagnostic certainty is far greater than that due to a negative laparotomy.* Most lacerations have stopped bleeding by the time operation is performed. These should not be sutured, because stagnation of blood and serum in the closed space thus created could lead to abscess formation. Active bleeding may be managed by ligation or suture of bleeding points. If the hepatic flexure of the colon is also injured the bowel should be exteriorized, i.e. a colostomy performed.

Cases with extensive damage to the liver parenchyma are difficult to manage. Debridement involves piece-meal removal of dead tissue rather than lobar resection. However, a particularly severe crushing injury may require lobectomy. At the end of the operation suction catheters should be placed and brought out through separate incisions.

A few other points to remember are the following:

1. The body temperature must be maintained, if necessary by having the room temperature above 26°C from the start. The core temperature will then remain within a physiological range, allowing normal enzymatic processes to work, particularly those responsible for coagulation of blood.
2. If bleeding persists and the site of origin cannot be found, it should be remembered that a tear in the inferior vena cava could be responsible.
3. An effort should be made to get the liver on to the abdominal wall for better exposure, by dividing the falciform and triangular ligaments.
4. If more than 5 units of blood have to be given, 10 packs of platelets and 5 units of packed cells should be given for every additional 5 units of blood transfused.

If all else fails or the patient's condition deteriorates rapidly, the bleeding area should be packed and the abdomen closed. A day or two later, when any coagulopathy, hypothermia or acidosis has been dealt with, the abdomen can be re-opened and the packs removed.

Prognosis. The mortality rate after liver injury is about 10%. Only 1% of stabs are lethal, but as many as 20% of blunt injuries result in a fatality. This is because stabs result in a puncture-like wound in the liver, whereas blunt injuries produce more widespread disruption of the hepatic tissue. If three major organs are damaged, the death rate is as high as 70%. Most deaths are due to bleeding.

TUMOURS OF THE LIVER

Benign tumours. The most common benign hepatic tumour is *cavernous haemangioma*. Women are affected 6 times more commonly than men. These tumours are solitary subcapsular growths. Spontaneous rupture may cause severe haemorrhage. A large haemangioma may occasionally behave like an arteriovenous fistula and produce cardiac hypertrophy and congestive heart failure. Small symptomatic haemangiomas can be excised, but this is rarely necessary. If large they may be dealt with by radiotherapy, because resection can be dangerous, unless the tumour is localized to a segment or lobe.

Primary malignant tumours. Primary carcinoma of the liver is common in parts of Africa, and also in China and Japan. Elsewhere in the world it is an uncommon tumour. It arises mostly as a complication of cirrhosis resulting from Hepatitis B virus or secondary to haemochromatosis. The histological varieties are hepatoma (80%) and cholangiocarcinoma (20%).

A hepatoma can take one of three forms:

1. A single large mass.
2. Multiple nodules, commonly in cases with cirrhosis.
3. Infiltration of tumour throughout the liver.

In 70% of patients distant spread has already occurred when the condition is first diagnosed. The tumour may be highly vascular. This sometimes leads to massive intraperitoneal haemorrhage from rupture of the tumour.

Clinical findings. The diagnosis is not easy. Abdominal pain and distension are the most common symptoms. Pain may be felt in the epigastrium and right hypochondrium, and may be referred to the tip of the right shoulder. Weight loss and jaundice are common. The liver is enlarged in 80% of cases, and a mass is palpable in most of the rest. An arterial bruit may be heard over the liver, and is a good clue to the diagnosis. Ascites or gastrointestinal bleeding from varices may occur. Fever may be present, and in tropical countries a diagnosis of amoebic liver abscess may be made. A primary site should be looked for, because secondary carcinoma of the liver is very much more common than the primary variety.

Investigations. *Alpha-fetoprotein* may be present in the urine. This protein is normally present only in the plasma of the foetus. It is produced by the cells of carcinoma of the liver because they have de-differentiated and reverted to their foetal type of metabolism.

Radio-scanning and ultrasound are very useful investigations. *Radio-isotope* scanning distinguishes between functioning and non-functioning areas in the liver. *Ultrasound* examination distinguishes between solid and fluid-containing areas, and also between solids of different densities. These two investigations taken together help greatly in arriving at the correct diagnosis. *CT scan* and *MRI* give an even better image than ultrasound. *Needle biopsy* establishes the histological diagnosis, but care must be taken not to cause a secondary haemorrhage, which can assume dangerous proportions in occasional cases.

Complications. The complications that can arise in cases of hepatic carcinomas consist of sudden intraperitoneal haemorrhage and portal hypertension from portal vein obstruction. Liver failure is a common cause of death.

Treatment. Only surgical resection offers a possibility of cure. *Hepatic lobectomy* can be carried out if the tumour is localized. If the tumour extends to the opposite lobe or if cirrhosis is present, which increases the risk of liver failure, resection is not feasible, but transplantation can be considered. Many 5 year survivals have been reported after hepatic lobectomy. Ligation of the hepatic artery with perfusion of cytotoxic agents through its distal end has also helped patients survive for 2 to 3 years. Otherwise the average life expectancy after diagnosis is only 6 months.

A small primary carcinoma of the liver occurring in the presence of cirrhosis, which precludes even partial resection of the liver, is an indication for total hepatectomy and *transplantation*. If the effects of chronic hepatic failure and portal hypertension are absent, the patient is a good surgical candidate. Cancer recurs in about half the patients within 1 year of liver replacement; long-term disease-free survival is seen in the other half.

Metastatic tumours. Metastatic tumours are 20 times more common in the liver than primary tumours. Cancers of the breast, lung, pancreas, stomach, large intestine, kidney, ovary and uterus account for most of the cases. Weight loss, fatigue and anorexia are the common complaints, with right upper abdominal pain, ascites and jaundice. The liver is usually enlarged and may be nodular. If ultrasound scanning is used to direct the needle, biopsy can establish the diagnosis.

Cases amenable to effective *treatment* are rare. However, if confined to one lobe, lobectomy may be considered, and 40% 5 year survival rates have been reported if the primary tumour was in the colon. Systemic chemotherapy does not improve survival. Hepatic artery perfusion by cytotoxic agents has benefited some patients temporarily.

LIVER ABSCESS

Hepatic abscesses may be bacterial, parasitic or fungal. Pyogenic abscesses are common in the advanced countries, and amoebic abscesses in the poorer communities.

Pyogenic liver abscess. The incidence of pyogenic liver abscesses has not changed much over the last 50 years. However, fifty years ago most patients were under the age of 40 and the most common cause was appendicitis. Today the average age lies between 50 and 60, and the most common cause is biliary tract disease, with an increasing incidence of malignant disease in these cases. Pyogenic abscesses may be solitary or multiple, are distributed throughout both lobes of the liver, and usually follow suppuration elsewhere. Examples of some conditions resulting in pyogenic liver abscesses follow:

1. *Cholangitis,* whenever bile flow is obstructed: typically, total obstruction raises the pressure in the biliary tree, producing an acutely septic course and miliary micro-abscesses throughout the liver — 'acute suppurative cholangitis'. Incomplete obstruction usually results in a subacute course and a single abscess.
2. *Suppurative thrombophlebitis* in the *portal* venous system secondary to appendicitis, diverticulitis, infected haemorrhoids, etc.
3. *Direct extension* from infections involving the gallbladder, subphrenic space or pleural cavity, and sites of bowel perforation.
4. In *trauma* to the liver, haemorrhage or bile extravasation into liver tissue, or areas of hepatic necrosis, produce devitalized tissue which can become infected.
5. *Hepatic arterial infection.* In leukaemias and chronic granulomas, systemic bacteraemias may seed the liver. Again, in liver transplantation in children the hepatic artery anastomosis may become thrombosed with local or systemic micro-organisms.

Clinical findings. Irregular fever with spikes occurs. The liver is usually enlarged and tender. Leucocytosis is commonly present. Serum alkaline phosphatase and bilirubin levels may be raised in multiple abscesses. On x-ray the right dome of the diaphragm may be raised, with basilar atelectasis or pleural effusion. CT scan (Fig. 2, Chapter 16) and ultrasound are extremely useful and accurately indicate the presence, size, number and location of the abscesses. Special needles passing through the centre of the ultrasonic probe are available for aspiration of abscesses under ultrasound control. The radio-isotope scan gives less clear-cut demarcation.

Treatment. The classical treatment of pyogenic liver abscesses consisted of *open* drainage of the abscess, correction of the underlying pathology if possible, and a 4- to 6-week course of antibiotics, usually a beta-lactam, an aminoglycoside and metronidazole. However, in the past decade most patients have been treated by antibiotics and *percutaneous* drainage with benefit. Firstly, the extensive abdominal wall wound with its attendant pain and likelihood of involvement in the suppurative process is avoided. Secondly, contamination of the peritoneal cavity is avoided. Thus, further surgery is dispensed with in an individual who is usually immunocompromised due to extensive sepsis.

Percutaneous drainage is carried out under ultrasound or CT guidance. Samples of pus are taken for microbiological examination, the cavity is gently irrigated with saline, and the catheter left in place to provide continuing drainage. It should be remembered that in about 15% of patients percutaneous drainage fails. This may be due to incorrect placement of the catheter, excessive viscosity of the pus plugging the catheter, or thick abscess walls that do not collapse with drainage. Open drainage is then necessary.

The overall mortality rate is high, and is due to delay in diagnosis and the presence of multiple abscesses. If jaundice is present, and if the serum albumin level is falling, the prognosis is bad. Even if the abscess is solitary and is treated promptly there is still a significant mortality rate, upto 10%.

Amoebic liver abscess. Amoebic dysentery is endemic in most underdeveloped countries. In a few cases of amoebic dysentery the amoeba passes into the radicles of the portal vein and lodges in the liver to produce an amoebic liver abscess. The amoebae produce liquefaction necrosis. A proteolytic enzyme produced by the amoeba causes coalescence of the invaded areas and abscess formation. 80% of the abscesses are located in the right lobe, probably because venous return from the right side of the colon, where the amoeba commonly lodges, is predominantly delivered to the right lobe. The pus is not yellow but brown or chocolate-coloured. It consists of broken-down liver cells, leucocytes and red blood cells. In many cases the pus contains staphylococci, streptococci and *Esch. coli* in addition to the amoebae. If the freshly aspirated pus is examined under the microscope for the presence of motile amoebae, usually none are seen; they are mostly to be found in the walls of the abscess.

The *further course* may be along any one of the following lines:

1. The abscess may resolve under treatment with metronidazole.
2. It may continue to enlarge.
3. It may become encapsulated.
4. It may rupture into the right lung, the peritoneal cavity or the pleural cavity.
5. Secondary bacterial infection may occur, specially if the abscess is treated by open drainage.

Clinical findings. There may or may not be a history of recent dysentery. Young males are the most common sufferers.

In early cases the patient complains of discomfort and fullness in the liver region. The liver enlarges and becomes tender. Fever develops, at first intermittent, later remittent. Sweating is severe specially at night. The patient loses appetite and weight. The enlarged liver may cause bulging of the chest wall. Chest movement is restricted on the affected side and deep breathing is painful. The liver dullness is increased upwards. Jaundice is uncommon but may occur.

Diagnosis. The diagnosis of hepatic amoebiasis may be difficult, as dysentery is present only occasionally. *Chest x-rays* often show changes: raised diaphragm with reduced movement on screening, basal collapse and pleural effusion. *Utrasound* examination is invaluable both in diagnosis and aspiration, and serial ultrasound scanning is used to monitor the progress of healing. It can diagnose liver abscess with a sensitivity of 98% and an accuracy of 99%, and is as good as a CT scan. A polymorph leucocytosis is nearly always present. The *stool* may show amoebae or cysts, and sigmoidoscopy may sometimes show the ulcers. *Liver function tests* are not often helpful. *Serological tests* are accurate. The indirect haemagglutination test is positive in 95% of patients with an amoebic liver abscess, and in areas of low prevalence a positive result strongly suggests the presence of acute infection. However, antibody levels remain elevated for many years after infection; therefore, the test is not of much use in endemic areas, as nearly half the general population may be seropositive. On the other hand levels of antibodies detected by indirect immunofluorescence and counterimmunoelectrophoresis become undetectable within a few months of acute infection; these tests are therefore more useful in the endemic areas.

Treatment. The treatment of choice is metronidazole 750 mg orally or intravenously three times daily for 10 days, although there are still a few failures. In those cases dihydroemetine is given in a dose of 1 mg/kg/day intramuscularly four times daily for 5 days. This should be accompanied by chloroquine phosphate 600 mg base/day orally four times daily for 4 days, followed by 300 mg/day for a total of 14–21 days. Small abscesses respond to this regimen. If an abscess does not resolve on medical treatment alone it will require percutaneous drainage or repeated aspiration, under ultrasound or CT guidance. A smaller volume of pus is obtained at each successive aspiration until the cavity completely dries up. The abovementioned medical regime must be followed by treatment with an agent that can eradicate cysts which persist in the intestine after treatment with metronidazole. Such *intraluminal* agents include:

1. Iodoquinol 600 mg daily three times a day for 20 days.
2. Diloxanide furoate 500 mg orally three times a day for 10 days.
3. Paromomycin 25 to 30 mg/kg/day orally three times a day for 7 days.

In deep-seated abscesses a long needle must be used at a level below the pleural reflection to avoid infection of the pleural cavity. The needle is passed under ultrasound control. Ultrasound probes are now available which feature a track for the needle down the middle of the probe, for extremely accurate placing of the needle. After aspiration a full course of specific antiamoebic drug therapy should be used. If the abscess cannot be reached by the needle, a laparotomy has to be performed. In that case, after evacuation of the pus the incision must be completely closed. If a drain is left in place, the amoeba can colonize its track, causing a spreading infection, *amoebiasis cutis*, which is very difficult to eradicate. Treatment requires injections of emetine hydrochloride, which are not easily procured these days.

It should be stressed that as far as possible an amoebic liver abscess should be treated by drug therapy plus aspiration, or at most percutaneous drainage. Open drainage should be reserved for those cases where aspiration has failed. It is interesting to mention that even aspiration needle tracks sometimes get infected by amoebiasis cutis.

HYDATID DISEASE OF THE LIVER

Hydatid disease is common in sheep-rearing areas e.g. Australia, South America, Greece, Turkey, Iran and Iraq. The most common form is caused by *Echinococcus granulosus* which occurs in the form of a cyst in the liver or lung. *E. multilocularis* is uncommon. It occurs in an invasive form in the liver. The lesions do not have a well-demarcated cystic structure, may spread via the blood vessels, and in fact behave like a malignancy, with a much worse prognosis.

Life-cycle. The hydatid has two forms, the adult and the larval. The adult is a short flat worm in the primary host, usually a dog. It lives in the small bowel of the host, and has 3 to 5 segments. The last is the gravid segment, containing a few hundred ova which are shed in the faeces. The ova resist drying and remain viable for weeks. A grazing animal like sheep swallows the ova. The outer coating of the ovum is digested, allowing an embryo to hatch in the small intestine of the sheep, penetrate the bowel wall and enter the portal circulation. Most embryos are trapped in the liver and grow into cysts; some pass into the lungs and onwards to other parts of the body (Plate II-I). The life-cycle is completed when a dog eats the contaminated liver of the sheep.

Human beings usually contract the disease during childhood or adolescence, when ova are swallowed after contact with an infected dog. The embryo reaches the portal circulation and develops into a cyst. Man is an occasional intermediate host, and represents a dead end for the parasite, since dogs seldom have access to human viscera. Although patients suffering from hydatid disease are often segregated, it should be remembered that human beings are not infective to other humans.

Pathology. A hydatid cyst has three layers:

1. It is lined inside by a single layers of cells, the germinal epithelium *(endocyst)*. This secretes internally the hydatid fluid, which is a crystal-clear watery fluid. Brood capsules develop from the germinal epithelium and are attached to it by stalks. Within these capsules the heads of future worms *(scoleces)* develop. Spillage of the fluid into the peritoneum or pleural cavity can allow further hydatids to develop.

2. On its outer aspect the germinal epithelium secretes the laminated membrane *(ectocyst)* which looks like a water-filled balloon.

3. The outer adventitia *(pseudocyst)* consists of fibrous tissue produced by the reaction of the liver to the parasite. It is not really a part of the cyst proper.

Clinical features. The patient commonly presents with a painless, symptomless mass in the right upper abdomen, which has been present for many years, as this cyst grows very slowly. If it ruptures into the bile duct, biliary colic and jaundice can occur. Rarely, secondary infection occurs in the cyst with fever as the presenting symptom. Hydatids can cause allergic phenomena like urticaria, pruritus, asthma and anaphylaxis.

Complications. *Secondary infection* may occur into the cyst, as in any other collection of relatively stagnant fluid in the body. *Rupture* may result from trauma, operative intervention or infection. Severe allergic manifestations may occur as a result of rupture, and constitute a grave complication of abdominal hydatid disease. Rupture may also occur into the gallbladder, biliary tree, pleural cavity or hepatic veins.

Laboratory. Although the cyst is isolated from the liver by an adventitial layer, there is an absorption of parasitic products which acts as an antigenic stimulus. This is manifested by *eosinophilia* in as many as one fourths of the patients. The *Casoni intradermal test* is 80% accurate. The *haemagglutination* test is even more reliable. The detection of circulating scolex antigen by counter current immunoelectrophoresis *(CIE)* or the enzyme-linked immunosorbent assay *(ELISA)* give the most reliable results. The cyst is readily and clearly demonstrated both by *ultrasound* and *CT scan*. *Scintiscanning* shows a large filling defect.

Treatment. ***Medical.*** Although the only effective treatment is surgical, albendazole (10 mg/kg/day in two divided doses for 4 weeks) is specifically available for hydatid. After liver function tests and blood counts have been checked, the cycle is repeated after an interval of two weeks. Penetration of the cyst by the drug is uncertain and although many cysts decrease in size, not all scoleces are killed. In Australia the drug is used only for disease which is recurrent or surgically inaccessible, or if there are serious associated medical conditions.

Surgical. If the cyst ruptures and the hydatid fluid spills into the peritoneal cavity, it can produce anaphylactic shock and implantation of cysts throughout the abdomen. Therefore surgical treatment involves removing the cyst *without contaminating the patient*. The cyst is exposed at laparotomy. A long transverse or oblique abdominal incision gives wide exposure. Coloured drapes soaked in hypertonic saline isolate the cyst from the peritoneal cavity. The cyst fluid is aspirated and replaced by a scolicidal agent like hypertonic sodium chloride. Formalin or phenol, which were used previously, should not be injected into the cyst, because they can severely damage the bile ducts if a communication exists. In any case there is little evidence of the effectiveness of these fluids. They would have to reach an adequate concentration within the cyst, and it is impossible to predict the degree of dilution caused by residual cyst contents. The cyst can usually be shelled out intact by developing a plane of cleavage between the ectocyst and pseudocyst. Otherwise the contents have to be removed piecemeal. After evacuation the cavity should be examined for any bile leaks which should be closed. The best way of dealing with the cavity left behind in the liver is omentoplasty. The greater omentum is mobilized from the transverse colon preserving its blood supply, and is laid into the cavity.

Complicated cysts. Cysts *superinfected* with bacteria are best considered as abscesses and treated by drainage and antibiotic therapy. For *E. multilocularis,* hepatic resection is the best treatment, as there is no central cavity to be emptied, nor is there a clear margin for pericystectomy. Cysts with *extensive calcification* are usually sterile and are probably best left alone. If jaundice develops due to *intrabiliary rupture*, the common bile duct needs to be opened with clearance of cysts followed by T-tube drainage.

Hydatid cysts in other organs. In the *brain* hydatid cysts usually present as space-occupying lesions. Hydatid disease of the *heart* may be discovered at autopsy. During life the cysts may rupture into the chambers of the heart with pulmonary metastases or systemic embolization causing infarction. In the *kidney* the cysts may rupture into the renal pelvis producing renal colic and dysuria with the passage of hydatid material into the urine. Finally, echinococcus may rarely involve other sites like orbit, ovaries, broad ligament and uterus, and even the limbs (Plate II-I).

CIRRHOSIS OF THE LIVER

Cirrhosis is defined as diffuse fibrosis with nodule formation in the liver. The common causes of this condition are different in children and adults:

In children. 1. *Congenital atresia of the bile ducts.* Most survive only a few months.

2. *Nutritional.* This occurs in protein-deficient infants. Examples are found in Africa among the undernourished infants of very poor parents, and in India among the babies of high-caste Hindu vegetarians, whose religion does not allow them to eat meat.

3. *Infective* i.e. viral hepatitis. A history of severe jaundice in early infancy is obtained.

In adults. 1. Overindulgence in alcoholic beverages.

2. Virus hepatitis, particularly of the B & C classification.

3. Chronic (surgical) biliary obstruction.

4. Schistosomiasis (in Egypt, etc.).

The outlook in cirrhosis depends upon the severity of the associated hepatocellular disease.

PORTAL HYPERTENSION

If the flow of blood through the portal system is obstructed it may lead to an increase in portal venous pressure. The obstruction may be classified as follows:

1. Prehepatic (20%). Most patients are children. The common causes are the following:

1. Congenital absence of portal vein.

2. Thrombosis of the portal vein due to extension of the normal obliterative process of the umbilical vein at birth or secondary to a hypercoagulable state.

2. Intrahepatic (80%). *The most common cause is cirrhosis.* In a few countries schistosomiasis is a very important cause. Idiopathic fibrosis may rarely be the cause.

3. Posthepatic. The common conditions responsible are constrictive pericarditis, veno-occlusive disease, thrombosis of hepatic veins or vena cava, or congenital caval valve.

Due to the raised pressure in the tributaries of the portal vein, blood flows across anastomotic channels to areas of lower pressure. When the portal vein is absent or thrombosed collaterals proximal and distal to the vein enlarge. When the obstruction is intrahepatic, anastomotic channels between portal and systemic veins become engorged. The only anastomoses which are dangerous to life are those in the submucosa of the lower oesophagus (oesophageal varices). The haemorrhoidal veins do not get engorged in portal hypertension. Even if haemorrhoids are present they are idiopathic, and not caused by the raised portal venous pressure.

Clinical features. Portal hypertension is responsible for some of the most severe cases of haematemesis. If the patient is known to have cirrhosis, haemorrhage should be assumed to be coming from oesophageal varices until proved otherwise. In most cases the spleen is palpably enlarged.

Prehepatic. The patient is usually a child or a young adult. He may be brought for a sudden haemorrhage or for weakness due to anaemia. The liver is impalpable but the spleen is obviously enlarged. Anaemia is due partly to hypersplenism. Liver function tests remain normal as the disease advances. Splenoportography displays the site of the block.

Intrahepatic. The patient is normally an adult and suffers from hepatic cirrhosis. The varices can be shown on x-ray or seen through an oesophagoscope. Enlargement of the veins of the abdominal wall radiating from the umbilicus may be present (*Caput medusae*). As long as hypertrophy of liver tissue is sufficient to compensate for cellular destruction by cirrhosis the liver function tests remain normal.

Investigations. ***Laboratory.*** Operative procedures in patients with compromised liver function carry significantly increased risk. Therefore, evaluation of the patient's hepatocellular reserve is important when selecting treatment for bleeding varices. Recommended laboratory investigations include the following:

1. Full blood count for anaemia, leucopenia and thrombocytopenia.

2. Liver function tests to indicate primary cause of liver disease.

3. Serum albumin and prothrombin time to determine efficacy of synthetic function.

4. Autoantibodies: in primary biliary cirrhosis and chronic active hepatitis.

5. Serological markers of hepatitis B and C.

6. Blood grouping.

Endoscopy not only confirms the presence of varices but also determines whether or not they are bleeding, and therefore removes any doubt about the source of the haemorrhage. It is of vital importance in excluding other causes of bleeding, such as peptic ulcer, gastritis, duodenitis, or an oesophageal tear. At the same time sclerosing agents can be injected into the varices to cause them to fibrose.

Imaging. Numerous imaging methods help the clinician in cases of portal hypertension. If endoscopy is not available, *barium studies* are useful in demonstrating oesophageal varices as irregular filling defects in the distal third or more of the oesophagus. They may also show up other causes of bleeding such as peptic ulceration. When operative intervention is planned, information about the anatomical details of the portal circulation is needed. Classically this has been obtained by angiography, but non-invasive methods like ultrasound, CT and MRI are being increasingly employed.

Angiography. *Coeliac* and *superior mesenteric angiography.* Using a transfemoral Seldinger catheter the coeliac trunk and superior mesenteric artery are selectively cannulated. Contrast medium is injected. X-rays are taken while the medium is in the arteries and also when it enters the veins. The arterial phase can show up haemangiomas as well as tumour circulation in the case of liver malignancies. The venous phase allows evaluation of the splenic vein and can demonstrate oesophageal varices.

If imaging by angiography is inadequate, *splenic venography* can be performed. Under local anaesthetic infiltration, a fine bore catheter is passed into the spleen and contrast medium injected into the splenic pulp. While withdrawing the needle, the track is sealed by injection of pledgets of gelatine foam. Even so, there is a slight risk of significant haemorrhage. Because of the risk of bleeding this test is reserved for patients in whom imaging is inadequate.

Ultrasound. Because it is non-invasive and provides detailed and accurate information, ultrasound scanning is now the first-line investigation in portal hypertension. It clearly shows up thrombosis of the portal vein and its tributaries, as well as the resulting large collateral veins. Portasystemic shunts can be measured and graft occlusion demonstrated.

CT scanning can also demonstrate the above lesions, but ultrasound and MRI can do so more easily and accurately, therefore it is rarely the procedure of choice.

MRI allows excellent parenchymal visualization, imaging in any plane and better blood vessel imaging than CT. It is limited by long imaging times. However, it gives better definition of soft tissues than computed tomography, and is displacing it in this as in many other fields.

TREATMENT OF OESOPHAGEAL VARICES

The following methods of treatment are available for dealing with oesophageal varices resulting from portal hypertension:

1. *Oral propranolol* in a dose sufficient to reduce the resting pulse rate by 25% reduces portal pressure, both by a decrease in cardiac output and by causing constriction of the splanchnic arteries. It reduces the frequency of rebleeds and some studies show it to be as effective as sclerotherapy.

2. *Vasoconstrictor therapy.* The main use of this is for emergency control of bleeding while waiting for endoscopic sclerotherapy. Vasoconstrictors restrict portal inflow by splanchnic arterial constriction:

i. Vasopressin is given by intravenous drip, 25 units/hour, preferably by a central venous catheter to avoid local spill and necrosis. It is contraindicated in patients with angina, as generalized vasoconstriction results.

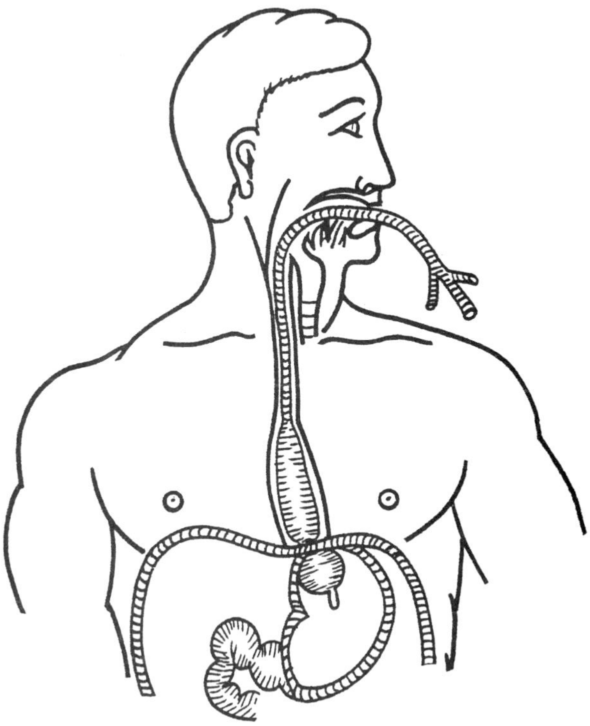

Fig. 1 Balloon tamponade by a Sengstaken tube.

ii. Octreotide, a somatostatin analogue, 50 mg bolus followed by 50 mg/hour for 48 hours, produces splanchnic vasoconstriction without systemic effects, and therefore should now be used as first-line treatment.

3. *Sclerotherapy.* A sclerosing agent is injected into the varices through an endoscope, the commonly used chemical being ethanolamine. This may be repeated at intervals. The procedure is associated with many complications, and *banding* of oesophageal varices, as practised in the case of haemorrhoids, is considered by some to be safer.

4. *Balloon tamponade.* This is carried out by a *Sengstaken* tube. This tube has a rounded inflatable balloon near its tip and a long cylindrical balloon just proximal to it. The tube is passed into the stomach and the distal balloon inflated. The tube is now gently withdrawn until the balloon impinges on the cardia. The long proximal balloon is now lying in the distal oesophagus. It is inflated, causing pressure on the varices and arresting haemorrhage. When the oesophageal balloon is deflated after some hours bleeding has often stopped (Fig. 1). The *Linton* tube has only a single large balloon in the stomach. Traction has to be applied to this tube, and pressure necrosis can therefore occur if it is left in place for more than 18 hours. *Balloon tamponade is used only if sclerotherapy and vasoconstrictor therapy are unavailable or have failed.*

5. *Transjugular intrahepatic portacaval shunt* (TIPS). This is an ingenious method to reduce the portal venous pressure and is used with local anaesthesia. A guide wire is passed from the jugular vein into the liver and an expandable metal shunt is forced through the liver substance to form a channel between the portal and systemic venous systems. It is used in cases where the bleeding cannot be stopped by any other method.

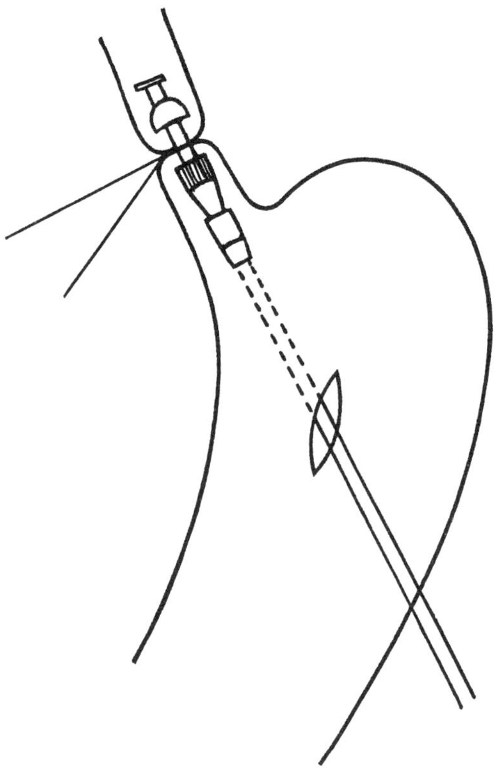

Fig. 2 Oesophageal transection with circular stapler.

6. *Oesophageal transection and reanastomosis.* Through a gastrotomy a cylindrical stapler is passed up the lumen of the oesophagus. A thread is tied around the oesophagus opposite the groove in the stapler. When the stapler is fired, the instrument divides the oesophagus and re-anastomoses it with a circular row of staples, so that the vessels across the anastomosis are disconnected (Fig. 2). With this, the high-pressure portal system of veins is disconnected from the low-pressure systemic veins. It is used as an emergency surgical procedure in bleeding varices.

7. *Porta-systemic shunts.* These shunts drain the high pressure portal system into the low-pressure systemic veins. They represent the definitive surgical procedures for portal hypertension. They can be carried out at three sites (Fig. 3):

i. Porta-caval shunt: the portal vein is anastomosed end-to-side or side-to-side to the inferior vena cava.

ii. Spleno-renal shunt: the spleen is removed. The proximal end of the splenic vein is anastomosed end-to-side to the left renal vein.

iii. Mesocaval shunt: the superior mesenteric vein is anastomosed to the inferior vena cava, the distance between the two being bridged by a Teflon vascular graft. Physiologically and haemodynamically this is similar to the side-to-side portacaval shunt.

Emergency treatment. If the patient comes into the emergency department *with massive haemorrhage from varices*, initial resuscitation is carried out by rapid transfusion of large volumes of blood. Vasoconstrictor therapy using vasopressin appears to be valuable. The addition of nitroglycerine is advantageous, as it reverses the adverse systemic cardiovascular effects of vasopressin. Ideally,

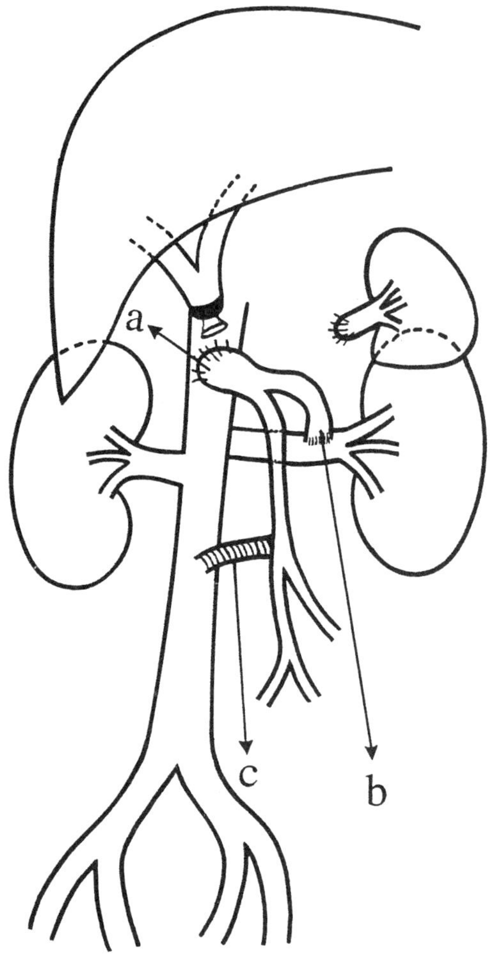

Fig. 3 Different kinds of porta-systemic shunts: (a) Portacaval, (b) Splenorenal, (c) Mesocaval.

emergency endoscopy should be available round the clock. This is required for confirming the diagnosis of bleeding varices, and a sclerosing agent should be injected into the varices at the time of the emergency endoscopy. If this successfully controls haemorrhage a Sengstaken tube will not be required, and the patient will be spared the inconvenience and the dangers of balloon tamponade by this tube. If emergency sclerotherapy fails to control the haemorrhage a Sengstaken tube should be inserted to arrest the bleeding. It is only rarely that oesophageal transection will be required for emergency control of variceal haemorrhage; usually sclerosing injection treatment suffices for this purpose.

Long-term control of varices. For the long-term control of varices, oral propranolol on a daily basis has been suggested. Repeated sclerotherapy into varices is the most popular method today. However if this fails transection, or one of the shunts, can be used. Generally speaking, shunts are used in the better-risk patients, and transection in the poorer-risk cases.

Of the various shunts the portacaval shunt is the most effective. However, it diverts the venous drainage of the intestine away from the liver and prevents prompt metabolism of the products of digestion, such as ammonia and the various amines; it therefore results in a high incidence of encephalopathy, with confusion, drowsiness, jaundice, and hypoglycaemia. The more peripheral shunts, i.e. lienorenal and mesocaval, are less often followed by encephalopathy. However, they are also somewhat less effective in reducing portal pressure and the frequency of variceal bleeds. In children with portal vein thrombosis only the peripheral shunts can be utilized.

In patients with end-stage liver disease and marked hepatic dysfunction, after the bleeding has been controlled with sclerotherapy or TIPS, liver transplantation is often appropriate.

22 *Gallbladder*

CONGENITAL ANOMALIES

Embryology. The hepatic diverticulum arises from the ventral wall of the foregut and elongates to form the bile duct. This divides into many branches which join up with the canaliculi attached to the liver cells. At the same time the bile duct gives off a lateral bud which forms the gallbladder.

Anomalies. The gallbladder may be *absent.* It may have a *mesentery.* In rare cases there may be a *double* gallbladder. *The cystic duct may be absent.* In such cases injury to the common duct can occur during cholecystectomy. An *accessory cholecystohepatic duct* may be present. If it remains unnoticed and is not ligated it may result in bile leakage after cholecystectomy.

BILIARY ATRESIA

In this condition the bile ducts are obliterated and the newborn suffers from obstructive jaundice. Two types of atresia occur, the 'correctable' and the 'incorrectable'. In the 'correctable' type the intrahepatic bile ducts are normally formed but the extrahepatic ducts are either partially or completely absent. In the 'incorrectable' type the intrahepatic ducts are also missing; only microscopic bile ducts are present at the liver hilum (Fig. 1).

Management of suspected biliary atresia. The common causes of jaundice in the newborn are three: physiological jaundice, neonatal hepatitis and congenital biliary atresia. If the jaundice is physiological it should clear up in two or three weeks. If it persists after that period it can either be neonatal hepatitis or atresia. Laboratory differentiation is difficult. *Therefore, if jaundice has not cleared up in 4 to 6 weeks the abdomen should be explored.* The biliary tract is examined and an operative cholangiogram carried out. If the whole biliary tract is present the case is not of biliary atresia but of neonatal hepatitis or some other hepatic pathology. A liver biopsy is taken and the abdomen closed.

If atresia is present it can belong to one of two types. In the *'correctable'* type (only 10%) the proximal hepatic duct is patent. Therefore the obstruction can be relieved by joining the hepatic duct with a loop of jejunum, i.e. a *hepaticojejunostomy*. In the *'non-correctable'* type of atresia there are no extrahepatic bile ducts at the porta hepatis. This situation used to be considered as incurable. However,

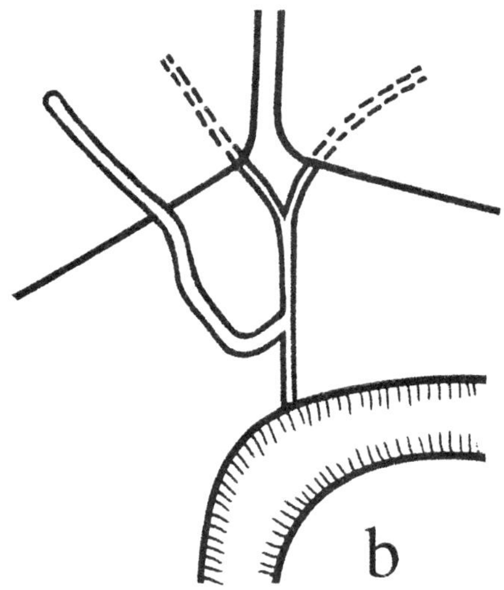

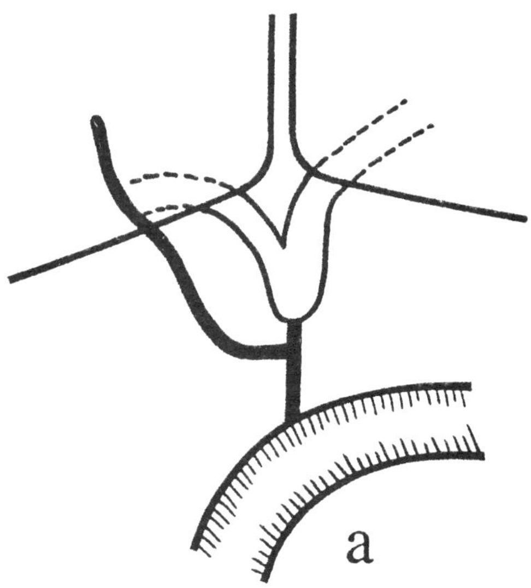

Fig. 1a 'Correctable' biliary atresia.

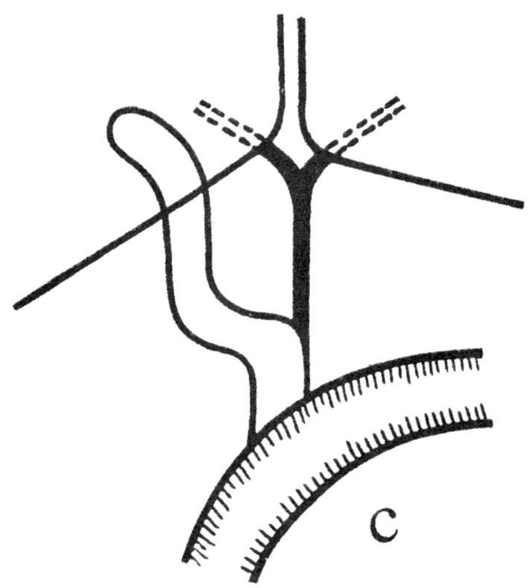

Fig. 1b and c 'Incorrectable' biliary atresia.

Kasai from Japan has shown that the porta hepatis can be transected to demonstrate bile passages of a diameter of about 200 microns. A loop of jejunum is anastomosed to the porta (*portoenterostomy*). As bile starts to flow the bile passages gradually dilate. After this operation there is no guarantee that bile will flow in sufficient quantities to eliminate jaundice. However, a small percentage of previously hopeless cases can be saved by this technique.

Portoenterostomy is successful only if carried out within the first six weeks. After this, so much cirrhosis has taken place that the previously existing bile passages inside the liver have become obliterated. Thus awareness of this condition is important, because only then can diagnosis be made early enough to be of any use. Both undergraduates and paediatricians should be taught that *if a case of neonatal jaundice has not been sorted out by the age of six weeks the abdomen should be explored.*

Prognosis. Although bile drainage is expected when the operation is carried out early, decompression of the bile ducts does not necessarily imply cure. Hepatic fibrosis may progress even when bile drainage is achieved. Postoperative cholangitis continues to plague infants having successful portoenterostomy procedures. At the same time, cirrhosis and portal hypertension have emerged as new problems in these children, who have been relieved of jaundice by functioning biliary conduits. Haemorrhage from oesophageal varices has been managed successfully by endoscopic sclerotherapy or portasystemic shunts. However, in these days of liver transplantation, shunt procedures have become less desirable alternatives. If the Kasai operation fails, liver transplantation remains the final hope for salvage. Biliary atresia is the most common indication for transplantation in children, with the 1-year survival rate now approaching 70 percent.

JAUNDICE

Jaundice is caused by an increase in the level of bilirubin in the serum so that the tissues, including the conjunctivae, become stained yellow. This can arise in five different ways:

1. Increased bile pigment load on the liver cells (haemolytic jaundice).
2. Disturbed diffusion of bilirubin from the sinusoids into the liver cells (caused by some drugs).
3. Defective conjugation of bilirubin (e.g. Gilbert's syndrome).
4. Defective transport of bilirubin to the cell membrane for excretion into the bile canaliculi (intrahepatic cholestasis).
5. Obstruction of the large bile ducts, e.g. from a gallstone or cancer of the head of the pancreas (extrahepatic cholestasis). *Only this last type of jaundice can be relieved surgically.*

In many instances, e.g. in viral hepatitis or cirrhosis, the exact defect concerned cannot be pinpointed, and many steps in bilirubin metabolism may be abnormal.

Symptoms. A carefully taken history helps in indicating the cause in certain cases. Drug addiction may suggest serum hepatitis from shared hypodermic syringes. In some patients with cirrhosis chronic alcoholism is responsible. Obstructing gallstones or tumours are more common in older people. Patients with gallstone jaundice may have attacks of biliary colic, fever and chills. On the other hand, the pain in malignant obstruction is deep-seated and dull. In extrahepatic obstruction the stool is light in colour and the urine dark. Pruritus also occurs and causes discomfort. It is caused by an excess of bile salts in the system.

Signs. The liver is enlarged in both hepatic and posthepatic jaundice. Secondary stigmas of cirrhosis are spider angiomas, ascites, caput medusae and splenomegaly. If the gallbladder is enlarged and non-tender this suggests malignant obstruction of the common duct. Conversely, if in a case of obstructive jaundice the gallbladder is not palpable this suggests that the cause of the obstruction is a stone in the common bile duct, the gallbladder having contracted in size due to chronic cholecystitis (*Courvoisier's law*). However, this law does not hold good in every case, so that absence of a palpable gallbladder does not rule out malignancy.

Laboratory tests. *Serum bilirubin level.* In *haemolytic* disease the increased bilirubin is mainly in the unconjugated indirect fraction. Because it is insoluble in water it does not pass into the urine (*acholuric* jaundice). The total serum bilirubin rarely exceeds 5 mg/dl, because the rate of excretion in the stool increases as the bilirubin level rises, and a plateau is reached. Higher values suggest that parenchymal disease is also present. In *hepatic* jaundice both unconjugated and conjugated bilirubin are increased. An increase in the conjugated fraction always means disease within the hepatobiliary system. Since direct bilirubin is water soluble it is excreted in the urine. With complete *extrahepatic obstruction* the total bilirubin may rise upto 30 mg/dl. At this point loss in the urine equals the additional daily production. If the values are still higher it suggests that either haemolysis is occurring so that a very large quantity of bile pigment is being produced, or the renal function is impaired so that these pigments are not being excreted. Obstruction of a single hepatic duct does not usually produce jaundice. In malignant extrahepatic obstruction the serum bilirubin level usually exceeds 10 mg/dl and may go upto 30 mg/dl. On the other hand in gallstone obstruction the values are rarely above 15 mg/dl.

Serum levels of other substances. As far as the level of faecal *urobilinogen* is concerned, haemolysis increases it; on the other hand complete biliary obstruction decreases both faecal and urinary urobilinogen. In extrahepatic obstruction the serum *transaminase* levels are raised only slightly. High levels may occur, but only for a few days. Transaminase levels above 1,000 units suggest viral hepatitis.

Hepatic *alkaline phosphatase* is produced by the epithelial cells of the cholangioles. The raised level is due to overproduction and not under-excretion. So it may occur even with focal hepatic lesions, e.g. solitary metastasis or abscess, and in the absence of jaundice. Alkaline phosphatase is also produced by bone. Therefore bone disease may complicate the interpretation of abnormal alkaline phosphatase levels. In such a case serum calcium and phosphorus levels should be determined. In cirrhosis the serum *albumin* level falls and the level of *globulin* rises, so that the albumin/globulin ratio is abnormal.

Imaging. In patients with persistent jaundice an *ultrasound* and *CT scans* are carried out first, which may show dilated intrahepatic bile ducts or gallstones. If hepatic parenchymal disease is suspected a *liver biopsy* should be carried out. If on the other hand a ductal obstruction is more likely a percutaneous transhepatic cholangiogram or endoscopic retrograde cholangiopancreatogram may be performed.

Percutaneous transhepatic cholangiogram (PTC). A 22-gauge flexible Chiba needle is advanced through the skin and well into the liver under local anaesthesia. Contrast medium is gently injected as the needle is slowly withdrawn. The procedure is watched on an image intensifier; when contrast enters a bile duct withdrawal is stopped. More contrast medium is then injected to fill the biliary tree. If the ducts are dilated the test is successful each time; if not, about two-thirds of the time. Major complications include bile leakage into the peritoneum, cholangitis and haemorrhage. Therefore, it is best to plan to relieve any obstruction immediately or soon after the examination. The mortality rate associated with the procedure is about 0.5 percent.

Endoscopic retrograde cholangiopancreatogram (ERCP). The sedated patient lies on his right side. The duodenoscope is introduced into the stomach, passed along the greater curvature, and its the tip lifted and passed into the duodenum. The ampulla is found on the medial wall of the duodenum. The pancreatic and bile ducts are cannulated in turn. Contrast medium is injected and x-rays taken.

Management. The foremost objective in the diagnosis of jaundice is to distinguish surgical (obstructive) from non-surgical jaundice. In most cases the history, physical examination, laboratory data and minimally invasive imaging tests allow a diagnosis to be made without invasive tests like liver biopsy or direct cholangiogram. Once obstruction is definitely demonstrated, either open operation or an appropriate minimally invasive procedure is employed for its relief.

Gallstones

Gallstone disease is one of the most common major surgical illnesses affecting the abdomen. It occurs mostly among women. Gallstones usually consist of cholesterol or calcium bilirubinate, or much more commonly alternate layers of these. Protein is another constituent.

A *cholesterol* stone is usually single (cholesterol solitaire). It is oval or rounded, 1–2 cm diameter, pale yellow and translucent. On section it shows radiating crystals. About 6% of gallstones are of this type. They form in aseptic but static bile. Sometimes cholesterol stones are numerous; in that case they look like mulberries (Fig. 2).

Pigment stones are composed of calcium bilirubinate. They are black, irregular shaped small concretions 5 mm or less in size. On section they are amorphous. They form in haemolytic jaundice.

Mixed stones constitute the majority of gallstones (80%). They are multiple and faceted due to mutual pressure (Plate VI-II). Dozens or hundreds may pack the gallbladder to capacity (Plate I-II). On section each one is laminated. Alternating layers of cholesterol and calcium bilirubinate/calcium carbonate are seen around a central nucleus of debris or bacteria.

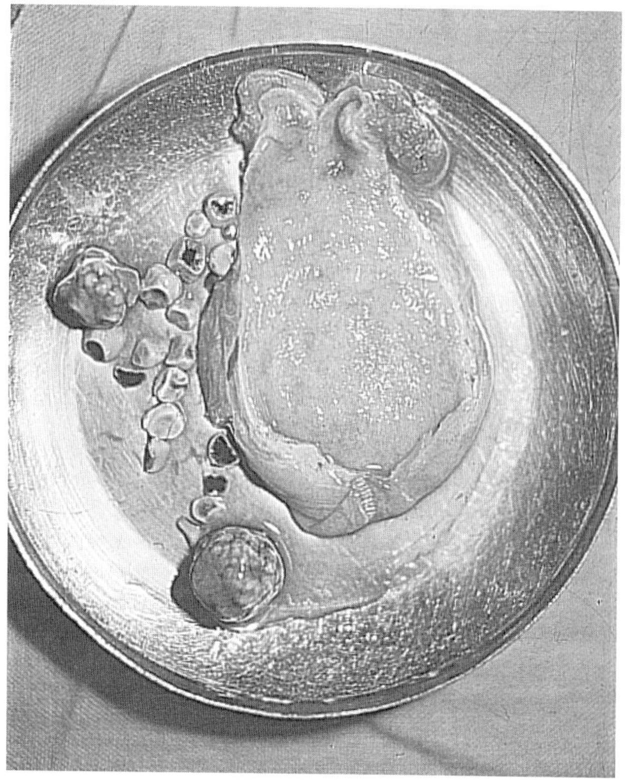

Fig. 2 Gallbladder with two large, rounded cholesterol 'mulberry' stones and numerous faceted mixed stones.

Age and sex distribution. A fat, fertile, flatulent female, forty years of age is the classic patient. However, gallstones form in both sexes. They may form at a much earlier age, and they are also common in old age. They are said to occur in 20% women in the child-bearing period. In advanced old age upto 20% persons of both sexes have gallstones.

Factors in the causation of gallstones. *Metabolism.* Bile salts keep cholesterol in solution in the bile. When the quantity of cholesterol in the bile increases, or that of bile salts diminishes, it precipitates out and forms calculi. In different haemolytic anaemias excessive haemolysis may lead to the formation of pure pigment stones.

Infection. Organisms have often been found in gallstones and have long been blamed as a cause. However, gallstones can develop in the absence of infection; this shows that infection cannot be an essential factor in their development.

Bile stasis. Without stasis stones would not grow to the sizes commonly found. They would be voided while still in particulate or gravel form. Stasis is usual during pregnancy. In the formation of gallstones in multiparae, stasis probably plays an important part.

Clinical findings. Gallstones may remain *silent* for long periods, and are often found only at autopsy after death from some other cause. They may cause *flatulent dyspepsia*, which usually improves after cholecystectomy.

The most characteristic symptom is *biliary colic* due to gallstone obstruction of the cystic duct. Severe pain starts abruptly in the right hypochondrium, lasts for a few minutes to several hours and subsides gradually. It may also be felt in the epigastrium. It very often radiates around the costal margin to the inferior angle of the right scapula. In many cases it radiates to the tip of the right shoulder. In a severe attack the patient usually curls up in bed in agony. During an attack of biliary colic it is difficult to examine the patient properly. Later, palpation may reveal an enlarged gallbladder. If pressure is exerted over the right hypochondrium while the patient takes a deep breath, there is a catch in the breath just before the end of inspiration (*Murphy's sign*).

Fatty food intolerance, dyspepsia, indigestion, heartburn, flatulence, nausea and *eructations* also occur in gallstone disease. However, they are also frequent in the general population. Therefore their presence in any given patient is not necessarily due to the gallstones.

Investigations. *Plain x-ray* shows radiopaque gallstones in only 10% of cases, because most gallstones are radiolucent.

Oral cholecystography. Oral cholecystography visualizes the gallbladder. Tablets of Telepaque, a radiopaque medium, are taken the evening before the x-ray about 3 hours after a meal. Nothing is taken by mouth after that, and the patient is x-rayed next morning, about 14 hours after ingestion of the dye. After this a fatty meal is given to stimulate gallbladder contraction, and another x-ray is taken:

1. The normal gallbladder concentrates the dye and is visualized on the cholecystogram. Any radiolucent stones can be seen as negative shadows. After the fatty meal the normal gallbladder contracts down in size.
2. In mild degrees of dysfunction the gallbladder is outlined but does not contract in size after the fatty meal.
3. A pathological gallbladder is not visualized on the x-ray.

Intravenous cholangiography. The radiopaque dye may also be injected intravenously. It outlines the intra and extra-hepatic bile ducts. This test is used to outline residual stones in the common bile duct after cholecystectomy. The dye used in this test contains iodine and can cause a severe reaction with shock and cyanosis. A test dose should be given an hour or two earlier, to see if any reaction is likely to occur. The treatment of such a reaction is by nikethamide, antihistaminic drugs and oxygen.

These investigations are useless in jaundice (serum bilirubin above 3 mg/dl) and in acute cholecystitis.

Ultrasound examination. This method has revolutionized investigation of gallbladder disease. It has replaced oral cholecystography. The cavity of the gallbladder appears black on the screen, while stones and debris look white. The ultrasound waves cannot penetrate the stone, therefore a linear shadow is seen on the side of the stone away from the ultrasound beam (an *acoustic shadow*). The thickness of the gallbladder wall can be measured to assess the degree of any inflammation, the maximum normal being 3 mm. Carcinoma of the gallbladder shows up as an irregular thickening of the wall. The test takes only a few minutes, is non-invasive and without the hazard of radiation or iodine sensitivity. It is therefore the first investigation to be undertaken in a patient suspected of suffering from gallstone disease.

TREATMENT

Medical treatment. *Chenodeoxycholic acid* is one of the bile salts. When given orally it expands the bile salt pool to normal, desaturates the bile with respect to cholesterol, and slowly dissolves gallstones. After a year or more of continuous treatment total dissolution occurs in one-third of the radiolucent stones. However, after treatment is stopped the stones recur in many cases. The treatment is ineffective in radiopaque stones and in a non-functioning gallbladder. In any case the argument against using this drug is that even if after 18 months of treatment and after risk of hepatic toxicity by the drug the stones are all dissolved, one would still be leaving behind a diseased gallbladder, where stones can form again. Therefore the drug is not commonly employed.

Surgical treatment. Cholecystectomy should be performed in most patients with symptoms. This operation removes not only the stones but also the gallbladder. If the gallbladder was left behind the stones would form in it again.

Cholecystectomy. A Kocher's or right paramedian *incision* can be used. If stones have been shown on ultrasound, the author's preference is for a Kocher's incision because it gives a more direct exposure, and is associated with a reduced incidence of incisional hernia. Also, because it opens the abdominal cavity on one side and not in the middle, it results in less handling of the intra-abdominal viscera with a reduced degree of postoperative paralytic ileus. It is therefore not necessary to pass a nasogastric tube for aspiration in the postoperative period; this fact expedites the recovery and also makes this incision popular with patients.

The intestines are displaced downwards and to the left by the assistant's hand placed over an abdominal pack. A haemostat is applied to the fundus of the gallbladder, which is drawn up. A second haemostat is applied over Hartmann's pouch and draws it up. The T-junction between the cystic duct and the common bile duct is exposed. This is important, in order to avoid ligating the common bile duct by mistake. The cystic duct and cystic artery are ligated and divided. The gallbladder is dissected away from its bed in the liver, and the resulting raw area is closed by suture.

The common bile duct is explored:

1. If stones have been shown in the duct on ultrasound examination.
2. If stones can be palpated in the duct.
3. If there is jaundice or a history of jaundice.
4. If the duct is dilated to a diameter of 10 mm or more.

If during operation a *per-operative cholangiogram* is carried out through a catheter in the cystic duct, it shows up any stone in the common bile duct clearly. Routine use of this investigation is desirable. Although it adds a few minutes to the operating time, it reduces the incidence of overlooked common bile duct stones considerably.

Laparoscopic cholecystectomy. This operation was first carried out in France in 1987. Since then, an ever-increasing number of surgeons around the world have learned this method and are utilizing it, so that in the near future it promises to become the method of choice everywhere. In this technique, cholecystectomy is carried out without making a full abdominal incision. Three, or sometimes four, small incisions, only 5 to 10 mm in length, are made, one each in the epigastrium and umbilical scar, and two in the right hypochondrium. The umbilical scar is punctured by a Veress needle (designed to prevent injury to the gut), and the abdomen insufflated with CO_2. A laparoscope is now introduced through the umbilical port. The hypochondrial ports are used to introduce forceps to hold up the fundus and the Hartmann's pouch respectively. Through the epigastric port a dissecting forceps exposes in turn the cystic duct and the cystic artery, which are divided between clips. Small blood vessels are sealed by diathermy. The gallbladder is finally dissected off its bed, and removed through the umbilical wound, after sucking out the bile from it.

The advantage of the procedure lies in the avoidance of an abdominal wound with its attendant pain and possibility of infection. The patient can usually go home on the first or second postoperative day. The disadvantages include: insufflation with carbon dioxide with a possibility of embolism, the inability to dissect formally in the region of the porta hepatis, and the fact that the method cannot be used in cases where the area of the hilum is obscured by dense adhesions and fibrosis.

During the few years since its introduction, laparoscopic cholecystectomy has firmly established itself as a surgical technique which has come to stay. However, a few gallbladders cannot be removed by this method, namely those with very severe acute cholecystitis, or those with excessively dense fibrosis. For such cases, open cholecystectomy still remains the technique of choice. Finally, laparoscopic cholecystectomy should only be employed by those who have received proper training in the method.

Extracorporeal shock wave lithotripsy (ESWL). This method, which has proved successful in the case of kidney stones, has also been tried in gallstones. However, it has not had the same success. If the gallbladder is not functioning it has clearly no place in management, as the viscus cannot contract to empty itself and will become a storehouse of biliary sludge. Another argument against its use is this: in the case of the kidney all we want to remove is the stone and not the kidney, because the kidney is a vital organ. On the other hand because the gallbladder is not a vital organ and can be dispensed with, it is far better to remove it along with the stones, to obviate any possibility of recurrence of the stones. ESWL cannot do this. Therefore, cholecystectomy is the more effective and preferred treatment.

Asymptomatic gallstones. What advice should be given to the patient who undergoes medical examination for some other condition and where gallstones are found incidentally? The presence of any of the following indicates a more serious course and should serve as a reason for cholecystectomy:

1. Non functioning gallbladder, as it is more likely to be the seat of infection due to stasis.
2. A calcified gallbladder, because it is sometimes associated with carcinoma.
3. Diabetes mellitus, because of the high morbidity and mortality in acute cholecystitis.

In general the tendency is to operate on most patients but to treat the very elderly patients conservatively. If coexistent cardiopulmonary or other problems greatly increase the surgical risk, operation should be avoided. In young patients with a long life-expectancy the possibility of development of carcinoma of the gallbladder due to the stones should not be lost sight of.

COMPLICATIONS OF GALLSTONES

If stones remain in the gallbladder for any length of time, the following complications can arise: acute cholecystitis sometimes leading to perforation, chronic cholecystitis, stones in the bile ducts leading to jaundice, and occasionally carcinoma.

ACUTE CHOLECYSTITIS

If a stone gets impacted in Hartmann's pouch the gallbladder becomes intensely inflamed, with its mucous membrane swollen and wall thickened. Occasionally, gangrene occurs in patches. The further course of the illness may be along one of the following lines:

1. The stone may get *disimpacted* as the gallbladder distends further. The mucopurulent contents of the gallbladder escape via the cystic duct and the inflammation subsides.
2. Less frequently, the impaction persists and an *empyema* of the gallbladder results.
3. Rarely the distended inflamed gallbladder *perforates*, with the formation of a local abscess. Unlike the situation in appendicitis, perforation into the general peritoneal cavity is fortunately rare (only 0.5% of cases), probably because the intestines and omentum get adherent to the inflamed gallbladder before it perforates, and localize the infection so that an abscess results.

Clinical findings. The onset of acute cholecystitis is sudden. Agonizing pain occurs in the right hypochondrium. Severe nausea and vomiting occur. Fever is usual, and in fulminating cases rigors also occur. There is marked tenderness, and may be some rigidity, in the right hypochondrium. The inflamed, tender gallbladder may be palpable. Differential diagnosis is from leaking duodenal ulcer and high retrocaecal appendicitis. Acute pancreatitis and coronary thrombosis should also be considered.

Treatment. In 90% of cases symptoms of acute cholecystitis subside with conservative treatment. The stomach is continuously aspirated through a nasogastric tube to give rest to the biliary and pancreatic systems. Fluids and electrolytes are given intravenously. Analgesics e.g. morphine or pethidine with atropine are administered, along with broad-spectrum antibiotics. When the temperature, pulse and physical signs show that the inflammation is subsiding, the nasogastric tube is removed. Glucose drinks are started, going on to clear fluids and to a fat-free soft diet within a few days. About two months later when the inflammation has subsided and the adhesions resolved, cholecystectomy is carried out.

If one of the following conditions is present *immediate operation* is advised:

1. If there is uncertainty about the diagnosis e.g. when perforated duodenal ulcer or acute appendicitis cannot be ruled out.

2. In typhoid cholecystitis, because perforation is common in this condition.

3. If pain and tenderness spread across the abdomen, or the pulse rate rises, conservative treatment is abandoned and cholecystectomy performed. However, in the very ill and the elderly cholecystostomy may be preferred, in order to shorten the operative procedure.

Prognosis. The overall mortality rate in acute cholecystitis is 3–5%. Nearly all the deaths are in patients over the age of 60 or those with diabetes mellitus. In the older age groups secondary cardiovascular or pulmonary complications contribute to an increased mortality rate.

CHRONIC CHOLECYSTITIS

In this condition the gallbladder wall is thickened, with loss of the normal mucosal pattern. Stones are usually present. The function of the gallbladder may be impaired. In these cases symptoms of dyspepsia become more persistent.

GALLSTONES IN THE BILE DUCTS

Most stones in the ducts have arisen in the gallbladder; a very few (usually sludge or concretions) have formed in the bile ducts.

Clinical findings. There is no great difference between the biliary colic due to gallbladder stones and that due to stones in the common bile duct. However, in the latter condition obstructive jaundice may supervene. The urine becomes dark with bile, and the stools become pale. The skin starts itching. The patient loses weight. There may be tenderness in the epigastrium. Usually the gallbladder cannot be felt because it is shrunken due to repeated attacks of inflammation. After an attack the patient may remain well for many months or may get another attack soon.

Charcot's triad of symptoms is characteristic of common bile duct stones: intermittent jaundice, intermittent pain and intermittent fever. These recurring symptoms are produced as follows: the stone becomes impacted, it floats free when the duct dilates, but later impacts again.

Differential diagnosis of a stone in the common bile duct is from viral hepatitis and carcinoma of the pancreas or ampulla of Vater.

Complications. If obstruction of the bile duct is unrelieved, the following complications may ensue:

1. *Worsening liver function.* When the bile duct remains obstructed the pigments in the bile are absorbed by the mucosa of the bile ducts, which secretes some mucus. The resultant clear mucoid fluid is called *white bile*, and its presence is a bad sign as it indicates long-standing biliary obstruction. However, brisk recovery may occur after relief of the obstruction. Unrelieved obstruction lasting over four weeks causes liver damage, and the operative mortality rises greatly.

2. *Suppurative cholangitis.* Due to stagnation of bile in the ducts infection occurs, and pus spreads in the whole biliary tree. This is a dangerous complication causing liver failure, septicaemia and death, and requires timely surgical drainage of the biliary tree along with antibiotic therapy.

Treatment. The treatment of calculous obstruction of the biliary tract is by operation. In jaundice the prothrombin level in the blood is low, due to failure of absorption of vitamin K^1, therefore this vitamin is given intramuscularly or intravenously before operation. Antibiotics are administered. Mannitol is given intravenously to promote diuresis and prevent the renal failure which can occur in obstructive jaundice. If the jaundice is subsiding a few days may be allowed before operation. If jaundice is increasing and specially when there is fever, operation should be performed within a day or two. In cases with an advanced degree of jaundice the postoperative course is usually stormy.

At operation it is advantageous to mobilize the duodenum by incising the posterior parietal peritoneum lateral to it, so that it can be lifted forwards (Kocher's manoeuvre). The common bile duct is opened in its supraduodenal part. Bougies are first passed gently upwards and downwards to detect any stones. Next, stone-removing forceps (of the Desjardin type) are passed in both directions. They are advanced with their jaws open to catch any stones, and then withdrawn with the stone or stones. The bile ducts are finally flushed out, using normal saline as irrigating fluid. A choledochoscope is passed in to ensure that all stones have been removed. The common bile duct is closed around a T-tube, the short limb of which lies in the bile duct, while the long limb is led via a tubing to a bag suspended from the side of the bed.

An important reason for not closing the common bile duct (CBD) primarily but draining it via a T-tube is that the wall of the CBD is quite thin, and sutures applied in it can therefore leak. The T-tube provides a safety valve. By the time the tube is removed after 10 to 12 days, adhesions have formed around the tube and therefore the bile does not leak into the peritoneal cavity.

Removal of stones from the common bile duct (choledocholithotomy) constitutes the most common operation on the duct.

Nd YAG laser has been used for lithotripsy in the endoscopic fragmentation of calculi in the common bile duct. Laser beams are transmitted down the flexible optical fibres, the ends of which are placed just touching the stone. The laser pulses produce a localized shock wave that can pulverize stones.

INJURY AND STRICTURE OF THE COMMON BILE DUCT

The most common cause of stricture of the common bile duct is *damage to the duct during cholecystectomy.* There are two ways in which this accident commonly takes place:

1. If the T-junction between the cystic duct and bile duct is not displayed, the ligature may be applied to the common bile duct by mistake.

2. If sudden haemorrhage occurs and an artery forceps is blindly plunged in to arrest it, the common hepatic duct may be damaged.

If the damage is *recognized at operation*:

1. There may be a short incision in the duct; this should be closed with fine absorbable sutures, over a T-tube if necessary.

2. The bile duct may be divided across but there is no loss of length. It should be repaired with fine absorbable sutures with a T-tube left through a separate stab incision, to minimize the chances of a stricture at the site of the division.

3. A portion of the duct may have been excised. Here the best course is a hepaticojejunostomy to a Roux loop of jejunum.

If the damage is *unrecognized at operation*:

1. Persistent bile leakage may occur from the wound.

2. If bile cannot escape through the wound, it may leak into the peritoneal cavity and produce bile peritonitis.

3. Deepening obstructive jaundice may follow due to complete blockage or stricture of the duct.

Treatment is by re-operation:

1. If the common bile duct or the common hepatic duct is divided, it is joined to a Roux loop of jejunum, which is prepared as follows: the jejunum is divided a suitable distance distal to the duodeno-jejunal flexure. The end of the proximal loop is anastomosed to the side of the distal, while the distal loop is brought up to the hilum of the liver and joined to the divided bile duct.

2. If the duct injury is very high, there is no duct available to which the jejunum may be anastomosed. In such cases the best results are obtained when the left hepatic duct, which is dilated due to the obstruction, is exposed by dissection in the groove behind the quadrate lobe and joined to a Roux loop of jejunum. Because mucosa-to-mucosa union is brought about, there is no chance of fibrosis occurring and causing jaundice due to stenosis at the anastomosis. In these cases it is no use trying to bring up the divided distal end of the common bile duct for anastomosis. The loop of jejunum is much more easily mobilized, has a much wider lumen and better blood supply. As such, it provides the best available replacement for the common bile duct.

CARCINOMA OF THE GALLBLADDER

This tumour occurs mostly in cases with gallstones. Therefore it is most common in women. The longer the history of stones the greater the chances of development of carcinoma. Most primary tumours of the gallbladder are adenocarcinomas: scirrhous, papillary or mucoid. Spread occurs early, directly to the liver and hilar structures, and by metastases to the liver and lungs. Nearly all cases have spread before symptoms appear. This tumour is not as uncommon in the East as in some western countries.

Clinical findings. There is pain in the right hypochondrium similar to the previous episodes of biliary colic, but more persistent. Obstructive jaundice may arise from involvement of the common bile duct. A hard mass is usually palpable in the gallbladder area. Ultrasound examination or CT scan may show gross and irregular thickening of a part of the gallbladder wall.

Treatment. If a localized carcinoma is found at laparotomy the gallbladder is removed with en bloc removal of an adjacent 2 cm of normal liver and dissection of the lymph nodes in the hepatoduodenal ligament. If malignancy has not penetrated the muscularis mucosa (as rarely happens) cholecystectomy is enough.

Surgery cannot offer much in most cases with liver metastases or distant spread. Nor is radiotherapy or chemotherapy effective. 90% of patients die within a year of diagnosis.

MALIGNANT TUMOURS OF THE BILE DUCT

These tumours are less common than carcinoma of the gallbladder. They are not more common in patients with gallstones. Most are adenocarcinomas. Obstructive jaundice due to these tumours is painless and progressive; in gallstone disease it is intermittent, with pain and fever. Hepatomegaly is common. If obstruction is due to a common bile duct tumour the gallbladder is enlarged and palpable; if due to a hepatic duct tumour, it is not. If the biliary obstruction remains unrelieved cirrhosis, splenomegaly, ascites and bleeding varices may be seen.

Treatment. Tumours of the distal common duct should be treated by *pancreaticoduodenectomy* i.e. removal of the head of the pancreas and duodenum. This is difficult surgery, with a high mortality rate due to breakdown of the anastomosis between the body of the pancreas and the jejunum. At operation, it has to be decided first of all whether the tumour is resectable or not. If the growth is adherent to the portal vein, the operation has to be abandoned because this vein cannot be sacrificed.

If the tumour is unresectable, obstruction to the flow of bile is bypassed by anastomosing the fundus of the gallbladder to a loop of jejunum *(cholecystojejunostomy)*. Life expectancy in such cases is only for a few months, death taking place due to distant secondaries.

23 Pancreas, peritoneum and mesentery

Pancreas

CONGENITAL ANOMALIES

Annular pancreas. The pancreas develops from a dorsal and a ventral segment. Normally the ventral segment also rotates and comes to lie dorsally. If it fails to do so a collar of pancreas surrounds the second part of the duodenum and may constrict it.

Clinical features depend on the extent of the obstruction. There may be complete or partial duodenal obstruction in the newborn, or obstruction arising later in life. Because of the duodenal obstruction the infant cannot absorb the amniotic fluid swallowed by him and maternal polyhydramnios results. Therefore if polyhydramnios is present one of the conditions which should be kept in mind is obstruction of the gastrointestinal tract at some level. If, as is usual, the constriction is distal to the entrance of the common bile duct, there is bile in the vomitus. X-rays show a dilated stomach and proximal duodenum (*double-bubble* sign).

Treatment. Fluid and electrolyte depletion is corrected, and the obstruction is bypassed by a *duodeno-duodenostomy*. The pancreas should not be divided or dissected, as a pancreatic fistula often develops.

ACUTE PANCREATITIS

Acute pancreatitis is a serious illness with a mortality rate which may be as high as 20%.

Aetiology. In acute pancreatitis, due to some unknown cause the trypsinogen and phospholipase in the pancreas get activated and cause auto-digestion of the organ. A number of factors can initiate acute pancreatitis:

1. Activation of pancreatic enzymes may occur due to *reflux* of bile or duodenal contents into the pancreatic duct.
2. Many cases are probably due to *a gallstone* impacting in the ampulla of Vater and obstructing the bile and pancreatic ducts.
3. A large number of cases occur in *alcoholics* after heavy use of hard liquor. Alcohol stimulates pancreatic secretion and induces spasm in the sphincter of Oddi, when reflux of bile may occur into the pancreas.
4. Certain *drugs* can cause acute pancreatitis: corticosteroids, contraceptives containing oestrogens, thiazide diuretics, tetracycline etc.
5. The pancreas is the only exocrine gland in the body which is so delicate that it can rupture due to *excessive production* of its own hormone, after over-eating.
6. Acute pancreatitis may be the first evidence of a *tumour* obstructing the pancreatic duct.
7. Pancreatitis may follow *cardiopulmonary bypass*.

Pathology. Acute pancreatitis may take one of two forms, the oedematous and the haemorrhagic. In oedematous pancreatitis there is mainly oedema and inflammatory cell infiltration. In haemorrhagic pancreatitis there is bleeding into the pancreas and peripancreatic tissues, and extensive pancreatic necrosis. When pancreatic lipase is liberated it splits fats into glycerol and fatty acids. The fatty acids combine with calcium to form soaps. These calcium soaps get deposited on the peritoneum and omentum, so that these surfaces are studded with small white tubercles, which are called areas of *fat necrosis*. In severe cases the pulmonary alveolar capillary membrane is rendered excessively permeable. This damage is supposed to occur either from fatty acids generated from serum triglycerides by lipase, or because of destruction of pulmonary surfactant. Finally, activated pancreatic proteolytic enzymes are capable of initiating intravascular coagulation.

Clinical findings. The attack usually begins after a large meal. There is severe epigastric pain which radiates to the back. The pain is persistent. Vomiting and retching usually occur. *In severe cases the patient collapses from shock.* There is profound dehydration, hypotension and tachycardia. Tenderness is most marked over the epigastrium, but may be generalized. Rigidity develops slowly. Bowel sounds are decreased or absent, and the abdomen slowly distends because of the paralytic ileus. If a mass is felt it may be the swollen pancreas or an abscess. In haemorrhagic pancreatitis the blood may dissect retroperitoneally into the flank *(Grey Turner's sign)* or into the periumbilical area *(Cullen's sign).*

Laboratory findings. There is commonly a moderate *leucocytosis. Liver function* studies are usually normal, but serum bilirubin is slightly elevated (below 2 mg/dl). The serum *amylase* rises above 200 i.u./dl within a few hours, and remains high for about 2 days. However, acute pancreatitis can occur without a rise in serum amylase. At the same time, the level of this enzyme can be raised in other acute abdominal conditions. Therefore, the value of this test is limited. *Isoamylase* analysis can distinguish pancreatic from non-pancreatic sources of amylase, but is not available everywhere. Unlike amylase, the pancreas is the only known source of lipase. Therefore the recently developed rapid accurate *lipase* assay is a more specific test for pancreatic disease. The serum *calcium* level may fall due to a combination of calcium with fatty acids (liberated from retroperitoneal fat by lipase).

Imaging. ***X-rays signs.*** There may be an air-fluid level due to a dilated loop in the region of the duodenojejunal junction (*sentinel loop*). One may sometimes see gas distending the right colon but stopping abruptly at the mid-transverse colon, the *colon cut-off sign*. This appearance is

Table 1 Ranson's criteria of severe acute pancreatitis.

On admission	
Age greater than 55 years.	
White cell count > 16 000/mm^3.	
Fasting blood glucose > 11.2 mmol/l (200 mg%).	
Serum LDH > 350 iu/l.	
SGOT > 250 S.F. Units%.	
Within 48 hours of admission	
A haematocrit decrease > 10%.	
BUN increase > 1.8 mmol/l (5 mg /dl).	
Serum calcium < 2 mmol/l (8 mg /dl).	
Arterial pO_2 < 7.98 kPa (60 mm Hg).	
Base deficit > 4 meq /l.	
Estimated fluid sequestration > 6 l.	
The *mortality* rates are as follows:	
< 3 signs:	1%
3–4 signs:	18%
5–6 signs:	50%
> 6 signs:	90%

produced by spasm of the colon adjacent to the inflamed pancreas. X-ray changes in the lungs are non-specific: from raised diaphragm, atelectasis and pulmonary infiltrates to pulmonary oedema.

Ultrasound. Ultrasound examination may show a swollen pancreas and gallstones, but gives abnormal findings in only about 40% of patients with acute pancreatitis. In the rest, the pancreas cannot be adequately seen because of gas in the overlying intestines.

CT scan visualizes retroperitoneal structures including the pancreas better than ultrasound, regardless of the presence of intestinal gas. However, both CT and ultrasound are usually normal in cases of mild pancreatitis.

Diagnostic paracentesis can help demonstrate the presence and severity of pancreatitis. The amylase concentration in the peritoneal fluid is of no value, but the physical properties are of interest. In a severe attack the fluid is dark, while in a mild attack it is straw-coloured.

Differential diagnosis. *Acute pancreatitis should be remembered as a possible cause in every case of upper abdominal pain,* and a serum amylase estimation carried out. Coronary thrombosis, high intestinal obstruction, perforated peptic ulcer and gallstone colic may have similar clinical features.

Prognostic markers. The risk of complications or death may be calculated by Ranson's parameters (Table 1).

Complications. The important complications of acute pancreatitis include *abscess formation* and *pseudocyst* of the pancreas. *Hypoxia* develops quite often, and in severe cases respiratory insufficiency may occur. Early endotracheal intubation, assisted ventilation, attention to fluid and acid-base balance, and peritoneal lavage to wash out the exudate may improve the prognosis.

Treatment. *Medical treatment.* Most attacks of acute pancreatitis are self-limited and subside spontaneously. The goals of medical treatment are: reduction of pancreatic secretory stimuli, and correction of fluid and electrolyte derangements. Oral intake is withheld and nasogastric aspiration started. This reduces the secretion of cholecystokinin and secretin. Thus it avoids pancreatic stimulation and hastens resolution of the disease. H_2-receptor blockers or antacids are given as prophylaxis against haemorrhagic gastritis to which these patients are prone.

Patients with severe pancreatitis lose much *fluid* into the retroperitoneal tissues. Therefore, large amounts of saline or colloid solutions are necessary to maintain the circulating blood volume, and measurement of cardiac output and pulmonary capillary wedge pressure with Swan-Ganz catheters may be required. In haemorrhagic pancreatitis blood transfusion may also be required. The volume and specific gravity of the urine should be monitored. This is a good way of judging the adequacy of fluid replacement.

For *analgesia* morphine or pethidine are given with atropine. In severe attacks *hypocalcaemia* requires parenteral calcium for its correction. In severe refractory cases *peritoneal lavage* is used to remove toxins in the peritoneal exudate; in fact peritoneal lavage should be used more often.

Hypoxaemia is common in acute pancreatitis, the Po_2 being less than 50 mm Hg in nearly half the patients. The airways should be humidified and tracheal suctioning carried out, with ventilatory exercise to keep the alveoli open. In pulmonary oedema diuretics should be used carefully because of potential renal compromise. If severe pulmonary oedema supervenes, endotracheal intubation and positive-pressure ventilation is required. However, the need for ventilatory support indicates the likelihood of a fatal outcome.

Total *parenteral nutrition* should be started and continued till the patient starts looking well. It provides a sufficient number of calories without stimulating the pancreas and increasing its secretion, which may leak and aggravate the peritonitis. In severe pancreatitis secondary infection is likely, therefore *antibiotics* are used to prevent it; in mild cases they are not required.

Surgical treatment. No single operative treatment and no operation cures pancreatitis. The role of surgery is reactive and responsive to particular complications as they evolve in a minority of patients. In fulminant pancreatitis, during the first few days *peritoneal lavage* can remove the dark brown toxic ascitic fluid which contains kinins and other vasoactive amines, and this frequently leads to rapid improvement.

At operation if there is any suggestion of biliary obstruction, choledochotomy and T-tube drainage is used. In patients with haemorrhagic pancreatitis the necrotic parts of the pancreas are removed. Large drains are laid down to the pancreas and the abdomen closed with non-absorbable materials. It is best to use the method of mass closure. This greatly reduces the incidence of wound dehiscence. No attempt is made to manipulate near the ampulla of Vater, because the oedema due to dissection may precipitate biliary and pancreatic obstruction.

PANCREATIC PSEUDOCYST

In acute pancreatitis part of the exudate may collect in the lesser sac. In some cases the opening into the sac may get closed by oedema. The closed lesser sac then distends with more exudate and produces a rounded swelling which is dull on percussion. This is called a pseudocyst because it is devoid of any epithelial lining. An ultrasound scan can show that the swelling contains fluid. A barium meal x-ray shows the lesser curvature of the stomach to be stretched out by a large rounded soft tissue shadow.

Such a collection may get absorbed spontaneously within a few weeks. If it does not, it should be drained, either to the exterior, or into a Roux loop of jejunum (cystojejunostomy). It can also be opened into the stomach (*cystogastrostomy*). In this method the stomach is opened and its posterior wall incised over the cyst. The fluid is sucked out, and sutures placed all around the edges of the opening to join the gastric mucosa to the wall of the cyst. The anterior wall of the stomach is then closed. After such free drainage the pseudocyst seldom causes any trouble.

CHRONIC PANCREATITIS

The most common *cause* of chronic pancreatitis is chronic *alcoholism*. However, a few cases are due to *metabolic* disorders e.g. hypercalcaemia and hyperlipidaemia. Gallstone disease can cause repeated attacks of acute pancreatitis, but rarely does it cause chronic pancreatitis. Two types of chronic pancreatitis are commonly recognized; a common 'calcific' form and a less common 'obstructive' form. The former type is associated with alcohol abuse.

The parenchyma of the pancreas is destroyed and replaced by fibrous tissue, with formation of calculi in the ducts, which show areas of stenosis and dilatation.

Clinical findings. Chronic pancreatitis may produce no symptoms. Alternatively, there may be abdominal pain, malabsorption with steatorrhoea, or diabetes mellitus. The pain is felt deep in the upper abdomen radiating through to the back. It may last for days or weeks and may come on after intervals lasting many months.

Investigations. ***Laboratory findings.*** Serum and urinary amylase may be elevated. Due to damage to the islets, insulin-dependent diabetes mellitus occurs frequently. Due to fibrosis around the lower end of the bile duct the serum alkaline phosphatase and bilirubin levels may rise. Splenic vein thrombosis may occur due to the proximity of the vein to the chronically inflamed pancreas, and may produce features of hypersplenism. Pancreatic pseudocyst and abscess may cause leucocytosis and elevated amylase levels.

Ultrasonography is inexpensive and non-invasive, and should be carried out first. Pancreatic size is assessed; in the early stages inflammation causes enlargement with an irregular outline, while in the advanced stages atrophy may ensue. Calculi produce bright echoes.

CT scan is more sensitive than ultrasound in the diagnosis of chronic pancreatitis, and may distinguish between pancreatitis and pancreatic cancer.

Endoscopic retrograde pancreatography helps establish the diagnosis by outlining the pancreatic ducts which are irregular, with stenoses and dilatations. However, it can itself aggravate pancreatitis.

Treatment. *Medical treatment.* Diabetes and malabsorption are treated. An enteric-coated pancreatic enzyme tablet is given with each meal to improve digestion by making good the deficiency of pancreatic ferments. Anaemia is corrected. The patient should be strongly advised against the continued use of alcohol, and if he heeds the physician's advice, he will find considerable relief from pain. When there are also problems arising from alcoholism, social deprivation and personality disorders, management can be very difficult.

Surgical treatment. Surgery is required if pain still persists after alcohol has been abandoned. The aim of surgery is to facilitate drainage of the pancreatic duct, or to resect diseased pancreas. For better drainage the *duct can be opened* along the whole body of the pancreas and *anastomosed* to a loop of jejunum. If the disease is even more widespread, a *subtotal pancreatectomy* is occasionally performed, leaving a remnant of the head of the gland attached to the duodenum.

CARCINOMA OF THE PANCREAS

This is a moderately common tumour which usually occurs in middle-aged people, specially in their fifties. The better established risk factors include cigarette smoking, intake of fats, diabetes mellitus, chronic pancreatitis, and prior gastrectomy and cholecystectomy. The neoplasm may arise in the head, the body, or the tail of the gland. Two thirds of the tumours are located in the head, the rest in the body and tail. Most are scirrhous adenocarcinomas, and at the time of diagnosis 85% have extended beyond the limits of the organ, most commonly to liver and peritoneum. The tumour spreads early to adjacent structures, to regional lymph nodes and to the liver. Distant spread occurs late. Carcinoma of the ampulla of Vater is also considered with pancreatic carcinoma, due to the fact that both the clinical features and treatment of the two conditions are similar.

Carcinoma of the head of the pancreas. As this carcinoma arises close to the termination of the common bile duct, it may present with *painless, progressive jaundice*. Sometimes pain in the back occurs due to infiltration of the tumour into the surrounding structures. There is also usually some loss of weight. The liver is enlarged, being distended with bile.

When the tumour obstructs the common bile duct, the gallbladder being normal distends greatly. On the other hand in obstructive jaundice due to gallstones the gallbladder being the seat of chronic cholecystitis cannot distend. Thus in jaundice due to carcinoma of the head of the pancreas the gallbladder is palpable, whereas in calculous jaundice it is not *(Courvoisier's law);* however, there are exceptions to this rule.

Laboratory findings. Alkaline phosphatase and bilirubin levels are raised due to common bile duct obstruction. The bilirubin levels average 18 mg/dl, being higher than those seen in benign bile duct obstruction. Serum transaminase levels are only slightly raised.

Imaging. *X-ray.* Barium meal x-ray may show a filling defect in the duodenum. *CT scan* is very useful in diagnosing small pancreatic tumours. *Ultrasound examination* can also help, but the image of the pancreas may be obscured by gas in the overlying intestines. *Endoscopic retrograde cholangiopancreatography* (ERCP) may demonstrate common bile duct obstruction. *Laparoscopy* can demonstrate even 2-mm nodules on the surface of the liver, peritoneum or omentum, which cannot be shown up by any other method.

Carcinoma of the ampulla of Vater. Ampullary adenocarcinoma accounts for only a small percentage of the tumours that obstruct the common bile duct. Its history and clinical presentation are similar to those of carcinoma of the head of the pancreas. However, it differs from the latter in the following respects:

1. It occurs at a somewhat earlier age.
2. It spreads locally and metastasizes more slowly.
3. Jaundice occurs early, so the tumour is often diagnosed while still curable.
4. Weight loss and pain are less prominent.
5. The stool often contains occult blood due to ulceration of the tumour.

Treatment. The only treatment offering any prospect of cure for either carcinoma of the head of the pancreas or periampullary carcinoma is removal of the head of the pancreas. As the duodenum is so intimately related to, and has a common blood supply with, the head of the pancreas, it has to be removed with it. The operation is called *pancreaticoduodenectomy.* After the excision the stomach is joined to a Roux loop of the jejunum, to which the pancreatic and bile ducts are also anastomosed. The operation carries a high morbidity and mortality rate. Therefore if all the gross tumour cannot be removed the operation should not be attempted. At the same time if the portal vein is infiltrated by the tumour the operation is abandoned, because this vessel cannot be sacrificed. The cure rate after surgery is unfortunately quite low. In the case of carcinoma of the head of the pancreas it is only about 10%; even with periampullary carcinoma it is not more than 30%.

Carcinoma of the body and tail. As these carcinomas lie at a distance from the common bile duct, jaundice is uncommonly seen in these cases. The presenting features are pain, weight loss, and finally the appearance of a mass. Unfortunately, by the time a mass becomes palpable it is too late. If the patient has only vague pain and weight loss he may be labelled a psychoneurotic. If back pain dominates the clinical picture, orthopaedic or neurological illness may be suspected.

If a pancreatic mass is detected on ultrasound examination, *percutaneous fine needle aspiration biopsy* may be carried out under ultrasound or CT scan control, for evaluation by cytological examination. Although this needle goes through the stomach the hole made by it is so small that after withdrawal of the needle the tissues of the stomach wall come together and no leakage of gastric contents takes place. However, for employing this method the help of a competent cytologist is required.

PANCREATIC ISLET CELL TUMOUR: INSULINOMA

The islets of Langerhans contain 5 types of cells. α-cells produce glucagon, β-cells insulin, and γ-cells somatostatin. F cells produce pancreatic polypeptide, and enterochromaffin cells produce serotonin.

The most common tumour arising from the islet cell of the pancreas is an *insulinoma.* It arises from the beta cells, produces insulin, and gives rise to signs of hypoglycaemia. Symptoms arise due to the brain being deprived of glucose: bizarre behaviour, lapses of memory, and unconsciousness. The patient may be diagnosed as suffering from a psychiatric illness. Profuse sympathetic discharge may cause palpitations, sweating, and tremulousness. The classic diagnostic criteria *(Whipple's triad)* are:

1. Hypoglycaemic symptoms produced by fasting.
2. Blood glucose level below 50 mg/dl during symptomatic episodes.
3. Relief of symptoms by intravenous glucose.

Since most insulinomas are less than 2 cm in diameter, CT scan and ultrasound fail to detect about half of them. Arteriography demonstrates upto half of the tumours.

Treatment. Surgery should be performed promptly, because with hypoglycaemic attacks permanent cerebral damage occurs, and also the patient becomes very obese. If a tumour is found it is enucleated. If not, the body and tail of the pancreas are excised and multiple sections made to detect the tumour. If a tumour is still not found, additional pancreas is resected until four fifths of the gland has been removed. This strategy is successful in 80% of cases. If hepatic metastases are present, chemotherapy with streptozotocin and 5-fluorouracil causes regression in half the cases, with complete remission in one-fifth.

Peritoneal cavity

ACUTE PERITONITIS

Nearly all varieties of peritonitis are due to bacterial infection of the peritoneum. This is so true that when the term peritonitis is used without qualification, bacterial peritonitis is normally meant.

Bacteriology. Acute peritonitis is commonly caused by bacteria which normally reside in the alimentary tract. However, a few cases occur due to non-enteric bacteria.

Bacteria from the alimentary canal. This variety is many times more common than the other. Bacteria may enter the peritoneal cavity from an inflamed organ, e.g. in acute appendicitis or cholecystitis; by perforation of a viscus, e.g. in a case of doudenal or gastric ulcer; or along the track of a penetrating abdominal wound. Usually the infection is a mixed one. The most common invaders are *Escherichia coli,* aerobic and anaerobic streptococci, and the bacteroides. Less often *Clostridium welchii* is found, besides staphylococci and *Klebsiella pneumoniae.* Many strains of E. coli, bacteroides and *Cl. welchii* produce toxins which cause severe illness or even death when they are absorbed from a large area like the peritoneum.

Bacteroides are Gram-negative non-sporing bacilli resident in the lower intestine. They are strictly anaerobic and grow slowly on culture media unless there is sufficient CO_2 tension in the anaerobic apparatus. As anaerobic cultures were not carried out in the past, their frequency and importance in the causation of peritonitis has only recently been recognized. They are resistant to penicillin and other commonly used antibiotics but sensitive to metronidazole, clindamycin and lincocin.

Bacteria not from the alimentary canal (Primary peritonitis). Examples of such bacteria include pneumococcus, beta-haemolytic streptococcus and gonococcus. If the infecting organism is the pneumococcus, the pus is slimy due to the mucopolysaccharide of the bacterial capsule. Such infection occurs mostly in patients with *impaired immunity*, specially those with ascites or with renal failure that is being treated with peritoneal dialysis. It is also seen in poorly nourished young girls who squat naked on the floor; the infection is presumed to reach the peritoneal cavity by ascending via the genital tract. Primary peritonitis can be treated with antibiotics and other medical measures.

Spread of the infection. Infection tends to spread widely if:

1. An inflamed appendix or other hollow viscus perforates before localization has taken place.
2. A purgative induces violent peristalsis.
3. The organisms are very virulent.
4. The omentum is small, e.g. in children.

If peritoneal defences cannot completely eliminate the bacteria but succeed in localizing the infective process, an *abscess* results. Mechanical barriers also help prevent the spread of the exudate. For example, the transverse colon and mesocolon divide the abdomen into supracolic and infracolic compartments, and discourage spread of infection from the one to the other.

Clinical findings. Severe *pain* of a cutting or burning type occurs, and is made worse by moving or breathing. The patient therefore lies still. The pain is at first localized to the site of the lesion, but soon spreads out from this point. Vomiting may occur. Marked *tenderness* and board-like *rigidity* are present if the peritonitis affects the anterior abdominal wall, otherwise both these signs are present to a lesser degree. The abdomen is *silent* due to paralysis of the intestines from the toxins of the bacteria. The pulse rises gradually.

Multiple organ dysfunction syndrome. Without treatment acute generalized peritonitis may rapidly progress to marked ileus with increasing abdominal distension, hypotension and septicaemia, with ultimately respiratory, renal, hepatic and cardiac failure. This condition is called multiple organ dysfunction syndrome. In such a case death may occur even after the primary focus of infection has been controlled.

On the other hand the condition may resolve. The pulse rate falls and the pain and tenderness diminish. The condition may localize, producing one or more abscesses, or may completely clear up. The peritoneum heals very rapidly after injury, so that mesothelial regeneration is complete within a week to ten days.

In localized peritonitis the initial symptoms and signs are those of the causative lesion. If inflammation is under the *diaphragm*, pain is felt at the tip of the shoulder. In *pelvic peritonitis* from a pelvic appendix the abdominal signs are often slight, but a rectal or vaginal examination reveals tenderness in the pouch of Douglas. With proper treatment localized peritonitis usually resolves. In 20% cases an abscess forms.

Investigations. Diagnostic aspiration of the peritoneal cavity may be helpful but is usually unnecessary. Plain x-ray of the upper abdomen in the erect posture may show gas under the diaphragm. Very high serum amylase levels support the diagnosis of pancreatitis, but can also occur in other acute abdominal conditions.

Treatment. If the cause can be established with certainty as primary peritonitis the treatment is conservative. If not, as in the vast majority of cases, operation is necessary. In early peritonitis treatment consists of removing the source of infection by operation. Thus the most common operations in the control of early peritonitis are appendicectomy, cholecystectomy, closure of perforated peptic ulcer and resection of gangrenous intestine. Combined with antibiotic therapy, early operation is associated with a very low mortality rate in this situation.

Advanced and established peritonitis also requires surgery for its control. Sometimes, however, patients are seen in whom the peritonitis is localizing, and a period of careful observation and conservative treatment may be advised.

The very advanced case. Rarely, specially in the aged and debilitated, the patient's condition has deteriorated to the point where anaesthesia and surgery would be lethal. In such cases it is a good plan to place a corrugated drain into the peritoneal cavity at the flank on either side through a small incision, under local anaesthesia. In some cases a large quantity of pus is thus drained away. If this happens, it reduces the toxaemia sufficiently to save the patient's life, and render him fit in a day or two for laparotomy under general anaesthesia to carry out the full surgical treatment of the condition. This method is not stressed as much as it should be in various textbooks. This is probably because such advanced cases of peritonitis are not nowadays seen in the developed countries, where most textbooks are written.

The essential *principles in the treatment* of peritonitis are the following:

1. *Intravenous fluids.* These patients have a great deficit of fluids. The peritoneal exudate contains nearly the same electrolytes as plasma, so replacement should be by lactated Ringer's solution. Inflamed peritoneum leaks proteins, and thus plasma proteins may need to be given. In countries where plasma is difficult to procure, blood transfusion is the cheapest and most readily available method of replenishment of plasma proteins, and may have to be used.

2. *Nasogastric tube aspiration* is carried out until the paralytic ileus resulting from the peritonitis has recovered. In seriously ill patients the aspirate is chocolate-coloured. This colour originates as follows: in the dilated stomach and intestine, due to hypoxia and toxaemia, minute erosions form in the mucosa. Small quantities of blood are lost into the lumen from these. The haemoglobin is broken down by the gastric and intestinal enzymes. Haematin is produced, which has a dark brown colour. When the patient's condition improves and the hypoxia and toxaemia are corrected, the above process is halted. No more blood leaks into the gut, so that the colour of the nasogastric aspirate changes back from chocolate to the normal green or yellow. *This is an extremely important sign of recovery.* Enough stress is not placed on this fact in the literature.

3. *Antibiotics* prevent the multiplication of bacteria and the release of endotoxins. As the infection is usually a mixed one, initially parenteral gentamycin, metronidazole and cephradine may be given.

4. *Surgical correction* of the cause should be carried out as soon as the patient is fit for operation. At surgery, after the cause has been dealt with, the pus in the peritoneal cavity is all sucked out. The cavity is then irrigated liberally with normal saline and sucked dry.

With modern treatment diffuse peritonitis carries a mortality rate of 10%. The lethal factors include bacterial toxaemia, paralytic ileus, electrolyte imbalance, and bronchopneumonia.

Complications of peritonitis. Besides the complications of any bacterial infection, there may be:

1. *Intestinal obstruction* due to adhesions. Gas and fluid levels are usually confined to the upper part of the small bowel.

2. *Paralytic ileus.* Air-fluid levels are distributed throughout the small and large intestine. If organic obstruction is clearly shown to be absent, the following regimen should be employed. The serum electrolytes are estimated. If the potassium level is low, the deficiency is made good. Any other electrolyte imbalance is also dealt with. Now a series of neostigmine 0.5 mg injections are given intramuscularly every hour for 4–6 hours. In a very significant number of cases wind is passed and the distension subsides.

3. *Residual abscesses.* The common sites are subphrenic, pelvic and midabdominal (paracolic and central). The abscess may gradually become smaller and subside. If it becomes larger it must be drained.

Peritonitis after abortion. The abortionist has usually pushed an instrument through the uterine vault and streptococcal peritonitis occurs. If the infection is confined to the pelvis the treatment is conservative with antibiotics, nasogastric aspiration and intravenous fluids. If a pelvic abscess forms it is drained through the vagina. If peritonitis is generalized a laparotomy is required. Commonly a loop of small or large intestine has been perforated, and requires repair or resection. As the treatment of the generalized peritonitis is sometimes neglected because of social factors, multiple organ dysfunction syndrome sometimes supervenes.

Meconium peritonitis. This is the term applied to any antenatal intestinal perforation. When the perforation occurs early in intrauterine life the meconium causes an inflammatory reaction and calcification within the peritoneal cavity. The baby vomits bile and shows all the signs of intestinal obstruction. X-ray shows air-fluid levels and calcification. At operation there are widespread adhesions and a localized mass of intestines encased in a dense inflammatory reaction. The bowel has to be dissected out of the adhesions and the perforated loop exteriorized.

When the perforation occurs late in intrauterine life there is no calcification. The infant is born with a hugely distended abdomen which interferes with respiration. X-ray shows an opaque abdomen with little gas. Prompt paracentesis is performed to decompress the abdomen and relieve the respiratory distress. The perforated loop of intestine is resected. The prognosis is bad, but recovery has followed prompt operation in some cases.

TUBERCULOUS PERITONITIS

Tuberculous peritonitis is commonly a chronic condition. It presents with abdominal pain, fever and night sweats, loss of weight, ascites or an abdominal mass. The infection originates from tuberculosis of mesenteric lymph nodes, caecum or fallopian tubes. It may take the form of an encysted or generalized ascites, or may present as a plastic peritonitis. In cases with *ascites* the peritoneal cavity becomes filled with pale, straw-coloured fluid. The fluid is rich in lymphocytes, and *Mycobacterium tuberculosis* can be cultured in it. The onset is gradual. There is loss of energy, pallor and loss of weight. The patient seeks advice because of enlargement of the abdomen. A transverse solid mass can often be palpated in the abdomen. This is thickened and rolled up greater omentum. Treatment is by a full course of antituberculosis chemotherapy.

In the *encysted* form the fluid is walled off in a part of the abdomen. A diagnosis of mesenteric or ovarian cyst may be made. In the *plastic* form there are widespread adhesions which cause coils of intestine, specially ileum, to become matted together and distended. These distended coils act as 'blind loops' and give rise to steatorrhoea, wasting and attacks of abdominal pain. The first indication of disease may be subacute or acute intestinal obstruction. At operation adhesions are divided and stenosed segments of gut resected. Antituberculosis drugs are used for the full prescribed period.

INTRA-ABDOMINAL ABSCESSES

Subphrenic abscess. There are four important intraperitoneal subphrenic spaces, two on either side. On the right side there are the right subphrenic and the right subhepatic spaces. On the left side lie the left subphrenic space and the lesser sac. Besides these there is an extraperitoneal space, the bare area of the liver.

The right subphrenic space lies between the liver and diaphragm, bounded posteriorly by the coronary and right triangular ligaments. Abscesses here are commonly due to a perforated duodenal ulcer, a perforated gallbladder, and appendicitis.

The right subhepatic space (Morrison's pouch) lies between the liver and the right kidney, with the duodenum medially and the hepatic flexure below. It is the most common site of a subphrenic abscess, which usually arises from appendicitis, cholecystitis, perforated duodenal ulcer, and after upper abdominal surgery.

The left subphrenic space. This space lies between the diaphragm and liver, bounded posteriorly by the triangular ligament. Common causes of an abscess here include complications after operations on the stomach, tail of pancreas, spleen or splenic flexure of colon.

The lesser sac. This cavity lies below the liver, with the lesser omentum and stomach lying in front. The causes of abscesses here include pancreatitis and perforated posterior gastric ulcer or cancer.

Clinical findings. The symptoms and signs of a subphrenic abscess are often obscure. The old saying 'pus somewhere, pus nowhere, pus under the diaphragm' is often appropriate.

Commonly the history is as follows: after an infective focus in the abdomen has been dealt with, the patient's condition improves temporarily, but after a few days symptoms of toxaemia reappear. The condition steadily deteriorates. Sweating, wasting and anorexia are present. There may be epigastric fullness and pain, or pain in the shoulder from irritation of the phrenic nerve referred to the cervical plexus.

Signs. If the abscess is anterior, the abdominal examination will reveal tenderness, rigidity or even a palpable swelling. Examination of the chest may reveal collapse of a lower lobe or a pleural effusion.

Course. If left unrecognized and untreated, a subphrenic abscess may rupture into a bronchus, or the peritoneum or pleura, with serious consequences. The mortality rate in neglected cases is very high.

Investigations. A leucocytosis is usually present. A plain x-ray may show an air-fluid level below the diaphragm with a pleural effusion above it. Ultrasound and CT scans are diagnostic.

Treatment. The treatment of subphrenic abscess is surgical. The best route for drainage of *right* subphrenic and right subhepatic abscesses is the lateral subcostal approach. The incision is started at the tip of the eleventh rib and carried obliquely forward along the costal margin. The advantage of this approach is that it is possible to drain all the subphrenic and subhepatic spaces while avoiding contamination of the general peritoneal cavity. A *left* subphrenic abscess is also best drained through a similar incision on the left side. An abscess in the lesser sac requires an upper abdominal incision, either vertical or transverse.

During recent years ultrasound-guided *percutaneous catheter drainage* has found favour in the management of subphrenic abscesses, and a transperitoneal approach is often used. With this method the risks associated with open transabdominal drainage have diminished greatly.

Pelvic abscess. The common causes of a pelvic abscess include pelvic appendicitis, salpingitis and diffuse peritonitis from any cause. *Neisseria gonorrhoeae* and *C. trachomatis* are the primary pathogens responsible for salpingitis in sexually active women. This abscess is easily recognized if suspected. There is fever, lower abdominal discomfort, and diarrhoea with passage of mucus. Rectal examination discloses tenderness and a fullness in the pouch of Douglas. The abscess may subside or progress to a tense mass bulging into the vagina or the anterior rectal wall. Pelvic ultrasound is valuable in corroborating the diagnosis and distinguishing an abscess from a phlegmon. In patients with a ruptured tubo-ovarian abscess, laparotomy with unilateral salpingo-oophorectomy is required. A pelvic abscess may be drained through the rectum or the vagina. In general such drainage provides a very gratifying result with rapid recovery.

Midabdominal abscess. These abscesses may occur anywhere within the abdomen from just below the transverse colon to the pelvis. The right and left paracolic gutters are the most common sites but an abscess may form wherever a collection of blood or foreign material has occurred. Midabdominal abscesses are particularly difficult to identify. Repeated gentle palpation for a developing mass may give the first clue. X-ray shows a persistently dilated loop of bowel. Ultrasound and CT scan help greatly in localizing the fluid collection, and should be utilized in every case of suspected abdominal abscess. A progressively enlarging mass is an indication for drainage. In other cases the patient may become so ill, with high fever, chills and hypotension, that laparotomy becomes essential even without definitive localization of the abscess. In such cases a paramedian incision is commonly used, and the whole of the abdomen should be thoroughly explored so as not to miss an abscess in any part. However, since the availability of ultrasound examination such a situation should be rare.

A word of warning about ultrasound: the person carrying out the examination must be properly trained and skilled. Otherwise his report may be worse than useless; it may be misleading. Ideally the surgeon should be present during the ultrasound examination, so that he can note the location of the abscess himself. Surgeons can profitably use ultrasound machines themselves for getting a better orientation of the lesions they have to operate upon.

Mesentery

Tuberculosis of mesenteric lymph nodes. Tubercle bacilli are ingested and reach the mesenteric lymph nodes by way of Peyer's patches. In the advanced countries following universal pasteurization of milk the bacilli are usually human, in the underdeveloped countries usually bovine. Sometimes only one lymph node may be infected, usually there are several. Occasionally massive involvement occurs. Abdominal tuberculosis is a common cause of a 'chronic abdomen' in the less affluent countries. Tubercular mesenteric lymph nodes may present clinically in one of many forms:

1. A *calcified lymph node* may be seen on x-ray. The shadow is round or oval and mottled. The infection may still be active, because other uncalcified nodes may also be present. The x-ray shadow may look like that due to a stone in the ureter. However, the shadow of a calcified lymph node is stippled. In doubtful cases pyelography clarifies the diagnosis.

2. Less often the *general symptoms* of evening pyrexia, pallor, anorexia and weight loss occur.

3. In other cases central abdominal pain may be seen. If there is tenderness in the right iliac fossa, *appendicitis* may be impossible to exclude, and operation may occasionally be performed.

4. A coil of intestine may become adherent to a caseating lymph node and be angulated to cause *intestinal obstruction.*

5. Tuberculous pus from caseating mesenteric nodes may collect between the leaves of the mesentery and be mistaken for a *mesenteric cyst.*

Mesenteric cysts. These cysts are common during the first two decades of life:

1. The cyst may produce a painless, fluctuant abdominal *swelling* which moves freely in a plane at right angles to the attachment of the mesentery.

2. There may be attacks of abdominal *pain* due to impaction of a food bolus in a segment of bowel narrowed by the cyst.

3. The cyst may *rupture,* or *infection* or *haemorrhage* may occur into it.

These cysts resemble enteric duplications in their location within the mesentery. However, they do not have any mucosa or muscular wall. Chylous cysts probably arise from congenital lymphatic obstruction, and contain milky chylous fluid (Plate III-I). Treatment is by surgical resection. Because of the intimate proximity of the cysts to the bowel, a segmental resection of the involved loop of intestine is usually required.

24 Spleen

Anatomy. The spleen is covered on all its surfaces by peritoneum. However, its hilum is connected to the kidney by a fold of peritoneum, the lienorenal ligament, which contains the splenic artery and vein. Similarly it is connected to the stomach by the gastrosplenic ligament, which contains the short gastric vessels. During splenectomy each of these ligaments has to be divided and the vessels contained therein ligated.

Physiology. The endothelial macrophages in the spleen remove from the circulation worn-out and damaged red cells, as well as particulate foreign matter, microbes, antigens and cellular debris. At the same time, the spleen contains the largest collection of both T and B lymphocytes in the body. Antigen is taken up by follicular cells and presented to immunocompetent cells leading to antibody production by the plasma cells. Further, the normal spleen contains about 8 percent of the red cell mass, which is discharged into the circulation during emergencies such as anoxia. Finally, the spleen is a center of haematopoiesis, although a minor one.

TRAUMA TO THE SPLEEN

Rupture of the spleen most often occurs in industrial or traffic accidents of the crushing or run-over type. Other organs may be injured at the same time. The spleen may also be injured during operations on the stomach, oesophagus, vagus nerves etc.

Clinical findings. The symptoms vary from minimal or no symptoms to hypovolaemic shock. There may be severe left upper abdominal pain. Referred pain may be felt in the left shoulder due to irritation of the diaphragm *(Kehr's sign).* The signs indicate low-grade peritoneal irritation, i.e. tenderness and slight rigidity. Abdominal distension occurs due to intestinal paresis. The area of splenic dullness may be increased. With marked bleeding there is tachycardia, hypotension and shock. Tenderness may be present over the left ninth and tenth ribs.

In a few cases a subcapsular haematoma forms. The red cells gradually disintegrate and the haematoma liquefies. Increased osmolarity of contents causes expansion of the cavity and finally rupture. This is probably how *delayed rupture* takes place days or weeks after the injury.

On *x-ray* there may be obliteration of the splenic outline and of the psoas shadow, and indentation of the left side of the stomach air-bubble. Fracture of one or more ribs on the left side may be seen.

If the diagnosis of splenic trauma is suspected in a patient whose cardiovascular system is stable, an ultrasound or CT scan can be carried out to obtain information about the presence and severity of the splenic injury.

Treatment. In the past immediate laparotomy was regarded as the only reliable course of action whenever splenic injury was strongly suspected. The ruptured spleen was removed, blood evacuated, injury to other viscera excluded and the abdomen closed.

However, in due course it was found that after splenectomy the patient, specially if a small child, is very vulnerable to overwhelming infections, particularly with pneumococci. Therefore the recent trend is to treat minor injuries non-operatively and moderate injuries with suture (*splenorrhaphy*) or partial splenectomy, reserving splenectomy for extensive lacerations of the spleen. If this course is followed, different measures can be employed at operation to achieve haemostasis:

1. For trivial trauma pressure can be combined with topical agents to arrest bleeding. *Fibrin glue*, a highly concentrated form of fibrinogen and clotting factors, can be sprayed onto the injury or over a fractured surface. It can also be used along with sutures to seal the splenic surface after a partial resection. *Microfibrillar collagen* forms a firm, adherent coagulum which traps and activates platelets. It can be packed into cracks and fissures.
2. If the short gastric vessels are intact, the splenic artery can be ligated in continuity for haemostasis without infarction of the spleen.
3. Sutures tend to cut through, but can be applied over collagen or teflon pledgets, or over omentum. The spleen may also be wrapped in omentum.

It should be stressed that such a patient must be nursed in a critical care unit for a few days and a close watch kept for recurrent bleeding.

Rupture of a malarial spleen. If the spleen is greatly enlarged as a result of malaria in a tropical country, even minor trauma can result in its rupture. Bleeding may be extremely profuse. The operation of splenectomy in this condition is much more difficult than in a ruptured normal spleen. To avoid going through the haematoma the splenic vessels may first be ligated as they run along the upper border of the body of the pancreas.

CONDITIONS REQUIRING SPLENECTOMY

In certain haematological and other disorders the surgeon may be called upon to remove the spleen as part of the management of the illness. It is essential that he has an understanding of these conditions and the effect of splenectomy on their course, as well as any contraindications to removal of the spleen.

HAEMATOLOGICAL DISORDERS

Splenectomy may be required in idiopathic thrombocytopenic purpura, certain haemolytic anaemias, and in hypersplenism from different causes.

Idiopathic thrombocytopenic purpura (ITP). This is a syndrome characterized by a low platelet count. The platelets of affected patients become sensitized by antiplatelet IgG autoantibodies and are then removed from the circulation. The term ITP should be applied to a haemorrhagic disorder only if the subnormal platelet count is found in the presence of bone marrow containing normal or increased numbers of megakaryocytes, and in the absence of any systemic disease or history of ingestion of drugs capable of inducing thrombocytopenia. There is a greatly reduced number of platelets, so that purpuric haemorrhages take place. The increased platelet destruction takes place in the macrophage phagocyte system, specially the spleen. As a response to this shortage of platelets, and in an effort to make good the deficiency, the number of megakaryocytes is increased.

Clinical findings. Most patients are young women. The onset may be *acute,* with ecchymoses, petechiae, and bleeding from gums, vagina, urinary tract or gastrointestinal tract. In the intestine the swollen, haemorrhagic mucosa may lead to the development of intussusception or intestinal obstruction. In some patients symptoms regularly get worse during menses. The spleen is rarely palpable and if it is enlarged, the diagnosis should be reconsidered. The *chronic* form may occur at any age. There is a gradual onset. The patient bruises easily, and may have menorrhagia.

The platelet count is always below 100×10^9/l, and at times approaches zero. Many patients need no treatment if the platelet count remains over 50×10^9/l. If the count falls below 20×10^9/l the risk of bleeding increases. Because of the thrombocytopenia, the bleeding time may be prolonged, but the clotting time remains normal. The bleeding results in an iron deficiency anaemia. The marrow shows large numbers of abnormal megakaryocytes. Before a definitive diagnosis of ITP can be made, different causes of nonimmunologic thrombocytopenic purpura, such as leukaemia and aplastic anaemia, must be ruled out.

Treatment. If the thrombocytopenia is secondary, the underlying cause must be removed. If the patient has only *mild* symptoms, he should avoid rough sports, elective surgery and non-essential drugs. In *moderate* or *severe* cases corticosteroids are used, when 80% of patients go into remission on 60 mg prednisolone/day. Steroids make the capillaries less permeable. However, if the disease does not respond to corticosteroids, or relapses after a remission, splenectomy is required. Although the platelet count is low, platelet transfusion is not commenced until the splenic vessels have been ligated, when 6 to 8 units of platelets may be transfused. In children with acute ITP, as many as 80% have a complete and permanent spontaneous remission; this occurs in only 25% of adults. Overall, splenectomy is successful in 85% of patients, but more often in idiopathic cases than in those secondary to another disorder.

Haemolytic anaemias in which splenectomy may be helpful include hereditary spherocytosis, β-thalassaemia, and autoimmune haemolytic anaemia.

Hereditary spherocytosis is the most common congenital haemolytic anaemia. It is transmitted as an autosomal dominant trait. In this condition the red cell membrane is more permeable to sodium ions than normal. As the sodium leaks into the cell it swells and becomes more rounded and therefore more fragile. Thus a large number of red cells are destroyed. Significant red cell destruction takes place only in the presence of the spleen. The haemolysis results in the production and excretion of excessive amounts of bilirubin, so that bile pigment stones often form in the bile ducts. During infancy the condition may resemble haemolytic disease of the newborn due to ABO incompatibility.

Clinical findings. As a result of the excessive haemolysis the patient is jaundiced. Due to the anaemia he is pale and gets tired easily. The spleen is enlarged. Exacerbations of haemolysis may occur from time to time. During a crisis there is sudden fever, abdominal pain, nausea, vomiting and extreme pallor with increased jaundice. The red cell count may fall to 1.5 million/cu mm.

In adult cases there is often a history of attacks of gallstone colic. The gallbladder may contain pigment stones. *Whenever gallstones are seen in a child the patient should be investigated for presence of hereditary spherocytosis.*

Laboratory findings. The diagnosis is made on examination of a peripheral blood film where spherocytes and reticulocytes are seen. The red cells are more *fragile* than normal. Haemolysis occurs in 0.6% saline or even stronger solutions, whereas normally it occurs only in much more dilute solutions of saline. The reticulocyte count is high. The patient's own red cells are *labelled with* ^{51}Cr and reinjected; scanning over the spleen shows increased radioactivity due to sequestration of red cells.

Treatment. The spleen does not allow the defective red cells to survive long enough to be of much use, therefore it must be removed. After splenectomy the abnormally shaped cells have a normal life span, so that the anaemia is rectified.

In children the optimum age for operation is about 7 years. Before this age splenectomy is followed by a greatly increased vulnerability to infections; after this age gallstones start to form. At operation if gallstones are present, the gallbladder is also removed. Following splenectomy the anaemia and jaundice disappear. It should be remembered that *special care must be taken to treat infections in the splenectomized child promptly.*

Thalassaemia. The thalassaemias are anaemias originally found in people living on the shores of the Mediterranean (Greek *thalassa* = sea) but now affect people throughout the world. This is an autosomal dominant disorder. One of the globin chains of the haemoglobin molecule is defective. Foetal haemoglobin (HbF) persists, and can be detected by serum electrophoresis; its presence is diagnostic. This produces abnormal red cells.

Heterozygotes have only mild anaemia *(thalassaemia minor).* On the other hand homozygotes have severe chronic haemolytic anaemia with jaundice, gross splenic enlargement and retarded growth *(thalassaemia major).* The peripheral blood film reveals target cells, nucleated red cells and a hypochromic microcytic anaemia. The haemolysis produces an excess of bile pigments, so that 25% of patients have gallstones.

Treatment. Minor thalassaemia requires no treatment. In major thalassaemia, due to excessively rapid haemolysis, blood transfusion may be required every few weeks. In order to prevent immunization to leucocyte antigens as a result of frequent transfusions, leucocyte-depleted red cell

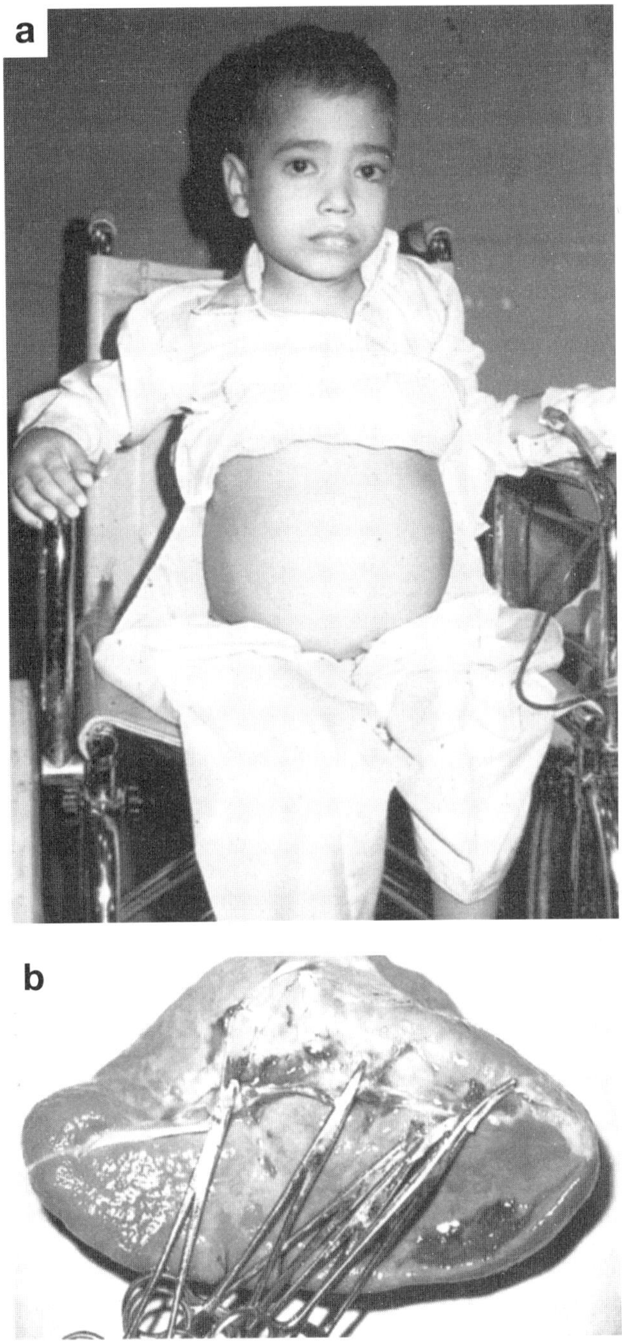

Fig. 1 (a) Young boy with major thalassaemia. The abdomen is enlarged due to the splenomegaly. (b) The spleen removed.

concentrates may be employed. When haemolysis becomes so severe that transfusion has to be given every 7 to 10 days, recourse must be had to splenectomy. The operation reduces haemolysis and transfusion requirements, and removes an enlarged, uncomfortable spleen (Fig. 1).

Autoimmune haemolytic anaemia. If a patient develops antibodies against his own red cells, the condition is called *autoimmune haemolytic anaemia.* Both warm and cold antibodies have been described. Only patients with warm antibodies (IgG) require splenectomy. Those with cold (non-gamma) antibodies do not benefit from this operation.

Autoimmune haemolytic anaemia can occur due to high doses of penicillin, quinidine or methyldopa, besides other chemical and physical agents and bacteria. Antibodies are produced which are haemagglutinins. The immunologically altered red cells are trapped in the macrophage phagocyte system, including the spleen, and are destroyed.

Clinical findings. The condition is most common after the age of 50. There is an acute onset of anaemia, mild jaundice and sometimes fever. The spleen is usually enlarged, and pigment gallstones are often present. Coombs test is positive.

Treatment. This includes removal of the offending drug or other agent, administration of corticosteroids, and blood transfusions. Associated diseases responsible for the condition are sought and treated. Corticosteroids produce a remission in 75% of patients, but only 25% of remissions are permanent. Splenectomy is indicated in the following situations:

1. If there is no response to 6 weeks of high-dose corticosteroid therapy.
2. If the condition improves with treatment, but a relapse occurs.
3. For patients in whom corticosteroid therapy is contraindicated.

Hypersplenism. One of the important functions of the spleen is to destroy worn-out blood cells. If the spleen enlarges greatly for whatever reason, this function is greatly exaggerated and there is excessive destruction of the different blood cells leading to anaemia, leucopenia and thrombocytopenia. Such a state is called hypersplenism, which is nearly always secondary to some other condition:

1. It may result from *excessive destruction* of red cells from one of the following causes:
   i. The red cells may be defective in structure, as in hereditary spherocytosis.
   ii. Autoimmunity may result in excessive destruction of red cells in auto-immune haemolytic anaemia.
2. In many diseases the spleen may be greatly enlarged for *different reasons:*
   i. In portal hypertension, due to venous congestion.
   ii. In various neoplastic conditions involving the spleen, e.g. Hodgkin's disease, lymphomas and leukaemia, due to deposition of the malignant tissue.

The common indications for *splenectomy* for hypersplenism include lymphoma and chronic lymphatic leukaemia. After splenectomy for these conditions about 80% of cases achieve haematological correction; this allows chemotherapy to be commenced and partial or complete remission to be obtained. α-Interferon is used for patients with little or no splenomegaly or in those in whom splenectomy is contraindicated.

Lymphoma. In lymphomas splenectomy may be required to arrive at a diagnosis (if there are no palpable lymph nodes), to correct cytopenia arising due to hypersplenism, to relieve the symptoms of gross splenomegaly, and to allow staging of Hodgkin's disease.

Staging. To plan the treatment of Hodgkin's disease a precise knowledge of the extent of the disease is essential, because the outcome depends greatly on the recognition and treatment of all sites of the disease. A staging laparotomy is therefore sometimes performed. The spleen is removed for histology and biopsies are taken from the liver and the para-aortic lymph nodes. Such a laparotomy is not necessary if the bone marrow or viscera other than the spleen are involved, because this means that the disease is diffuse, cannot be cured by x-rays, and should be treated by chemotherapy. In any case, since the advent of ultrasound, CT scans and MRI, the need for a staging laparotomy for Hodgkin's disease has been very considerably reduced, as these tests provide most of the information which is obtained by laparotomy.

OTHER INDICATIONS FOR SPLENECTOMY

The spleen may be removed for hydatid cyst of the spleen; for schistosomiasis, and as part of a cancer operation because of local extension of tumours of the stomach, colon or pancreas. Splenectomy is no longer practised for immunosuppression after renal transplantation, because of the resulting increased death rate from overwhelming infection in immunosuppressed recipients of transplants.

Schistosomiasis is common among Egyptian peasants in the Nile delta and elsewhere in Africa, as well as in Venezuela. It is caused by *Schistosoma mansoni* or *S. haematobium*. Periportal fibrosis in the liver occurs first. The spleen then enlarges due to the portal hypertension and the products of disintegrated worms and ova which are filtered by the spleen. In advanced cases the liver is shrunken with ascites, and the spleen may be so large as to extend to the pelvic brim. The urine and faeces should be examined for ova. Early cases of schistosomiasis respond to treatment by antimony salts. In advanced cases, after careful preoperative preparations with blood transfusions and antibiotics, splenectomy is undertaken and confers a great deal of benefit.

SPLENECTOMY

Preoperative preparation. In view of the risk of post-splenectomy sepsis, all patients should receive vaccines against the pneumococcus, meningococcus and *Haemophilus influenzae type b.* In patients with idiopathic thrombocytopenic purpura, platelets should be available for use after splenectomy if thrombocytopenic bleeding occurs. The blood and blood products should be warmed before use, specially in chronic lymphocytic leukaemia and lymphoma, because the patient may have developed cold haemagglutinin disease and may have an increased risk of haemolysis.

Technique. Either a subcostal or midline incision can be used to expose a spleen. A midline incision is preferred in two situations:

1. In a ruptured spleen because it allows a better examination of other viscera which may have been injured at the same time.
2. In a case where the spleen is huge, because the incision can be extended greatly if required.

The spleen is mobilized by dividing its posterior ligamentous attachments, which may contain blood vessels requiring electrocautery or ligation. The short gastric vessels are next divided and ligated. Finally, the hilum of the spleen is dissected, and the splenic artery and vein ligated and divided individually, to avoid the possibility of the development of an arteriovenous fistula. In a case with a huge spleen, it is desirable to reduce its blood supply before mobilizing it. This can be achieved by exposing the artery through the gastroplenic ligament and ligating it as it runs along the upper border of the pancreas. When splenectomy is carried out for a haematological disorder, a careful search should be made for accessory spleens, which should be removed. The left upper quadrant is not drained routinely. If there has been injury to the tail of the pancreas or if haemostasis is incomplete, closed suction drainage should be employed.

Complications. Most patients tolerate the operation well. The most common postoperative complication of splenectomy is collapse of the lower lobe of the left lung. Other more serious complications include postoperative haemorrhage, subphrenic abscess, injury to the pancreas causing fistula or pancreatitis, wound infection, and portal and mesenteric vein thrombosis.

25 Small intestine

In the intestines food is digested and absorbed. In the small intestines the various enzymes break down the constituents of food into smaller molecules which are then absorbed. In the large intestine some further absorption of nutrient materials takes place, and water is absorbed so that the residue is firm and relatively dry for easier disposal. In such conditions of the intestines where digestion or absorption is at fault, malnutrition results.

Investigation of small bowel disease. The function of the small intestines being digestion and absorption, this is the aspect which is the subject of most tests carried out in small gut disease.

Radiology. Plain erect and supine films are useful mainly in acute intestinal obstruction and perforation. For the chronic disorders, barium meal follow-through is more useful. To increase the diagnostic yield, specially for small bowel tumours, Crohn's disease and in patients with occult gastrointestinal haemorrhage, the barium may be instilled directly via a tube into the upper jejunum (*small bowel enema).* In malabsorption the contrast medium appears flocculated and segmented, the mucosal folds thickened, and the intestinal loops dilated. However these changes are non-specific and must be confirmed by other more specific tests.

Selective splanchnic angiography is the best method of detecting angiodysplastic lesions (vascular malformations) which present with occult gastrointestinal bleeding. A Seldinger catheter is passed up from the femoral artery. Its tip is placed opposite the origin of the coeliac artery and the dye injected. *Digital subtraction angiography* can also be employed. For *computed tomography* (CT) of the small intestines, barium sulphate suspension is administered. The distance between the shadows of barium in adjacent loops is due to the two thicknesses of bowel wall between them. Thus, CT helps in detecting thickening of the bowel wall by disease. However, the same information can also be obtained by ordinary contrast studies. In intestinal obstruction *ultrasound scan* can distinguish between fluid-filled dilated bowel loops and other cystic structures.

Isotope scintigraphy. In patients with intestinal bleeding due to a suspected Meckel's diverticulum, polyp or tumour, a small bowel enema may not help. In such cases, isotope methods are helpful. *Technetium pertechnetate* is injected intravenously. The ectopic gastric mucosa in Meckel's diverticulum excretes it into the lumen, where it appears as a hot spot in the scan. In active bleeding in an emergency situation, ^{99m}*sulphur-colloid* (Tc Sc) is preferred. After intravenous injection, Tc Sc is cleared from the circulation by the macrophage system within 15 minutes, so that radioactivity at the bleeding site increases, allowing its detection as a hot spot.

Small bowel transit time can be estimated by administering isotope-labelled meals. The end-point is reached when radioactivity is detected over the caecum.

Faecal fat. Quantitative estimation of faecal fat is the most sensitive and reliable test of disorders of digestion and absorption, the normal upper limit of faecal fat output on a standard diet, containing 80 to 100 g of fat, being 6.0 g/day.

Jejunal biopsy. This is the definitive test for most cases of mucosal malabsorption. It is essential for the diagnosis of coeliac disease, tropical sprue, amyloidosis and giardiasis. Endoscopic biopsies from the distal duodenum have been shown to be as useful as jejunal biopsies. The steerable Medi-tech biopsy capsule is much quicker than the Crosby capsule and two or three biopsies can be taken.

SMALL BOWEL OBSTRUCTION

Many diseases of the intestines, both congenital and acquired, end up by obstructing the passage of intestinal contents and present to the clinician as cases of intestinal obstruction. This results in an emergency situation which requires prompt treatment. For appropriate management one has to decide whether obstruction is present and if so, what is the likely cause. In many cases the exact cause is found only at operation.

Intestinal obstruction may be classified into two types, mechanical and paralytic:

Mechanical. There is a mechanical block to the passage of intestinal contents. The latter may be:

1. In the lumen, e.g. inspissated faeces or gallstones.
2. In the wall, e.g. inflammatory or malignant stricture.
3. Outside the wall, as in hernias or adhesions.

Paralytic. In this condition peristalsis ceases. This is called *paralytic ileus* (ileus means colic), e.g. in mesenteric vascular occlusion, peritonitis, etc.

Clinically, there are three types of mechanical obstruction:

1. *Acute obstruction*, with severe pain, vomiting, distension and absolute constipation (i.e. no faeces and no flatus) coming on suddenly.
2. *Chronic obstruction*, with abdominal colic at first, and absolute constipation and distension after a few weeks.
3. *Acute-on-chronic obstruction*, in which acute (complete) obstruction supervenes on a longstanding chronic i.e. incomplete obstruction.

PATHOLOGY

The intestine *above* the obstruction undergoes vigorous peristalsis to overcome the obstruction. If this is unrelieved for several days the increasing distension causes the peristalsis to diminish and finally cease, the intestine now being flabby and toneless. When a smooth muscle fibre is rapidly stretched beyond a certain limit, it loses the power to contract. The intestine *below* the obstruction shows normal peristalsis and absorption. When the residue of its contents has been passed onwards, it becomes immobile, contracted and pale.

Distension occurs proximal to the obstruction due to both gas and fluid. *Gas* is derived from swallowed air, diffusion from the blood, and products of digestion. The carbon dioxide and oxygen get absorbed into the blood-stream, leaving behind nitrogen and foul-smelling hydrogen sulphide. As far as *fluid* is concerned, it must be remembered that every day many liters of fluid are secreted into the upper part of the gastrointestinal tract as follows: saliva (1,500 ml), gastric juice (2,500 ml), bile (500 ml), pancreatic juice (1,000 ml), and succus entericus (3,000 ml). When the intestine is obstructed this secretion persists, but absorption from the gut is very greatly reduced. Therefore body fluid volume is depleted.

This reduction in extracellular fluid volume occurs due to:

1. Vomiting.
2. Defective absorption.
3. Loss of the above-mentioned secretions into the lumen of the bowel. This fluid, although within the body, is outside both the compartments of body fluid i.e. the intracellular and extracellular spaces. It is therefore said to be *sequestrated* into a *third space.*

Fluid depletion is severe and occurs early in high small intestinal obstruction, later in ileal obstruction, and even more slowly in colonic obstruction. This is because the lower the obstruction the greater the absorptive area available above it.

Strangulation of the bowel occurs when its blood supply is interfered with due to its being trapped in a hernia or involved in a volvulus or intussusception. It is a dangerous condition and demands early treatment. First the veins are compressed and the gut becomes blue or purple. Later the arterial supply is affected. The peritoneal coat loses its shine, the mucosa is ulcerated, and gangrene is imminent. Loss of blood volume into the congested segment is proportional to the length of the segment. If a long loop of intestine is strangulated, the patient may go into oligaemic shock, and his life may be in danger.

When the wall of the gut is devitalized, first bacterial toxins and later bacteria pass into the peritoneal cavity and are absorbed into the circulation. Therefore strangulation in an external hernia is far less dangerous than intraperitoneal strangulation, because in the former case the toxic transudate is confined to the relatively small hernia sac. It should be remembered that in most cases of strangulation the obstruction is of the closed-loop type. After relief of strangulation, toxic substances in the strangulated loop may pass on to normal intestine and become absorbed. This may cause a deterioration in the patient's condition or even death.

CLINICAL FEATURES

The clinical features of intestinal obstruction consist of pain, vomiting, distension and absolute constipation.

Acute obstruction. *Abdominal pain* is the first symptom, and it starts suddenly. It recurs at intervals of a few minutes. These colicky attacks spread all over the abdomen, but are localized mainly at the umbilicus. Such attacks of pain are absent only in paralytic ileus.

Vomiting. In high jejunal obstruction vomiting starts after several hours of pain, except that the first attack of pain may be accompanied by a vomit. As the obstruction progresses the character of the vomiting changes. First it contains partly digested food, then mucoid gastric juice, then yellow fluid from regurgitation of bile, and finally faeculent fluid. The lower down the gut the site of obstruction, the later does vomiting commence.

Distension. This takes several hours to develop. Visible peristalsis may be seen in thin individuals. Peristaltic sounds may be loud enough to be audible *(borborygmi).* The hernial sites must be examined to exclude strangulated hernia.

Constipation. After the contents of the bowel below the obstruction have been evacuated, there is absolute constipation i.e. neither faeces nor flatus is passed.

Dehydration. Loss of absorptive power by the intestine and repeated vomiting leads to dehydration. The skin and the tongue are dry, the eyes are sunken, the urine is small in amount and concentrated.

Chronic obstruction. The common cause of chronic obstruction in the small intestine is a tubercular stricture, in the large intestine a carcinoma. Constipation appears, increases gradually over weeks or months, and finally may become absolute. Abdominal distension then occurs. In small gut obstruction intestinal loops are seen lying one above the other – the *ladder pattern.* In large gut obstruction, on palpation a tumour can occasionally be felt in the line of the colon. Pain occurs as bouts of colic.

Acute-on-chronic obstruction. This condition starts as chronic obstruction, but the narrowing of the lumen increases so much that it ends up as acute obstruction.

Strangulation. This must be distinguished from non-strangulating obstruction, because strangulation requires immediate operation to avoid gangrene. The picture is usually that of an obstruction together with a degree of shock. Pain is more severe and constant. Tenderness and rigidity may be present. If strangulation occurs in an external hernia, the lump is tense, tender and irreducible, with no cough impulse.

X-rays. A plain x-ray of the abdomen is taken with the patient erect and supine. Distended jejunum shows closely packed transverse lines due to the valvulae connivantes. In contrast, the haustral folds of the colon are spaced further apart and the indentations are not placed opposite each other; at the same time these lines do not extend right across the shadow of the bowel loop. Fluid levels appear at a late stage (Fig. 1). The lower the site of obstruction in the small bowel and the longer its duration, the larger the number of fluid levels. Obstruction low in the colon does not commonly produce fluid levels in the small gut.

TREATMENT

This resolves itself into three steps:

1. Gastroduodenal suction.
2. Replacement of fluid and electrolytes.
3. Relief of the obstruction, usually by operation.

The first step is to empty the stomach and keep it empty by an indwelling *nasogastric tube.* By relieving distension and reducing the size of the distended coils of intestine, aspiration facilitates the operation and closure of the wound. Also, toxic intestinal contents, which would have been

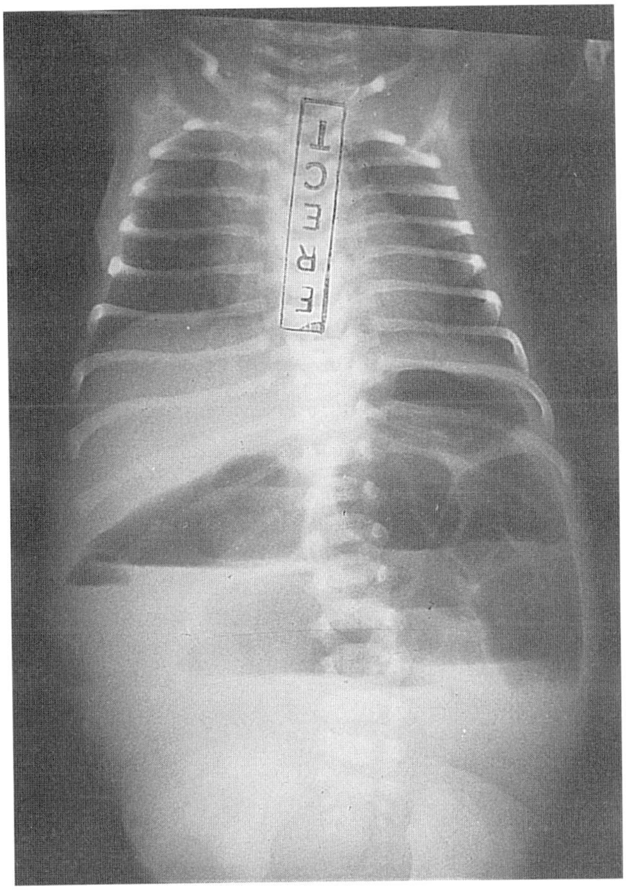

Fig. 1 Multiple air-fluid levels in acute intestinal obstruction due to ileal atresia in a newborn.

absorbed after the relief of obstruction, are evacuated beforehand. The outer end of the nasogastric tube should not be closed but left open, so that air continues to escape constantly, as the air pressure in obstructed intestine is higher than the atmospheric pressure. The end should be connected to the tubing of a collecting bag, which should be cut open near the top so that pressure does not build up inside it.

The fluid and salt lost must be replaced. If signs of dehydration are present, three to four liters of normal saline are commonly required. A fluid balance chart must be maintained. When the stomach has been deflated and as soon as any fluid deficit has been made good, operation for the relief of the obstruction is usually carried out.

INTESTINAL OBSTRUCTION IN THE NEWBORN

The common causes of this condition are congenital anomalies. These include atresias at various levels, arrested rotation, volvulus of the midgut and meconium ileus.

Atresia and stenosis of the duodenum. In atresia the duodenum is completely blocked; in stenosis its lumen is greatly narrowed. Vomiting starts immediately after birth. If the atresia lies below the duodenal ampulla the vomitus is bile-stained, otherwise it is colourless. Visible peristalsis may be seen in the epigastrium passing from left to right. A plain film shows a large bubble in the stomach and a smaller one in the duodenum (*double-bubble sign*). To relieve the obstruction the dilated proximal duodenum is anastomosed to the most proximal loop of the jejunum (*duodenojejunostomy*).

Jejunal and ileal atresia. In this condition either the ileum is blocked by a septum, or a whole segment of the gut is missing. Vomiting starts within a day or two after birth. If not diagnosed early, the increasing distension impairs the blood supply of the gut, causing gangrene and perforation. Central distension comes on within 24 hours of birth. Plain x-ray shows many more fluid levels than in jejunal atresia. The grossly distended ileal segment does not function, due to its smooth muscle having been overstretched and put out of action. Therefore it must be resected before anastomosis is performed. Before this point was appreciated, newborns usually suffered continuing obstruction even after anastomosis, and often died of it.

Malrotation. In this condition, after the midgut returns to the abdomen, it fails to undergo rotation. The caecum remains in the left hypochondrium. A peritoneal band runs from it to the right across the duodenum and obstructs the latter. At the same time the caecum and the whole of the small intestine, which has a narrow attachment, may revolve around its pedicle resulting in a volvulus of the midgut.

Midgut volvulus is a dangerous condition. If it remains untreated it results in gangrene of the whole small gut, a condition which is incompatible with life. At the same time it leads to serious hypovolaemia due to loss of fluid into the very long segment of gut. *Therefore recurrent obstruction in the newborn should be carefully investigated.*

Meconium Ileus. This is the neonatal presentation of mucoviscidosis of the pancreas. Due to the absence of pancreatic enzymes from the gut, the terminal ileum is filled with meconium mixed with viscid mucus to produce a hardened mixture which may be felt as a rubbery mass. The infant is born with intestinal obstruction. At operation the affected coil of gut is irrigated with 1% hydrogen peroxide through a short incision to loosen the glue-like mass. If this method fails, the coil is resected.

Meconium peritonitis. This is the term applied to any antenatal intestinal perforation. When the perforation occurs *early* in intrauterine life the meconium causes an inflammatory reaction and calcification within the peritoneal cavity. The baby vomits bile and shows all the signs of an intestinal obstruction. X-ray shows air-fluid levels and calcification. At operation there are widespread adhesions and a localized mass of intestines encased in a dense inflammatory reaction. The bowel has to be dissected out of the adhesions and the perforated loop exteriorized. At a later stage continuity of the bowel can be restored.

When the perforation occurs *late* in intrauterine life there is no calcification. The infant is born with a hugely distended abdomen which interferes with respiration. X-ray shows an opaque abdomen with little gas. Prompt paracentesis is performed to decompress the abdomen and relieve the respiratory distress. The perforated loop of intestine is resected. The prognosis is bad, but recovery has followed prompt operation in some cases.

ACUTE INTUSSUSCEPTION

In this condition a segment of the gut becomes invaginated into the one immediately distal to it. There may be an obvious cause which initiates the intussusception, e.g. a polyp, a submucous lipoma, an inverted Meckel's diverticulum, etc. The outer tube is called the intussuscipiens, the inner and middle layers together from the intussusceptum. The blood supply of the inner layers may be impaired due to pressure, resulting in gangrene. The ileocolic type accounts for about 77% of cases, other types being ileo-ileo-colic, ileo-ileal, colo-colic etc.

INTUSSUSCEPTION OF INFANTS

In the intussusception of infants there is no obvious cause. It is thought that a change in the diet predisposes to inflammation of the intestine and causes swelling of Peyer's patches. Such a swollen patch becomes the focus of commencement of the intussusception.

Clinical features. Usually the patient is a male child aged six to nine months. The reason for this particular age incidence is probably to be found in the fact that the lymphoid tissue in the submucosa of the small gut is most plentiful at this time. The onset is sudden with attacks of severe abdominal pain each lasting a few minutes, the baby lying pale and listless between the attacks. He may vomit at the onset, but only after twenty-four hours is vomiting a conspicuous feature. In the early stages a normal stool may be passed; later, blood and mucus are evacuated. On examination the abdomen is not distended. A lump may be felt if the child is quiet or asleep, and if the swelling is not lying under the costal margin. The right iliac fossa may feel empty. In the few cases where the intussusception has travelled far enough, its apex may be felt by rectal examination, otherwise blood and mucus are found on the examining finger.

After twelve to twenty four hours the abdomen starts to distend. If untreated, death may occur due to the obstruction or due to peritonitis secondary to the gangrene. Very rarely a natural cure occurs after sloughing of the intussusceptum.

Plain films of the abdomen reveal increased gas shadows. *Barium enema* may show up an ileocolic intussusception. The column of barium ends abruptly in a convex filling defect occupying the whole lumen of the gut.

Differential diagnosis. Acute intussusception must be distinguished from the following conditions:

1. In acute *enterocolitis* diarrhoea is a leading symptom, and faecal matter or bile is always present in the stools.
2. In *prolapse* of the rectum the mucosa can be felt to be continuous with the perianal skin.
3. In *purpura* with intestinal symptoms intussusception often coexists.

Treatment. After rehydrating the baby with saline, laparotomy is carried out. The lowest part of the sausage-shaped mass is squeezed to reduce the intussusception. The last portion is the most difficult to reduce, and should be gently compressed in a warm saline pack to reduce the oedema. If reduction proves impossible the affected loop is resected, with end-to-end anastomosis. Postoperatively, gastric aspiration and intravenous fluids are continued for a day or two, after which sips of water and later mother's milk are started. Recurrent intussusception is very rare but does occur.

In Australia some surgeons reduce an intussusception of a few hour's duration by administering a barium enema under hydrostatic pressure, the procedure being controlled by flouroscopic screening. This method should only be employed by experienced personnel and in case of failure to reduce the intussusception, immediate operation must be carried out. In certain parts of the world the opportunities for using this method are few because the infants are brought late, when the employment of this technique would be dangerous.

BLIND (STAGNANT) LOOP SYNDROME

If a blind loop of small intestine is formed, or is made at operation, stasis is the result. This can happen when a loop of gut is bypassed at operation. Stasis produces an abnormal bacterial flora which leads to defects of absorption. If the blind loop is in the jejunum the defect is of fat absorption leading to pale, bulky, greasy stools (steatorrhoea); if it is in the ileum vitamin B_{12} deficiency results, with macrocytic anaemia. Sometimes bacterial overgrowth develops in the absence of a local cause. This may occur in patients with malnutrition or immune deficiency.

The *clinical features* are non-specific and include weakness, nausea, vomiting and weight loss. Diarrhoea is frequent. Other features include stomatitis, anaemia, hypoproteinaemia, oedema, tetany, rickets and osteomalacia, and retardation of growth in children.

Treatment. Cure is obtained only by surgical removal of the blind loop. However, in certain situations removal is not feasible, for example in cases where the underlying disease is either systemic like scleroderma, or very extensive like jejunal diverticulosis. In these cases temporary improvement follows the use of antibiotics to destroy the abnormal bacteria. Tetracycline and metronidazole are the common agents used, for about two weeks at a time. Soon after the antibiotic is stopped, bacteria again colonize the gut. However, symptomatic relief lasts for many months. This is fortunate because intermittent therapy can be employed, obviating the need of continuous long-term treatment with its side-effects.

SHORT-GUT SYNDROME

This is the most serious form of intestinal decompensation, and is seen after massive *resection* of the small bowel and in some patients subjected to jejuno-ileal *bypass* for morbid obesity. The conditions which may necessitate extensive removal of the small gut include Crohn's disease, mesenteric infarction, radiation enteritis, midgut volvulus and small bowel tumours. Crohn's disease is the most common cause, requiring repeated resections over a number of years culminating in the short-gut syndrome; therefore resections for this condition should be as conservative as possible.

An assessment of how much length of gut *remains* behind is more important than knowing how much has been removed. As a general rule 50 percent of the small intestine can be resected without causing severe or persistent malabsorption. As more intestine is removed the effects of malabsorption become more severe, but life can be continued more or less normally if more than 100 cm remains. Below this figure, the patient requires life-long home parenteral nutrition. It is important to retain the last few centimetres of the terminal ileum as well as the ileocaecal valve; the former because vitamin B_{12} is absorbed in this part, the latter because it both slows down the transit time and limits colonization of the residual intestine by an overgrowth of colonic bacteria.

The short-gut syndrome may be followed by malabsorption of fats and proteins as well as lactose intolerance. Other *sequelae* may also result: gallstones and urinary stones may form, the levels of hepatic enzymes may be raised, and renal excretion may be impaired. With time, structural and functional changes occur in the residual bowel as an adaptation to the reduced absorptive area. The remaining intestine gets dilated and lengthened, and the villi enlarge in size.

Treatment. *Enteral or parenteral nutrition* is provided according to the situation as indicated above. *Antidiarrhoeals* are prescribed.

Surgical. *Reversed intestinal segment.* A segment of small intestine about 10 cm in length is isolated, its direction *reversed*, and continuity restored. It delays transit and allows more time for absorption from the gut proximal to it.

Bianchi's *intestinal lengthening* operation is ingenious, and has been used on a number of infants. It relies on the fact that each side of the small gut is supplied independently by alternating terminal branches of the mesenteric arteries. The leaves of the mesentery, each with its contained vessels, are separated and the intestine divided longitudinally by a stapling device. The two tubes are joined end-to-end to double the length of the intestine which also dilates in due course, increasing its absorptive surface.

The future. Small bowel *transplantation* has been carried out successfully from an HLA compatible sibling. Multiple rejection episodes requiring aggressive immunosuppression and life-threatening infections were encountered. However, long-term survival and health independent of parenteral nutrition has been achieved. This is a major breakthrough and points towards the likely developments in the future.

MECKEL'S DIVERTICULUM

This is the most important intestinal diverticulum, being present in 2% individuals. It is a remnant of the vitello-intestinal duct, and is situated on the antimesenteric border of the ileum about 60 cm from the ileo-caecal valve. In a few cases the diverticulum contains abnormally located epithelium, which may be gastric or colonic, or sometimes pancreatic tissue.

Complications. A Meckel's diverticulum usually remains symptomless throughout life. If encountered during an operation it should be removed, because the following complications can arise in it:

1. *Bleeding* per rectum due to peptic ulceration in abnormally placed gastric mucosa. This can pose a difficult problem in differential diagnosis.
2. *Intussusception*, which can occur at any age, and result in intestinal obstruction.
3. Meckel's *diverticulitis* due to lodgement of coarse food residue etc. Symptoms are very similar to those of appendicitis. If perforation occurs, the very severe peritonitis may simulate perforated peptic ulcer.
4. *Intestinal obstruction.* If a band connects the diverticulum to the umbilicus, a coil of intestine may get twisted around it.

SURGICAL COMPLICATIONS OF TYPHOID

Because of poor food hygiene typhoid fever is still common in certain parts of the world. Therefore, from time to time surgeons receive patients where a typhoid ulcer has perforated or bled. At the same time, acute typhoid cholecystitis and a chronic carrier state is occasionally seen.

Perforated typhoid ulcer. A typhoid ulcer develops over a Peyer's patch in the terminal ileum. In cases of typhoid the wall of the bowel is extremely friable due to the effect of the bacterial toxins. It is not surprising therefore that it sometimes breaks down at the site of an ulcer. Such a perforation usually occurs during the second week of the fever, and the patient presents with severe abdominal pain and tenderness, along with some rigidity. The diagnosis is relatively easy, and can be made fairly confidently if the usual course of the disease is remembered and the history taken carefully. *This is the only type of peritonitis where abdominal pain and tenderness are* ***preceded*** *by a few days of high fever.* In all the other forms of peritonitis, whether due to a perforated peptic ulcer, a perforated appendix, etc., fever comes on *after* the onset of pain. *The occurrence of many day's fever before pain is diagnostic of typhoid.* Although the Widal test is usually positive in these cases, it is not required for diagnosis. Patients are usually critically ill with septicaemia from the generalized peritonitis, dehydration and electrolyte imbalance, specially potassium deficiency. They should be resuscitated in an intensive care unit. Blood transfusion may be required to correct severe anaemia.

Treatment. The treatment of any perforation of the small intestine is closure of the opening by surgical operation, and this is carried out. However, as mentioned above, the wall of the bowel is as friable as wet blotting paper. Therefore the incidence of breakdown of the repair with formation of an ileal fistula is fairly high. Various measures have been employed to prevent this serious complication:

1. Unabsorbable sutures are used.
2. An omental patch may be sewn over the repair.
3. The worst affected segment of ileum may be resected.
4. A temporary catheter ileostomy may be carried out proximal to the repair, to decompress the ileum.

The results of closure of typhoid perforations are so poor that some advise a conservative management for this condition. Many surgeons, including the author, feel this is too extreme a view. Specially in gravely ill patients, a compromise between operative repair of the perforation and conservative treatment can be arrived at. Under local anaesthesia a corrugated drain is placed into the peritoneal cavity on each side in the paracolic gutter. Large quantities of pus are evacuated and the fever and toxaemia subside. As the patient's general condition improves very greatly, the perforation often gets walled off and closes itself; if it does not, surgical repair is carried out.

Bleeding typhoid ulcer. Very occasionally a typhoid ulcer may bleed massively. Blood transfusions along with antibiotics effective against typhoid are indicated. The situation where resection of the terminal ileum has to be carried out for uncontrollable haemorrhage is very rare indeed.

Typhoid cholecystitis. *Acute* typhoid cholecystitis occurs from time to time and perforation can occur. Ultrasound examination is helpful in these cases. If in a case with fever and tenderness in the right hypochondrium the wall of the gallbladder is thick indicating acute cholecystitis but no stones are seen, this is strong evidence in favour of typhoid cholecystitis, as this is the only common cause of acalculous cholecystitis. *Chronic* typhoid cholecystitis can result in a carrier state, with bacteria being discharged with the faeces from the gallbladder reservoir. If such a carrier state is proved by examination of the stools, ciprofloxacin is a useful drug. If gallstones or chronic cholecystitis are present, cholecystectomy is the treatment of choice, but cholecystectomy alone is inadequate if there is associated infection in the biliary tract.

INFLAMMATORY BOWEL DISEASE

The term inflammatory bowel disease includes two major entities, namely ulcerative colitis and Crohn's disease. Although these two diseases differ from each other in many ways, they also have common features. Both conditions are common in the West, specially among Jews, and uncommon in the Eastern and developing countries. The lymphoid tissue of the gut is active in both conditions: in Crohn's disease as a granuloma, in ulcerative colitis in the form of an Arthus reaction. Both conditions show autoantibody production and raised serum levels of gammaglobulins. Finally, the extraintestinal manifestations of inflammatory bowel disease are present in other immunologically mediated diseases. However, rather than an autoimmune assault on a target cell, recent work suggests that these conditions arise due to a *hyperactivation of the immune response*, including lymphocyte proliferation, cytokine release, excessive neutrophil products, specially leukotrines and reactive oxygen metabolites, and ultimately tissue injury. The actual tissue damage is probably in the nature of a nonspecific injury to an 'innocent bystander'. Crohn's disease is described next, while ulcerative colitis is discussed in the succeeding chapter.

CROHN'S DISEASE

Crohn's disease consists of a chronic inflammation involving the gut. It may affect any part of the alimentary canal from the mouth to the anus, but is seen most often in the ileum and colon. This condition which is very common in the West specially among Jews, is encountered less often in the underdeveloped countries. The cause is not known. *Mycobacterium paratuberculosis* has been suspected but not proved. Some constituents of the intestinal contents may be responsible, as elemental diets are as effective as steroids in providing relief. At the same time, defunctioning of the colon by an ileostomy helps the condition to subside. There is much evidence to show that immunological mechanisms play a role in pathogenesis. Intestinal macrophages and T lymphocytes are activated within the inflamed intestine and release cytokines and inflammatory mediators, which alter epithelial permeability, damage endothelium, activate fibroblasts and initiate fibrosis.

The disease is characteristically discontinuous, affecting a number of segments with normal mucosa in between. The mucosa undergoes inflammation and fibrosis, accompanied by ulceration. The inflammation is predominantly submucosal although it often goes right through the bowel wall. It usually commences at the ileocaecal junction and extends proximally for an average distance of 30 cm. Above this there may be another separate area of diseased intestine — a *skip* lesion. The intestine is swollen and bright pink with a fibrinous exudate. The mesentery is thickened and its lymph nodes are fleshy.

Clinical features. In the *acute* condition, which is seen in only 5% of cases, the appearances are similar to those of acute appendicitis, except that diarrhoea nearly always commences before the attack of pain.

The *chronic* condition is divided into three stages:

In the *1st* stage there is prolonged diarrhoea and colic, with fever and a tender mass. Stools show mucus and occult blood.

The *2nd* stage presents as acute or chronic intestinal obstruction.

In the *3rd* stage adhesions develop and sometimes slow perforation occurs, which may result in fistulae into surrounding viscera e.g. pelvic colon or bladder, or to the exterior through the scar of a previous operation e.g. appendicectomy.

Complications include perforation, acute dilatation and haemorrhage, as well as uveitis and arthritis, but less often than in colonic disease. Gallstones and renal stones occur more commonly than in the general population. Amyloidosis occurs rarely.

Diagnosis. ***Barium meal x-ray.*** This shows straightening of the valvulae conniventes. If ulcers are present, multiple specks of barium are left behind after the gut segment has emptied of barium. In advanced cases the terminal ileum is stenosed — the *string sign* of Kantor. If available, a *small bowel enema* allows a much better definition of the mucosal pattern, as well as of strictures, than a conventional barium meal follow-through. If this confirms the diagnosis of Crohn's disease a full examination of the colon should be made by colonoscopy and biopsies. *CT scan* and *MRI* are useful in the assessment of fistulae and pelvic abscesses.

Laboratory data, specially haemoglobin, platelet count, albumin, ESR and serum levels of the acute-phase proteins, help assess the severity of the disease.

White-cell scan. If technetium-labelled granulocytes are injected intravenously, they collect at the sites of inflammation, i.e. the loops of the ileum and the colon, and show up on the scan.

Treatment. Since Crohn's disease cannot be cured, the clinician's role is to control the inflammation, correct the nutritional deficiencies, and ameliorate the symptoms. Surgery is often required in this connection, and most patients undergo at least one operation during their lifetime. In general, medical treatment should be dictated by symptoms. If the activity of the disease is shown only by laboratory data, large doses of corticosteroids or immunosuppression are not indicated. In the early stages medical treatment is given a trial with bed rest, a diet rich in proteins and vitamins, and iron. Oral iron is poorly tolerated by these patients and the total dose may have to be given intravenously, with preparations to deal with the rare case of anaphylaxis. Magnesium and zinc deficiencies can also occur, and serum concentrations should be measured in patients with extensive chronic disease.

Patients with mild disease are given sulphasalazine 1 g twice a day or oral prednisolone 20 mg daily for 6 weeks. Those with severe disease require intravenous hydrocortisone, 100 mg every 6 hours, intravenous fluids and blood. If such a patient goes into relapse on reducing the dose, it means he has chronic active disease, and immunosuppression by azathioprine 2 mg/kg/day should be employed over a long period, with regular blood counts to monitor possible marrow suppression.

Surgical treatment is indicated for the following situations:

1. If medical treatment fails to arrest the disease.
2. If intestinal obstruction supervenes. The most common indication for surgery in Crohn's disease of the small intestine is recurrent intestinal colic provoked by solid food, so that the patient is afraid to eat.
3. If a fistula forms which causes disability.

As this condition recurs over a period of time, resections of intestines should be very conservative. At the same time, bypass operations should be avoided as they result in malabsorption by creating blind loops. If the abdomen is opened on the mistaken diagnosis of appendicitis and Crohn's disease is found instead, the appendix should not be removed, otherwise often an external fistula develops.

ABDOMINAL TUBERCULOSIS

This term includes tuberculous infection of the gastrointestinal tract, mesentery, peritoneum, liver and spleen. Genitourinary tuberculosis is a separate entity and is not discussed here. The primary type of intestinal disease is caused by ingestion of milk contaminated by *Mycobacterium bovis*. The secondary type is due to swallowing of sputum infected with *Mycobacterium tuberculosis* from an active primary focus in the lung. In the advanced countries abdominal tuberculosis is nowadays rarely seen because of tuberculin testing of cows, pasteurization of milk, effective treatment of pulmonary tuberculosis and improvement in living conditions and nutrition. However, elsewhere in the world it is still common.

TUBERCULOUS PERITONITIS

In most cases *chronic* tuberculous peritonitis results from reactivation of a primary peritoneal focus, and is therefore

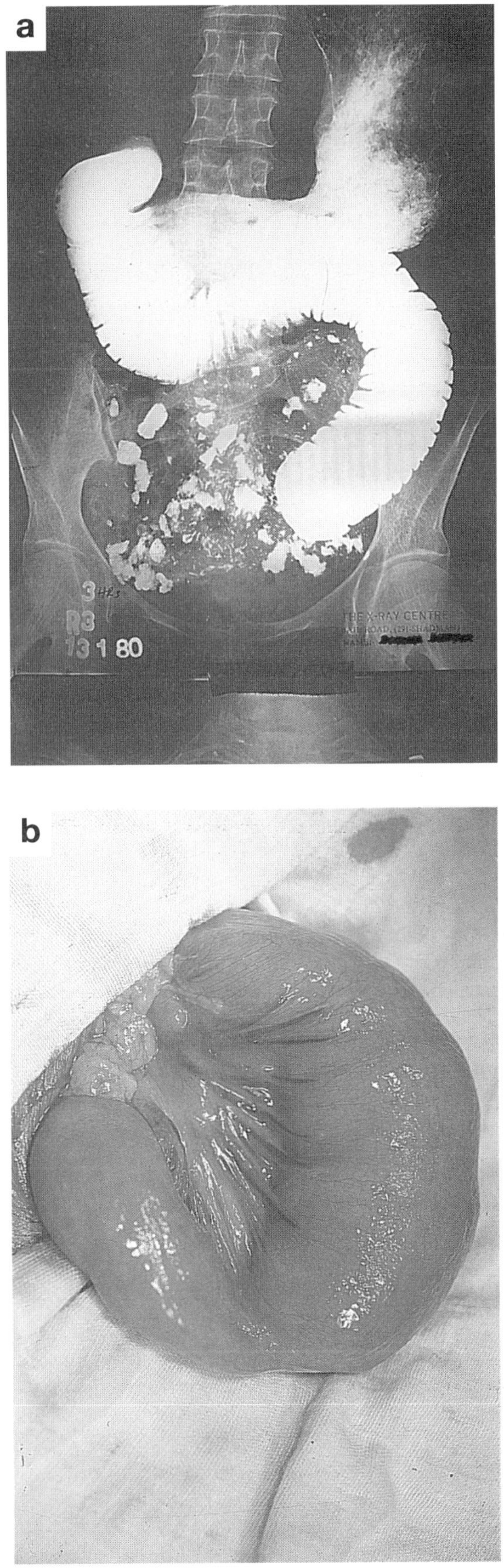

Fig. 2 (a) Barium meal x-ray showing most proximal loop of jejunum grossly dilated due to tuberculous stricture of the jejunum. (b) Distended loop delivered at operation. The stricture was resected and an end-to-end anastomosis carried out.

haematogenous in origin. It causes malaise, weight loss, fever and ascites. Active intestinal infection is usually not present, but infections of other serous cavities, e.g. the pleura and pericardial cavity are commonly seen. The dry plastic type of disease which gives a doughy abdomen is rare.

Acute tuberculous peritonitis is sometimes seen, as part of miliary disease or following rupture of a tuberculous mesenteric lymph node.

INTESTINAL TUBERCULOSIS

This condition occurs in two main forms, the ulcerative and the hyperplastic.

Ulcerative tuberculosis. This is secondary to pulmonary tuberculosis due to swallowing tubercle bacilli. Ulcers form in the terminal ileum, the long axis of the ulcers lying transversely along the lymphatics. Diarrhoea with pus and blood occurs. Often the patient has had treatment for pulmonary tuberculosis. Barium meal may fail to visualize the terminal ileum and caecum due to hypermotility. A prolonged course of chemotherapy heals the ulcers. However, if a stricture forms operation may be required for intestinal obstruction (Fig. 2).

Hyperplastic tuberculosis. This occurs most often in the ileocaecal region. There is much thickening of the wall of the caecum and consequent narrowing of the lumen. Besides fibrous tissue there is a great deal of fatty tissue. This accumulation of fibrofatty tissue around the gut is a characteristic but non-specific feature of chronic disease of the large bowel. Lymph nodes enlarge, and may caseate. Abscess and fistula formation is rare. Although this condition is usually called ileocaecal tuberculosis, the lesion is in fact confined to the caecum and should therefore be called tuberculosis of the caecum.

Clinical features. Attacks of abdominal pain with stoppage of wind occur. Stasis and infection of the ileal contents may cause steatorrhoea, anaemia and loss of weight. A firm mass is palpable in the right iliac fossa. This has to be differentiated from an appendix mass, a carcinoma of the caecum, Crohn's disease and an actinomycotic granuloma. A mass in the epigastrium may be due to thickened and rolled up omentum.

Barium meal x-ray shows a long narrow filling defect, consisting of terminal ileum and ascending colon. The latter is shortened due to fibrosis and the caecum lies at a high level.

Treatment. If obstructive symptoms have not developed and the diagnosis is certain, *chemotherapy* may completely cure the condition. The current World Health Organization regimen for a patient weighing 40 to 60 kg consists of a daily intake of isoniazid 300 mg, rifampicin 450 mg, pyrazinamide 1.5 g, with streptomycin 0.75 g intramuscularly or ethambutol 25 mg/kg. This is continued for 2 months, followed by twice weekly administration of 600 mg each of isoniazid and rifampicin for 4 months. The patient is monitored periodically for hepatotoxicity. Pyridoxine 10 mg /day must be given with isoniazid to prevent peripheral neuropathy.

On the other hand isoniazid 300 mg and rifampicin 600 mg are sometimes given for as long as 18 to 24 months, with streptomycin 1 g/day being added for 2 to 3 months only if the sputum reveals large numbers of bacilli.

If obstruction is present *resection* of the involved segment of gut is the treatment of choice. Occasionally in a poor-risk patient an ileocolostomy allows improvement of health. A resection can then be carried out a few months later.

TUMOURS OF THE SMALL INTESTINE

BENIGN TUMOURS

Adenoma, lipoma or leiomyoma are rare. They may produce intussusception. The first-named may also produce melaena.

Peutz-Jegher's syndrome consists of:

1. Familial intestinal polyposis of the jejunum, causing melaena or intussusception,
2. Melanosis of the oral mucosa and lips.

MALIGNANT TUMOURS

Carcinoid tumours. These occur in the gastrointestinal tract and also in the bronchus, testis and ovary. The appendix and the ileum are the most common sites. Carcinoids are seen in about 0.5% of appendicectomy specimens. The tumour produces 5-hydroxytryptamine, which is responsible for various symptoms, including the following:

1. Reddish blue cyanosis and flushing attacks of the face.
2. Loud peristaltic sounds with bouts of diarrhoea.
3. Asthmatic attacks and ultimately pulmonary and tricuspid stenosis.

The tumour, specially if it has arisen from the ileum, may metastasize to the liver.

Treatment. As carcinoids are tumours which metastasize, a *radical operation* e.g. right hemicolectomy should be performed.

If metastases have occurred to the liver:

1. Considerable palliation can be obtained by reduction of the tumour burden by either *surgical extirpation* or *hepatic arterial embolization*. In the latter procedure, a Seldinger catheter is passed up percutaneously from the femoral artery until its tip lies in the origin of the hepatic artery. The arteries supplying the metastases are blocked by injecting bits of gelatin sponge.

26 Appendix

Anatomy. The vermiform appendix is inconstant in position, the common positions being the retrocaecal (74%) and pelvic (21%). The other positions are paracaecal, subcaecal, preileal and postileal (Fig. 1). *Mc Burney's point* lies at the junction of the lateral with the middle third of a line joining the anterior superior iliac spine and the umbilicus. The grid-iron incision in appendicectomy is commonly centred around it. The appendix is usually looked for by following one of the taeniae coli downwards on the caecum until the appendix is reached.

ACUTE APPENDICITIS

Aetiology. Appendicitis is more common in the developed countries. It is thought that this is due to the change from a traditional diet rich in bulky cellulose to one rich in meat and fats, so that constipation is common, with its resulting stagnation of large bowel contents. Quite often the actual precipitating cause is a faecolith, which consists of inspissated faecal material. The infection in the appendix is usually a mixed one, the most common organisms being *Esch. coli* (85%), enterococci, and streptococci. Anaerobic organisms, specially Bacteroides often play an important role in the infection.

Pathology. Appendicitis may be non-obstructive or obstructive. In the *non-obstructive type* the inflammation varies from quite mild to really severe forms. In the mild form the appendix looks virtually normal from outside, but on being slit open the mucosa is unmistakably inflamed; it is purple in colour, with blood, blood clot, and sometimes pus in the lumen. *Specially in the milder cases the appendix should be split open* to confirm or exclude the presence of inflammation. In the *obstructive* type of appendicitis the products of inflammation become pent up. Therefore inflammation proceeds more rapidly to gangrene and perforation, adhesions have no time to develop, and generalized peritonitis often results.

Clinical features. Rare before the age of two, acute appendicitis is common during childhood, adolescence and adult life, being less common in advanced age. More than half the patients give a history of previous, though usually milder, attacks. Usually the first symptom is *pain*, which may be umbilical, epigastric or generalized. This pain is mediated through the visceral nerves. It is colicky in obstructive cases, but constant in the non-obstructive type. After a few hours it shifts to the right iliac fossa, where the inflamed appendix irritates the parietal peritoneum. This latter pain is mediated through the somatic nerves, and is therefore accurately localized and constant. In a few cases the pain is located in the right iliac fossa from the start. In *obstructive appendicitis* the symptoms are more severe, and their onset more sudden. There may be generalized abdominal colic with vomiting. Pylorospasm occurs and may cause *anorexia, nausea, vomiting, a furred tongue* and a foul breath. The *temperature and pulse* usually remain unaltered during the first few hours after the onset of the attack. Later, they are both raised slightly, or in severe cases moderately.

Tenderness occurs at McBurney's point or elsewhere according to the site of the appendix. In the case of a pelvic appendix the tenderness may be confined to the pelvis, so *rectal examination should be carried out in every case of lower abdominal pain.* A high retrocaecal appendix may cause pain and tenderness in the right flank and loin. If after deep palpation in the right iliac fossa the pressure is suddenly released by lifting the hand, pain may be felt. This is called *rebound tenderness* and is elicited in cases where the parietal peritoneum is irritated by an inflamed appendix.

With a retrocaecal or pelvic appendix it may be difficult to elicit the signs of peritoneal irritation. If the inflamed appendix is lying over the psoas there may be spasm of this muscle, so that extension of the right hip causes pain *(Psoas test)*. Similarly, if a pelvic appendix is lying over the obturator internus muscle, pain may be produced when the right hip is flexed and internally rotated *(Obturator test)*. If a pelvic appendix is lying over the bladder there may be dysuria. Similarly, an appendix lying over and irritating the rectum may result in *diarrhoea* with mucus and tenesmus. Diarrhoea is also seen in cases where the appendix is lying behind the terminal ileum and irritating it (post-ileal appendix).

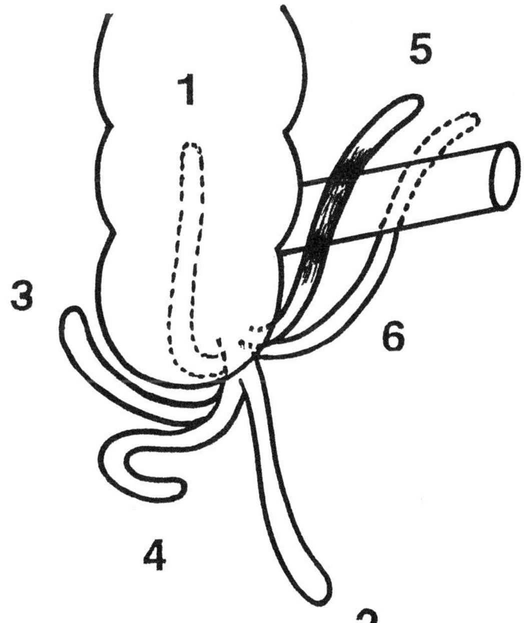

Fig. 1 Positions of appendix. 1. Retrocaecal, 2. Pelvic, 3. Paracaecal, 4. Subcaecal, 5. Preileal, 6. Postileal.

In elderly patients the diagnosis of appendicitis may be missed. There are two reasons for this: firstly, as the condition is uncommon at this age, it may not be suspected. Secondly, as the abdominal wall is lax, rigidity may not be present even though the appendix is gangrenous. In *obese* patients the signs of an inflamed appendix may be masked. If serious doubt exists operation should be carried out.

Appendicitis in pregnancy. The treatment of appendicitis at any stage of pregnancy is apendicectomy. However, the following points may be mentioned in this connection: during the first 6 months of pregnancy symptoms of appendicitis do not differ from those in the non-pregnant woman. During the third trimester the enlarged uterus displaces the appendix, so that it lies at a higher position, and this fact should be kept in mind. At the same time the abdominal wall is lifted from the appendix by the gravid uterus; the signs of peritoneal irritation may therefore be minimal. Also, leucocytosis is a normal response to pregnancy and cannot be relied upon to help confirm the diagnosis. If appendicectomy is carried out before the appendix perforates, upto 30% of cases could proceed to premature labour. If it has already perforated this figure rises as high as 50%. Therefore, if acute appendicitis develops during pregnancy it should be diagnosed and treated promptly.

Differential diagnosis. The conditions from which acute appendicitis commonly requires to be distinguished include the following:

Acute cholecystitis. If the appendix is highly placed it may be confused with acute cholecystitis. However, in the latter condition the pain commonly radiates to the inferior angle of the scapula, and to the right shoulder.

Perforated peptic ulcer. In this condition pain starts in the epigastrium and quickly spreads to the right iliac fossa, because the irritating stomach contents spill over into the right paracolic gutter. However, here the pain is diffuse, with board-like rigidity.

Enterocolitis. In dysentery there may occasionally be pain in the right iliac fossa. However, diarrhoea is the most important feature of dysenteries, whereas it is normally absent in cases of appendicitis.

Non-specific mesenteric lymphadenitis. This condition is supposed to be responsible for pain in children in those cases where operation is carried out but a normal appendix is found, and mesenteric lymph nodes are seen to be enlarged. It is difficult to be certain whether such an entity actually exists.

Ectopic gestation. A ruptured ectopic gestation is associated with signs of severe internal haemorrhage, and is unlikely to be mistaken for appendicitis. However, unruptured tubal pregnancy may cause pain in the right iliac fossa. *Thus if the patient is a female in the childbearing period, the menstrual history must always be enquired into.* In cases of ectopic gestation usually only one period has been missed.

Ruptured ovarian follicle. When an ovarian follicle in the right ovary ruptures, it may produce pain in the right iliac fossa. This always comes on in the middle of the menstrual period. Occasionally, when operation is carried out the appendix is seen to be normal and a ruptured follicle is found, having caused diagnostic confusion.

Salpingitis. In this condition the pain is usually bilateral; in cases of doubt an ultrasound examination can show up the distended fallopian tubes.

Intestinal obstruction. Here the pain usually remains around the umbilicus. Bowel sounds are loud and plain x-ray in the erect posture shows many fluid levels.

Right ureteric colic. In this condition pain often radiates down to the groin. Coughing does not cause pain. Microscopy of the urine reveals red blood cells. Ultrasound examination or plain x-ray may show a stone in the line of the ureter.

'Diabetic abdomen'. In diabetic ketosis severe abdominal pain and vomiting sometimes come on before coma sets in, and cause confusion. The urine should therefore be tested in every acute abdominal emergency.

Right-sided pneumonia or pleurisy. The lower part of the chest wall is supplied by the 7th to the 12th thoracic nerves. These nerves then proceed onwards to supply the abdominal wall. Therefore in basal pneumonia or pleurisy pain is sometimes felt in the abdomen. However, in pleurisy the respiratory rate is increased, inspiration causes severe pain, a pleural rub may be heard, and a chest x-ray may show up the effusion or consolidation.

A word of caution. When a clinician receives a patient suffering from an acute abdominal condition about whom a diagnosis of acute appendicitis, ureteric colic, or other acute condition has been made by someone else, he should consider the patient as suffering from an 'acute abdomen' until his own interrogation and investigation reveals the exact diagnosis. He should not rely on a diagnosis made elsewhere, because having undertaken the patient's treatment he is personally responsible for the accuracy of the diagnosis and the correctness of the management. *In fact this rule should be followed throughout one's clinical practice*; otherwise one will be treating patients on the basis of diagnoses made by other people, which may or may not be correct.

The appendix mass. If a severely inflamed appendix remains untreated for a few days the oedematous omentum and intestines adhere to the appendix and result in the formation of an inflammatory mass, the appendix mass. The presence of the mass indicates that the infection has become walled off and that generalized peritonitis is unlikely to supervene. If left alone an appendix mass can follow one of two courses: it can enlarge and become an appendix abscess, or it can become smaller and subside slowly as the inflammation resolves.

Appendix abscess. If an appendix perforates but the infection remains confined to the right iliac fossa, an appendix abscess may result. If the pus is under tension there may be a swinging temperature. If the pus is 'pointing' through the abdominal wall, there may be overlying oedema, with induration and greatly increased tenderness. A marked polymorphonuclear leucocytosis is the rule.

Diagnosis. Appendicitis is most reliably diagnosed by a carefully taken history and by physical examination to elicit tenderness. Leucocytosis is common, but occurs once the condition is well established, and the illness should generally be diagnosed before it develops. Plain x-rays are so non-specific as to be of no value, and a barium enema would be wholly meddlesome, apart from being useless. Similarly, ultrasound and CT examinations have very limited value in appendicitis, although they are useful in the diagnosis of appendix abscess. *In short, physical signs are the mainstay of diagnosis, and the above-mentioned imaging methods have created avoidable confusion in the minds of clinicians.* Even in very straightforward cases of appendicitis precious time is sometimes wasted while awaiting the results of these quite unnecessary tests.

TREATMENT OF ACUTE APPENDICITIS

The treatment of acute appendicitis is appendicectomy. If the case is seen before a mass has formed, there is universal agreement that the appendix should be removed urgently.

Appendicectomy. If the diagnosis is certain, it is best to use a grid-iron incision for this operation. If doubt exists the midline incision is to be preferred; in the female it can be extended downward to deal with pelvic pathology, in either sex it can be extended upwards to deal with a perforated peptic ulcer. In the *grid-iron* incision each of the three muscles of the anterolateral abdominal wall are split along the line of their fibres. Therefore in theory the overlying skin incision can be made in any direction. It is best placed parallel to the skin creases in this region, when it results in a more inconspicuous scar.

After the peritoneum has been opened the caecum is withdrawn and the appendix hooked out by the finger and held in a Babcock forceps. If any difficulty is encountered, the taenia coli on the caecum are traced downwards, and will lead the operator to the base of the appendix. The mesoappendix is clamped in an artery forceps, divided and ligated. The base of the appendix is crushed in a haemostat, which is removed and reapplied a little distal to the crushed portion. A chromic catgut or polyglactin ligature is tied round the crushed portion near the caecum. A purse-string suture is applied to the caecum around the appendix base. The appendix is amputated with a knife, and the lumen of the appendix stump cleaned out with a small swab on a holder. The stump is invaginated and the purse-string suture tied, burying the appendix stump. The peritoneum and abdominal wall muscles are repaired in layers with unabsorbable sutures, usually employing chromic catgut for the peritoneum and polyglactin for the muscles. The skin is sutured using fine polypropylene or silk. In an occasional case, if there is much pus in the peritoneal cavity, a drain may be placed through a separate stab incision. This ensures that the main wound heals undisturbed.

The bacterial flora in the appendix are the same as in the colon. The use of *antibiotics* effective against both aerobic and anaerobic organisms therefore reduces the incidence of postoperative wound infection. In early acute appendicitis without pus and gangrene, a short course consisting of the first dose before operation followed by 24 to 48 hours of antibiotics should suffice. In perforated appendicitis 7 to 10 days of antibiotic therapy is advisable. Effective regimens include cefoxitin alone, ampicillin-sublactam, an aminoglycoside with metronidazole, and imipenem.

If the diagnosis is in doubt, it is best to admit the patient overnight for observation. During this period it should be possible to determine whether exploration for appendicitis should be carried out or the patient discharged. If the diagnosis is still doubtful, laparoscopy may very occasionally be indicated to help determine the cause of the illness.

The treatment of an appendix mass. If an appendix mass has already formed before the patient presents, the treatment is normally conservative. This is because an attempt at appendicectomy at this time would require separation of the adhesions; this could result in perforation of the intestine and lead to the formation of an intestinal fistula. Besides, it may be impossible to find the appendix in the inflammatory mass. The patient is placed on an *Oschner Sherren regimen.* Antibiotics are started parenterally in full doses. For example, ampicillin may be given for the Gram-positive organisms, gentamicin for the Gram-negative, and metronidazole for the anaerobes. Fluids are given intravenously, though plain water may be allowed by mouth. The pulse, temperature, degree of tenderness and rigidity, and size of the mass are recorded every few hours. Normally the symptoms and signs abate in a day or two, and the inflammation subsides over a few weeks. 'Interval appendicectomy' is then carried out after two or three months. However, if the abdominal pain spreads widely, vomiting becomes copious and chocolate-coloured, the pulse rate continues to rise, and the size of the mass increases, operation has to be carried out. The causes of failure of conservative treatment of an appendix mass include abscess formation and small bowel obstruction from adhesions.

The treatment of an appendix abscess. If in a case of appendix mass the temperature continues to swing, the pulse rate remains high and the swelling becomes larger and more tender it means that an abscess has formed, and incision-drainage should be carried out. During this operation no effort should be made to remove the appendix unless it is lying free in the abscess cavity. If a CT scan shows the abscess to be lying immediately deep to the abdominal wall, CT-guided catheter drainage can be carried out. After successful drainage of an appendix abscess appendicectomy must be carried out after 3 or 4 months, as otherwise the patient will remain prone to further attacks of appendicitis.

CARCINOID TUMOUR OF THE APPENDIX

This tumour arises in the Kulchitsky cells of the crypts of Lieberkuhn. These cells have a special affinity for silver stains, therefore they are called argentaffin tissues (L. argentum = silver), and the tumour is called an argentaffinoma. It can arise anywhere in the gastrointestinal tract; however, the most common site is the appendix, followed by the small intestine. The tumour is found once in about 200 appendices submitted for histology. Most patients are female. Most carcinoid tumours of the appendix are found incidentally at the time of appendicectomy, usually at the tip of the organ. The muscular coat of the appendix is often involved, but more distant metastases are quite rare. Appendicectomy is curative, unless the tumour arises from the base of the appendix, in which case right hemicolectomy is the operation of choice. A carcinoid syndrome has never been reported following such a tumour of the appendix.

Adenocarcinoma is a rare tumour of the appendix. It presents as acute appendicitis or intestinal obstruction, and is best treated by right hemicolectomy.

27 Colon and rectum

Absorption of foodstuffs takes place mainly in the small gut; the colon is primarily a receptacle and conduit for the products of digestion. However, sodium and chloride are absorbed in the colon, and potassium, bicarbonate and mucus are secreted. Certain carbohydrates and proteins are also digested, and an environment provided for the production of vitamin K by bacteria. Water is absorbed along the whole length of the colon. The fibrous residue is thus rendered firm and dry for easier disposal, and is stored in the descending and sigmoid colon before being expelled at the time of defaecation.

MEGACOLON

Megacolon is defined as an abnormally large or dilated colon. It may be primary or secondary.

PRIMARY MEGACOLON — HIRSCHSPRUNG'S DISEASE

In this condition there is delay in passing meconium after birth, followed by severe constipation. This is due to complete absence of parasympathetic ganglion cells in the wall of the rectum and sigmoid colon, which arises as follows: the ganglion cells of the bowel migrate from the neural crest along the vagus nerves within the bowel wall to reach the anus by birth. If this migration fails to reach the anus, the result will be a segment of bowel without ganglion cells. This segment extends upwards from the anus for a varying distance. The segment of bowel without proper innervation by the autonomous nervous system cannot conduct a peristaltic wave and acts as a physiological obstruction to the onward passage of bowel contents. The more proximal colon becomes greatly dilated and hypertrophied. The mucosa of the dilated intestine is chronically inflamed due to the stagnant contents, and often ulcerated. The aganglionic bowel contracts down to a small size. This is the *narrow segment* seen on barium enema.

Clinical features. The condition is much more common in males, with a familial tendency. Symptoms always appear within a few days of birth. The baby fails to pass meconium during the first two or three days of life. He suffers from severe constipation, and passes meconium only after the passage of a finger into the rectum. The infant strains to bring out toothpaste-like stools in small amounts. Abdominal distension appears within the first few days of life, with loud borborygmi and visible peristalsis. The rectum is empty and grips the examining finger. Complete intestinal obstruction may occur. The baby fails to thrive, with malnutrition and stunted growth. *Severe constipation in the newborn is a very serious condition, and could be due to Hirschsprung's disease.* If this fact is overlooked the consequences can be grave.

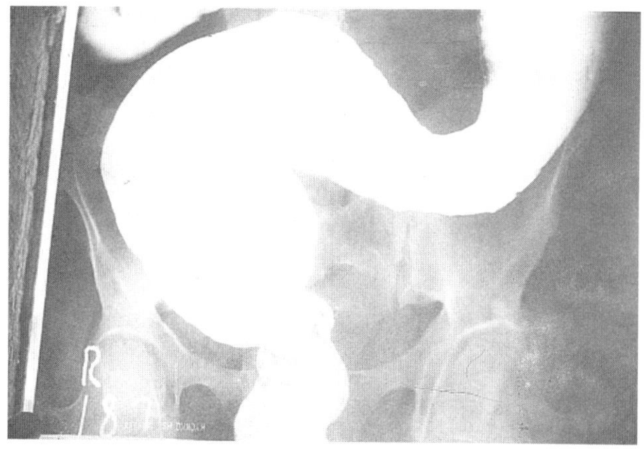

Fig. 1 Hirschsprung's disease in an adolescent. Contracted aganglionic rectum and dilated colon are clearly seen. The patient suffered from severe constipation since birth.

Investigations. *Gastrografin enema.* X-ray of the abdomen and pelvis is taken after giving an enema of barium or Gastrografin solution. A lateral view of the pelvis is also taken, as it shows the rectum better. The enema shows the dilated colon and the contracted aganglionic segment of the rectum (Fig. 1).

Rectal suction biopsy. If Hirschsprung's disease is suspected on the basis of the contrast enema, a rectal suction biopsy should be performed. This can be carried out without anaesthesia as an outpatient procedure. The cylindrical suction biopsy instrument (Fig. 2) is passed into the rectum. When suction is applied a small piece of mucosa of the rectum is sucked into the lumen through a side opening. The built-in blade is now advanced forwards. This cuts off the mucosa, which is sucked into the bottle attached to the biopsy instrument. As serious bleeding can occasionally occur, the infant should be kept in hospital for a few hours after the procedure. Only mucosa and submucosa can be obtained by this method. The tissue is examined microscopically after paraffin section and staining. If ganglion cells are present this means that the bowel wall is normal and Hirschsprung's disease is not present. If on the other hand, ganglion cells are absent and there is hypertrophy of the nerve fibres, the case could be one of Hirschsprung's disease. Recently, some surgeons have started using *punch biopsy* forceps to obtain rectal biopsies under local anaesthesia.

However, a firm diagnosis cannot be made on the basis of suction biopsy alone. For this purpose:

1. A *full-thickness rectal biopsy* has to be carried out under general anaesthesia, in order to prove that ganglion cells are absent from the muscle layers also.

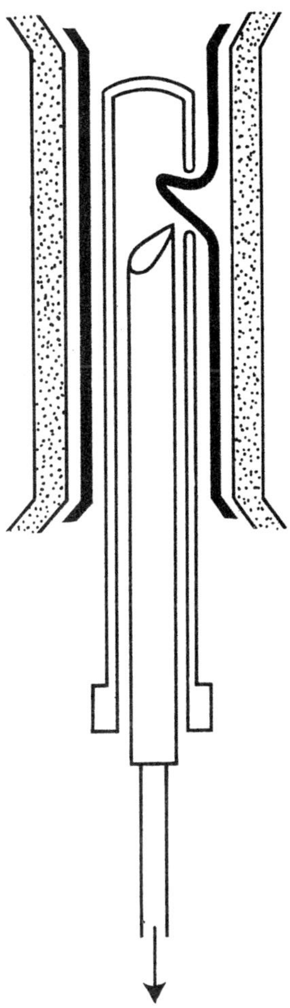

Fig. 2 Rectal suction biopsy instrument.

2. The tissue is examined *histochemically* for the presence of increased acetylcholine esterase activity.

3. In normal persons if the rectum is distended the internal sphincter is reflexly inhibited. In Hirschsprung's disease this inhibition does not occur, and this can be demonstrated by *anorectal manometry*.

Treatment. Although the severe constipation of Hirschsprung's disease can be temporarily tided over by repeated enemas, the only curative treatment is excision of the non-functioning aganglionic segment which acts as a peristaltic block. In the newborn, a loop colostomy is carried out just above the cone area to relieve the obstruction.

When laparotomy is carried out for resecting the aganglionic area, the only way in which the upward extent of the aganglionic segment can be determined with certainty is by frozen-section examination of biopsies taken at different levels, which should be carried out. When the upper limit of resection has been decided upon, the further operative procedure can take one of three forms:

1. In the *Swenson operation* the entire aganglionic segment of large bowel is removed, and the normal ganglionic colon anastomosed to the anal canal.

2. In the *Duhamel procedure* the lower part of the rectum is preserved. The ganglionic colon is brought down behind the rectum and out through the internal sphincter. To the adjoining walls of the colon and rectum is applied a specially designed stapler, which crushes, staples and divides them to produce a single cavity. The posterior part of this tube consists of ganglionic colon, providing propulsive activity. The anterior part is rectum which, although it is aganglionic, provides the rectal sensation of fullness.

In both the above operations the nervi erigentes are in danger of damage leading to impotence; this is prevented by staying close to the colonic wall during the pelvic dissection.

3. During the 1980's *Soave's operation* had become the most popular procedure. In this operation the muscular tube of the rectum is left in place, while its mucosal layer is excised. The normal colon is passed down through the rectal muscular sleeve, and sutured to mucosa at the anorectal junction. Any possibility of damage to the nervi erigentes is thus eliminated by dissecting inside rather than outside the rectum. The Soave operation is best carried out in early infancy, when it can be performed without a covering colostomy. The other two operations normally require a preliminary colostomy. Recently, the Soave operation has gone out of favour because the rectal muscle sleeve often contracts around the pulled-through colon to produce a severe stricture of the new rectum. Its place is again being taken by the Duhamel procedure. If Hirschsprung's disease is treated promptly and by correct surgery, the prognosis is excellent. If it remains undiagnosed the infant gets severely malnourished, or dies of enterocolitis.

SECONDARY (ACQUIRED) MEGACOLON

Acquired megacolon usually results from faulty bowel care and training. Symptoms can be traced from infancy, but never from birth. In this way it differs from Hirschsprung's disease. In contrast to the situation in Hirschsprung's disease, the rectum and sigmoid are also dilated, and barium enema shows no contracted rectal segment. Similarly, rectal biopsy shows normal ganglion cells, i.e. the rectum is developmentally normal.

If the bowel wall is normal, what then is the cause of acquired megacolon? Inadequate toilet training in infancy and emotional deprivation are probably responsible. Both these factors are often present in orphans, and in children from broken homes. As the infant is not made to pass stools at the normal times, he does not develop a regular bowel habit. The stools accumulate in his bowels and lead to their chronic dilatation. An important cause of an emotional disorder is seen when another child is born into the family, the family moves to a new town or a different house, or the child is shifted to a new school. When the history is being taken this aspect should be carefully enquired into.

Treatment. Treatment consists of emptying the greatly dilated colon of its contents by repeated enemas or, if that is not feasible, by manual evacuation under anaesthesia. This should be followed by careful toilet training, along with as much emotional support and encouragement as possible.

DIVERTICULAR DISEASE OF THE COLON

This condition is relatively uncommon in the East, possibly because the diet contains natural fibre which has been removed from the food consumed in the more advanced countries. It is commonly seen in middle and old age. The diverticula protrude outwards through the circular muscle coat at the point where blood vessels penetrate the colonic wall. In the vast majority of cases the sigmoid colon is involved. 5% of the patients have associated gallstones and hiatus hernia.

Diverticulosis is probably caused by muscular incoordination and hypertrophy resulting in increased intraluminal pressure. Diverticulitis involves inflammation of one or more diverticula due to stagnation of their contents. These episodes may occur at varying intervals, but symptoms usually get worse with the passage of time. Diverticulitis is not precancerous, but cancer can coexist with it.

Clinical features. *Diverticulosis* may be symptomless, or there may be distension and heaviness in the lower abdomen, with pain off and on. *Diverticulitis* causes more persistent pain. Fever, malaise and leucocytosis may be present. There may be diarrhoea or constipation. The left iliac fossa is tender, and the sigmoid colon may be thickened with overlying fibro-fatty tissue. Diverticular disease occurs predominantly in the elderly who often have associated diseases that complicate diagnosis and influence treatment. Diverticulitis has to be distinguished from carcinoma. As compared to carcinoma, in diverticulitis the history is longer and pain and bleeding more common.

Complications. The complications to which sigmoid diverticula are prone include the following:

1. Recurrent inflammation.
2. Perforation with generalized or localized peritonitis and septic shock.
3. Intestinal obstruction from progressive fibrosis.
4. Haemorrhage.
5. Fistula formation with bladder, vagina, small bowel or skin.
6. Intractable disturbance of bowel function (distension, cramps, diarrhoea, or constipation) and persistent pain, occasionally requiring surgical treatment even in the absence of the more defined complications listed above.

Investigations. Often, diverticulosis of the sigmoid colon is present without causing any symptoms. Therefore, symptoms should be ascribed to diverticulosis only if other causes have been excluded by colonoscopy and barium enema. The latter confirms the presence of diverticula, provides evidence for or against the diagnosis of diverticulitis, and helps exclude the presence of carcinoma. In diverticular disease the length of the affected segment is greater, the mucosa is intact, spasm is often present and the ends of the narrowed segment are tapering rather than blunt. In diverticulitis barium enema should be carried out only when the inflammation has subsided, in order to avoid perforation. The diagnosis can be confirmed by colonoscopy.

Treatment. *Diverticulosis* should be managed with a high residue diet. When the large gut is well filled with abundant residue it functions better, and the mild symptoms of diverticulosis disappear. If necessary, supplementary bulk may be added by about 20 g of wheat bran daily. The stool may be softened and moisturized by powdered psyllium seed husks (5–10 g daily). Drugs that inhibit peristalsis (such as propantheline bromide 7.5 mg thrice daily) may give symptomatic relief.

Diverticulitis requires bed rest, fomentation, antispasmodic drugs and a week-long course of broad spectrum antibiotics, usually a cephalosporin and metronidazole. Only a few patients require resection of the sigmoid colon. If obstruction is present, the faeces are first diverted by a transverse colostomy. This gives rest to the sigmoid and allows the inflammation to subside. After a few weeks resection is carried out, and after another few weeks the colostomy is closed.

INTESTINAL AMOEBIASIS

Amoebiasis is defined as infestation with *Entamoeba histolytica* with or without overt clinical symptoms. In countries where the condition is endemic there are innumerable carriers of the disease, because the vast majority of infestations are asymptomatic. The disease is contracted by consuming food or drinks contaminated with the cysts of the parasite. The active form of the amoeba lives in the mucous membrane of the large intestine, where it ingests red blood cells. If it becomes pathogenic it invades the submucosa and produces ulcers with undermined edges and a necrotic floor. These ulcers are usually confined to the rectum and sigmoid colon. Some of the amoebae migrate to the surface, become transformed into cysts and pass out with the faeces. The most common symptom is dysentery, with or without blood and mucus.

Diagnosis. The stool should be examined for amoebae. At the same time the suspected area of rectal mucosa may be scraped and the tissue examined immediately for the presence of amoebae.

Treatment. Metronidazole is the drug of choice for amoebiasis. Asymptomatic intestinal amoebiasis can be treated by diloxanide furoate 500 mg orally thrice daily for 10 days, or di-iodohydroxyquinoline 600 mg thrice daily for 21 days. Attacks of acute amoebic dysentery are treated by metronidazole 400 mg orally thrice daily for 5 days. An alternative regimen consists of emetine hydrochloride 1 mg/kg intramuscularly in two divided doses daily for 4 to 10 days. This drug should not be used in cases of cardiac disease, and the patient should be confined to bed.

Surgical complications. From time to time a case of intestinal amoebiasis may present with one of the following complications:

1. *Typhlitis* (i.e. inflammation of the caecum). This may be mistaken for appendicitis.
2. *Perforation of the colon with peritonitis.* The wall of the colon becomes a white slough and multiple perforations result. The commonly affected sites are the caecum and the ascending and sigmoid colon. The condition has a very high mortality rate. Three types of perforation occur: extraperitoneal; perforation of a granuloma or ulcer without acute dysentery; and perforation in a case of fulminant disease.

Anti-amoebic therapy is commenced. If the patient's condition deteriorates and rupture appears imminent, an ileocolostomy may be carried out to divert the faecal stream. However, if perforation is associated with gangrene, resection is the best course of treatment.

3. *Granuloma or 'amoeboma'*, i.e. a mass of amoebic granulation tissue. This may need to be distinguished from

an appendix mass, a neoplasm, ileocaecal tuberculosis and an actinomycotic granuloma.

4. *Fulminant amoebic colitis.* This type of colitis is seen in malnourished individuals and in patients with co-incident debilitating disorders, also in patients on steroids and other immunosuppressive therapy. If the patient's condition deteriorates in spite of medical therapy (with severe diarrhoea, toxicity and abdominal tenderness) with x-ray evidence of toxic colonic dilatation, or the onset of an acute episode of perforation or bleeding, surgical treatment is indicated. The best operative treatment is primary resection with exteriorization of the bowel ends. In the past the mortality rate was nearly 100%; this has been reduced to about 50% with improved medical treatment and early and aggressive surgery.

5. *Massive haemorrhage* from erosion of a large vessel in the bowel wall; this complication is quite rare.

6. *Amoebiasis of the skin.* If an amoebic abscess is treated by open drainage the amoeba may colonize the drainage tract, and can be quite difficult to eradicate even with intensive anti-amoebic therapy. In fact, even if the abscess is treated with closed drainage by aspiration, the needle track may not heal because of amoebiasis cutis.

7. *Amoebic liver abscess* is described in Chapter 21.

ULCERATIVE COLITIS

Ulcerative colitis is a condition in which the mucosa and submucosa of the colon are the seat of chronic inflammation, with the formation of large numbers of ulcers over wide areas of the mucosa. The cause of this condition is not known. It may be related to the autoimmune diseases but this is not certain. There is some evidence that the patient may be prone to allergic reactions in the gastrointestinal tract. At the same time, in the mucous membrane there is a deficiency of type IV mucin and hydrolase, both of which have a protective function. Therefore the mucosa becomes more susceptible to injury by intraluminal irritants. When ulcers develop, secondary infection plays a large part in the disease process.

Pathology. In early cases haemorrhagic inflammation is seen, with petechial haemorrhages and bleeding. In more advanced disease, small ulcers form all over the mucosa of the colon and later join up to form larger ones. When they extend into the submucosa they cause reflex muscle spasm, and the false appearance of a stricture. When fibrosis occurs during the process of healing, the epithelium gets piled up between the ulcers, producing the so-called pseudopolyps, and also permanently shortening the affected part of the colon. When remission takes place, the normal structure of the mucosa may be restored, but some atrophy of the mucosa is often seen. In the long term certain areas in the mucosa become dysplastic; this is an important change, as it predisposes to the development of carcinoma of the colon.

Clinical features. Ulcerative colitis is a disease of adult life, women being affected more often than men. The first symptom is watery diarrhoea occurring day and night. Mucus with pus or blood is very common. The symptoms come and go.

The disease is defined as *mild* if fewer than 4 motions are passed daily, and there are no systemic symptoms or signs. This is the most common form of the disease, and the inflammation is usually confined to the rectum and sigmoid. The long-term prognosis is good, the patients rarely requiring admission to hospital, and the life expectancy is not affected by the disease.

If between 4 and 6 stools are passed daily, the disease is defined as *moderate*. The stools invariably contain blood. Abdominal pain, low grade fever, and iron-deficiency anaemia are in evidence, with loss of appetite and weight. The disease responds well to corticosteroids, but the long-term prognosis is not good, and rapid deterioration with the development of local complications e.g. toxic megacolon, massive bleeding and colonic perforation may occur at any time.

Severe ulcerative colitis is responsible for most of the deaths from the disease. The diarrhoea is accompanied by tenesmus and rectal bleeding, with severe dehydration, electrolyte depletion, acidosis and anaemia.

A *fulminant* type of disease also occurs. In this type there is fairly high temperature, continuous diarrhoea with blood, mucus and pus, and a toxic appearance. Toxic paralysis of the colon may produce abdominal distension (*toxic megacolon*). This condition must be distinguished from dysentery and typhoid by examination of the stool and by blood culture or Widal test.

The *chronic* type of disease is much more common. The initial attack is moderately severe, but exacerbations occur at variable intervals. The patient is wasted and anaemic. The greater the area of colon affected the more frequent the motions, and the greater the degree of ill-health due to protein loss and the toxaemia of bacterial infection. When the whole colon is involved the patient may be bedridden, due to the combined effects of malnutrition, electrolyte depletion and toxaemia. A bad prognosis is indicated in the following situations:

1. If the initial attack is severe.
2. If the disease involves the entire colon.
3. If the age is above sixty.

Investigations. The earliest *x-ray* sign is loss of haustrations in the distal colon. Later changes include a narrow contracted colon, ulcers with undermined edges, and pseudopolyposis. In long-standing cases the acute angles of the hepatic and splenic flexures are lost, resulting in a rounded course for the colon due to its shorter length. On *sigmoidoscopy* and *colonoscopy,* at first the mucosa is hyperaemic and bleeds on touch, and there is a good deal of exudate. Later, tiny ulcers form and may join up. In amoebic dysentery, on the other hand, there are large deep ulcers with fairly healthy mucosa in between. *Rectal biopsy* establishes the diagnosis and shows the effects of treatment.

Complications. ***Systemic.*** These are common to both ulcerative colitis and Crohn's disease. They include liver changes e.g. cirrhosis, skin lesions e.g. pyoderma gangrenosum, arthritis, and anaemia.

Local. *Carcinoma.* If the patient has suffered from ulcerative colitis for 10 years the risk of carcinoma developing is 1%; if for 10 to 20 years, then as high as 5%. Therefore, if the disease has been present for over ten years, regular colonoscopy should be carried out. Cancer in cases of ulcerative colitis occurs at a younger age than in non-colitic patients. The tumours tend to be less well differentiated and are more often multiple.

Dysplasia is now regarded as indicative of neoplastic change. However, dysplasia has to be differentiated from regenerative changes in the epithelium. For this purpose, several 'mucosal markers' have been developed to detect dysplasia, for example enzyme activity (G6-PDH), and antigen expression by the epithelial cells, like carcino-embryonic antigen. If moderate to severe dysplasia is present, prophylactic proctocolectomy is advised because of the risk of malignant change.

Other local complications include massive haemorrhage, toxic megacolon, perforation, perianal suppuration, fibrous stricture and haemorrhoids.

In *toxic megacolon* the inflammation spreads to all coats of the colonic wall, with gross distension and resultant thinning of the bowel wall. The patient's general condition deteriorates, with absent bowel sounds due to paralytic ileus, severe toxicity, fever, tachycardia, and fluid and electrolyte depletion leading to hypovolaemia. The risk of perforation is very high; therefore, most cases are treated by emergency colectomy after resuscitation. Toxic megacolon is sometimes also seen in Crohn's disease and in the pseudomembranous colitis which occasionally follows antibiotic therapy.

Treatment. Mild and moderate cases of ulcerative colitis often respond to medical treatment; severe cases usually require surgery.

Medical treatment. The type of measures required depend on the severity of the disease.

Mild disease. These patients require sulphasalazine in a daily dose of 3–4 g, along with steroid enemas containing 20 mg of prednisolone-21-phosphate. Some add low-dose oral prednisolone (20 mg/day). For *maintaining a remission* low-dose steroid therapy is ineffective, and sulphasalazine is the most effective agent in a dose of 2 g daily; in fact this is the most important indication for the use of this drug. Its side effects include headache, vomiting, diarrhoea, skin rashes, male infertility, and haemolytic and aplastic anaemia.

Moderate disease. Here, suphasalazine and steroid enemas should be accompanied by 40 mg daily of oral prednisolone. If a remission is not achieved within two weeks, the patient should be hospitalized and treated as a case of severe disease.

Severe disease. Intensive medical therapy and monitoring should be provided. The fluid and electrolyte losses, the acidosis, and the hypovolaemia are corrected. Blood transfusions and human albumin solutions are often required to restore the haemoglobin level and protein content.

Intravenous prednisolone-21-phosphate is given in a dose of 64 mg/day. Hydrocortisone drip enemas (100 g in 100 ml of water) are administered twice daily. Some add tetracycline and metronidazole to the regimen. Codeine phosphate, belladona etc. are not recommended. Not only are they ineffective, they may also contribute to the development of toxic megacolon by aggravating any paralytic ileus.

Daily clinical and radiological assessment enables the clinician to monitor the progress of the case. Sudden deterioration of the general condition, increasing abdominal girth and absent bowel sounds indicate failure of medical therapy and the need for an emergency colectomy. If improvement is not obvious within a few days, surgery is indicated. The factors suggesting a poor prognosis include a fever higher than 38°C, a pulse rate greater than 100, motions more frequent than 12 per day, and a serum albumin level lower than 30 g/liter. About 70% of patients respond favourably. However, in the long term as many as 50% require proctocolectomy.

Surgical treatment. Surgery may be indicated:

1. As an *elective* measure where medical therapy has failed, or where the colon has to be removed as a prophylactic against the development of cancer, e.g. if dysplasia or villous adenomas are seen during follow-up colonoscopy.
2. As an *urgent* measure in a severe attack if medical therapy has failed to bring about an improvement within 5 days.
3. As an *emergency* measure for toxic megacolon, colonic perforation or massive haemorrhage.

The different operations for ulcerative colitis. The operations commonly performed for ulcerative colitis include the following:

1. ***Total proctocolectomy and ileostomy.*** The ideal operation is removal of the whole colon and rectum in one stage. As the entire large bowel has to be removed, a permanent ileostomy has to be made.

Continent ileostomy. The ordinary ileostomy requires an ileostomy bag to keep the patient dry. If it is desired to avoid wearing one, an ileostomy is required which contains a reservoir to store the intestinal contents and a valve to prevent them from spilling out. A reservoir is made by turning a segment of ileum on itself and joining the limbs by anastomosing them throughout their length. A valve is created by intussuscepting the efferent loop into itself. The result is a 'continent' ileostomy, which can be emptied every few hours by passing a catheter into it. In practice, unfortunately, the pouch encourages bacterial overgrowth and ileitis, and is therefore not very popular.

Ileostomy alone. An ileostomy may occasionally be indicated in a desperately ill patient who is not fit for any longer procedure. If he survives and his condition improves, colectomy is undertaken later.

2. ***Total colectomy with ileorectal anastomosis.*** In a few patients where the rectum is not diseased, the whole colon is removed but the rectum is preserved, with ileorectal anastomosis. After operation the patient passes stools through the normally placed anus. However, because of the absence of the colon the frequency of the stools is greater than normal. The operation has lost a good deal of its popularity since the advent of restorative proctocolectomy.

3. ***Restorative proctocolectomy.*** The whole of the colon and rectum are removed. To replace the rectum a pouch of ileum is formed by folding the ileum on itself and anastomosing the limbs together *(J and S pouches)*, and this is joined to the anal canal (Fig. 3). Not only is the patient spared the need for an ileostomy; the pouch also acts as a reservoir, so that the number of movements of the bowel is reduced, making life more comfortable.

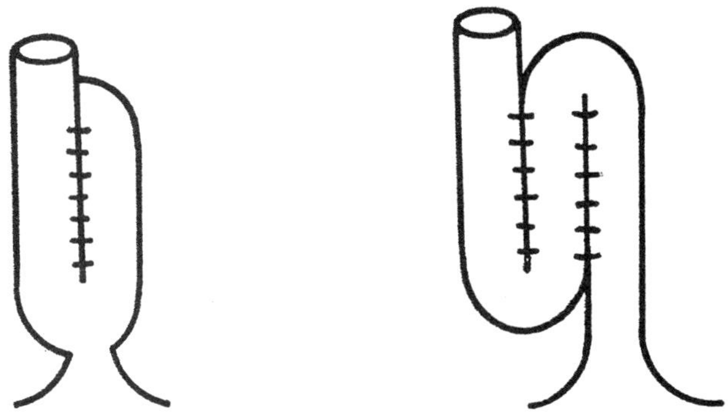

Fig. 3 J and S ileal pouches to increase the capacity of the new 'rectum'.

Care of ileostomy. There are thousands of patients all over the world who are living with permanent ileostomies. If the ileal stoma is made properly and looked after with due care, a fairly reasonable life can be led by the patient. The patient can also benefit by joining one of the *ileostomy associations* in his area. These groups, which are quite active in some countries, provide very useful literature, besides much-needed support in the form of comradeship.

ISCHAEMIC COLITIS

Ischaemic colitis is an inflammatory condition of the mucous membrane of the colon produced by interruption of its blood supply insufficient to cause full thickness tissue death. It commonly affects those in the seventh and eighth decades of life. Its causes include occlusion of a major artery, minor vessel disease, venous obstruction, 'low flow' states and intestinal obstruction. Ischaemia reduces the integrity of the mucosa and allows invasion by pathogenic organisms such as clostridia, which are normal constituents of the colonic flora. Inflammation and ulceration result, which may resolve completely, or may cause permanent injury with healing by fibrosis and stricture formation.

The patient complains of acute pain starting in the left iliac fossa, with loose stools containing dark blood as well as clots. There may be low grade fever. The affected colon is tender and may be palpable. Submucosal oedema and haemorrhage produce swellings that bulge into the bowel lumen and are seen on barium enema as 'thumb printing.' Mucosal ulcers develop.

If a stricture results, it may be difficult to distinguish it from carcinoma. In ischaemic colitis strictures are often long, uniform and smooth. If doubt exists colonoscopic biopsy should be carried out.

Conservative *management* with bed rest, analgesics and intravenous fluids is the mainstay of treatment for those presenting with acute symptoms. In the rare case of stricture a resection and end-to-end anastomosis should be carried out.

RECTAL PROLAPSE

Prolapse of the rectum is a relatively rare condition in which some or all of the layers of the rectum protrude through the anus. The prolapse may be partial or complete.

Partial prolapse. In partial prolapse only the mucous membrane prolapses out, for a distance of not more than 3.5 cm. When it is palpated between finger and thumb it becomes obvious that it consists of no more than a double layer of mucosa. A partial prolapse can be easily distinguished from prolapsed internal piles. Firstly, prolapse forms a continuous ring all round, whereas piles constitute three or more separate masses. Secondly, prolapsed mucous membrane is pink, whereas piles are purple in colour.

Complete prolapse. In complete prolapse the full thickness of the rectal wall comes down. It is more than 3.5 cm in length, and may be as long as 10–15 cm.

Rectal prolapse occurs at the extremes of life; on the one hand in children below the age of 5, on the other in elderly females. In *children* it often follows a bout of diarrhoea, and may disappear spontaneously. Simple bowel training is adequate treatment. Complete prolapse in *adults* may be due to muscular degeneration in the elderly. There is weakness of the pelvic fascia, the muscles of the pelvic floor, and the anal sphincter.

The prolapsed mucous membrane may be oedematous or ulcerated. It secretes mucus, which soils the clothes and causes perianal dermatitis. On examination the sphincter is lax. The majority of cases are incontinent of faeces. They regard themselves as social outcasts, and are ashamed to mention this symptom unless asked.

Treatment. *Partial prolapse* requires submucosal injections of a sclerosing solution e.g. 5% phenol in almond oil, to cause the submucosa to undergo fibrosis and adhere to the underlying muscle layer. Injections are quite adequate treatment for this type of prolapse.

For *complete prolapse* various operations have been devised:

1. The simplest procedure, which is used only in the elderly and poor-risk patient, is the *Thiersch operation.* A circumferential suture of nylon is placed subcutaneously around the anal canal. The anal orifice is left large enough for the faeces to pass, but not enough for the rectum to prolapse. It is effective provided the patient empties the rectum adequately; however, impaction often develops.

2. For good-risk patients many operations have been devised but none is perfect. In the most popular operation the rectum is wrapped in a *polyvinyl alcohol sponge* which is fixed to the front of the sacrum. Alternatively, the redundant sigmoid and upper rectum may be excised in a *rectosigmoidectomy.* The success rate of these repairs is upto 80%.

In children, even complete prolapse can be managed by submucosal injections of phenol in almond oil. However, unlike the injections given for the treatment for piles in adults, these are given under general anaesthesia. Injections are given into each quadrant, a longer needle being used so that the oil can be deposited in the submucosa upto higher levels.

FAECAL IMPACTION

Hard dried stools impacted in the rectum and unable to pass through the anal canal are commonly seen in elderly and debilitated patients. This may be seen after orthopaedic, pelvic or abdominal operations. A painful anal fissure may also inhibit defaecation to the extent that overloading occurs.

The *symptoms* are those of chronic intestinal obstruction. Liquid stool passes around the faecal mass and leaks out in an uncontrolled manner (*spurious diarrhoea*). Faecal masses may be palpable in the abdomen and can be distinguished from other abdominal lumps by the fact that they can be indented. On rectal examination the single large rock-like mass of stool can be felt.

Treatment. Enemas are usually insufficient. A stool softener, like dioctyl in mineral oil solution, can be left in the rectum overnight and may disimpact the faeces. If it does not, the anal sphincter must be stretched under general anaesthesia and the mass removed manually. Enemas are then given for a few days to allow any remaining hard stools to be expelled. After the evacuation, advice is given about diet. Foods containing roughage, e.g. salads, vegetables and fruits should be taken in abundant quantities. Their bulk provides the most effective stimulus to peristalsis, so that the gut empties efficiently.

RADIATION PROCTITIS

Exposure to radium, ^{60}Co or x-rays during treatment of carcinoma of the cervix, uterus or bladder may cause inflammation in the adjacent rectum. This may subside, or may persist in a chronic form for many years and lead to stenosis. Treatment is rarely required. Occasionally a stricture requires dilatation, or a rectovaginal fistula needs repair.

VOLVULUS

Volvulus means axial rotation of a portion of the alimentary tract. It occurs occasionally in the small intestine and caecum, more commonly in the pelvic colon. As both ends of the twisted loop are closed it behaves as a closed loop obstruction.

VOLVULUS OF THE SIGMOID COLON

This condition is common in Eastern Europe, Peru, Uganda, and in Pakistan among the Pathans. Elsewhere in the world the condition is uncommon, except in inmates of mental institutions, in whom the enlargement of the sigmoid colon occurs due to neglect of regular evacuation of the bowel. The sigmoid colon is long with a narrow attachment of the pelvic mesocolon. The patients are adult, often middle-aged, and mostly males. There may be a previous history of attacks of left-sided colicky pain. When volvulus occurs there is sudden severe abdominal pain, with rapid onset of marked distension. There is absolute constipation. Vomiting occurs late. Plain x-ray shows the immensely distended loop of pelvic colon.

Treatment. If the diagnosis is certain and the case is of only a few hours' duration, a sigmoidoscope should be passed into the rectum, and an attempt made to pass a flatus tube into the distended sigmoid loop through the sigmoidoscope. If this is successful a great deal of wind is passed and the obstruction is relieved. If the flatus tube fails to pass into the sigmoid, immediate laparotomy should be carried out and the obstructed loop untwisted to allow the wind to pass. However, this is not the end of the matter. Due to the greatly increased length of the sigmoid, the patient remains liable to repeated attacks of volvulus. Therefore, a few weeks after untwisting the volvulus, the gut should be prepared and the sigmoid colon resected, eliminating the possibility of further attacks.

If *gangrene* has already set in before the patient presents, immediate resection of the gangrenous sigmoid colon must be carried out. In such a case the ends are not anastomosed together; they are brought out i.e. exteriorized, because if they were joined together, this would result in a high incidence of leakage at the anastomosis and spell disaster for the patient. The resulting colostomy is closed a few weeks later. In cases of gangrene the operative mortality rate is very high, due mainly to the toxaemia of anaerobic infection.

TUMOURS OF THE COLON

Benign. Adenomatous polyps are dark red pedunculated neoplasms. They are common.

Malignant. Carcinoma.

CARCINOMA OF THE COLON

Pathology. Microscopically, the tumour is a columnar-celled carcinoma. Macroscopically, it assumes one of the following forms:

1. Annular.
2. Tubular.
3. Ulcerative.
4. Cauliflower.

The annular variety causes early obstructive symptoms and is treated promptly, so the prognosis is good. The cauliflower type often commences as a benign adenoma. The most common sites are the pelvic colon and the rectosigmoid junction.

Spread. The neoplasm grows slowly, and if it is removed thoroughly at an early stage, a cure can be hopefully expected.

Local spread. The growth spreads at a slow rate, and usually causes intestinal obstruction before it has penetrated adjacent structures. Penetration may produce an internal fistula, or a local abscess and an external fistula.

Lymphatic spread. This occurs first to the epicolic lymph nodes lying on the colonic wall, and then successively to the paracolic, intermediate and 'main' lymph nodes. Blood spread occurs late, and to the liver.

Grading. Dukes has classified colorectal cancers into the following histological grades:

1. Low grade i.e. well-differentiated tumours.
2. Average grade tumours.
3. High grade i.e. poorly-differentiated tumours.

The more differentiated the tumour, the better is the prognosis.

Staging. As regards the extent of spread of the tumour, Dukes has also provided a system of staging of colorectal cancers:

A: Growths limited to the rectal wall: the prognosis in these cases is excellent.

B: Growths extending into the extra-rectal tissues, but with no metastases to the lymph nodes: here the prognosis is good.

C: Growths with secondary deposits in the lymph nodes: the prognosis in this stage is bad. This stage is further subdivided into two:

C1: Only local para-rectal nodes are involved.

C2: Nodes accompanying the supplying blood vessels are implicated.

In recent years a stage D has been added which was not described by Dukes; it signifies the presence of metastases, usually hepatic.

The TNM staging is more precise, and allows useful division into subsets without being unduly complex. For this reason it is the most suitable system for clinical trials. Yet, because of its great simplicity Dukes' classification is attractive for clinical practice. As the next generation of surgeons will use the TNM system from the beginning, they will find it easy to work with. Therefore this system is likely to displace all other methods of staging in times to come.

Clinical features. Except for occasional cases the patient is over fifty years of age. Over a quarter of the patients present with intestinal obstruction or peritonitis.

In carcinoma of the *left colon* the symptoms are often those of increasing intestinal obstruction due to the narrower lumen and more solid faecal contents. Pain is usually of the nature of a colic. Increasing constipation may be present with distension. The carcinoma itself, or impacted faeces, may be palpable. Carcinoma of the *caecum* may present as an undiagnosed anaemia, a mass, or an intussusception. Carcinoma of the *transverse colon* may be mistaken for a neoplasm of the stomach due to its position. In the *sigmoid* colon a papilliferous growth may produce a feeling of the need for evacuation, tenesmus, mucus and blood.

Investigations. *Radiography.* X-ray after *barium enema* may show a constant irregular filling defect (Fig. 4). If the barium is partly evacuated and air injected into the colon *(contrast enema)* the walls of the colon become delineated, and even a small lesion may be shown up. Early growths in the lower pelvic colon may be missed by radiography, but are shown up on *sigmoidosocopy.* Modern fibreoptic *colonoscopes* can go all the way to the caecum. *Exfoliative cytology* of the colon is a laborious procedure, but successful diagnoses have been made in growths situated in all parts of the colon. Since the advent of colonoscopy exfoliative cytology has lost much of its popularity.

Treatment. The treatment of carcinoma of the colon is by operation, to remove the segment of colon carrying the lesion as well as the whole of the primary lymphatic field draining the area of the lesion.

Preoperative preparation. For 48 hours before the operation the patient is allowed only clear fluids by mouth, and enemas are given twice daily to cleanse the bowel. At the same time metronidazole plus a cephalosporin are given during this period, to reduce the number of pathogens normally present in the colon. Stronger antibiotics sterilize the gut more effectively, but risk dangerous staphylococcal enterocolitis due to overgrowth of antibiotic-resistant staphylococci.

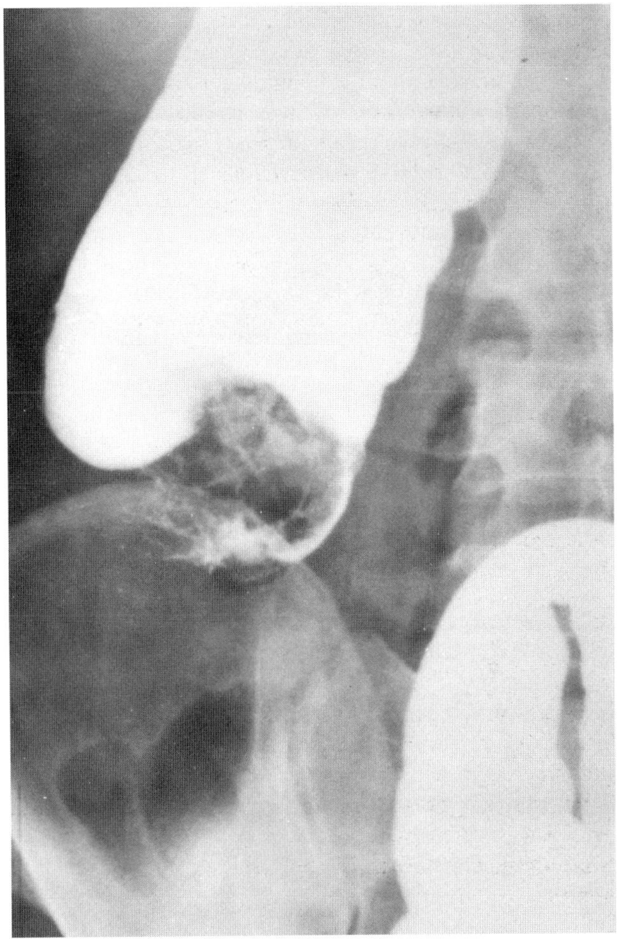

Fig. 4 Barium enema x-ray showing irregular filling defect in caecum due to a cauliflower carcinoma.

At operation the first job is to ascertain the extent of spread of the tumour by examining the liver, the lymph node groups and the peritoneum to detect any secondaries, and the tumour to determine whether it is fixed or free. While removing the colonic cancer the lymph nodes which drain the tumour must be removed, because they may be involved by metastases. As these lymph nodes lie along the regional veins and arteries those vessels, and therefore obviously the whole segment of colon supplied by them, has to be removed.

Thus it comes about that during any particular resection a segment of the colon supplied by one of the following arteries is removed: the ileo-colic and right colic, the middle colic, the left colic and the sigmoid arteries. If the tumour lies at the junction of segments supplied by two different arteries, both segments are removed.

If a growth is *inoperable* surgery may still be carried out to relieve or prevent obstruction. In the ascending colon an ileo-transverse colostomy is carried out. In the upper left colon a transverse colostomy, and in the pelvic colon a high left iliac colostomy is performed. This provides for unhindered passage of faeces for the remaining period of the patient's life.

If the patient has advanced metastatic spread or severe concomitant disease that render him unfit for surgery, *laser* therapy can be employed. It aims at removing all of a cauliflower tumour, improving bleeding, discharge and obstructive symptoms. Treatment is entirely local and is used to coagulate and vaporize the tumour.

Metastases in the liver. Colorectal cancer metastatic to the liver is highly resistant to systemic chemotherapy. However, postoperative portal venous perfusion of 1 g of 5-FU has been shown to reduce the risk of development of hepatic metastases.

TUMOURS OF THE RECTUM

Rectal tumours may be benign or malignant.

BENIGN TUMOURS

Juvenile rectal polyp. If an infant between 2 and 4 years of age passes bright red blood per rectum, without pain and in the absence of dysentery, it is very likely a case of rectal polyp. It commonly arises from the posterior wall of the rectum as a pedunculated bright red rounded mass. The diagnosis is easily confirmed by digital rectal examination, which is best carried out after giving the infant a sedative like tricloryl syrup. A juvenile rectal polyp does not exhibit any tendency to become malignant, but should be removed by operation under general anaesthesia. Incidentally, sometimes it falls off itself, but one should not wait for that to happen.

Pseudo-polyps. These are just tags of mucosa which have hypertrophied due to chronic inflammation, commonly in ulcerative colitis.

Villous adenomas. These adenomas are often very large, and contain villi on the surface. They tend to become malignant, when the tumour becomes hard. These polyps secrete a good deal of mucus, which has a high potassium content. If the tumour is large, potassium depletion may result.

Familial polyposis coli. In this condition multiple polyps develop in the colon during adolescence and cause rectal bleeding. The polyps in the rectum and sigmoid can be seen by the sigmoidoscope. However, to assess the full extent of the disease and the total number of polyps, either colonoscopy or an air-contrast barium enema are required. In time some of these polyps become malignant. The malignant potential of any one polyp is very small. However, when it is remembered that in these cases there may be hundreds of polyps, it becomes obvious that the chances of any one of them becoming malignant are very great. In fact if left untreated, the patient is sure to develop a carcinoma in one of the polyps.

Treatment. In view of the above, the only proper treatment for familial polyposis coli is removal of the whole colon and rectum *(total proctocolectomy).* However, if the polyps in the rectum are regularly excised by diathermy the rectum can be preserved, sparing the patient the inconvenience of life with a colostomy. If malignancy develops in one of the rectal polyps in spite of repeated diathermy, the rectum would require to be removed.

CARCINOMA OF THE RECTUM

Rectal carcinoma is one of the most common malignancies in both men and women. It used to occur only in middle and old age; however, during recent decades younger and younger patients are being seen, some even in their twenties.

Pathology. The tumour commonly starts as a nodule. The less malignant of these nodules project into the lumen, the more malignant tend to infiltrate the wall and ulcerate. The ulcer feels hard and has everted edges like malignant ulcers elsewhere (Plate II–II). When a segment of large bowel is removed for carcinoma often there are in addition one or more adenomas or papillomas. This suggests that these latter are pre-malignant lesions.

Histological sub-types. Dukes has classified colorectal carcinomas into the following grades:

1. Well-differentiated adenocarcinomas.
2. Averagely-differentiated adenocarcinomas.
3. Anaplastic, undifferentiated adenocarcinomas.

The more differentiated the tumour, the better is the prognosis.

Spread. Carcinoma of the rectum spreads locally, via the lymphatics, via the blood-stream, and by peritoneal dissemination.

Local spread occurs circumferentially rather than longitudinally. It takes a tumour about six months to spread around a quarter of the circumference, and about two years to go all round. Spreading outwards, the tumour infiltrates through the muscle of the rectal wall, then fat, then perirectal fascia. If the tumour is located anteriorly, in the male the prostate, seminal vesicles or bladder become involved, in the female the vagina or uterus. In either sex a lateral tumour may infiltrate into a ureter; similarly, extension backwards may involve the sacrum and the sacral plexus. *Spread in a downward direction is uncommon.*

Lymphatic spread. From the upper and middle thirds of the rectum lymphatic spread occurs almost entirely upwards along the inferior mesenteric vein and artery. From the lower third spread can also occur laterally along the middle rectal vein. Downward spread to the groin lymph nodes is very uncommon.

Venous spread. As a rule spread via the veins occurs late. However, anaplastic and rapidly growing tumours in younger patients often spread in this way. The most common sites for blood-borne metastases are the liver (because blood from the rectum is drained via the portal system), the lungs, the adrenals, and the brain.

Peritoneal dissemination can occur when a high-lying rectal carcinoma penetrates the peritoneal coat. The malignant cells set free into the peritoneal cavity can lodge on the surface of any organ, so that there may be small nodules everywhere if the case comes late.

Staging of rectal carcinoma. As regards the extent of spread of the tumour, Dukes has classified rectal carcinomas into three stages:

A. Growths limited to the rectal wall: the prognosis in these cases is excellent.

B. Growths extending into the extra-rectal tissues, but with no metastases to the lymph nodes: here the prognosis is good.

C. Growths with secondary deposits in the lymph nodes: the prognosis in this stage is bad. This stage is further subdivided into two:

C1: Only local para-rectal nodes are involved.

C2: Nodes accompanying the supplying blood vessels are implicated.

Clinical features. *Rectal bleeding* is the earliest and most common symptom. Unfortunately, it often closely resembles the bleeding due to piles. Thus it is bright red in colour, and the blood is usually smeared on the surface of the mass of stools. Therefore it is often not taken seriously, and the rectum is not properly examined.

Sense of incomplete defaecation. After the patient has passed stools he still feels the desire to pass more faeces. This is because after defaecation the tumour is still present in the bowel, which cannot distinguish between the mass produced by faeces and that resulting from a tumour. The patient may try to empty the rectum several times a day, usually with the passage of some blood-stained mucus *(spurious diarrhoea).*

Increasing constipation may set in if the carcinoma is annular, i.e. one which has gone all round the rectum and is causing increasing constriction.

Pain. Colicky pain may be seen due to some degree of intestinal obstruction. Severe constant pain occurs when the tumour infiltrates the surrounding structures. For example, pain in the back or sciatica occurs when the growth invades the sacral plexus.

Abdominal examination is positive only in advanced cases. For example, distension may be present due to intestinal obstruction, ascites due to peritoneal deposits, and nodularity of the liver due to secondaries.

Rectal examination. Digital rectal examination is an *essential investigation in every case of rectal bleeding or unexplained alteration of bowel habit.* Most carcinomas of the rectum can be felt by the finger. In an early case a hard nodule may be felt; more commonly the tumour has already ulcerated, the ulcer having a raised and hard edge. If an ulcer is felt, the finger on withdrawal is usually found to be blood-stained. In females a vaginal examination should also be performed, to find out if the tumour is adherent to the vagina.

Investigations. *Proctosigmoidoscopy* should be carried out in the knee-elbow position, so that the rectum hangs forwards and straightens out and the endoscope can be passed up further. If a tumour is seen a *biopsy* should be taken using a biopsy forceps, usually including a portion of the edge of the tumour.

Barium enema or colonoscopy may be performed to rule out adenomas or synchronous carcinomas at higher levels in the large bowel.

Treatment. The only proper treatment for a carcinoma of the rectum is removal of the rectum along with its primary lymphatic field. Now, as mentioned before, the lymphatics and lymph nodes draining the rectum lie along the superior haemorrhoidal and inferior mesenteric vessels. As these vessels supply the sigmoid colon in addition to the rectum, the sigmoid must also be removed. Again, lymphatics from the rectum accompany the middle rectal arteries which pass in relation to the levator ani muscles; these muscles therefore have to be excised. Although the chances of downward spread of the cancer into the anal canal are few, yet when the levator muscles have been removed, the anal canal has no attachments left and no function to perform, and therefore has to be excised. Thus it comes about that the following structures are removed during an operation for rectal carcinoma: the sigmoid colon, rectum and anal canal; the pelvic mesocolon and inferior mesenteric artery upto its origin; and the levators ani. A permanent colostomy is now made in the left iliac fossa. As the operation requires dissection both in the abdomen and the perineum, it is called an *abdominoperineal resection.* This is the standard treatment for carcinoma of the rectum.

In tumours which lie in the *upper half of the rectum* there is a considerable length of normal rectum below the tumour. Further, spread of the tumour normally takes place in an upward direction. Advantage is taken of these facts in the operation of *anterior resection of the rectum.* Here the sigmoid colon and rectum are removed from above, leaving just a short segment of rectum below. The descending colon is mobilized and anastomosed to this fringe of rectum. In this way the sphincters are saved and the patient spared the very considerable inconvenience of life with a permanent colostomy.

More extensive operations. When the rectal carcinoma has spread to neighbouring organs, the radical operation can usually be extended to remove these structures. Thus, in the male a total cystectomy can be added to the operation where indicated, in the female a hysterectomy. If necessary, all the pelvic organs may be removed, together with the pelvic lymph nodes (*pelvic evisceration*). However, this operation is justified only when the surgeon is confident that the disease can be removed *in toto.*

More limited operations. In a very old and debilitated patient, who will not be able to withstand an abdominoperineal or anterior resection, a *Hartmann's excision* can be employed. Through an abdominal incision the rectum is excised down to within 2.5 cm of the anus and a colostomy performed. The peritoneal floor is closed and the perineal wound drained through the anal canal. In the elderly patient, where the tumour is usually slow-growing and spread is late, this is a most useful operation.

As in the case of the colon, if the patient has advanced metastatic spread or severe concomitant disease that renders him unfit for surgery, *laser* therapy can be used to coagulate and vaporize a cauliflower tumour improving bleeding, discharge and obstructive symptoms.

Prognosis. The 5 year survival rate for rectal carcinoma treated by radical surgery (total rectal excision or a restorative procedure) is about 50% in the advanced countries. In the underdeveloped countries due to late presentation the overall figures are more dismal.

FAECAL FISTULA

A faecal fistula usually results either from leakage of an intestinal anastomosis, or after operation on a case in which the gut wall is necrosed due to one cause or the other. Examples of the latter are found after surgery for the following conditions: gangrenous appendicitis, appendix abscess, strangulated hernia with gangrene of the gut, abscess connected with diverticulitis or colonic carcinoma, actinomycosis, amoebiasis, and regional enteritis.

The track of the fistula may be lined by granulation tissue or fibrous tissue, but in long-standing cases becomes epithelialized. The higher the fistula the greater the extent of both fluid loss and skin digestion, because the duodenum and jejunum contain large volumes of potent digestive enzymes. In fistulas of the ileum or caecum the discharge is fluid; in the distal colon it is solid or semi-solid faecal matter. In cases of doubt methylene blue given by mouth gives the discharge a blue colour. To determine the site of the leak and the length of the fistula a barium meal or barium enema may help, or lipiodol may be injected into the outer opening.

Treatment. Faecal fistulae tend to heal spontaneously if there is no distal obstruction. The abdominal wall should be protected by the use of disposable ileostomy bags. Duodenal and jejunal fistulae cause dehydration and hypoproteinaemia, and intravenous parenteral feeding is required. Pulv. cretae aromat makes the faeces more solid. In order for surgical closure of an intestinal fistula to be successful, three conditions must be met:

1. The patient should be in positive nitrogen balance.
2. There should be no infection.
3. There should be no distal obstruction.

A faecal fistula with an epithelialized track will not heal until the track is removed. At operation an incision is made around the track which is dissected up through the abdominal wall and peritoneum, and the segment of gut bearing the fistula is resected.

28 Anal canal

ANORECTAL ANOMALIES

In the embryo the terminal part of the hindgut (before its division into rectum, bladder and genital primordia) is called the cloaca. The anal canal and rectum develop from the cloaca and proctodaeum in stages:

1. First the cloaca gets divided by a transverse septum into an anterior urinary and a posterior alimentary part.
2. Next the anus migrates backwards along the perineum.
3. Finally, the lateral genital folds or anal tubercles fuse at their posterior ends.

Arrested or distorted development at any of these stages can lead to an anorectal anomaly.

The anomalies fall into two main groups, the high and the low. In the high type the rectum ends above the puborectalis muscle. In the low type it has traversed this muscle and come down.

HIGH ANOMALIES

The common high anomalies include the following:

1. The undivided *cloaca* may persist as such. The bladder enters this cavity from in front, the rectum from behind and the uterus from above (Fig. 1). There is a single opening in the perineum from which greenish watery fluid (meconium plus urine) discharges. This is the severest form of anorectal anomaly, but is fortunately rare.
2. The cloaca may divide incompletely into its urinary and intestinal parts:

i. In the male this results in a *recto-urethral fistula* (RUF). The baby passes meconium in his urine (Figs. 2 & 3).

ii. In the female the Mullerian system comes to lie between the urinary and alimentary tracts. Therefore the rectum opens into the *vagina* instead of the urethra, and a rectovaginal fistula (RVF) results (Fig. 4).

In both these types the rectum does not develop. Therefore the complete anomaly is rectal agenesis with RUF or RVF.

LOW ANOMALIES

Low anomalies may take one of many forms:

1. If the anus fails to migrate backwards the anal orifice is located far forwards. The result is as follows:

i. In the male the anus opens far forwards in the perineum — *an anterior perineal anus* (Fig. 5).

ii. In the female the anus opens into the vulva or vestibule — *a vulvar or vestibular anus.*

2. If overfusion of the lateral genital folds or anal tubercles occurs, the anus becomes covered from behind by skin — a *covered anus*. There are various forms of this anomaly:

i. A *microscopic anus.*

ii. A *membrane* occludes the normal anal site.

iii. The fusion extends still further forwards:

(a) In the *male* it carries a *track* in the skin along the perineal raphe. In this track a streak of meconium may be seen extending onto the scrotum or even the penis.

(b) In the *female* the track may end in the vulva as a *vulval ectopic anus.*

In all these cases of overfusion the anus beneath is practically normal.

Clinical findings. *The most important method for establishing the type of anomaly is by physical examination of the perineum.* In low anomalies an ectopic opening of

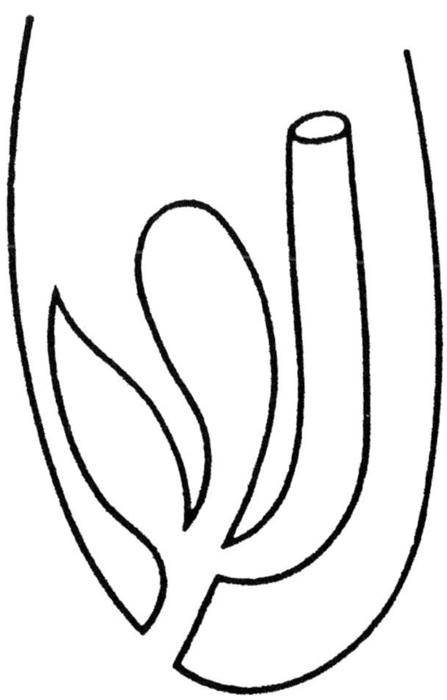

Fig. 1 Cloaca.

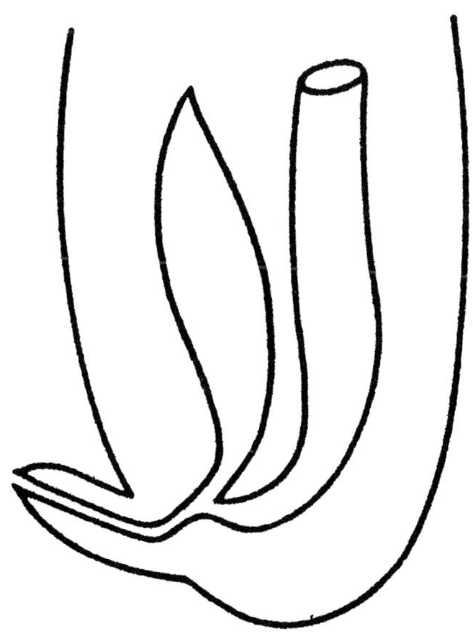

Fig. 2 Recto-urethral fistula.

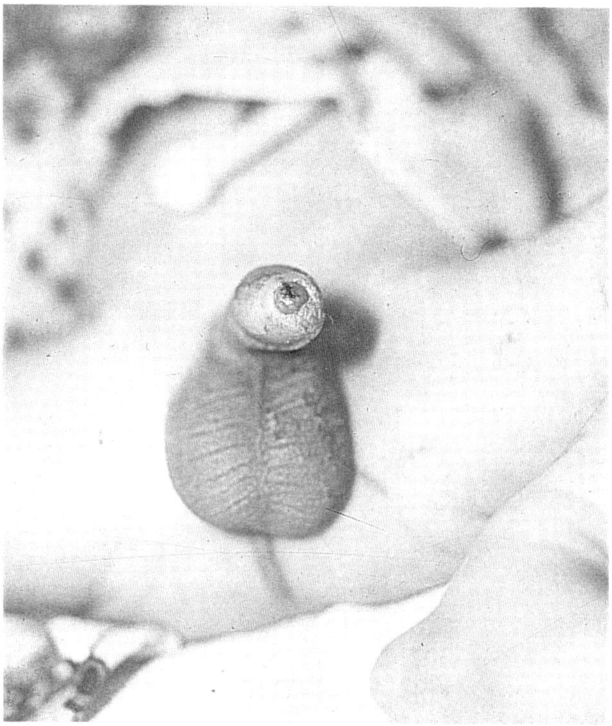

Fig. 3 Recto-urethral fistula. Note meconium at external urinary meatus.

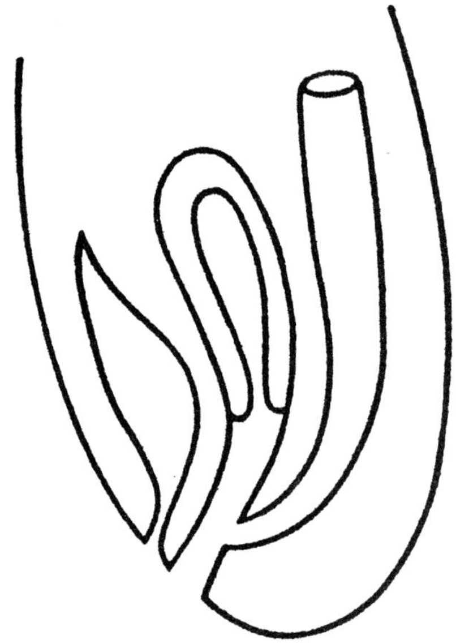

Fig. 4 Recto-vaginal fistula.

the rectum can be detected in the perineal raphe in males. In females this opening lies in the lower vagina, vestibule or fourchette. In many cases of anorectal anomalies other congenital abnormalities are also present, and should be looked for.

X-ray. It takes 12 to 18 hours after birth for swallowed air to reach the rectum. The baby is now held upside down to enable the gas to ascend to the rectum, and a lateral x-ray of the pelvis is taken *(invertogram).* The distance between the gas bubble in the rectum and the anal dimple (marked by a little barium paste) helps distinguish between high and low anomalies. For more exact differentiation, a straight line is drawn on the x-ray film joining the pubis with the coccyx. If the air bubble extends distal to this *pubococcygeal line* it is a low anomaly; if not, it is a high anomaly.

Treatment. *Low anomalies* are repaired by a simple perineal operation in the newborn. The microscopic anus needs dilatation. For the other varieties the orifice is cut backwards with a scissors blade in the opening. Daily dilatations are carried out for about 3 months after the operation.

In the *high anomalies* a colostomy is performed in the newborn. At the age of about one year the abdominoperineal pull-through procedure is performed. In this operation the bowel is mobilized, brought down anterior to the puborectalis muscle and sutured to the perineum. A few weeks after the pull-through operation the colostomy is closed.

In high anomalies the puborectalis muscle is poorly developed. Therefore after operation continence is not always perfect. Very many different operations have been tried; none has given complete satisfaction. The latest operation described consists of mobilization of the rectum through a posterior sagittal approach in the newborn without a covering colostomy. Better results have been obtained than with other methods.

PERINEAL WOUNDS

Wounds in the perineum are different from wounds elsewhere. Whether they result from trauma or surgery, they heal slowly and with difficulty. The reasons are not far to seek. As the buttocks come together, the secretions of the skin are retained. At the same time the stools, which soil the perianal skin daily, contain millions of anaerobes, as well as both Gram negative and Gram positive bacteria. A few clinicians close perineal wounds with suture in an effort to obtain prompt healing. Most others consider this too risky in the unhygienic environment of the anus, and leave the wounds open to granulate. After operation sitz baths* are employed twice daily. The wound is dressed with a cotton pad, which should be changed by the patient himself every 3 to 4 hours, as otherwise it gets soggy and foul-smelling. Elastic underpants can be worn over the pad to keep it in place. The surgeon must personally inspect the wound about once weekly. If the granulations are oedematous, a 15% solution of silver nitrate may be applied to the wound as an astringent. The wounds normally granulate and epithelialize in three to four weeks.

HAEMORRHOIDS

Haemorrhoids arise as follows: in normal individuals a plexus of veins lies under the mucosa in the lower rectum above the mucocutaneous junction. They form vascular *anal cushions* at three, seven and eleven o'clock. These provide a spongy 'washer' on which the sphincter can act, assisting its closure and playing an important role in con-

*Greek *sitzen,* to sit; sitz bath, a bath tub in which one sits up and cannot recline.

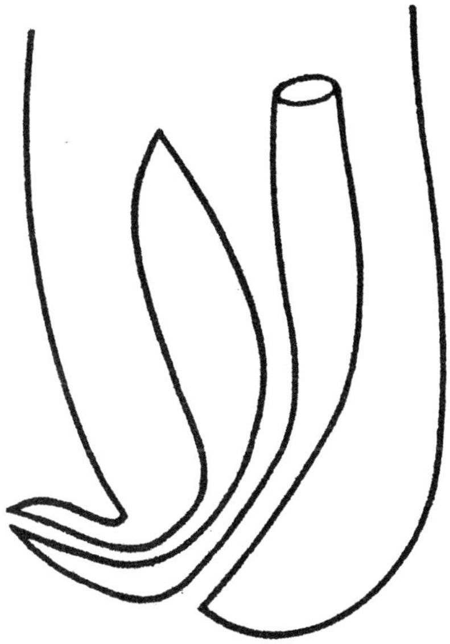

Fig. 5 Anterior perineal anus in male.

tinence with respect to flatus and faeces. Over a period of time the shearing force of hard stools can cause their disruption, engorgement and downward displacement. They then constitute internal haemorrhoids. Important factors in the development of piles include chronic constipation and pregnancy. Constipation is often due to the low-fibre diet which is popular in modern societies. Finally, haemorrhoids are frequently seen in members of the same family. Here a congenital deficiency in the supporting tissues of the anal cushions is probably at work.

The term 'external haemorrhoids' causes some confusion. It is used to signify pile masses that lie below the mucocutaneous junction underneath the anal epithelium and the perianal skin. It is better to regard the piles as disrupted vascular cushions, and observe whether the anodermal part is also involved.

The reason why the main pile masses always arise at 3, 7 & 11 O'clock is probably as follows: the superior rectal artery divides into a left and a right branch. The left branch runs down along the left side of the rectum (at 3 O'clock with the patient in the lithotomy position). The right itself divides into two branches which descend at 7 and 11 O'clock respectively. Because the corresponding veins accompany the arteries, internal haemorrhoids occur at 3, 7 and 11 O'clock, with the branches of the artery. In between these three primary haemorrhoids there may be smaller secondary haemorrhoids.

Clinical findings. *Bleeding* is the first and most important symptom. At first it is slight. It is bright red and occurs during defaecation. Drops of blood may fall into the pan. Haemorrhoids that bleed but do not prolapse out of the rectum are called *first degree* haemorrhoids. One type of bleeding is very typical of piles. When the stool mass passes over a pile it compresses it, so that blood spurts out through a tiny puncture in the mucosa as if it was being ejected from a syringe, and gets sprinkled around the inside of the commode. This kind of bleeding is rarely seen except in cases of haemorrhoids, and makes the diagnosis of piles virtually certain.

Prolapse usually starts later. At first prolapse occurs only at stools and reduces itself; these are *second-degree* haemorrhoids. At a more advanced stage the pile masses protrude with straining and have to be reduced manually; these are called *third-degree* haemorrhoids. *Fourth-degree* haemorrhoids are those that are permanently prolapsed.

Mucoid discharge occurs only when the piles are prolapsed and the mucosa exposed to the exterior. The discharge is followed by pruritus due to irritation of the skin. It should be remembered that *pain* is always absent in haemorrhoids unless complications e.g. strangulation or thrombosis occur. The presence of pain in the history should make one think about fissure, abscess, fistula or strangulated piles. Physical examination easily settles the matter. *Anaemia* may be caused rarely if the bleeding is persistent and profuse.

On *inspection* of the anal region external haemorrhoids may be seen as skin tags; internal haemorrhoids are not visible. On digital rectal examination internal haemorrhoids cannot be felt unless they are thrombosed.

Proctoscopy. The patient lies down in the left lateral position. He is asked to draw his knees up and advised to breathe gently though his open mouth and relax. A gloved and lubricated finger is always passed first. A proctoscope is next passed to its fullest extent and the obturator removed. The instrument is slowly withdrawn. Just above the anorectal ring haemorrhoids, if present, bulge into the lumen of the proctoscope. If the patient is highly strung, one or two tablets of diazepam 5 mg administered an hour before the examination allow the procedure to be carried out smoothly.

Complications of haemorrhoids. *Profuse bleeding* with anaemia is rare.

Strangulation. One or more haemorrhoids prolapse and are gripped by the sphincter. Venous return is impeded and congestion follows. There is considerable pain. Unless the haemorrhoid can be reduced within an hour or two thrombosis may result, the haemorrhoids becoming purple with considerable oedema. *Ulceration* and *gangrene* with sloughing may follow. After thrombosis the pile gets fibrosed. Due to repeated traction at defaecation a *fibrous polyp* may form.

Treatment. In very early cases a high-fibre diet (vegetables, salads, fruits) helps. It softens the stools, so that there is no need to strain. If active treatment is required, it takes the form of injection, band-ligation or haemorrhoidectomy.

Injection treatment. This treatment is ideal for first-degree haemorrhoids. Early second-degree haemorrhoids are also usually cured, but a few of them relapse later. 5% phenol in almond oil is used. 3 to 5 ml is injected into the submucosa at the upper pole of each pile (Fig. 6). Usually a second and a third set of injections have to be given, with intervals of a month between injections. The second set of injections is commonly given into the pile masses themselves, and the third set into the submucosa at a higher level between the necks of the piles. Injection is performed with a long needle through a proctoscope.

The injection leads to inflammation, followed by fibrosis and shrinkage of the piles. At the same time, due to the

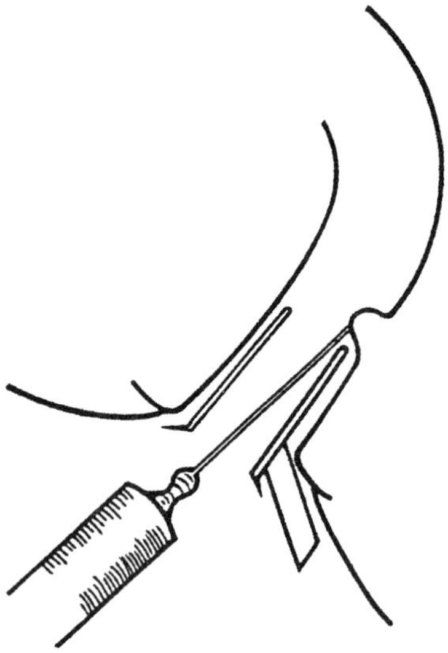

Fig. 6 Injection into a haemorrhoid.

fibrosis surrounding the submucosal veins the bleeding stops. Complications are rare but include local sloughing of the mucosa, infection, and sensitivity reaction to the injected material.

Rubber band ligation. This is an effective simple outpatient procedure. It has gained in popularity and has partly replaced injections. A constricting rubber band is placed around the upper part of the haemorrhoid (Fig. 7). The tissue distal to the rubber band undergoes necrosis and sloughs off in a week's time. The result is more permanent than that of injection therapy, because there is precisely controlled loss of redundant mucosa. The patient should be warned that some bleeding occurs when the sloughs separate in 7 to 10 days.

Haemorrhoidectomy. This is usually reserved for patients with third or fourth degree piles. Thrombosed haemorrhoids should be treated by haemorrhoidectomy after a few weeks, after the oedema has subsided. At operation each haemorrhoid is dissected from the underlying tissues. Its pedicle is securely ligated and the haemorrhoid excised. Adequate columns of mucosa must be left behind between adjacent piles, otherwise stenosis results. Margins of the skin wounds are trimmed so as not to leave overhanging edges. After operation sitz baths should be employed twice daily and the cotton pad changed every 3 to 4 hours. The wounds granulate and epithelialize in three to four weeks.

Postoperative complications. Retention of urine occurs rarely. Reactionary and secondary haemorrhage can occur, but with careful technique are quite uncommon. Stricture results only if an excessive amount of mucosa is removed, which should be avoided.

Treatment of thrombosed piles. Bed rest with frequent sitz baths cause the pile mass to shrink in size in a few days. Haemorrhoidectomy is then carried out two to three weeks later. However, in the rare event of necrosis supervening, debridement haemorrhoidectomy (cutting away the dead tissue) speeds recovery.

Thrombosed external haemorrhoid. This is also called a *perianal haematoma.* It is a small clot occurring in the perianal subcutaneous tissues. It arises due to rupture of a small vein while straining at stool. It is a tense, tender, hemispherical swelling about 1 cm in size. Untreated it usually resolves and undergoes fibrosis, and may or may not produce a skin tag. Occasionally it suppurates, or extrudes the clot. It has been called a 'five-day, painful, self-curing lesion'. If seen within 24 hours of onset the haematoma is best evacuated under local anaesthesia. However, even if left alone it usually resolves.

Conditions which simulate external haemorrhoids. The differential diagnosis of external haemorrhoids includes the following:

1. *Anal warts.* These are raised above the level of the skin and have a dry tufted surface (Fig. 8). They are best removed by diathermy.
2. *Condylomas* have a smooth surface and are moist.

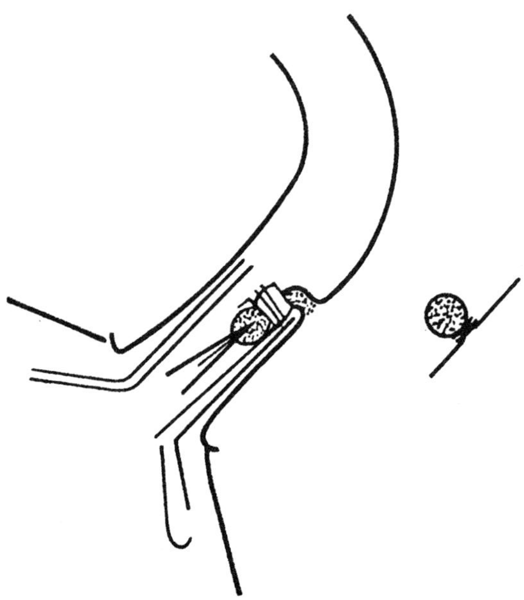

Fig. 7 Rubber band ligation of a haemorrhoid.

ANAL FISSURE

An anal fissure is a longitudinal tear of the skin-lined part of the anal canal. It commonly occurs in the posterior midline. The angle between the rectum and the anal canal causes the mass of stool to damage the anal epithelium at this site. A few anal fissures occur at the anterior midline.

Pathology. *An acute anal fissure* is a tear through the skin of the anal margin. There is severe spasm of the internal sphincter, but as yet little inflammatory reaction. *A chronic anal fissure* has indurated margins and a base consisting of scar tissue. In some cases the lowermost fibres of the internal sphincter may be seen running transversely across its floor. At the lower end of the fissure small bits of faeces burrow under the skin. An oedematous tag of skin forms, which is called a *sentinel pile,* because it stands as a sentinel below the fissure. In long-standing cases the internal sphincter muscle may be organically contracted by fibrous tissue. Infection spreading from the fissure may cause abscess or fistula formation.

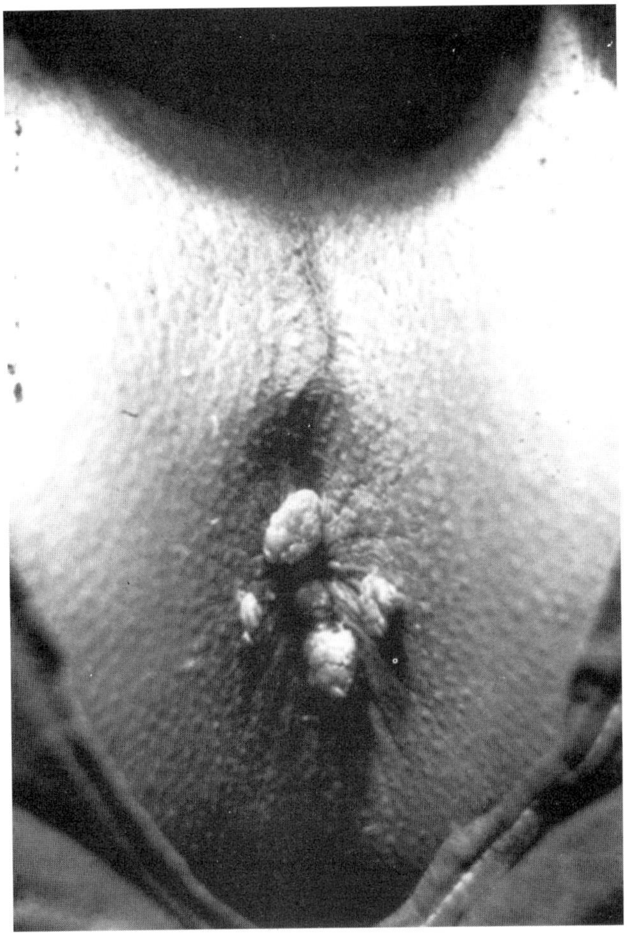

Fig. 8 Anal warts.

Clinical findings. Anal fissures are commonly seen in adults. They are very painful because they lie below the mucocutaneous junction. Occasionally in an infant a fissure may cause severe constipation due to the pain, and result in acquired megacolon. During examination the buttocks have to be separated gently to display the fissure. In chronic cases the sentinel pile may be seen. Rectal examination cannot be carried out in acute cases because of the pain. In chronic cases the examination may be carried out, when the indurated edges of the ulcer can be felt.

Differential diagnosis. Very early *carcinoma* of the anus may simulate a chronic fissure. Excision-biopsy should be carried out. In *procto-colitis* multiple fissures are seen.

Treatment. The patient demands relief from pain. *Conservative methods* are first tried. Warm sitz baths and a local anaesthetic ointment give some relief. The stool is made soft by a bulky diet and by hydrophilic laxatives.

Surgical treatment is considered if the fissure remains unhealed after a week or two of supervised conservative treatment. The lowermost fibres of the internal sphincter from the dentate line distally are divided under general anaesthesia *(internal sphincterotomy).* This abolishes the spasm of these fibres and allows the fissure to heal promptly. Sphincterotomy was in the past carried out in the posterior midline. Recently a lateral subcutaneous sphincterotomy has usually been carried out; this is followed by less post-operative pain and more rapid wound healing. Forceful stretching of the anal sphincter has also been used in the treatment of anal fissure, but is losing its popularity.

ANORECTAL INFECTION

Anorectal infection has two phases: an acute phase i.e. anorectal abscess formation, and a chronic phase i.e. fistula-in-ano.

ANORECTAL ABSCESSES

An anorectal abscess results from the invasion of a pararectal space by pathogenic micro-organisms. A mixed infection usually occurs, mostly with *Escherichia coli, Proteus vulgaris,* streptococci, staphylococci and bacteroides. Anaerobes are often present. The abscess contains a good deal of foul-smelling pus. Anorectal abscesses are much more common in men.

Sources of infection. Infection usually extends from an anal crypt into an anal gland, and thence into one of the pararectal spaces. A perianal abscess may result from a thrombosed external haemorrhoid, or an infection of a hair follicle or sweat gland.

Classification. Anorectal abscesses are classified according to the anatomical space they occupy:

A *perianal abscess* lies immediately beneath the perianal skin (Fig. 9 i). *This is the most common anorectal abscess.* Constitutional symptoms are less severe than in an ischiorectal abscess because the pus can expand the walls of the space easily. It forms a tender rounded cystic mass about 1.5 cm in size at the anal margin.

An *ischiorectal abscess* lies in the ischiorectal space (Fig. 9 ii). The fat in this space has a poor blood supply, therefore the whole space becomes involved soon. The ischiorectal fossa communicates with that of the opposite side via a passage just behind the anal canal. Therefore if untreated, infection spreads to the fossa on the opposite side. A tender, firm swelling may or may not be seen, but *constitutional symptoms are severe* with fever upto 39°C.

A *submucous abscess* lies in the submucosa above the dentate line (Fig. 9 iii). It usually results from injection for haemorrhoids, and nearly always resolves itself; if not, it requires incision.

A *pelvirectal abscess* lies above the levator ani and below the peritoneum (Fig. 9 iv). *It is really a pelvic abscess* and usually secondary to appendicitis, salpingitis or parametritis.

Intermuscular abscess. As mentioned above, in anorectal abscesses the infection starts from an anal gland, which lies in the intermuscular space. If infection remains confined to this site, an intermuscular abscess is the result (Fig. 9 v). It can cause severe throbbing pain like that of a fissure. On examination no fissure is present, and the *diagnosis may be overlooked because of the deep location of the pus.*

Treatment. The management of anorectal abscesses is relatively straightforward. They should all be drained as soon as diagnosed. In the case of perianal and ischiorectal abscesses a cruciate incision is made and the flaps of skin over the whole abscess are excised. If a fistula track to the anal canal is found leading from the inner wall of the

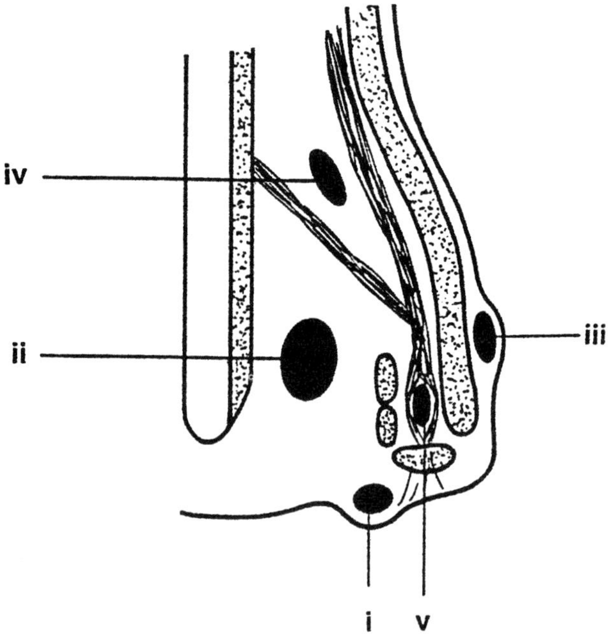

Fig. 9 Anorectal abscesses. i. perianal, ii. ischiorectal, iii. submucous, iv. pelvirectal, v. intermuscular.

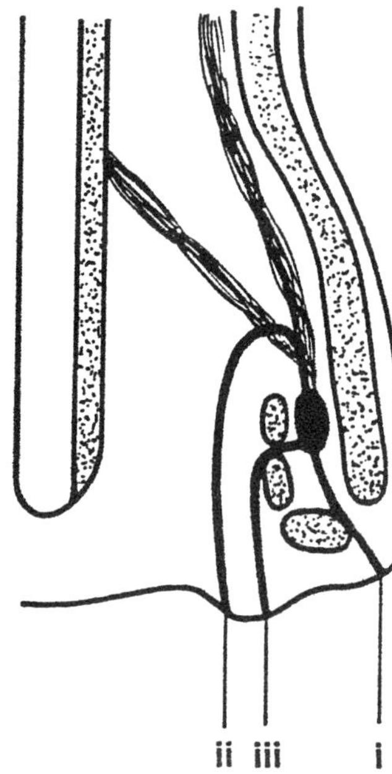

Fig. 10 Anal fistulae. i. Intersphincteric, ii. Suprasphincteric, iii. Transsphincteric.

abscess it is opened, provided too much of the sphincter does not lie below it. In other words fistulotomy is performed at the same time. If no fistula track is found and opened up, the patient should be warned that after the wound fills up there may be a persistent discharge due to the unopened track, which may require a second operation. This will ensure that the patient is not disappointed and demoralized if this should happen.

FISTULA-IN-ANO

A fistula-in-ano is a track lined by granulation tissue which opens internally into the anal canal or rectum, and externally onto the skin around the anus. It usually results from an anorectal abscess which either burst spontaneously or was opened without laying open the entire track, as mentioned above.

Origin of anal fistulae. Infection enters through an anal crypt. An abscess forms in an anal gland which lies between the external and internal sphincter muscles (intersphincteric abscess). From this abscess pus can spread in various directions, producing the different types of fistulae.

Clinical findings. The main symptom of an anal fistula is a persistent discharge of a mixture of pus and serum which irritates the perianal skin and causes discomfort. If the opening gets closed, pain and sometimes fever occur till the collection of exudate bursts and discharges itself. The subcutaneous fibrous track can often be palpated under the skin, specially in low fistulae. For this purpose *the finger should be moved firmly across a line joining the fistula opening to the anal orifice.* The track is easier to feel in its outermost part where it lies close to the skin; in the inner portion it usually lies more deeply. The author has found this method of palpation very useful; however it is not stressed sufficiently in textbooks.

Goodsall's rule helps in predicting the site of the internal opening in cases of anal fistulae. It states that fistulae with the external opening in front of a transverse line drawn through the anus proceed in a straight line towards the anus. Those with the external opening behind this line have curved tracks and open into the anal canal in the posterior midline.

On digital examination an internal opening may sometimes be palpated as a nodule. On proctoscopy the same opening may be seen. If a probe is passed one must be very gentle, otherwise a simple transsphincteric fistula may be converted into an extrasphincteric fistula, with serious consequences for the patient.

Classification. The most widely used classification is that by Parks:

1. *Subcutaneous.* This uncommon type of fistula runs just beneath the perinanal skin.

2. *Intersphincteric.* This is the most common type of fistula; the track runs through the lower part of the internal sphincter (Fig. 10 i).

Treatment. The above two types can be treated simply by laying open the track. In the intersphincteric fistula the lower fibres of the internal sphincter are divided, but this does not lead to incontinence.

3. *Transsphincteric.* The track runs across both sphincters (Fig. 10 iii).

4. *Suprasphincteric.* Here the track passes upwards in the intersphincteric space over the puborectalis and down through the ischiorectal fossa to the skin (Fig. 10 ii).

Treatment. In both the preceding types laying open the fistula would lead to incontinence as it divides the sphincters. Therefore, a method has to be found to avoid such an eventuality:

i. A silk or soft plastic thread may be passed through the fistula and left in place; to prevent it from getting dislodged its ends are tied together. A thread utilized in this manner is called a seton. The mechanism of its action is often not clearly understood. *It allows constant drainage of the discharge of the fistula*, and in this way usually leads to healing.

ii. A *flap* technique may be employed. The external part of the track is first cored out. Inside the anal canal a flap of mucosa is now raised and advanced over the orifice of the fistula, thus closing down its internal opening.

Postoperative care. Fistulotomy leaves behind a wound looking like a groove, which is packed and allowed to heal from the floor and the edges. The wound takes three to six weeks to fill up with granulations and epithelialize, depending upon its size. One of the important reasons for *recurrence* of anal fistulae after operation is the lack of meticulous postoperative care. Usually the margins of the innermost part of the wound come together before the groove itself has filled up with granulations, so that the fistula is formed again. Therefore it is important that the surgeon should carry out the postoperative dressings himself; if this is not possible he should inspect the wound at least once a week.

The *recurrence rate* following fistulotomy is high. Failure of treatment may be due to one of the following reasons:

1. The internal opening of the fistula is not laid open.
2. Collateral tracts are missed.
3. Postoperative care is inadequate.

PILONIDAL SINUS

A pilonidal sinus presents either as a sinus or an acute abscess over the coccyx and lower sacrum. There is granulation tissue, fibrous tissue, and often a tuft of hair. The sinus extends into the subcutaneous tissues. Branching side channels are frequent. Stratified squamous epithelium is found in patches along the walls of the sinus. Some believe this to be a congenital condition. However, the general opinion is that most cases are acquired due to trapping of hair which fall down along the midline groove at the back. Some arguments in favour of the acquired theory are the following:

1. The disease mostly affects men, and specially hairy men.
2. The common sites apart from the natal cleft are between the fingers, specially in barbers.
3. Hair follicles have never been demonstrated in the wall of the sinus.
4. Recurrence is common even after adequate excision of the track.

Clinical findings. Symptoms usually start in the third decade. There is a persistent or recurring sinus in the midline at about the level of the first piece of the coccyx. Typically, a tuft of hair projects from its mouth. The discharge is often foul-smelling due to stagnant contents and may contain hair. Secondary openings may be present on the sides where recurrent abscesses have burst through the skin.

Treatment. Both the acute abscess and the chronic sinus can be dealt with similarly with excision of half a centimeter of skin on either side of the sinus tract. This allows full drainage and formation of healthy granulation tissue, resulting in healing from the depths of the cavity. The wound edges are kept apart by an acriflavine gauze roll which is left in place for a day or two. During this time the patient takes baths. When the dressing is removed, a clean granulating wound is found. This allows healing from the bottom by contraction of the wound. The skin edges must be kept apart by daily packing with a gauze roll by a nurse, or by the patient at home if he is provided with a silastic foam dressing prepared to size. These methods prevent the edges coming together until the wound has filled up with granulation tissue. The wide excisions of the past are no longer practised. They used to leave behind large raw areas which took a long time to heal. Some surgeons apply skin grafts to expedite healing. If the graft takes there is nothing like it; if it is rejectecd it delays healing further. *Whichever way the wound is managed, its healing must be personally supervised by the surgeon.* Otherwise a fair number of recurrences will occur.

PRURITUS ANI

Pruritus is defined as itching of the skin, specially without visible eruption. When this is confined to the perianal area it is known as pruritus ani. The skin may be thickened, red and moist. The causes are numerous:.

1. *Skin diseases.* Psoriasis, seborrhoeic dermatitis, atopic eczema, fungus infections, pinworm, scabies.
2. *Drugs.* Local anaesthetic ointments used over long periods; prolonged use of oral antibiotics which encourage the growth of *Candida.*
3. *Systemic diseases.* Diabetes, liver disease.
4. *Anal diseases.* Draining fistulae, skin tags.
5. *Poor hygiene.* Warm bedclothes, obesity, excessive trauma by toilet paper.
6. *Psychoneurosis* is suspected as a cause in some cases.

Treatment. Any underlying cause is treated. Soap should not be used in the perineum. Soap is alkaline, whereas the perineal area is slightly acid. The area should be cleaned after each bowel movement by washing with plain water. A water-soluble corticosteroid cream with acid pH may be applied thrice daily. Consultation with a dermatologist may be required.

NON-MALIGNANT STRICTURES OF THE ANAL CANAL

Anal canal strictures may be congenital or acquired.

Congenital. 1. A *microscopic anus.*

2. *Postoperative.* After operation for an anorectal deformity the anal canal may be narrow and require repeated dilatation.

Acquired. 1. A chronic anal *fissure* produces some fibrosis in the sphincter.

2. If during an operation for *piles* adequate vertical columns of mucosa are not left between the haemorrhoidectomy wounds, stenosis may result.

3. *Irradiation* for carcinoma of the cervix or bladder can produce fibrosis in the anal canal.

Clinical features. There is increasing difficulty in defaecation with toothpaste-like stools, and the patient requires increasing doses of laxatives. Rectal examination reveals the stricture, when biopsy should be undertaken.

Management. *Prevention.* Strictures following operations for haemorrhoids and low ano-rectal anomalies can be prevented by meticulous technique and by regular dilatations carried out a few weeks after the operation if required.

Treatment. In the case of many benign strictures of the anal canal repeated dilatations at regular intervals prove adequate. If dilatations fail or are judged to be unsuitable, the stricture may be *incised* and the resultant wound covered by a *split-skin graft*, which is sutured in place. If a stricture has caused intestinal obstruction, *colostomy* has to be undertaken, specially in strictures complicated by anal fistulas. If a stricture is located in the lowermost part of the rectum and the anal canal is normal, it may be excised and a colo-anal anastomosis performed.

MALIGNANT TUMOURS OF THE ANAL CANAL

Epidermoid carcinoma. This is the most common tumour of the anal canal. However, it is much less common than adenocarcinoma of the rectum. The tumour starts as a hard nodule which may be ulcerated. Rectal pain and bleeding are the most common symptoms. *Many cases are misdiagnosed as benign lesions, e.g. haemorrhoids or anal fissure, and treatment delayed.* Early diagnosis is made by careful examination of the anal canal and is confirmed by biopsy. Ultrasound, CT scan or MRI can be used to assess muscle invasion. Anal carcinoma spreads to the superior rectal, pelvic and inguinal lymph nodes.

Treatment. The anal canal extends from the anorectal ring to the dentate line; the area from then onwards to 5 cm beyond the anal verge is properly called the anal margin.

With early epidermoid carcinoma of the *anal margin,* local excision is sufficient treatment. If recurrence occurs, irradiation with external beam or implant is required. However, if the tumour has infiltrated deeply abdominoperineal resection is indicated.

Epidermoid carcinoma of the *anal canal* has a worse prognosis and requires more complex treatment. Abdominoperineal resection is the standard treatment, with a 5-year survival of 50%. Primary megavoltage radiotherapy produces similar survival figures, with the added advantage of allowing anal sphincter preservation. A combination of chemotherapy and radiotherapy before operation is followed by a complete response in most cases, when the residual fibrous tissue can be treated by local excision. For those who fail to respond, abdominoperineal resection is required. Simple local excision is generally not recommended, being possibly suitable only for superficially invasive tumours less than 2 cm in diameter.

Malignant melanoma. Malignant melanoma of the anal canal has a very poor prognosis. Fortunately it is rare. It presents as a dark mass protruding from the anus, and *may be mistaken for thrombosed haemorrhoids.*

29 *Hernia and abdominal wall*

Hernia

A hernia is the protrusion of a viscus or part of a viscus through an abnormal opening. It is a very common condition, so that 2% of the population suffer from hernias. The most common hernias are inguinal and umbilical.

Aetiology. Indirect inguinal hernia probably occurs in a congenital preformed sac which develops as the peritoneum accompanies the testis during its descent through the inguinal canal into the scrotum. Predisposing factors in the formation of other acquired hernias include the following:

1. Increased intra-abdominal pressure, e.g. in chronic cough or urethral obstruction.
2. Stretching of the abdominal muscles, e.g. in pregnancy and obesity.
3. Degenerative changes in muscles in middle and old age.

COMPLICATIONS OF HERNIAS

If left untreated, hernias are subject to the complications of irreducibility, obstruction and strangulation.

Irreducibility. This usually occurs due to adhesions between the sac and its contents, or from overcrowding within the sac. It predisposes to obstruction and strangulation.

Obstruction. The intestine in the hernia is obstructed, but the blood supply to the bowel is not interfered with. There is vomiting, abdominal distension and absolute constipation, i.e. no passage of flatus or faeces. The symptoms are less severe than in strangulation. *However, the safe course is to assume that strangulation is imminent, and to operate at once.*

Strangulation. In this condition the intestine is obstructed, and at the same time its blood supply is constricted. First the veins are obstructed, so that the intestine becomes congested and purple. Later, the arteries are also blocked. The serosa now becomes dull and covered by a fibrinous exudate. The intestine feels flabby and friable. The lowered vitality of the intestine allows bacteria to pass through its wall. Gangrene appears at the constriction rings (the points where the intestine is being constricted at the tight neck of the sac) and spreads, resulting in perforation.

Clinical features. There is sudden, severe pain over the hernia, spreading to the whole abdomen, with forceful, repeated vomiting. The hernia is tense, tender and shows no cough impulse. The patient is seriously ill and operation should be carried out urgently. If the constriction remains unrelieved, ultimately pain disappears due to the onset of paralytic ileus and endotoxic shock.

Treatment. The treatment of a strangulated hernia is by immediate operation to avoid ischaemic necrosis of the gut. However, if the case comes within about four hours, it is legitimate to try conservative measures first, as follows:

1. The patient is nursed in a warmed bed, specially in winter, for muscular relaxation.
2. The foot end of the bed is raised to reduce venous congestion.
3. Morphine injection is given subcutaneously.
4. An effort is very gently made to push the hernia back. If it gets reduced, the operation is performed at the next convenient date. If reduction does not take place, operation must be carried out at once.

At *operation* for a strangulated hernia the sac is first exposed and opened. Usually some blood-stained or dirty coloured fluid escapes, which has oozed out from the congested intestines; this is mopped up. The constricting neck of the sac is now divided, and the intestines drawn gently downwards. 100% oxygen is administered and the gut examined. Viable gut is pink and undergoes peristalsis, and its arteries throb briskly. Gut which has lost its blood supply looks purple or black, does not exhibit peristalsis, and the mesenteric arteries do not pulsate; in fact thrombi may be palpated in them. If the gut is found to be viable it is returned to the abdomen. If it is decided that the intestine is non-viable, the dead portion is resected and an end-to-end anastomosis carried out. Finally, the sac is ligated and hernia repair carried out. After operation, fluids are administered intravenously. Oral fluids are started only after flatus starts passing freely.

INGUINAL HERNIA

There are two kinds of inguinal hernia, the indirect and the direct. Indirect hernias come out through the internal inguinal ring. Direct hernias come out through the lower part of *Hasselbach's triangle*, which is bounded by the inguinal ligament, inferior epigastric artery, and the lateral margin of the rectus muscle.

INDIRECT INGUINAL HERNIA

This is by far the most common of all the hernias. The sac into which this hernia descends is probably always congenital i.e. present at birth, due to non-obliteration of the processus vaginalis. However, intestine cannot descend into the sac because its neck is very narrow. During childhood or early adult life a bout of straining stretches the neck. Intestine or omentum comes down and a hernia is the result. An indirect (oblique) inguinal hernia comes out through the internal inguinal ring, which lies 1.5 cm above the midpoint between the anterior superior iliac spine and the pubic symphysis (not the pubic tubercle). Its coverings include skin, subcutaneous tissue, external spermatic fascia (from the external oblique aponeurosis), cremaster muscle and fascia, and transversalis fascia.

Clinical features. An indirect inguinal hernia can appear at any age, and males are twenty times more com-

Section 2

Genitourinary tract

tigations for the urinary tract. It can tell us about the location and the different dimensions of the kidneys, the thickness of their cortices, any dilatation of the pelves and calyces, any stone in the pelvis, and any abnormality of the ureter, and can give us similar information about the bladder. However, unlike intravenous urography it cannot tell us anything about the function of the kidneys.

Computerized tomography (CT scan). Like ultrasonography, a CT scan provides us with images of sections through the body. However, these sections are all taken at right angles to the long axis of the body. Therefore they are more reproducible, and comprise a more accurate and complete record. Again, as each of the different tissues has a different and defined density in the CT scan, it is easier to distinguish the one from the other on the basis of a CT scan report. As against this must be mentioned the ability of the ultrasound probe to be tilted and thus provide a perspective from many different angles. Ultrasonography is very much cheaper than a CT scan, and much more widely available. Therefore it can be regarded as a poor man's CT scan, although this is not to underestimate the considerable value of the information it provides.

Magnetic resonance imaging (MRI) is particularly valuable in the investigation of masses in the adrenal, uterus and adnexa, and the staging of cancers of the kidney, bladder, prostate and uterus.

Isotope renogram. Dimercaptosuccinic acid (DMSA) labelled with Technetium 99 m is injected intravenously. The findings are as follows:

1. In a *normal* kidney radioactivity on the Gamma camera rapidly reaches a high peak, and within 10 to 15 minutes most of it has disappeared due to the isotope having been excreted in the urine.
2. In acute urinary *obstruction* a high peak is attained rapidly, but the isotope cannot be excreted so the level remains high.
3. In *renal artery stenosis* a low peak is followed by rapid excretion.
4. When the kidney function is *impaired* the peak is low, and excretion also takes place slowly.

This study is thus very useful in distinguishing between different types of dysfunction of the kidneys. Further, DMSA has a prolonged transit time through the renal cortex and can be used to define renal masses. At the same time DTPA (Technetium 99 d-t-pentaacetic acid) is entirely excreted by glomerular filtration and is used to measure relative renal perfusion and glomerular filtration rate.

Endoscopy. ***Urethroscopy and cystoscopy.*** With cystourethroscopes the interior of the urethra and bladder can be visualized, and a diverticulum, a stone, a ureterocele, and an enlarged prostate can all be seen.

Ureteroscopy. The interior of the ureter and of the renal pelvis can be visualized through a *ureteroscope* and a *nephroscope* respectively. Ureteroscopes comes in sizes 7 through 12 French. The larger sizes require dilatation of the ureteric orifice by an angioplasty type of balloon.

Endoscopes give us very direct and first-hand information about the interior of the urethra, bladder and ureter. Bleeding points can be identified, tumours localized and biopsied, and stones and strictures treated.

CONGENITAL ANOMALIES OF THE KIDNEY AND URETER

Congenital anomalies in general. Sometimes a baby is born with an organ either missing or imperfectly formed. It is then not an easy matter to create an exact replica. The reasons are not far to seek. Nature takes a period of nine months i.e. 7000 hours working round the clock to produce and perfect each organ in the mother's womb; the surgeon has only an hour or two in the operation theatre. Again, as nature works at the molecular level, her tools of the trade are infinitely more sophisticated than the surgeon's. It should not surprise anyone, therefore, if the organs constructed by the surgeon, usually from adjacent but different tissues, are sometimes not as perfect in form or in function as those created by nature. This fact should be clearly explained to the baby's parents in advance of the surgery, to avoid raising hopes of a perfect result and subsequent disappointment.

Absent kidney. About once in 2,000 persons one kidney may be absent, so that pyelography demonstrates only one kidney and cystoscopy shows one ureteric orifice.

Ectopic kidney. An ectopic kidney occurs once in 1,000 cases, when the kidney is arrested during its normal ascent, usually at the pelvic brim. If such an abnormally placed kidney becomes the seat of a pathological process, the diagnosis is difficult, and may be missed. An ectopic kidney lying in the pelvis in a female patient may cause obstructed labour.

Horse-shoe kidney. The kidneys and ureters develop from the mesonephros and metanephros. Each ureteral bud arises from the mesonephric duct of the same side, and penetrates the metanephros. The mesonephros contributes the ureters, pelves, calyces and collecting tubules; the metanephros supplies the nephrons. If the lower medial portions of the two kidney anlages get fused together, the result is a horse-shoe kidney. Such a kidney fails to ascend all the way to its adult position, and therefore lies at a lower level than normal. The bridge joining the lower poles lies in front of the 4th lumbar vertebra. Stasis of urine occurs due to two factors. Firstly, as the lower poles of the kidneys are joined together, the pelves face upwards rather than downwards, so that drainage is impaired. Secondly, the ureters are kinked as they pass over the isthmus.

Clinical features. These are due to stasis of urine. Infection, stone formation and tuberculosis can all occur. A firm, immobile mass below the umbilicus can be a horse-shoe kidney. However, the diagnosis can be confirmed only by ultrasonography or intravenous urography. With urography the lowermost calyx can be seen to be pointing medially. At the same time the ureters curve outwards in the upper part of their course.

Treatment. In the past the isthmus of a horse-shoe kidney was divided to improve drainage. Nowadays this is not considered to be necessary, and surgery is carried out only if indicated by the development of hydronephrosis or a calculus.

Crossed ectopia. Crossed ectopia or *unilateral fusion* of the kidneys is rare. If both pelves face medially the result is a *unilateral long kidney.* If the pelvis of the crossed kidney faces laterally, an *S-shaped kidney* results.

Congenital cystic kidneys. In this condition the kidneys are greatly enlarged, and are riddled with cysts of varying sizes. The condition is inherited as an autosomal dominant, so the risk of transmitting the disease to the offspring is fairly high, and this fact should be mentioned during genetic counselling.

Clinical features. The disease rarely manifests itself before adult life, and is slightly more common in women. If both kidneys are large and nodular, the diagnosis is most likely congenital cystic kidneys. Most of the renal parenchyma is replaced by the cysts. As such, the urine secreted by these diseased kidneys is of a poor quality, having a low specific gravity. There may be a dull *ache* in the loin, probably from tension inside one of the cysts. A cyst may rupture producing *haematuria*, but the most common complication encountered is *pyelonephritis*. The majority of adults with this condition suffer from *hypertension*. In later years chronic *renal failure* supervenes, with anorexia, headache, dyspepsia and anaemia. Very few patients survive beyond the age of fifty-five years.

Diagnosis. In the past diagnosis used to require intravenous urography, when the calyces were seen stretched over the cysts like the legs of a spider (*spider-leg deformity*). Nowadays the diagnosis is more easily made by ultrasonography, which shows up the cysts to good advantage.

Treatment. In order to avoid burdening the poorly functioning kidneys, the patient should take a low-protein diet, and to prevent anaemia he should take iron. If infection occurs it should be treated appropriately. If the different cysts are punctured, renal function is improved somewhat. Nowadays this can be done percutaneously under ultrasound control. When renal failure supervenes it is managed by dialysis, or by bilateral nephrectomy and renal transplantation.

Other types of cystic kidneys. *Infantile polycystic disease* is rare. The kidneys are large and may obstruct labour. *Unilateral multicystic disease* presents as a mass in the flank, and after making sure that the other kidney is present and functioning well, it should be treated by nephrectomy. *Solitary renal cyst* may have a congenital origin, but its appearance in adult life suggests that it is acquired. It may produce a symptomless swelling, or be associated with loin pain. These days such a cyst is often found incidentally during an ultrasound examination for a different condition. If on aspiration the cyst contains clear fluid and no malignant cells, it may be watched. However, it should be kept under regular observation by ultrasound examinations. If it enlarges it is best operated upon and the needful done according to the situation found at operation.

Aberrant renal artery. Sometimes in a case of hydronephrosis the lowermost branch of the renal artery appears to be the cause, as it crosses over the pelviureteric junction (PUJ). In actual fact, however, in most cases the PUJ is already obstructed, and the artery merely accentuates the obstruction as the pelvis prolapses forwards over it. In such a case the artery may need to be divided to relieve the obstruction. However, it often supplies a large part of the kidney and cannot be sacrificed. In that case a dismembering type of pyeloplasty needs to be done, i.e. one in which the pelviureteric junction is divided across, the cut end of the ureter enlarged by slitting it open for some distance, and the pelvis and ureter re-anastomosed in front of the aberrant artery, so that the vessel need not be divided.

Duplication of the renal pelvis. In this condition the upper pelvis is the smaller one, and drains the upper major calyx. The lower pelvis drains the middle and lower major calyces. A double pelvis is more prone to develop the complications of stone formation, infection or hydronephrosis than a normal pelvis, because each of the two pelves, and specially the upper one, is smaller and narrower than the normal pelvis. If stones damage one calyx, that part of the kidney may have to be removed in a partial nephrectomy.

Duplication of a ureter. In this condition the two ureters usually join up in the lower third of their course. In other cases both open separately into the bladder. In that case the ureter draining the upper pelvis crosses its fellow and opens below it into the bladder.

Ectopic ureteric orifice. This is clinically important only if the orifice lies below the bladder sphincter, because in that case it results in incontinence of urine. It may not be easy to spot the opening at urethroscopy. If the urine is clear the ideal treatment is to reimplant this ureter into the bladder. On the other hand if repeated infections arise, the part of the kidney draining through this ureter should be removed by a partial nephrectomy.

Retrocaval ureter. In this condition the right ureter passes behind the inferior vena cava instead of lying to the right side of it. Sometimes, due to the distortion of its course and the pressure of the cava the ureter becomes obstructed. In such a case it should be divided across and re-anastomosed in front of the cava.

Ureterocele. A ureterocele arises when there is congenital stenosis of a ureteric orifice. The intramural part of the ureter dilates into a thick-walled cyst. The condition is usually not recognized till adult life. During cystoscopy the cyst is seen to enlarge with each efflux of urine, after which it slowly collapses. If the case is symptomless no *treatment* may be needed. If hydronephrosis, stone or infection arise, the ureterocele should be resected. The ureter is dissected upwards, its obstruction relieved, and it is reimplanted to create a non-refluxing tunnel.

INJURIES TO THE KIDNEY

A kidney may be injured by a blow to the loin or from in front, or by being crushed during a road accident. The extent of the injury varies a good deal, from a small subcapsular haematoma to a complete tear extending from the capsule to the pelvis. In such a case blood and urine collect in the retroperitoneal area.

Clinical features. There is usually pain and tenderness in the loin. A few hours after the accident haematuria may be seen, sometimes accompanied by clot colic. If the injury is severe, abdominal distension may appear after about forty-eight hours due to paralytic ileus from involvement of the splanchnic nerves. If a large perirenal haematoma forms, the contour of the loin may become convex.

Investigations. Despite advances in radiology, plain x-ray of the abdomen and intravenous urogram are the mainstay for evaluation of renal trauma. On plain x-ray obliteration of the psoas shadow, obscure renal outline, and scoliosis towards the side of injury all indicate fluid i.e. blood or urine in the pararenal space. Once the patient is hydrated an intravenous pyelogram determines the degree of injury as well as the function of the contralateral kidney. If the kidney is not visualized or a large volume of contrast medium is extravasated, selective renal angiography should be carried out. If this shows renal artery thrombosis operation must be carried out within about two hours to anticipate irreversible ischaemic damage.

Treatment. The great majority of injuries to the kidney settle down with conservative management. The patient should rest in bed until haematuria has been absent for a few days. Morphine is given for analgesia and sedation. The pulse and blood pressure are recorded every hour. A sample of each specimen of urine should be kept, to watch the progress of the haematuria. Blood should be grouped and cross-matched, so as to be available in case of continuing haemorrhage. An intravenous urogram is obtained urgently, in order to find out whether a normally functioning kidney is present on the other side. With such management haematuria often diminishes, pain and muscle guard decrease, and the pulse becomes normal.

Operation becomes necessary in a few patients. The indications for operation are the following:

1. If there is continuing blood loss.
2. If a gross swelling develops in the loin.
3. If selective renal angiography shows renal artery thrombosis.

In cases of renal trauma the kidney is best approached from in front, through a midline incision. Other viscera are first examined for evidence of injury. The peritoneum overlying the aorta is next incised and a vascular clamp applied to the renal artery. The kidney is now exposed by incising the peritoneum in the paracolic gutter and retracting the colon medially. Control of the renal pedicle allows the renal bed to be explored without excessive bleeding. Small tears in the kidney can be sutured over a piece of detached muscle. If the tears involve only one pole of the kidney a partial nephrectomy can be performed. If the kidney has multiple lacerations or the kidney pedicle is damaged, nephrectomy should be carried out.

INJURY TO THE URETER

The ureter is commonly injured by gunshot wounds, when primary repair is best. The lumen of the ureter being narrow, a circular anastomosis tends to stenose due to contraction of the fibrous tissue. To prevent this, each end of the ureter is slit down the side a short distance ('spatulated') to enlarge the opening. When the ends are now joined together, stenosis is avoided.

Injury to the lower end of the ureter occurs from time to time during the operation of hysterectomy, at the site where it crosses obliquely in front of the vaginal fornix to reach the bladder. Commonly the operator is a gynaecologist. If a surgeon is available, it is best to immediately reimplant the ureter into the bladder. If, on the other hand, the gynaecologist has to deal with the situation unaided, the best he can usually do is to tie a ureteric catheter or other fine tube into the ureter and bring its end outside. He can then request a surgeon to repair the ureter. If the lower end of the ureter has been divided during hysterectomy it can be reimplanted into the bladder. If, as happens rarely, the damage has taken place during oophorectomy, the divided ends of the ureter have to be anastomosed together.

HYDRONEPHROSIS

A hydronephrosis is an aseptic dilatation of the kidney due to a partial obstruction to the outflow of urine. If the pelvis is intrarenal, more damage is caused to the kidney by its dilatation than if it is extrarenal. In either case in advanced hydronephrosis the kidney may be reduced to a mere fibrous sac. Usually it takes years before this stage is reached. Hydronephrosis may be unilateral or bilateral.

UNILATERAL HYDRONEPHROSIS

When hydronephrosis is present on only one side the cause must lie in the ureter of that side, because if it was located at a lower level, i.e. in the bladder or the urethra, the pelvic dilatation would have been bilateral. The obstruction is commonly located at the pelvi-ureteric junction, but sometimes at a lower level.

Pelvi-ureteric junction obstruction. When the obstruction is at the pelvi-ureteric junction (PUJ), the cause usually lies in the wall of the ureter, but is not visible externally. It is commonly either *congenital stenosis* or *physiological narrowing* of the PUJ. A third suspected cause of PUJ obstruction is an *'aberrant renal artery'*. If an inferior branch of the renal artery happened to be crossing in front of the PUJ and a hydronephrosis developed, in the past it was thought that this was an abnormally placed vessel (an aberrant artery), and that it had produced the hydronephrosis by obstructing the outflow of urine from the pelvis. We know now that in most of these cases the cause of the hydronephrosis is an intrinsic PUJ obstruction, and the dilated pelvis is merely bulging forwards over this normally placed vessel.

Obstruction at a lower level in the ureter. Here the cause may lie in the lumen of the ureter, in its wall, or outside the ureter.

1. *Intraluminal.* A stone in the ureter may produce hydronephrosis by causing partial or intermittent obstruction.

2. *Intramural.* i. A *congenital small ureteric orifice* may result both in a ureterocele (cystic dilatation of the intramural ureter), and hydronephrosis.

ii. *Stricture* of the ureter may arise in a case of tuberculosis, or after damage to the ureter during a pelvic operation, usually hysterectomy.

iii. A *neoplasm* of the ureter, or a tumour of the bladder involving the ureteric orifice, may be the cause of the obstruction.

3. *Extramural.* The ureter may be involved by a *growth* arising in a neighbouring organ, e.g. carcinoma of the cervix, rectum or prostate.

Clinical features. Usually the patient complains only of a dull ache or a sense of weight in the loin, which may be aggravated by excessive fluid intake. An enlarged kidney may be palpated. On the other hand sometimes there may only be attacks of renal colic, without a palpable kidney.

BILATERAL HYDRONEPHROSIS

Bilateral hydronephrosis may be caused by any of the conditions mentioned above if they occur on both sides. However, much more commonly it is the result of some form of obstruction to the urethra. The conditions which may result in bilateral hydronephrosis include the following:

1. *Congenital.* i. Congenital valves of the posterior urethra.

ii. Congenital contracture of the bladder neck.

iii. Phimosis.

2. *Acquired.* i. Stricture of the urethra, either traumatic or gonorrhoeal.

ii. Enlargement of the prostate, usually benign but occasionally malignant.

iii. Carcinoma of the cervix or rectum involving both ureters.

iv. Carcinoma of the bladder involving the ureteric orifices.

Clinical features. Bilateral hydronephrosis commonly presents with symptoms of *uraemia*, i.e. polyuria with resultant thirst, along with loss of appetite. There may only be a dull ache in the loins. During *pregnancy* some dilatation of the ureters and renal pelves occurs, and becomes maximum by the fifth or sixth month. After delivery the situation returns to normal within a few weeks. It is due to the hormone progesterone producing atony of the ureters. In the dilated, atonic ureters urine does not drain freely and infection often results.

Investigations. Confirmation of the diagnosis of hydronephrosis can be obtained by an *ultrasound scan,* which shows up the dilated pelvis and calyces as black cavities. The dimensions of the pelvis and the thickness of the cortex should be measured and recorded for comparison with future scans. *Intravenous urography* is nowadays utilized mainly for assessing the functional state of each kidney. It should be noted that if the hydronephrosis is at an advanced stage, the 15 and 30 minute films will not be of much use, as the kidney function will be too poor for any excretion of the dye to take place so early. In such a case pictures should be taken at increasing intervals until the excretion of the dye is demonstrated. The length of time which elapses before sufficient dye is excreted for visualization gives a rough idea of kidney function on each side; the longer the time period the worse the state of kidney function. A *radioisotope renogram* assesses the function of each kidney, and helps in deciding about the type of operation to be performed.

Treatment. If the hydronephrosis is of a slight degree no treatment may be required. However, repeated ultrasound scans at yearly intervals are advised in order to monitor the progress of the condition. If on repeated ultrasound scans the dilatation is increasing, operation is usually the best course. Other indications for operation include repeated attacks of colic and recurrent bouts of infection. In bilateral cases when the cause lies in the bladder or urethra it should be removed; the hydronephrosis will then regress. At *operation* the aim should be conservation of renal tissue. Nephrectomy should be performed only if the renal parenchyma has been mostly destroyed.

Anderson-Hynes pyeloplasty. If surgery is required for PUJ obstruction, the most common procedure employed is the Anderson-Hynes operation. In this procedure the excess part of the pelvis is removed along with the pelvi-ureteric junction. The upper part of the remaining pelvis is now closed. The upper end of the ureter is slit down the side in order to enlarge its opening, and it is anastomosed to the lower part of the pelvis.

In other types of pyeloplasty the PUJ is not disconnected, but a flap is turned down from the pelvis to widen the pelvi-ureteric junction and improve drainage from the pelvis. The advantage of the Anderson-Hynes operation lies in the fact that it can be applied to every case, including cases where an artery is passing across the PUJ. In the other operations the artery would have to be divided, and this could result in ischaemic infarction in the part of the kidney supplied.

Surgery on the foetus. If severe bilateral hydronephrosis develops in the foetus, the foetal urine output is low, with resultant oligohydramnios. The cramped space in the uterus leads to pulmonary hypoplasia, which may be life-threatening. If the lungs are mature, immediate delivery and decompression of the hydronephrosis should be carried out; if the lungs are immature, the decompression can now be performed even *in utero.*

Renal calculus

Stone formation in the kidneys is a fairly common event. In the 'stone belt' of the world, which stretches across North Africa, Arabia and the southern parts of Iran, Pakistan and Rajasthan, the condition is extremely common. Whether this is due to the hot and dry climate of these areas resulting in underhydration, and leading to precipitation of crystals in the concentrated urine, is not certain.

Aetiology. Urinary calculi develop as a result of excessive excretion of calcium, oxalate, uric acid or cystine:

1. *Hypercalciuria* may be:

i. Idiopathic.

ii. Due to increased intestinal absorption of calcium (in hyperparathyroidism).

iii. Due to decreased renal reabsorption of calcium (calcium leak).

iv. Due to prolonged recumbency (e.g. in paraplegia) where bone reabsorption is increased.

2. *Hyperoxaluria* may occur as a result of increased intestinal absorption of oxalate after ileal resection or colon bypass surgery.

3. *Uric acid* stones are associated with hyperuricosuria, and may occur without a raised level of uric acid in the blood.

4. *Cystinuria* results from a disorder of cystine metabolism.

5. Magnesium ammonium phosphate stones occur due to the combined presence of obstruction (or a foreign body) and infection by a urea-splitting organism, usually Proteus.

6. Urinary calculi are also seen in patients with sarcoidosis, and with excessive intake of calcium and alkali in cases of peptic ulcer ('milk alkali syndrome').

However, in the above-mentioned regions of the world where urinary stones are endemic, in most cases none of the above causes can be found.

Varieties of urinary calculi. About 80% of all urinary calculi are composed of calcium oxalate. The other common types of stones include the following: magnesium ammonium phosphate (15%), uric acid (4%), and cystine (1%). The surface of a calcium *oxalate* stone is rough. The sharp projections damage the mucosa of the renal pelvis, so that haematuria results. Altered blood may be deposited on the surface of the stone, rendering it black in colour. An oxalate stone produces a dense shadow on x-ray. It is very hard, and on section it is laminated concentrically. 'Envelope-shaped' oxalate crystals are seen in the urine. *Phosphate stones* usually contain calcium magnesium phosphate. They are smooth and dirty white. If the urine is alkaline they enlarge rapidly and may fill the renal calyces, taking on their shape (Fig. 1). The surface of phosphate stones is smooth, so that they cause less pain and haematuria than oxalate stones. They are radiopaque, but less dense on x-ray than oxalate stones.

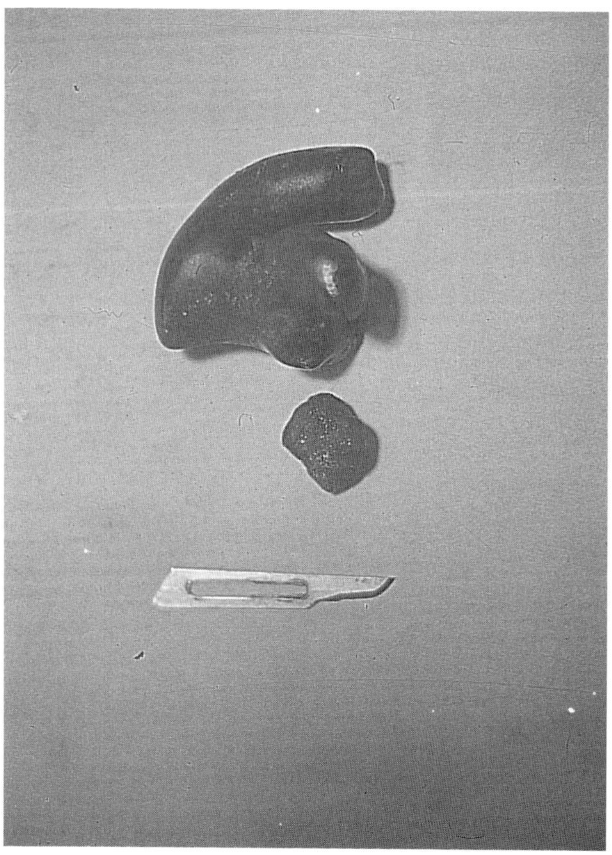

Fig. 1 Stone taking the shape of the renal pelvis, and black in colour due to altered blood on its surface. Note the second stone which lay in the lower calyx.

Uric acid and urate stones are yellow or brown in colour, and are smooth and hard. They are not opaque to x-rays. However, most of them contain a mixture of calcium oxalate, so that they show up on plain x-rays. Urate stones are more soft, and are commonly seen in children. In some persons there is greatly diminished resorption of *cystine* from the renal tubules, and excessive quantities of cystine are excreted in the urine; in such patients cystine stones can form. They are soft, and pink or yellow in colour. They may assume a cast of the renal pelvis. They are radiopaque due to the sulphur they contain. *Xanthine* and *indigo* calculi are very rare.

Clinical features. Most cases of calculi present between the ages of thirty and fifty years. Males are slightly more often affected than females. There may be no symptoms, specially in the case of the more smooth phosphate stones. In such cases *uraemia* may be the first indication of the presence of the stones.

Pain is the presenting and most important symptom in most cases. It can be of two kinds, fixed renal pain and ureteric colic. *Fixed renal pain* occurs when a stone is lying in the renal pelvis. It is located in the renal angle, or occasionally in the hypochondrium. It is usually made worse by movement. *Ureteric colic* is a very severe pain, which radiates from the loin to the groin. It comes suddenly and the patient rolls about in agony. If the stone is in the intramural part of the ureter there may be painful straining, followed by the passage of a few drops of blood-stained urine. This is called strangury. During the attack of renal colic there is tenderness over the renal angle — *Murphy's renal punch.* At the same time, the kidney may be tender on *bimanual palpation,* which is an important clinical method of examination of the kidney. If the stone leads to the development of a hydronephrosis or a pyonephrosis the kidney may become palpable.

Haematuria is not normally a leading symptom. Occasionally, small quantities of blood may render the urine 'smoky' in colour. Small amounts of pus may also be found in the urine.

Investigations. *Ultrasound examination.* This shows up every calculus, whereas x-rays show up only those stones which are radiopaque. Ultrasonography indicates the location and the dimensions of the kidney, the thickness of the cortex, the presence and the degree of any dilatation of the calyces and pelvis, and the number and sizes of stones in the pelves and ureters. The one thing which ultrasound cannot do is to tell us about the function of the kidneys. This information can only be obtained by employing either intravenous urography or an isotope renogram.

Plain x-ray. Plain x-ray should be taken after an overnight fast and after emptying the bowel by a laxative, otherwise the shadows of gas and minerals in the intestines obscure the picture. The appearance of a kidney stone can be mimicked by a calcified mesenteric lymph node, a gallstone, a phlebolith, and a calcified lesion in the kidney. Gallstones and mesenteric lymph nodes lie anteriorly, and a *lateral radiograph* can be taken, which will show that they are located anterior to the bodies of the vertebrae.

Intravenous urography. This is carried out by injecting intravenously such a radiopaque dye which is excreted and concentrated by the kidneys. Within a couple of minutes it accentuates the shadow of the kidney substance by getting concentrated in the renal tubules producing a 'nephrogram'. X-rays are commonly taken after 5, 15 and 45 minutes, and they outline the pelves, the ureters, and the bladder. Intravenous urography helps in confirming that the opacity due to a stone is intrarenal, and in showing in which part of the kidney it is situated. At the same time it reveals the function of both kidneys. A non-opaque stone may also be shown up as a filling defect in the pelvis.

TREATMENT OF KIDNEY STONES

The treatment of kidney stones resolves itself into the relief of renal colic and the removal of the calculi. For the *relief of pain* morphine, in a dose of 15 mg subcutaneously, and the antiprostaglandin agent diclofenac in a dose of 50 mg i.m., are effective.

METHODS OF REMOVAL OF STONES

Classically, stones in the kidneys were removed by open operation. Recently introduced methods include extracorporeal shock wave lithotripsy, percutaneous nephrostolithotomy and ureterorenoscopy. Since the last two decades these are being used with increasing frequency, so that in the major centres today only a very small percentage of all cases are removed by open operation. However, the modern methods are not only expensive but also require technology not available everywhere.

1. Open operations for removal of kidney stones. ***Technique.*** *Position.* The patient is placed on a four-piece table in the lateral position, with the affected side uppermost. The opposite lower limb is flexed, the limb of the same side being extended. The trunk is held in this position by a strap passing over the pelvis. The table is 'broken' opposite the patient's waist to open out the lumbar region and increase the space between the ribs and iliac crest.

Incisions. The nerves of the lateral abdominal wall run obliquely, from above downwards and forwards. Therefore, in order to avoid damaging them, most incisions in this area are made in the same direction. *Morris's incision,* which is the most popular, starts at the renal angle and runs downwards and forwards to a point about 3 cm above and medial to the anterior superior iliac spine. The external oblique is split along the direction of its fibres. The internal oblique and transversus muscles are then divided in the same line. The fascia of Gerota is now opened. Blunt dissection of the perirenal fat allows the kidney to be mobilized and delivered into the wound. It may be mentioned that the smaller stones in the pelvis can be removed without mobilizing the kidney, thus minimizing the dissection.

Drainage. After most operations on the kidneys a drain is placed inside the perirenal fascia, in order to allow egress to any urine which may leak from the pelvis. It is led out through a separate stab incision to allow the main wound to heal uninterruptedly.

Closure. The fascia of Gerota is closed by a few interrupted sutures of catgut. Each layer of muscles is sutured separately, using either polyglactin or monofilament polypropylene.

The ***different operations*** for removal of renal stones include pyelolithotomy, nephrolithotomy, partial nephrectomy and nephrectomy.

Pyelolithotomy. This is the most common open operation carried out on the kidney for the removal of calculi. The posterior wall of the pelvis is cleared of its surrounding fat. The pelvis is now incised along its long axis. The stone is removed with a suitable forceps. If a small stone is lying in a calyx and the neck of the calyx is wide enough, the stone can be removed by a forceps introduced through the pelvis. A bougie is now passed down the ureter in order to demonstrate free passage, and to detect any stone lying lower down. The pelvis is flushed with saline. In the case of multiple stones it is a great advantage if, at this stage, the kidney can be delivered outside the wound and x-rayed, to detect any small stones still remaining in the various calyces, so that they can also be removed. The pelvis is finally closed with interrupted sutures of fine plain catgut.

Nephrolithotomy. If a stone is lying in a calyx and cannot be removed via the pelvis due to the narrowness of the neck of the calyx, it can be removed by making a small incision in the renal parenchyma directly onto the stone. Interrupted catgut stitches passed through the kidney substance and tied over a piece of muscle help haemostasis.

Partial nephrectomy. If a stone is lying in the lowermost calyx, and the calyx is dilated and damaged so that it does not drain very well, it is necessary to remove the calyx in order to prevent the reformation of the stone. Now, it is self-evident that if the calyx is to be removed, the lower pole of the kidney must be excised. Thus it comes about that a stone in the lowermost calyx is often treated by a lower polar partial nephrectomy.

Nephrectomy. This operation is indicated if stones have destroyed most of the renal substance, and the other kidney has been proved by intravenous urography or radioisotope renogram to be functioning normally.

2. Extracorporeal shock wave lithotripsy (ESWL). If high energy shock waves (electrohydraulic, acoustic or piezoelectric) are concentrated onto a stone in the kidney, it disintegrates into small particles, which are then passed out with the urine. In this method the waves are focussed onto the stone with the aid of fluoroscopy or ultrasound. It used to be a requirement of this method to soak the patient in a tub bath, but this has become unnecessary. After being broken down, the small bits pass out with some colic.

The *advantage* of this method is that the kidney does not have to be exposed at open operation. As such, the pain and the problems associated with a major wound in the loin, e.g. infection, haematoma formation, etc., are avoided.

However, there are also important *drawbacks* to the method. Whereas in the case of open operation all the stones and pieces of gravel are removed completely and with certainty, with lithotripsy the gravel is left in the urinary tract to pass out. Specially if the stone was a large one, this mass of gravel can produce its own problems, the more important ones being obstruction and resulting infection. Small pieces of fragmented calculi collect in the distal ureter, like sand occluding a straw. This condition is called *steinstrasse* ('stone street'). A *double-pigtail* catheter is usually passed through a cystoscope up into the ureter to during pregnancy. This results in stasis of urine and infection.

Ascending infection is potentiated by any *obstructive* process, e.g. due to prostatic hypertrophy, stricture, stone or bladder tumour. *Quite often such infection is precipitated by the passage of a catheter, therefore full aseptic precautions should be taken during the procedure.*

It should be remembered that urinary tract infection *in childhood* may be overlooked, as there may be no symptoms referable to the urinary tract. Therefore one should be on the lookout for it in a child who fails to thrive or has a high temperature with rigors; the urine should be examined in such cases for pus cells. Most cases are due to congenital abnormalities producing *obstruction,* and usually require operative relief of the obstruction.

The other important cause of urinary infections in childhood is *reflux* of urine up the ureters. If conservative measures fail and renal scarring results, reimplantation of the ureter into the bladder is required, to put an end to the reflux by creating an oblique tunnel for the ureter through the bladder wall.

Clinical features. The illness starts suddenly with a rigor and vomiting. There is severe pain in the loin. The temperature rises, and is swinging in type. Cystitis develops, and leads to frequency of micturition. There is scalding pain on passing urine. The loin and the hypochondrium are tender. *If the infection is bilateral and severe, symptoms of uraemia may be present.* The urine is scanty and concentrated. If a centrifuged deposit is examined under the microscope, it is loaded with pus cells and bacteria.

Differential diagnosis. If the symptoms and signs are atypical the condition may be confused with *acute appendicitis, acute cholecystitis* or *pneumonia.* In pyelonephritis the pain does not start from the midline; this helps distinguish it from appendicitis. Intravenous urography will show no shadow, or a hazy shadow, of the renal pelvis on the affected side.

Treatment. If treatment is to be successful it must be started early and continued for a sufficiently long time; *brief courses of antibiotics allow the organisms to become resistant to them,* so that the treatment fails to eradicate the infection. After the course of treatment has been completed, follow-up with repeated cultures and white cell counts of the urine is necessary to ensure that the condition has been cured. Intravenous pyelography to exclude the presence of abnormalities in the urinary tract is an essential part of the follow-up of the case. Before any antibiotics are started a mid-stream specimen of urine should be taken and sent for culture and tests of the sensitivity of the organisms to antibiotics. After the specimen has been obtained, a broad-spectrum antibacterial e.g. ampicillin or co-trimoxazole, should be started pending the results of the tests. When these arrive, the antibiotic may have to be changed.

For *pain* an antispasmodic e.g. hyoscine, and an analgesic, e.g. paracetamol or metamizole, should be prescribed. Morphine or pethidine may sometimes be required. *Bed rest* is an important part of the treatment. In *E. coli* infections the urine is acid. In these cases *alkalinization* of the urine, using powders containing potassium citrate and sodium bicarbonate, helps not only in relieving symptoms but also in inhibiting the growth of the organisms by changing the pH of the urine. The patient should drink large quantities of fluids. If vomiting and dehydration occur, intravenous fluids may be required. When a course of an antibiotic has been started, the urine should be cultured about four and seven days later, to find out what effect the antibiotic is having. The antibiotic should be continued for at least three weeks. If a congenital abnormality is found which is causing obstruction, surgery will be required, as otherwise the infection will continue to recur.

Choice of antibacterial agent. No one agent is the drug of choice for all cases. A short-acting oral sulphonamide, like sulphisoxazole is preferred by many, in a dose of 1 gm 4 times a day. However, this drug cannot be used in newborns and pregnant women. Apart from this, equally effective alternate choices of antibiotic therapy include the following, the doses mentioned being administered 4 times a day:

1. Ampicillin or amoxicillin 500 mg.
2. Cephalexin or cephradine 250–500 mg.
3. Nitrofurantoin 100 mg.
4. Tetracycline 250 to 500 mg.

Co-trimoxazole in a dose of two single-strength tablets twice a day is another very useful addition to this list of drugs.

The use of these drugs is often associated with side effects. At the same time compliance with the doctor's instructions is often quite poor. Therefore the rate of treatment failure is quite high, upto 15%.

Gram-negative bacteraemia. In gram-negative bacteraemia the urinary tract often provides the portal of entry. Frequently the bacteraemia follows instrumentation in the presence of pre-existing urinary infection that has been ineffectively treated. The patient experiences a shaking chill followed by high fever, peripheral vasodilatation and hypotension. The organisms are frequently resistant to the usual drugs and require large doses of parenterally administered antibiotics. Drugs that are bactericidal are preferred, to prevent liberation of additional quantities of endotoxin by the multiplying bacteria. An aminoglycoside such as gentamicin, tobramycin, or amikacin, and amoxil or a similar drug in combination have proved effective. Vancomycin can be used as prophylaxis or therapy for staphylococcal infections. Drug dosage is carefully regulated according to renal function.

CHRONIC PYELONEPHRITIS

Repeated bacterial infections of the kidney cause chronic renal insufficiency. However, when such a case is investigated, underlying urinary tract disease is nearly always found, e.g. vesicoureteral reflux, stone or stricture. Most of the damage is caused to the renal tubules which are atrophic, dilated and sometimes cystic. In contrast, the glomeruli retain their structure till late in the disease. The histologic picture is non-specific: inflammatory changes, associated with fibrosis and scarring.

Clinical features. Chronic pyelonephritis produces few symptoms until it ends up in renal insufficiency, and then the symptoms are similar to those of any other form of chronic renal failure. Similarly, the physical findings are few. However, if the disease is the end result of many episodes of acute pyelonephritis, intermittent symptoms of fever, flank pain and dysuria may have occurred in the past.

Laboratory findings. Microscopic study of the urine is nonspecific. There may be an increased number of leucocytes, but their presence in the urine does not prove the existence of upper urinary tract infection. Bacteriuria alone is also not diagnostic of chronic pyelonephritis, and conversely, patients who have chronic pyelonephritis may have negative urine cultures.

X-rays show loss of cortical thickness, blunting of calyces, contracture, cortical scars with an irregular contour, and decreased excretion of contrast material. In the absence of stones, obstruction and tuberculosis, and without a history of ingestion of analgesics, chronic pyelonephritis is virtually the only disease that produces a localized scar over a deformed calyx. *Ultrasound examination* shows up blunted calyces with thinning of the overlying cortex, and aids in diagnosis.

Management. The management of chronic pyelonephritis should be directed towards treating infections if present, preventing future infections, and monitoring and preserving renal function. Investigations should be carried out to detect the underlying cause, which can usually be found. In advanced cases diminishing renal function may require recurrent haemodialysis. Transplantation of a kidney from a donor or a cadaver may be possible.

PYONEPHROSIS

In this condition the kidney is reduced to a sac containing pus and urine. A pyonephrosis can result from the following:

1. Infection in a hydronephrosis: in such a case the wall of the sac often consists of a thin shell of fibrous tissue, with very few remnants of renal substance.
2. Infection in a case of renal calculus (calculus pyonephrosis).
3. Acute pyelonephritis.

Clinical features. There is fever, anaemia, and a tender swelling in the loin. If the pyenophrosis is open, cystitis may result, producing frequency and dysuria; if it is closed the fever may be quite high, with a swinging temperature.

Imaging. *Ultrasound* examination shows the enlarged kidney containing fluid with echoes, i.e. turbid fluid. If the cause is a stone it is visualized, with an acoustic shadow underneath. *Plain x-ray* also shows up most stones. *Intravenous urography* shows absence of excretion of dye on the affected side. In open pyonephrosis *cystoscopy* may show efflux of pus from the ureter on the affected side.

ESR. If in a case with a renal swelling, kidney function on the affected side is absent as shown by the intravenous pyelogram, the differential diagnosis includes hydronephrosis and pyonephrosis. To distinguish between the two conditions, ESR plays an important part; in hydronephrosis it is normal, in pyonephrosis it is markedly raised.

Management. The appropriate antibiotics should be administered through the intravenous route for maximum effect. At the same time immediate drainage of the kidney must be carried out. This can take the form of either percutaneous or open nephrostomy. When the case has stabilized, either appropriate corrective surgery or nephrectomy should be carried out. Nephrectomy is indicated when obstruction is known to have destroyed most of the renal substance, and function on the other side is good. Corrective surgery can be undertaken if a remediable obstruction is found, and the kidney substance is in a good state of preservation.

PERINEPHRIC ABSCESS

A perinephric abscess consists of a collection of pus in the perinephric space due to rupture of an acute cortical abscess into this space. Patients with pyonephrosis are very susceptible to the formation of a perinephric abscess. In a few patients such an abscess arises due to haematogenous spread, usually from sites of skin infection. The *clinical presentation* of perinephric abscess is similar to that of pyelonephritis, but the symptoms come on more gradually. A mass in the flank can be felt in about half the cases. Laboratory findings include leucocytosis, raised serum creatinine, and pyuria in about 75% of cases. Pyelonephritis usually responds to appropriate antibiotic therapy in 4 or 5 days, while perinephric abscess does not. Therefore, if the condition does not resolve within that period, perinephric abscess should be suspected. On *plain x-ray* the psoas border is not visible, being obscured due to the inflammatory oedema. There may be a scoliosis towards the affected side.

Treatment. Antibiotics are commenced. Through a lumbar incision the abscess is incised and drained, any pockets of pus being opened. A large drain is placed in the perinephric space and the wound closed. The pus is sent for culture and sensitivity tests.

TUBERCULOSIS OF THE KIDNEY

Pathology. Tuberculosis of the urinary tract cannot arise except as a blood-borne infection. However, the distant focus from which the infection arrives at the kidney is normally not demonstrable. Microscopic lesions gradually enlarge and discharge pus and tubercle bacilli along the tubules, producing ulceration of the pyramid. The progress of the disease is slow. In the early stages *tubercle bacilluria* may be the only evidence of tuberculosis. However, it should be taken seriously and treated with the appropriate drugs. With the passage of time tuberculosis may produce one of the following lesions in the kidney:

A *caseous mass* may form in the cortex. This may rupture into the pelvis, discharging its contents and resulting in the formation of a cavity in communication with the pelvis. Alternatively, it may rupture into the perinephric space leading to a *perinephric abscess.* A stricture may form at the pelviureteric junction, leading to *hydronephrosis.* Secondary infection, usually with *E. coli*, may supervene, leading to the development of a *pyonephrosis.* The whole kidney may become a mass of *caseous* material. Finally, in generalized *miliary tuberculosis* the kidney may also be involved. Untreated, the disease spreads along the ureter to give rise to tuberculous cystitis. In the male it can also spread to the seminal vesicles and the epididymis.

Clinical features. Tuberculosis of the kidney occurs most commonly between the ages of twenty and forty, men being twice as often affected as women. The earliest symptom is increased *frequency* of micturition, both by day and by night. At the same time there may be *suprapubic pain* and *terminal haematuria.* These symptoms are due to tuberculous cystitis. In a few cases there may be *painless haematuria,* the blood coming from an ulcer situated on a renal papilla. In most other cases the blood is only detected on microscopic examination. There is usually slight *loss of weight* and some evening rise of temperature. On *examination* the kidney is usually not enlarged to such an extent as to be palpable. The prostate, seminal vesicles, vasa deferentia, and epididymes should always be examined for evidence of tuberculous involvement, which usually takes the form of one or more nodules in these structures.

Investigations. An early morning specimen of *urine* should be examined. It should be centrifuged and the sediment stained with Ziehl-Neelsen's stain for acid-fast bacilli. At the same time guinea-pig inoculation and Lowenstein-Jensen (LJ) culture should be carried out. Staining for acid-fast bacilli is usually negative, while LJ culture and guinea-pig inoculation are positive in a high percentage of cases. *Plain x-ray* may show calcification in healing foci, either in the form of specks or as broad dense areas. A chest x-ray should be taken to rule out pulmonary tuberculosis. In early cases *intravenous urography* may show absence or irregularity of a calyx. When a calyx is completely obstructed an abscess may form, which displaces adjacent calyces. The fibrosed ureter is shortened, and is therefore more straight than a normal ureter. If cystitis develops the bladder becomes more rounded due to spasm. On *cystoscopy* the earliest change takes the form of oedema around the ureteric orifice followed by the development of tubercles, and later ulcers, in the area. In long-standing cases as the ureter becomes shortened, its orifice remains open – the *golf-hole* ureter. In advanced disease the capacity of the bladder gradually diminishes.

Treatment. Anti-tuberculosis therapy is carried out. If the full course of medicines is given there is a high cure rate, with few recurrences. In certain situations operation may become necessary. For example if very advanced disease is present, nephroureterectomy may be carried out. For hydronephrosis, pyeloplasty may be employed. If a caseous mass is present in the renal cortex it may be deroofed (*cavernostomy*) and evacuated.

NEOPLASMS OF THE KIDNEY

Benign neoplasms are very rare. Adenomas usually produce no symptoms and are found incidentally at autopsy. Angiomas can produce haematuria.

Malignant neoplasms occur commonly either in infancy and early childhood, or after the age of forty. The common renal malignancy of childhood is Wilms' tumor. In adult life hypernephroma occurs commonly, and transitional cell carcinoma of the renal pelvis is seen from time to time.

NEPHROBLASTOMA (WILMS' TUMOUR)

Nephroblastoma (Wilms' tumour) is the most common intra-abdominal tumour of children. The incidence is 1/10000 live births. The peak incidence is between 2 and 4 years; very few cases occur after the age of 7. Very occasionally both kidneys are affected. An interesting feature of this tumour is that growths arising below the age of one year have a much better prognosis.

Aetiology. Knudson has explained the development of nephroblastoma on the basis of his two-hit hypothesis, namely that two separate factors act to cause the disease:

1. A tumour suppressor gene is normally present on chromosome 11; this is lost ('first-hit').
2. This then allows tumour development in the presence of any predisposing factor; this constitutes the 'second-hit'.

Pathology. On *section* the tumour is greyish or pinkish white in colour. As regards consistency, the slower growing tumours are firm, whereas rapidly growing tumours are soft. This is in fact a general rule among most tumours, of whichever organ.

Microscopically the tumour is unusual in having both epithelial and connective tissue elements; most other tumours have either the one or the other type. Histological markers of a poor *prognosis* include extreme cellular pleomorphism (anaplasia) and the presence of sarcomatous changes. Tumours with these characteristics are termed UH (unfavourable histology), while those without anaplasia and sarcomatous changes are called FH (favourable histology). Whereas the relapse-free survival rates in UH tumours are only about 30%, the same rates for FH tumours are as high as 75%. Therefore *the histopathology report is an important part of the data on which the estimate of prognosis is based.*

Staging by the National Wilms' Tumour Staging Group (NWTSG) is shown in Table 1.

Clinical features. *Swelling.* The infant is nearly always brought because the mother noticed a swelling in the abdomen, which has been enlarging rapidly. Along with this the general health deteriorates. On examination the swelling is found to be filling most of the abdomen; however, it can usually be shown that the tumour is arising from one side. This tumour usually grows within a capsule, pushing the rest of the kidney aside.

Fever. A number of patients run a slight temperature, which subsides when the tumour is removed.

Haematuria. Normally there is no blood in the urine, as the tumour is away from the pelvis. Haematuria is a bad sign, as it shows the tumour has burst through its capsule into the renal pelvis.

Table 1 Modified NWTSG staging of nephroblastoma.

Stage I	Tumour limited to kidney
Stage II	Tumour extends beyond capsule but completely excised
Stage III	Local spread of tumour in abdomen
Stage IV	Deposits in brain, lung or liver
Stage V	Bilateral renal involvement

Certain *anomalies* may occasionally be associated with Wilms' tumour: aniridia, hemihypertrophy and deformities of the external genitalia.

Metastases. Wilms' tumour metastasizes early by the bloodstream to the lungs, and less commonly to the liver and bones. Lymphatic dissemination is a great deal less common.

Investigations. *Ultrasound examination* is first carried out, and confirms that a solid mass arises from the kidney. The other kidney is examined, the liver checked for secondaries, and the renal vein imaged to exclude venous tumour extension. *Intravenous urography* shows the kidney displaced upwards or downwards by the tumour, with the calyces stretched out on the surface of the mass; it also indicates renal function. A *chest x-ray* may show cannon ball secondaries in the lungs. A *radioisotope skeletal scan* shows up any bony metastases. A *blood count* and *biochemical profile* are also performed.

Differential diagnosis. The only swelling with which a Wilms' tumour can be confused is a neuroblastoma. However, the treatment of both the tumours is similar. If x-rays show secondaries in the bones, this favours the diagnosis of neuroblastoma.

Treatment. The treatment of a nephroblastoma consists of urgent nephrectomy followed by radiotherapy. In contrast to renal cell carcinoma, radiotherapy and chemotherapy have much to offer after nephrectomy for nephroblastoma. During recent decades survival has improved dramatically due to improved surgical techniques as well as refinements in radiotherapy and chemotherapy.

Nephrectomy. Radical nephrectomy is carried out, through an anterior transperitoneal approach for better access to the renal vessels. It entails removal *en bloc* of Gerota's fascia (with its contents: kidney, adrenal and perinephric fat) along with the upper ureter and renal vessels. This *en bloc* removal is carried out because it has been shown that spread into the perinephric fat worsens the prognosis. The opposite kidney is palpated to exclude a bilateral tumour.

In *bilateral* tumours a radical nephrectomy is carried out on the side of the larger tumour, with partial nephrectomy on the other side. In these cases a *renal hyperperfusion syndrome* develops after operation, and can lead to chronic deterioration in renal function. This effect has stimulated a renal-sparing approach to surgery, particularly as effective chemotherapy is becoming available.

Extensive *lymphadenectomy* is not advised, but lymph node sampling probably improves staging. If venous *tumour thrombus* is found, it may recede after preoperative chemotherapy. If the tumour thrombus extends to the heart cardiopulmonary bypass may be required for its removal.

Chemotherapy and radiotherapy. A combination of radiotherapy and chemotherapy maximizes benefits and minimizes side effects. Again, combination chemotherapy is more effective than single agents, vincristine, actinomycin D and doxorubicin being commonly employed. However, the preoperative use of these therapies has been decried on two grounds:

1. Staging is more accurate in the untreated patient.
2. Upto 8% children prove, after nephrectomy, to be suffering from some other condition.

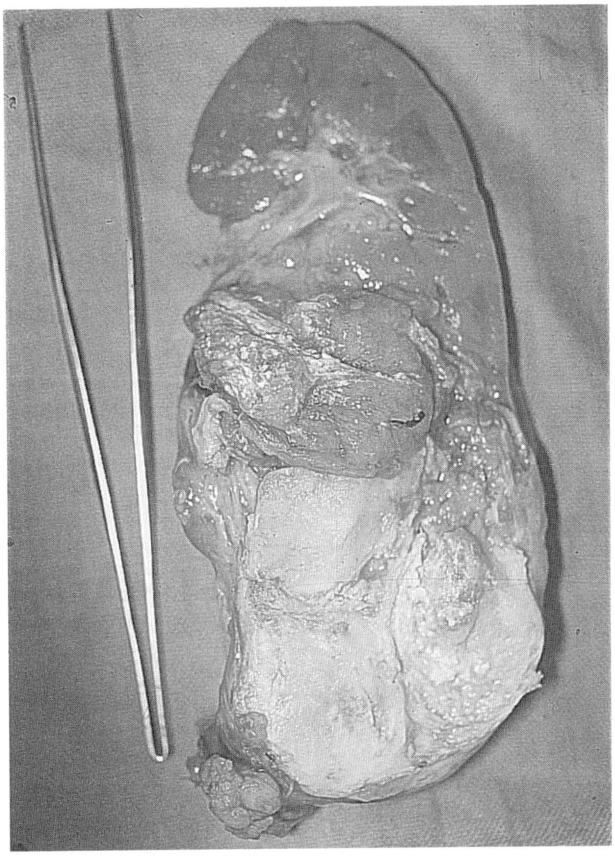

Fig. 3 Renal cell carcinoma occupying one pole of the kidney.

Recurrence after treatment is difficult to manage, and a multidisciplinary approach is best. Ifosfamide, cisplatin and etoposide are all effective and are used. The *prognosis* after nephrectomy and radiotherapy is much better under the age of 1 year; under this age 80% infants survive five years, over it only 30%.

RENAL CELL CARCINOMA

Pathology. This is an adenocarcinoma and is the most common neoplasm of the kidney. It is usually rounded in shape, and occupies one or the other pole of the kidney (Fig. 3). On section it is commonly yellow due to the fat content, often with haemorrhagic areas. Fibrous septa divide it into lobules. In the larger tumours the cells at the centre, being away from the blood supply, often undergo necrosis.

Microscopically, solid alveoli of cubical or polyhedral clear cells are seen, with deeply staining small rounded nuclei and abundant cytoplasm. There are numerous blood vessels, whose walls appear to be made up of tumour cells at places.

Spread. As the tumour enlarges it tends to grow into the renal veins. From the veins tumour emboli can lodge in the lungs to produce *cannon-ball* secondaries. The other common sites for metastases are the bones. At the same time spread by lymphatics occurs, first to the lymph nodes in the hilum of the kidney and from there to the para-aortic nodes.

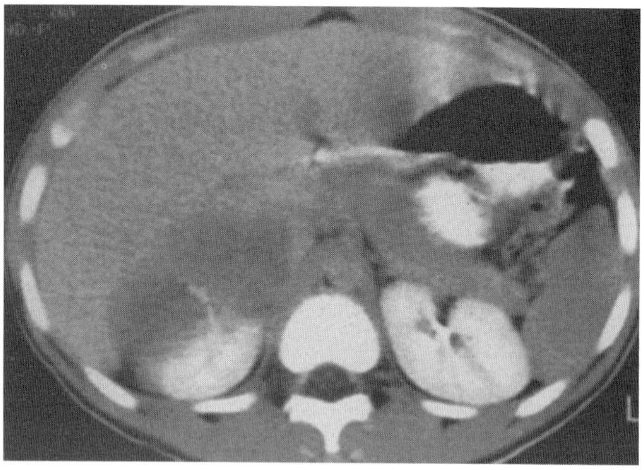

Fig. 4 CT scan: renal cell carcinoma right kidney.

Clinical features. Men are twice as often affected by renal cell carcinoma as women. The earliest sign is *haematuria*, which is usually intermittent. If the blood gets coagulated during its passage through the ureter it may produce *colic*. In other cases there may simply be a dull pain in the loin. Occasionally the patient comes with the complaint of a *swelling*. Unusual presentations include the rapid development of a *varicocele* due to blockage of the left spermatic vein by tumour cells; moderate *fever* due to absorption of blood and necrotic material; a spontaneous *fracture* due to a bone secondary; and cough or haemoptysis due to secondaries in the lungs. Finally, an increasing number of tumours is being detected *incidentally* because of the widespread use of CT scans.

Diagnosis. The presence of any of the above clinical manifestations may cause a clinician to suspect renal malignancy and to begin investigations. A *plain x-ray* is first carried out. Calcification of a renal mass seen on x-ray significantly increases the chances of its being a cancer. *Intravenous urography* is now carried out, preferably with nephrotomography. The intravenous urogram also shows the function of the opposite kidney. When a renal mass is seen on urography, the most common lesion responsible for it is a renal cyst.

If an *ultrasound scan* is now carried out, it shows whether the lesion is solid or cystic. If it is a *cyst* it can usually be left alone, but its progress should be monitored repeatedly by ultrasound scans, and in case of enlargement it should be aspirated for cytological examination. If the mass is *solid* the liver, renal vein and inferior vena cava should be examined to exclude the presence of hepatic metastases and spread via the renal vein. Finally, a *CT scan* (Fig. 4) or *MRI* confirms that the mass is solid and may give some indication of its nature and extent, which helps greatly in staging. Solid lesions can be *biopsied* under x-ray guidance, but most lesions are removed surgically because of the high likelihood of renal cell carcinoma, so biopsy is seldom performed. If there is doubt about spread via the renal vein, a *vena cavography* should be carried out.

At places where a CT scan is not available, *renal arteriography* should be carried out; it shows up the arrangement of blood vessels in the mass. The blood vessels in a tumour generally conform to a pattern, and this helps the diagnosis. However, angiography is an invasive procedure, and carries a small but definite risk of arterial embolism.

A *chest x-ray* should always be taken to show up or rule out lung secondaries. An *isotope bone scan* should be carried out, as it shows up bone metastases. If it is positive, the sites of metastases should be examined by radiography for details concerning the metastases.

Staging. As regards the extent of spread of the tumour, renal cell carcinomas are classified into four stages as follows:

Stage I: Tumour confined by renal capsule.

Stage II: Tumour confined by Gerota's fascia.

Stage III: Tumour involving renal vein and/or lymph nodes.

Stage IV: Spread to contiguous organs, or distant metastases.

Local clinical staging depends primarily on CT scan.

Treatment. *Nephrectomy.* If metastases are not present, the treatment of renal cell carcinoma is nephrectomy. Even if metastases are present, nephrectomy may still be performed to control local symptoms such as pain or haematuria. In order to provide for removal wide of the tumour, the perinephric fat is excised with the kidney. This operation is called *radical nephrectomy*. However, there is no evidence that radical nephrectomy confers a survival advantage compared to simple nephrectomy. Manipulation of the kidney or its veins during the operation can result in dislodgement of tumour emboli. To prevent this eventuality, the renal pedicle should be ligated first. The abdominal approach is best for accomplishing this. Removal of para-aortic nodes has been advocated; however, there is no evidence to confirm a survival advantage of this more extensive procedure. Upto 10% of patients have a vena caval tumour thrombus. If no metastases are present, removal of the thrombus can be followed by prolonged survival.

Partial nephrectomy may be employed in the following situations:

1. In a solitary kidney.
2. With bilateral tumours.
3. In cases where the tumour has been detected incidentally by radiology, and is quite small in size.

Embolization. In cases with advanced disease and a symptomatic primary tumour, embolization relieves symptoms with less morbidity than that associated with nephrectomy. At the same time, it can reduce the vascularity of very large tumours before surgery. The renal artery can be occluded by a variety of materials introduced via a percutaneous arterial catheter.

Radiotherapy does not improve survival, whether given pre- or postoperatively. However, it can relieve the pain of bone metastases.

Treatment of metastases. Renal cell carcinoma is unusual in that resection of solitary metastases (specially pulmonary or cerebral) can be followed on occasion by long-term survival. Radiotherapy relieves pain due to skeletal metastases in most patients, and internal fixation can stabilize long bones affected by metastatic disease.

No *cytotoxic* agent used either alone or in combination has shown more than a 10% response rate.

Immunotherapy. For metastatic renal cell carcinoma both interferons and interleukins have been used. Interferons have produced remissions in 13% of patients for about 8 months. Interleukins are lymphokines produced by T lymphocytes which enhance the killing of tumour cells. Interleukin-2 has elicited remissions in 20% patients for about 3 years. The two types of agents have also been combined with additive effects.

The latest approach is *adoptive immunotherapy.* This involves administration of cells which have antitumour activity. Initial reports have been encouraging.

Prognosis. This depends upon the histological type, the presence of local extension into the renal vein, perinephric tissues and lymph nodes, and distant metastases. The overall survival rate for renal tumours is about 50% for 5 years and 33% for 10 years. Stage-wise 5 year survivals are approximately as follows: stage I found incidentally, 85%; stage I, 65%; stage II, 55%; stage III 40%. This shows the importance of early diagnosis.

PAPILLOMA OF THE PELVIS

Papillomas of the renal pelvis are transitional cell tumours, which resemble bladder papillomas but are less common. They tend to invade the kidney and become malignant. Multiple tumours of the ureter and the bladder can arise due to seeding.

Clinical features. These tumours present with haematuria, which may continue for weeks. The kidney is usually not palpable. Clot colic may occur.

Investigations. The *urine* shows red cells, and may show exfoliated malignant cells. *Ultrasonography* and *CT scan* show a soft tissue mass in the renal pelvis, while on *intravenous urography* a filling defect is seen in the pelvis.

Treatment. Papillomas of the renal pelvis are treated by nephroureterectomy. The excision of the ureter should extend downwards to include the intramural ureter along with the ureteric orifice, to minimize the chances of leaving behind tumour implants.

SQUAMOUS-CELLED CARCINOMA OF THE RENAL PELVIS

This tumour is rare. It is usually preceded by leucoplakia, and in most cases a stone is present; these factors result in metaplasia of the transitional epithelium of the renal pelvis to squamous, predisposing the patient to the development of squamous-celled carcinoma. Symptoms are vague, so that the diagnosis is often missed. As the diagnosis is often made at a late stage, the prognosis is poor.

Operative steps of nephrectomy. The patient is placed on the table in the lateral *position* with the affected side uppermost. The leg on the affected side is fully extended, the other leg which lies underneath in this position is flexed at the hip and the knee. The patient is held in this position by a strap which passes over the pelvis, and is fixed at either side to the edges of the table. An arm rest supports the upper arm, so that it does not lie on the chest and embarrass respiration.

Morris's incision is the one most commonly employed to expose the kidney. It commences at the renal angle and runs forwards and downwards towards the anterior superior iliac spine. All muscle layers are divided in the line of the incision. If this is made with the use of a cutting diathermy current, it saves a good deal of both blood and time. Alternatively, the incision is made over the 12th rib which is resected subperiosteally avoiding the pleura. This allows the incision to be made at a higher level, providing for better exposure of the kidney. The perinephric fascia is now opened and the perinephric fat dissected away from the kidney all round, using mostly blunt dissection. The blood vessels at the hilum are exposed, ligated individually, and divided, and the kidney removed. The wound is closed in layers, leaving a suction drain in place.

31 Urinary bladder

Cystoscopy. In the diagnosis and management of diseases affecting the urinary bladder, cystoscopy plays a central role. Many conditions can only be diagnosed by direct visualization of the bladder mucosa, e.g. sources of bleeding, inflammatory lesions and bladder trabeculation. Tumours can be visualized as well as biopsied; they can also be resected through the working element of a cystoscope. Conventional cystoscopes are rigid and vary from 15 to 24 French in size. They have fibreoptic illumination which allows better visualization. The recently-introduced flexible cystoscopes result in less discomfort, specially in male patients, and provide visualization in all directions. In addition, they make the lithotomy position unnecessary; the examination can be carried out in the supine position and without anaesthesia.

ECTOPIA VESICAE (EXSTROPHY OF THE BLADDER)

Ectopia vesicae arises due to incomplete development of the infraumbilical part of the abdominal wall and of the anterior wall of the bladder. It arises once in 50,000 births. Intra-abdominal pressure causes the posterior bladder wall to protrude through the defect. The trigone is seen at the lower part, with spurts of urine being discharged from the ureteric orifices. The exposed bladder mucosa tends to become chronically inflamed. When the bladder wall is reduced backwards the edge of the abdominal wall defect can be felt. Umbilical and inguinal hernias may be present. The rami of the pubic bones are widely separated and the pelvic ring is 'open', affecting the gait. On the other hand in those females who become pregnant this separation of the pubes facilitates delivery. In the male child epispadias is present, and the penis is shorter and broader than normal. The unfortunate patient smells of urine and remains wet all the time. He suffers repeated urinary infections, and most such patients die of renal failure before the age of thirty.

Treatment. 1. In the past ectopia vesicae was treated by *diversion of urine*. This was achieved by one of the following two methods:

i. The classical method was *ureterosigmoidostomy*, i.e. implantation of both ureters into the sigmoid colon. The main problems associated with this operation were two:

(a) Urine refluxed up the ureter to cause recurrent urinary tract infections. This problem was partly overcome by creating a submucosal tunnel in the colon for the ureter, so that a valve was created and reflux prevented.

(b) Excessive absorption of chloride ions by the colonic mucosa produced *hyperchloraemic acidosis*. For this, powders containing sodium bicarbonate and potassium citrate were administered.

By this method of urinary diversion there was an improvement in the quality of life. The patient passed a mixture of urine and faeces per anum. He was no longer wet or foul smelling. However, most patients did not live beyond their teens or twenties.

ii. Later, in order to avoid hyperchloraemic acidosis, surgeons started diverting the urine to an *isolated loop of terminal ileum*, which was opened out in the right iliac fossa. Because disposable ileostomy bags become available about this time, this method become more popular than ureterosigmoidostomy. However, the life-long care of an *ileal-loop bladder* is no easy matter.

2. Recently, *closure of the bladder* and the abdominal wall has been tried. The urethral groove is also closed to make a tube, and is placed behind the pubis, which is brought together in the midline. The success of this operation is very variable, most patients failing to achieve continence. Although results in recent series are somewhat better than in the past, exstrophy of the bladder remains as one of the unsolved problems in surgery, posing a challenge to surgeons of the future.

RUPTURE OF THE BLADDER

The bladder may be ruptured in its intraperitoneal or extraperitoneal portion. *Intraperitoneal rupture* is usually caused by a blow on a fully distended bladder. Besides this gunshot and stab wounds, the passage of instruments, and diathermy coagulation of bladder tumours can also be responsible. Following the trauma there is sudden severe pain in the hypogastrium, with shock. However, soon the pain gets diminished due to wide distribution of the urine in the peritoneal cavity. If the quantity of urine is large, shifting dullness may be found. The abdomen distends due to paralytic ileus and is rigid. Because the bladder is collapsed after rupture, the patient has no desire to pass urine, and there is no dullness in the suprapubic region. *Extraperitoneal rupture* occurs after a fracture of the pelvis with penetration by bone spicules, as also after instrumentation and penetrating wounds. It cannot be differentiated from rupture of the posterior urethra, so it is discussed along with it.

The *diagnosis* of rupture of the bladder may be confirmed by passing a catheter and injecting a radiopaque dye. X-rays taken will show leakage of urine outside the bladder.

Treatment. If rupture of the bladder is strongly suspected operation should be carried out at once. A midline subumbilical incision is commonly used. The edges of the tear in the bladder wall are trimmed and repaired by two layers of catgut stitches, and a wide-bore catheter is sutured into the bladder, to be removed after about a week. Early operation is followed by a low morbidity and mortality rate.

Bladder injury during childbirth. The bladder may be injured during childbirth. The most common example of obstetric injury to the bladder is that which occurs in neglected obstructed labour. In this condition there is pressure necrosis of the anterior wall of the upper part of the vagina and the contiguous wall of the bladder due to prolonged and unrelieved pressure of the baby's head, and a vesicovaginal fistula results. This is a most distressing condition for the poor sufferer, with urine constantly dribbling from the vagina so that she is wet and foul-smelling all the time. The fistula requires very skilful repair of the walls of the vagina and bladder in layers. The incidence of vesicovaginal fistula can be reduced only by better obstetric care.

FOREIGN BODIES IN THE BLADDER

These are not common. Hairpins and similar assorted objects have been found in the bladder, which in most cases have been introduced during urethral masturbation. Occasionally a piece of tubing may be left behind after cystostomy. The foreign body may result in infection, perforation of the bladder or stone formation. A small foreign body can be removed by an operating cystoscope; a larger one requires a suprabupic operation.

RETENTION OF URINE

Retention of urine may be acute or chronic.

Acute retention. ***Aetiology.*** The *most common causes* of acute retention in the male are prostatic enlargement, urethral stricture, and postoperative retention. In the female retroverted gravid uterus and multiple sclerosis account for most cases.

Less common causes include: spinal anaesthesia or spinal cord injury, blood clot in the bladder, and faecal impaction in the rectum. Causes in the urethra include rupture of the urethra, urethritis, urethral calculus, and phimosis.

Clinical features. The patient is unable to micturate, although he has not passed urine for several hours. If the patient is slim the distended bladder may be seen, otherwise it can be palpated as a slightly tender swelling above the pubic symphysis which is dull to percussion. As the bladder muscle contracts, spasms of acute pain occur from time to time.

Examination. On *inspection* a tight phimosis, or in the case of a circumcised patient a meatal stricture, may be seen. On *palpation* along the urethra on the ventral aspect of the penis, an area of induration due to a stricture or a calculus in the urethra may be felt. *Digital rectal examination* may reveal an enlarged prostate. In order to exclude a neurogenic cause, the *reflexes* in the lower limbs and *sensations* in the perineum must be tested as a routine in all cases.

Treatment. If a patient presents with acute retention of urine he must be admitted and made comfortable. A few cases will pass urine just like that; most will require more active measures. A *sedative* injection and sitting in a tub or basin of *hot water* will sufficiently relax the sphincters in a few patients so that urine can pass. If this does not come about, a *catheter* will have to be passed into the bladder to evacuate the urine. This should be carried out under full aseptic precautions, i.e. mask, sterile gloves, cleansing of the genitalia with an antiseptic, use of a sterile catheter, etc. In the absence of a stricture the catheter should pass easily.

The common conditions in which the catheter will not pass are two:

1. If the middle lobe of the *prostate* is enlarged it may obstruct the passage of the catheter. In that case a coude' catheter, i.e. one with a bent tip, will usually pass. Alternatively, if the patient is fit, an immediate prostatectomy may be carried out.

2. In the case of *stricture* the catheter will be held up. Only a filiform bougie will be able to pass. These are fine bougies made of gum elastic. When one filiform has been made to pass, a series of follower bougies can be screwed onto it and the stricture dilated. A small catheter can now be passed and left indwelling.

If after two or three attempts the catheter refuses to pass, the urine may be evacuated by *suprapubic puncture*, e.g. with a lumbar puncture needle. Alternatively, a catheter is inserted into the bladder through a 1.5 cm incision made under local anaesthesia about 2 cm below the point where the bladder wall starts receding. The fibres of the linea alba are divided. The catheter on its introducer is passed until it meets the resistance of the muscle wall of the distended bladder. It is passed into the bladder with a short, sharp thrust downwards and backwards. The introducer is removed. The catheter is passed onwards and secured to the skin with a stitch (*suprapubic catheterization*).

Chronic retention. As chronic retention comes on gradually and the bladder distends slowly, the distension of the bladder is painless. If the blood urea is above 70 mg/dl, the bladder should be decompressed slowly, as bleeding can sometimes start from the rapid decompression of a chronically distended bladder.

MANAGEMENT OF THE BLADDER IN SPINAL INJURIES

Immediately after a spinal cord injury spinal shock occurs, from which the bladder may take weeks to recover. The detrusor muscle is paralysed, so that the bladder distends and overflow incontinence results. In the stagnant urine infection takes place, which gradually damages the kidney so much so as to end up in renal failure.

In order to assess the extent of the neurological damage the following examinations are performed:

1. The level of *sensory* and *motor* loss is charted, in order to find out the upper level of the neurological lesion. It may be mentioned that sacral segments S2, 3 and 4, which contain the bladder outflow, lie at the level of the T12 and L1 vertebrae. If the sensory loss below this level is total, recovery is unlikely. On the other hand if the lesion is incomplete, some recovery of bladder function may take place.

2. The *bulbo-cavernosus* and *anal reflexes* are tested. If these are present it indicates that the sacral cord is intact, and a reflex or automatic bladder will ultimately emerge. If the reflexes are absent and perineal sensation is lost, recovery is unlikely and the bladder will behave in an autonomous fashion.

3. A *full assessment* of the bladder function is carried out at the end of three months after injury:

i. Lesions *above cord segment D10* result in an upper motor neurone type lesion. All bladder reflexes are intact, but the bladder is separated from higher control and inhibition. Irregular detrusor contractions with spasm of the external sphincter produce the condition called detrusor sphincter dyssynergia. The intravesical pressure is chronically raised, so that the upper urinary tract suffers from back-pressure effects. Hydronephrosis may result, ultimately ending up in renal failure.

ii. Lesions involving *segments D11 to L2* involve the sympathetic outflow: the result is an upper motor neurone type of lesion, with the additional loss of sympathetic afferents and sensory efferents from the bladder.

iii. Damage to the *sacral centre S2, 3, 4* and cauda equina lesions: this type of damage results essentially in a lower motor neurone bladder. The detrusor is paralysed due to injury to the parasympathetic outflow. Abdominal straining and manual pressure on the bladder can produce emptying. If D11 and 12 segments are intact, sensations through the hypogastric nerves enable the patient to know when the bladder is getting full. Alternatively, intermittent catheterization may be employed.

INCONTINENCE OF URINE

Aetiology. 1. *The common causes of incontinence* in men differ from those seen in women:

i. *In the male* chronic retention with overflow is a very common cause of incontinence. This may be secondary to benign prostatic hypertrophy, hypertrophy of the bladder neck, or a urethral stricture. There is a long history of hesitancy (difficulty in initiating urination) with a poor stream, along with 'dribbling incontinence' at night. The bladder is usually visibly distended, and is palpable as a painless suprapubic swelling.

ii. *In the female* the most common cause of leakage of urine is *stress incontinence*, i.e. the involuntary loss of urine associated with an elevation of intra-abdominal pressure. The patient complains of leakage of urine when she laughs, coughs, sneezes, or even changes posture. Physical examination shows that the bladder is not distended. If a finger is placed on either side of the urethra and pushed upwards to support the pelvic floor, incontinence is prevented *(Bonney's test).* The most probable cause of stress incontinence is hypermobility of the urethrovesical junction which results in failure of transmission of increases in pressure equally to urethra and bladder.

Treatment. Minor degrees of stress incontinence can be controlled by alpha adrenergic drugs which tone up the bladder neck muscle. Faradic stimulation and exercises of the pelvic floor also help greatly. However, sometimes the bladder has herniated backwards through the damaged anterior wall of the vagina (cystocele). In such a case surgical repair of the vaginal wall (anterior colporrhaphy) is required. At the same time the neck of the bladder is slung up to the pubis by sutures.

2. *Other causes of incontinence* (common to both sexes) include the following conditions:

i. *Congenital.* Hypospadias, and an ectopic ureteric orifice below the level of the sphincter.

ii. *Trauma.* Injury to the urethra during pelvic surgery or from fracture of the pelvis.

iii. *Neurogenic.* Spinal cord injury, multiple sclerosis, cerebral vascular accident, and Parkinson's disease.

iv. *Psychogenic.* Hysteria and depression may be accompanied by incontinence of urine.

v. *Drugs.* Anticholinergic drugs, tricyclic antidepressants and some antihypertensives can induce incontinence.

VESICAL CALCULUS

A stone in the bladder is common at two ages: in childhood and in old age.

In *children*, bladder stone is very common in the poorer countries, where protein deficiency leads to endemic metabolic bladder stone disease. Elsewhere in the world, bladder stone in children is quite uncommon and occurs due to the same causes as in adults, i.e. obstruction, infection or a foreign body (urinary catheter). The child with a stone in his bladder suffers pain during micturition, and pulls on his penis. Terminal haematuria may be seen. Before the advent of x-rays the method of detecting a bladder stone consisted of the passage of a metallic 'bladder sound' and feeling and hearing the click resulting from its contact with the stone. Today ultrasonography is used to show up the stone. Classically, the stone was removed by open operation; these days it can be dealt with by ultrasound lithotripsy.

In *old age* the obstructive lesion responsible for a vesical calculus is usually an enlarged prostate. The stone is dealt with at the same time as the lesion causing it. A stone less than 2.5 cm in diameter can be fragmented during a transurethral procedure by using the electrohydraulic lithotriptor to fracture it. Stone-crushing forceps can then be used to fragment the stone to pieces that may be irrigated from the bladder. Calculi larger than 3 cm are more difficult to fragment and extract transurethrally and are best dealt with by suprapubic cystotomy. In such a case bladder outlet obstruction may be dealt with by simultaneous removal of the prostate. Alternatively, a suprapubic tube may be left indwelling and a transurethral resection of the prostate carried out as a secondary procedure. Complications include perforation of the bladder from the use of the lithotriptor, mucosal bleeding, and infection.

DIVERTICULUM OF THE BLADDER

A bladder diverticulum is an outpouching of the mucosa through the muscle wall of the bladder. If the protrusion passes outwards only through the inner muscular layers of the wall it should be called a saccule.

The most common *cause* of a diverticulum is an *obstructing lesion* at the bladder neck, examples of the same being congenital valves of the posterior urethra, bladder neck contracture, urethral stricture and benign prostatic enlargement. A *congenital* diverticulum occurs occasionally. In this variety, there is no vesical neck obstruction; it arises due to a developmental defect in the vesical musculature through which the bladder mucosa is protruded by the normal increase in intravesical pressure during micturition.

The most common site for a diverticulum is near a ureteric orifice, usually above and lateral to it. The diverticulum is lined by mucosa and its wall is formed of fibrous tissue. When it enlarges it may compress the ureter. Alternatively, it may incorporate the ureter into its floor, so that vesico-ureteric reflux develops.

The common *complications* of a diverticulum are four:

1. Stagnation of urine in the diverticulum leads to repeated infections.
2. Due to the same reason stones develop in the pouch.
3. Hydronephrosis may develop due to compression of the ureter by the diverticulum.
4. A carcinoma may arise in a small number of cases.

Clinical features. Most patients are males above the age of 50. The patient usually presents with symptoms of the bladder neck obstruction which caused the diverticulum. However, sometimes a patient reports with a urinary tract infection, or a calculus which has arisen due to a diverticulum. In many cases haematuria is a leading symptom. The blood comes from the mucosal lining of the diverticulum, which is inflamed due to the stagnation of urine in its lumen. In occasional cases micturition occurs twice, the second act being due to urine from the diverticulum.

Diagnosis. Diagnosis is usually by *cystoscopy*. The orifice of the diverticulum appears as a dark round hole. On the other hand a saccule, being shallow, is well illuminated. *Excretory* urography gives an indication about the size of the diverticulum, and also shows up any dilatation of the pelvis and ureter. However, if it does not give a good picture *retrograde cystography* may be employed, by emptying the bladder and filling it with a radiopaque medium.

Treatment. Unless the diverticulum is quite small is should be removed, because otherwise it keeps enlarging and causes recurrent infections. Usually the removal is carried out during the operation in which the bladder neck obstruction is treated. If the urine is infected preoperative antibiotics are required. A ureteric catheter is passed up the ureter on the affected side in order to avoid damage to it during dissection.

URINARY FISTULAE

A urinary fistula is an abnormal communication between any part of the urinary tract and the skin or some other internal hollow organ. If a fistula refuses to heal, this may be due to one of the following conditions:

1. Distal obstruction.
2. A foreign body.
3. A chronic infection, e.g. tuberculosis.

Causes of fistulae. ***Congenital.*** 1. *Patent urachus.* The urachus is a canal in the foetus which connects the urinary bladder with the allantois. Normally it closes down and is replaced by a fibrous cord – the median umbilical ligament. Occasionally it persists in its patent form. A patent urachus does not leak, because the contractions of the bladder start from the apex, where the urachus is attached to the umbilicus, and pass down the organ. It reveals itself usually in middle age, and then only if bladder neck obstruction from some cause arises. In such a case there may be leakage of urine from the umbilicus.

Treatment. The bladder neck obstruction is dealt with. If leakage still persists, the urachus is excised and the bladder closed.

2. In some cases of *anorectal anomalies* a fistula may be present between the rectum and the urethra, or the vagina in the female. In the newborn the faecal stream is diverted by a colostomy. Later, when the rectum is mobilized and brought down to the perineum, the fistula is also closed. Alternatively, the fistula can be closed during the operation of posterior sagittal anorectoplasty in the newborn.

Acquired. *Traumatic urinary fistula.* The common causes of this condition are the following:

1. Penetrating wounds.
2. Unrecognized division of ureter or bladder during surgery.
3. Avascular necrosis following radiotherapy for malignant disease.

Vesico-vaginal fistula. This is always a distressing condition because of uncontrolled leakage of urine, which causes dermatitis of the inner thighs with maceration of the skin. Some of its common causes are the following:

1. In areas with inadequate obstetric facilities this is one of the most wretched curses on women from the poorer sections of society.
2. This fistula may also develop due to injury to the bladder during *hysterectomy.*
3. In *carcinoma of the cervix* a vesico-vaginal fistula may develop due to ulceration of the carcinoma into the bladder or after radiotherapy to this lesion.

CYSTITIS

Aetiology. Infection may reach the bladder via the haematogenous route, from infected tonsils, carious teeth etc. Much more commonly, bacteria ascend to the bladder via the urethra. Finally, obstruction at the bladder neck results in infection in the stagnant urine. The most common organism involved is *E. coli,* others being Proteus, *Strep. faecalis* and staphylococci.

Clinical features. There is marked *frequency* of micturition during the day and at night. Lack of sleep produces exhaustion. *Pain* may be severe in the hypogastrium, or the penis or labia. *Pyuria* is always present, and the urine may be blood-stained. On *examination* there is tenderness over the suprapubic region. A midstream urine specimen should be examined microscopically and also cultured.

Treatment with a chemotherapeutic agent should be commenced as soon as the urine has been sent for culture. While awaiting the culture and sensitivity reports nitrofurantoin 100 mg q.i.d. may be started. If the infection recurs, the case must be investigated further to detect the underlying cause.

Tuberculous cystitis. Tuberculous cystitis is always secondary to renal tuberculosis. Cystoscopy shows tubercles around one ureteric orifice. In long-standing cases there is much fibrosis, and the *capacity of the bladder is reduced* resulting in greatly increased frequency of micturition.

The *treatment* of tuberculous cystitis is by antituberculosis drugs. If the bladder is greatly contracted, the marked frequency can be alleviated by ileocystoplasty. In this operation a segment of small intestine is isolated, its lumen is opened along the antimesenteric border, and it is sutured as a patch to the opened dome of the bladder to enlarge its cavity.

BILHARZIASIS OF THE BLADDER

This disease is prevalent in the valley of the Nile, and is also found in some neighbouring Arab countries.

Life cycle. Biharziasis is caused by a trematode called *Schistosoma haematobium*. It is acquired while standing in infected water. The embryos in the water cause infestation of the human being by penetrating the skin of the feet. They reach the liver through the blood-stream, where they mature into adult worms. From the liver they travel down the portal vein and the inferior mesenteric vein against the flow of blood. They cross the portal-systemic anastomotic channels and reach the plexus of veins in the urinary bladder. Eggs are shed in the urine. On reaching fresh water the miracidium emerges from the egg. It penetrates into a snail, reaches its liver, and leads to the development of daughter cysts. These are liberated on the death of the snail. They shed large numbers of embryos into the water, thus completing the life cycle.

Clinical features. When the embryos penetrate the skin urticaria develops. After a few weeks high fever with eosinophilia occurs. Finally, when ova are shed in the urine intermittent painless haematuria results, which is the classic symptom.

Investigations. The ovum is recognized in the urine without staining, under the low-powered *microscope*. *Cystoscopy* may show pseudo-tubercles, nodules, ulcers or papillomas, and in neglected long-standing cases, carcinomas.

Treatment is by niridazole or by compounds containing antimony, repeated courses being required. Bilharzial papillomas and carcinomas require surgical treatment.

TUMOURS OF THE URINARY BLADDER

Tumours of the bladder are moderately common, the vast majority being malignant. Males are affected about three times more often than females. Most patients are elderly, 75% being over 60 years.

Aetiology. In 1894 Rehn was the first to show a relationship between a chemical agent and cancer. He showed the very high incidence of cancer of the bladder among industrial workers exposed to arylhydrocarbon dyes. These dyes were formerly used in the paints, dyestuffs, rubber and chemical industries, but in the advanced countries none have been used since the 1960s. Other risk factors include the following:

1. Smoking: an average of 15 cigarettes a day doubles the risk, so that 40% of the patients are smokers.
2. Chronic over-ingestion of analgesics containing phenacetin.
3. Pelvic irradiation.
4. Bilharziasis, 80% of cases in Egypt being due to this cause.

Pathology. In the bladder the most common sites of occurrence of tumours are the lateral walls and the trigone. The overwhelming majority of bladder tumours arise in the mucous membrane.

Benign urothelial tumours are extremely rare. Malignant tumours are of three histological types:

1. *Transitional cell carcinomas* (95%). These are morphologically of three types:

i. Papillary tumours (70%) tend to be pedunculated and grow into the bladder lumen. They are usually superficial and well differentiated.

ii. Solid tumours (20%) are sessile with ulceration, necrosis and calcification. They tend to be invasive lesions and are usually less well differentiated than papillary lesions.

iii. Carcinoma *in situ* appears as flat, red, velvety patches in the bladder and may be difficult to distinguish from chronic infection. Histologically it is poorly differentiated. Most cases show malignant cells on cytological examination of the urine. If dysuria is present most cases go on to invasive cancer; if it is absent, most cases do not.

2. *Squamous tumours*. These account for only 1% of urothelial tumours. They are usually caused by chronic irritation of the bladder, from a calculus or an indwelling catheter. In Egypt these tumours constitute 80% of bladder cancers. They arise in patches of the bladder which have undergone squamous metaplasia as a result of infestation with *S. haematobium*. These bilharzial tumours are nodular lesions, are usually well differentiated, and carry a low risk of lymph node or distant metastases.

3. *Adenocarcinomas* are extremely rare.

Bladder tumours are *graded* into well differentiated, moderately differentiated and poorly differentiated tumours according to the degree of cellular anaplasia. There is a strong correlation between tumour grade and stage.

The important factors in *prognosis* include tumour stage, tumour grade, vascular invasion and the presence of associated carcinoma *in situ*. However, some tumours remain localized whereas others that appear identical recur or become invasive. Factors that result in a poor prognosis include: a high proliferative rate, aneuploidy, and the loss of expression of tumour suppressor genes.

Spread. So long as the tumour is confined to the mucous membrane or muscle coat distant metastases are uncommon. Once it has infiltrated into the perivesical fat, it spreads to the iliac and para-aortic lymph nodes. It can also spread via the blood-stream to the lungs, liver and bones.

Clinical features. The first symptom is intermittent *painless haematuria*. With the passage of time the intervals between the episodes of haematuria become shorter, and the bleeding more profuse. The anaemia may become so severe as to necessitate blood transfusion. Other patients may present with recurrent urinary tract infections or sterile pyuria. An obstructed ureter may result in pain in the loin. Similarly, infiltration of a nerve may cause pain referred to the perineum, the groins or thighs. The tumour may be detected incidentally, either during cystoscopy or on routine 'dip-stick' testing for haematuria: 10% of these patients will have a bladder cancer.

Investigations. ***A. Diagnostic.*** The clinical problem is usually of unexplained haematuria. A *urine* sample is obtained for culture and for examination for malignant cells. Urinary cytology is specially helpful if carcinoma *in situ* is suspected. In such cases 90% of specimens will be

Table 1 Modified UICC (TNM) staging system for bladder cancer.

Tis	Carcinoma *in situ*
Ta	Does not cross lamina propria
T1	Extends beyond lamina but does not infiltrate muscle
T2	Invades superficial muscle layer
T3	Invades deep muscle layer
T4	Fixed to adjacent viscera
N0	No nodes
N1	Single node
N2	Bilateral or multiple nodes
N3	Fixed mass of nodes
M0	No metastases
M1	Metastases

positive; in well-differentiated tumours only 50%. An *intravenous urogram* may show a filling defect within the bladder; however, its primary purpose is to exclude a source of bleeding in the upper urinary tract. *Cystoscopy* is carried out under local anaesthesia. A papilloma shows delicate villi which sway about in the fluid. On the other hand in the case of a more malignant papilloma both the stalk and the villi are more thick and short. Nodules may be present around the growth. At cystoscopy a *biopsy* of the tumour should always be carried out. Abdominal *ultrasound* shows up papillary tumours larger than 1 cm in diameter.

B. Staging. If histological examination shows the tumour to be superficial, no further staging is required. With invasive cancers it is necessary to distinguish between localized extension and advanced pelvic or disseminated disease. A modified UICC (TNM) staging system for bladder cancer is given in Table 1. For this purpose CT scan is better than bimanual examination, which often understages these tumours.

Treatment. All patients with bladder tumours should first undergo *transurethral resection (TUR)* of the tumour under general or local anaesthesia. Separate samples of the tumour and its muscle base should be sent to the laboratory to help in the detection of muscle invasion. A bimanual examination should be carried out both before and after resection in order to stage the tumour, as the further management depends upon the grade and stage.

Carcinoma in situ. All macroscopic disease should be resected first. With localized disease this is all that is required; with widespread disease this should be followed by intravesical instillations of *Bacillus Calmette-Guerin* (BCG) weekly for 6 weeks, with a similar course after 3 months. This treatment is highly effective. On the other hand systemic chemotherapy and radiotherapy are quite ineffective in treating carcinoma *in situ.*

Superficial bladder cancer. Here also, TUR should be followed by intravesical BCG. This should be followed by cystoscopy 3-monthly for 18 months, and yearly thereafter.

Invasive bladder cancer carries a poor prognosis, with 5-year survivals of 50%.

In all the above three types of case if the tumour fails to respond or relapses after treatment, cystectomy should be offered.

Radical cystectomy. The disappointing results of radiotherapy in the treatment of invasive bladder cancers have led some surgeons to turn to radical cystoprostatectomy and pelvic lymphadenectomy. Recently, nerve-sparing cystoprostatectomy has been employed. This has the advantage that sexual function is likely to be preserved. Whether the long-term results of this operation match those of the standard radical cystoprostatectomy remains to be seen.

Urinary diversion. Traditionally, the ureters are reimplanted into an ileal segment, which is used as a *urinary conduit* to an abdominal wall stoma. Urine drains continuously and is collected in a bag attached to the skin around the stoma. Recently, a *continent urinary diversion* has been described. An intra-abdominal pouch is fashioned from ileum (the Koch pouch), and can be catheterized intermittently by the patient through the abdominal stoma.

Neobladder. In this technique, after cystectomy a pouch of ileum, into which the ureters have been implanted, is sutured to the internal urethral meatus. The patient is continent because the external urinary sphincter is preserved. He can either void spontaneously by using the Valsalva manoeuvre, or catheterize the pouch intermittently via the urethra.

Chemotherapy. The poor results of radiotherapy are explained by the presence of unrecognized distant disease at the time of the initial treatment. Accordingly, urologists are turning increasingly towards chemotherapy, where the recent introduction of multiagent regimens has brought fresh hope. Methotrexate, vinblastine and adriamycin have shown good results. Such treatment *prior* to cystectomy *(neo-adjuvant chemotherapy)* can 'down-stage' the tumour in most cases, and make it more easily dealt with by surgery.

The treatment of *disseminated disease* is palliative, as median survival is only 6 months. Multiagent therapy can double the survival time, but the already debilitated patient has to face significant morbidity.

Treatment of recurrences. If a tumour recurs after a course of transurethral resections, it should be dealt with by irradiation. Conversely, if radiotherapy is followed by a recurrence, the patient should be a candidate for cystectomy. However, before this is carried out it should be ensured that there is no evidence of spread of the disease, and that the patient is fit for the operation.

32 Prostate

Benign enlargement of the prostate

Benign enlargement of the prostate is a very common condition. It occurs usually above the age of fifty, and specially after sixty. Over 80% of males above the age of 50 have various degrees of bladder outlet obstruction secondary to benign prostatic hyperplasia. The cause is unknown; the most popular theory considers it as due to a relatively greater quantity of oestrogens compared to the male hormone, as the quantity of the latter diminishes with advancing age.

Pathology. Both the glandular and connective tissue elements undergo hyperplasia, specially in the submucous area. These form nodular enlargements in each lateral lobe, and compress the outer part of each lobe into a false capsule. When the hyperplasia affects the subcervical area a 'middle lobe' develops, and projects upwards into the bladder. In such a case urine remains in this post-prostatic pouch after micturition, and calculi can form in it.

The urethra becomes stretched and elongated by the enlarging prostate, and is compressed from the sides into an antero-posterior slit. The bladder hypertrophies to overcome the obstruction; if the obstruction is unrelieved it ultimately undergoes atony and becomes a passive bag. Gradually, due to back pressure, hydroureter and hydronephrosis develop. Reflux may occur into the dilated ureters and result in damage to the kidneys. Ascending infection may produce pyelonephritis.

Clinical features. *Frequency* is usually the first symptom. In the beginning it is noticed only at night; later it occurs during the day as well. The following factors contribute towards its development:

1. Stretching of the sensitive bladder neck epithelium by the intravesical enlargement of the prostate.
2. Increasing amounts of residual urine, so that the bladder refills early and the patient has to void repeatedly.
3. Cystitis, by irritating the bladder mucosa.
4. Finally, due to prolonged back pressure the distal tubules lose their ability to reabsorb water and salt and polyuria results so that large volumes of urine have to be expelled, leading to even more frequent voiding.

The next most frequent symptom is *difficulty in micturition*. The patient has to wait for micturition to commence. Straining makes matters worse, whereas on the contrary in cases of stricture of the urethra straining facilitates micturition. The *stream* is thin and weak, with dribbling at the end. Cystitis and acute retention of urine result in *pain* in the hypogastrium. A dull pain in the loins may indicate the development of hydronephrosis.

Acute retention of urine may be the symptom which brings the patient to the doctor, and often results from postponement of micturition so that the bladder is overstretched. If the retention of urine is *chronic,* the gradual stretching of the bladder is painless and the distended bladder passes unnoticed. The only symptom is *dribbling*, which occurs due to overflow from the full bladder.

Haematuria may occasionally occur due to rupture of a prostatic vein from congestion. Finally, the patient may present with symptoms due to *renal failure,* e.g. anorexia, hiccups, vomiting, thirst and drowsiness.

Thc International Prostate Symptom Score is a useful new index for measuring the severity of symptoms of benign hyperplasia of the prostate. The patient is asked:

Over the last one month how often have you:

1. Had a sensation of incomplete emptying of the bladder?
2. Had to urinate again within two hours?
3. Stopped and started several times during micturition?
4. Found it difficult to postpone micturition?
5. Had a weak urinary stream?
6. Had to strain to begin urination?
7. Had to get up during the night to micturate (on average)?

If the answer to any question is 'not al all' the score is zero; if 'almost always' the score is 5. Intermediate replies get appropriate marks.

Symptom severity is determined as follows:

Score	Severity
1–7	Mild
8–19	Moderate
20–35	Severe

Clinical examination. During the clinical examination the tongue should be inspected for the presence of dryness, and the external meatus for stenosis. The hypogastrium should be palpated to detect bladder distension, and the renal areas for tenderness which may be present due to hydronephrosis.

A *rectal examination* is carried out. In benign enlargement the lobes of the prostate are found to be increased in size, smooth, convex and elastic. When pressure is exerted a slight degree of mobility of the gland is noted. Hardness and fixity of the gland suggest a carcinoma. The act of *micturition* should be watched, when the thin stream is obvious. Finally, the *nervous system* is examined to exclude a neurological lesion, e.g. spinal tumour or tuberculosis. For this purpose testing for the knee and ankle jerks, and for sensation in the lower limbs, is generally sufficient.

Investigations. The *urine* is examined for the presence of infection and is cultured. The *blood* is examined for the white cell count and urea and creatinine levels. A *plain* *x-ray* of the abdomen may show calculi in the urinary tract and sclerotic metastases in the pelvis and lumbar spine in case the enlargement is due to carcinoma.

As urinary symptoms are unreliable, it is useful to have objective information. The most useful is the *urinary flow rate*, in which the patient is asked to void into a machine from a 'comfortably full' bladder, and the flow is converted into a graph tracing. A maximum flow rate of less than 10 ml/second from a voided volume of more than 200 ml strongly suggests obstruction.

Ultrasound examination carried out over the hypogastrium along with ultrasonography using a transrectal probe provide an effective, reliable and non-invasive method of assessing the size of the prostate, the volume of the residual urine, and the size of the bladder. Evaluation of the upper urinary tract is indicated if haematuria is present.

Cystourethroscopy should always be carried out before a prostatectomy to detect a urethral stricture, a carcinoma, etc.

TREATMENT

The aim of treatment of benign prostatic hyperplasia is to improve the quality of life by removing outflow obstruction and restoring comfortable micturition. Because the disease is not associated with any risk of mortality, the patient's preference should be the dominant factor in the decision. Symptomatic patients should be given the option of immediate treatment or watchful waiting. Treatment options include drug therapy and surgical techniques.

Drug therapies. 1. *a-blockers* like terazosin relax the smooth muscle of the bladder neck; they thus improve micturition. Postural hypotension is a significant side effect. Young patients with small prostates derive the greatest benefit.

2. *Androgen withdrawal.* Androgens are necessary in the development of prostatic hyperplasia. Androgen withdrawal therefore causes regression of this condition; however, loss of libido and potency make this course of action unacceptable. Testosterone has marked effects on secondary sex characters; on the other hand, dihydrotestosterone stimulates hyperplasia of the prostate. The enzyme 5 a-reductase converts testosterone into dihydrotestosterone. Finasteride inhibits this enzyme and results in reduced production of dihydrotestosterone; it thus helps reduce the size of the prostate without producing loss of libido. After 6 months of administration of finasteride the size of the prostate is reduced by about 20 percent.

As the actions of the above two groups of drugs are complementary to each other, it is likely that the next important advance will come from using drugs from the two groups in combination. However, neither of the above groups of drugs are likely to replace surgical treatment of this condition in the near future.

Indications for operation. 1. *Dysuria.* As mentioned above, the mere presence of an enlarged prostate is not an indication for operation, because many old people have prostatic enlargement without any symptoms. Again, mild symptoms do not warrant surgery. However, increasing difficulty in micturition, with delay in starting the act and a poor stream, or very marked frequency which upsets the patient's life routine, are situations where prostatectomy is advised.

2. If acute urinary retention is present it has to be treated by catheterization. If *acute retention* recurs after catheterization, prostatectomy should be carried out.

3. *Chronic retention.* In the case of chronic retention, if the serum creatinine is normal and there is no infection prostatectomy can be carried out without catheter drainage. If uraemia is present decompression of the bladder is essential, to be followed in due course by prostatectomy. Such cases are often also dehydrated, and intravenous fluid replacement should be carried out.

4. *Complications.* The development of stones, diverticula, infection or persistent haematuria indicates the necessity of surgical treatment.

The operations available and their steps. The prostate may be approached transurethrally, transvesically, retropubically, or via the perineum. Perineal prostatectomy has never been popular, due to the high incidence of incontinence and fistula formation. Further, transurethral resection has all but replaced the older methods of open prostatectomy. Finally, minimally invasive surgical procedures have been introduced, including transurethral incision and ultrasonic aspiration of the prostate, cryosurgery, prostatic stents and laser prostatectomy. Except for the first method, their final position has yet to be established.

Transurethal resection and the newer methods are described first, to be followed by the older methods of transvesical and retropubic prostatectomy.

Transurethral prostatectomy. Fibreoptic resectoscopes have greatly facilitated transurethral resection. Strips of tissue are cut from the bladder neck down to the level of the verumontanum using a high frequency diathermy current. Accurate haemostasis can be achieved. Damage to the external sphincter is avoided by staying above the verumontanum. The strips of tissue are removed from the bladder by using a bulb evacuator. A 3-way Foley is left indwelling for constant irrigation.

This method has all but replaced the older methods of prostatectomy, mainly because the necessity of incising the abdominal wall and the bladder is dispensed with. In this way abdominal pain and paralytic ileus are prevented, the patient can get out of bed earlier, and convalescence is expedited. However, the method requires sophisticated equipment and specialized training, which is not available everywhere. Therefore the transvesical and retropubic methods still have a place in certain parts of the world.

Minimally invasive methods. *Transurethral incision of the prostate.* This simple operation, which has been introduced only recently, has been followed by good results in patients with an enlarged prostate weighing 30 g or less. At the same time surgery, hospitalization and convalescence all require a shorter period of time. The procedure is carried out under general or regional anaesthesia. Two incisions are made at the 5 and 7 o'clock positions. The incisions are begun distal to the interureteric ridge and extend across the bladder neck and prostatic urethra to the verumontanum. As the incisions are deepened the bladder neck and prostatic urethra spring open and the bladder outlet obstruction is relieved. This procedure is ideal for:

1. Men with small prostate glands.
2. Those in whom preservation of the capacity for normal ejaculation are important considerations.
3. Debilitated men in whom the risks of surgery and anaesthesia are considerable.

Transurethral ultrasonic aspiration of the prostate. Through a resectoscope, the tissues with a high water content are ultrasonically fragmented, irrigated and aspirated, sparing tissues with high collagen levels such as the prostate capsule. Initial reports are encouraging, though the procedure is not without its complications.

Hyperthermia. Heat can be selectively delivered to the prostate by microwave probes placed in the rectum or prostatic urethra. Several sessions lasting half an hour each are required. However, if the tissue is heated to a temperature higher than 45°C, a single session of one hour can suffice. Outpatient treatment can be carried out with minimal morbidity. However, although good symptomatic responses are obtained, there is very little improvement in minimal flow rate.

Prostatic stents. Short tubes made of titanium or a superalloy are now available for use in patients who are not fit for anaesthesia. They are placed in the prostatic urethra as stents. These endoprostheses have several advantages. They can be placed quickly under regional anaesthesia or only a prostatic block and intravenous sedation. The placement causes minimal bleeding. An indwelling catheter is not required after the procedure, and the patient can be discharged the same day. However, the stent is a foreign body and its long-term effects are not known. Besides, precise positioning to avoid the stent protruding into the bladder or the external sphincter may be tedious.

Laser prostatectomy is the method which probably holds the most promise for the future. The laser probe directly touches and vaporizes the prostatic tissue, the result being the immediate removal of obstructing tissue in a manner similar to transurethral prostatectomy. Improvement in the urinary stream is usually prompt. It is expected that diminished bleeding may lead to reduction in the requirements for transfusion and the possibility of avoiding catheterization. If this materializes, selected patients could be treated in this way in a day surgery unit.

The older methods. *Transvesical prostatectomy.* Classically, the method of prostatectomy has been through the transvesical route, mainly because it can be carried out without very specialized training. The bladder may be opened through a midline incision. Alternatively, a *Pfannensteil's incision* may be employed. This is made transversely just above the pubis, being convex downwards. The rectus sheath is divided in the line of the incision and the upper flap raised upwards. The rectus muscles are now separated in the midline. The peritoneum is displaced upwards, and the bladder opened. The bladder mucosa is incised around the prostatic swelling, preferably with cutting diathermy. The finger now sweeps all round the adenoma, between it and the false capsule. The urethra is divided, preferably with scissors, and the 'adenoma' removed. The prostatic arteries are suture-ligated at 5 and 7 o'clock at the bladder neck. In Freyer's technique the bladder is drained by a stout tube. In Harris's method the mucosa at the posterior lip of the internal meatus is sutured to the urethral mucosa, and the bladder is closed, a 3-way Foley catheter being left in place for continuous irrigation. For the first day or two after operation constant irrigation of the bladder is carried out till the fluid returned becomes pale pink.

Retropubic prostatectomy. This method is superior to transvesical prostatectomy as the bladder muscle is not incised and therefore the return of bladder voiding is more prompt. At the same time, haemostasis is achieved under vision. The prevesical space is opened through a Pfannensteil's incision. A self-retaining retractor is placed in position and the bladder retracted upwards by its third blade. The anterior capsule of the prostate is incised by diathermy transversely about 1 cm below the bladder neck. The prostatic adenoma is enucleated with the finger or by the use of a curved scissors. A wedge is removed from the posterior bladder neck to prevent a stricture. Haemostasis is obtained by diathermy under vision, an indwelling 3-way Foley catheter placed and the prostatic capsule closed.

Complications of prostatectomy. *Haemorrhage* is the most important complication after prostatectomy through any route. Clot retention is signalled by a distended bladder and a catheter that does not drain. The bladder should be washed out by a syringe. *Secondary haemorrhage* occurs during the second week, and may be associated with infection. If clots are present they have to be washed out, and an antibiotic should be started. *Infection* can occur, and should be treated with an appropriate antibiotic. If prostatectomy is to be carried out on a patient who has had an indwelling catheter for a prolonged period of time, parenteral antibiotics should be administered as a prophylactic measure.

Incontinence. The internal sphincter at the bladder neck is put out of action by every type of prostatectomy. However, if incontinence occurs it means the external sphincter has also been damaged; its treatment is quite difficult. *Stricture* may occur at the bladder neck or at the external meatus. At the meatus it may be due to an excessively large catheter left indwelling for a long period.

In transurethral prostatectomy *perforation* of the prostatic capsule, and *water intoxication* from absorption of excessive amounts of irrigating fluid, can occur. *Osteitis pubis* is a rare complication of prostatectomy. It should be remembered that after every type of prostatectomy retrograde ejaculation of the semen into the bladder occurs, rendering the patient *infertile.*

Distant complications. Pulmonary atelectasis, pneumonia, and deep vein thrombosis can all occur, so that *early ambulation* is important. Myocardial infarction can also be precipitated.

CATHETERIZATION

A catheter should be passed into the bladder only by a doctor or a trained nurse. Catheterization should only be carried out under full aseptic precautions i.e. mask, sterile gloves, sterile sheets etc. The glans or labia should be cleansed with a suitable antiseptic. Even so, a sterile catheter is best passed with a non-touch technique, i.e., being held with a sterile forceps. In an adult, the size of the catheter should not be larger than about 12 F, as it only increases the chance of urethritis and stricture formation. 7 to 10 ml of fluid in the balloon is enough to help retain the catheter in place; with larger volumes bladder spasms may be caused by the detrusor contracting to expel the balloon. The catheter should be connected to a closed system drainage bag. This bag should be emptied only by opening the outlet at its bottom; the connection with the catheter should be left undisturbed, as otherwise infection can be introduced. These points are stressed because careless technique can result in infection which, in the presence of stagnation and reduced general resistance of the patient, can run riot in the urinary tract.

BLADDER NECK CONTRACTURE

This condition may be due to congenital muscular hypertrophy, in which case it occurs in children. Alternatively, it may arise from fibrosis around the bladder neck, when it is seen during middle age. The former type is called Marion's disease. There may be difficulty in micturition or repeated urinary infections. A distended bladder may be visible or palpable. Reflux of bladder urine into the ureters may cause loin pain and pyelonephritis. A bladder diverticulum may develop due to raised bladder pressure, or a hernia may arise due to straining.

Treatment. Adrenergic alpha blockers, e.g. phenoxybenzamine, can be useful by producing relaxation of the bladder neck. In other cases bougie dilatation of the bladder neck may work. If these measures fail transurethral resection or simple incision of the bladder neck is effective.

CARCINOMA OF THE PROSTATE

Carcinoma of the prostate is the most common malignancy in men above the age of sixty-five years, the median age at clinical diagnosis being 72 years. However, the condition is very much less common than benign prostatic enlargement. The tumour arises in the external group of glands, so it can develop even after 'prostatectomy' for benign enlargement.

95% of the tumours are adenocarcinomas, the remaining few being transitional cell carcinomas, either as extension from a bladder tumour or arising in the prostate from its own transitional epithelium.

Risk factors. Prostate cancer is more common in the Western countries than in the East. It is endocrine dependent and requires testosterone to grow; thus it never occurs in eunuchs. High fat intake is associated with high prostate cancer rates. Finally, first degree relatives have an eightfold increased risk of developing prostatic cancer.

Grading. Gleason's system of grading is the most popular. It assigns a grade of 1 to 5 depending on degree of differentiation, gland formation, and the relation of cancer cells to stroma.

Recently, the use of *flow cytometry* to determine DNA ploidy has become an important prognostic tool. Cells with an abnormal number of chromosomes have a higher risk of progression and recurrence. On the other hand patients with diploid untreated, localized disease have a 90% 6-year survival rate. Apart from grade, the strongest predictor of tumour progression and metastases is *tumour volume.*

Table 1 American Urological Association classification of cancer of the prostate.

Stage A
Clinically unsuspected tumour found on pathological examination of TURP specimen

Stage B
Confined within capsule
B1 Involving one lobe, less than 2 cm
B2 " " " , more than 2 cm
B3 Involving both lobes

Stage C
Extension beyond capsule
C1 Minimal extension
C2 Bulky extension

Stage D
Metastatic disease

Spread. The fascia of Denonvilliers prevents backward growth, therefore the tumour usually spreads *upwards,* where it may involve the lower ends of the ureters, leading to anuria. *Blood* spread occurs to bones, particularly the pelvis and the lower lumbar vertebrae, probably due to connections between the prostatic and pelvic veins. Primary *lymphatic* spread occurs to both the internal and external iliac lymph nodes; the secondary field includes inguinal, common iliac and para-aortic nodes.

Staging. The American Urological Association of staging is given in Table 1.

Clinical features. Most sufferers are old men. The disease may present in various forms. A hard *nodule* may be felt in the prostate during rectal examination for dysuria. *Tissue* removed at prostatectomy may show features of malignancy on microscopic examination. The patient may present with *pain* in the lower back or sciatica. Bilateral sciatica in an old man is specially significant. A bleeding tendency may occur due to destruction of bone marrow from metastases.

Diagnosis. This requires careful digital rectal examination, followed by laboratory and imaging procedures, and biopsy.

Digital rectal examination. Signs of malignancy include asymmetry of the gland, induration and hard nodule formation. More than half the tumours detected in this way have spread beyond the prostate. The method has its limitations; a third of cancers less than 1.5 cm in size are missed. Further, only the peripheral zone is accessible to digital rectal examination, so that tumours confined to the central zone will be missed.

Prostatic acid phosphatase. This substance is produced by the lysosomal fraction of the epithelial prostate cells and is present in the blood of patients with stage C and D prostate cancer. However, the levels are also raised in osteosarcoma, deep vein thrombosis and cancers of the breast and pancreas. At the same time rectal examination and urethral catheterization can elevate the levels of prostatic acid phosphatase.

Prostatic specific antigen (PSA). The discovery of prostatic specific antigen has revolutionized the early detection as well as the monitoring of prostate cancer. This glycoprotein serine protease liquefies coagulated semen and is 100 per cent specific to the prostate. Both benign and malignant prostate cells produce PSA, but malignant cells produce about 15 times more per gram of tissue. Moderate elevation may therefore be due to a benign gland, but seldom above 10 ng/ml, and never above 20 ng/ml.

The PSA level is directly proportional to the stage and Gleason grade of the prostate cancer; 95% of patients with a PSA level below 10 ng/ml have disease confined to the prostate. At the same time, PSA is the best test for monitoring therapy of prostate cancer; following radical prostatectomy persistently elevated levels indicate residual or metastatic disease.

Other laboratory tests. If metastases are present, tests for *haemoglobin, white cells* and *platelets* are carried out, as any of these can be deficient due to replacement of the red marrow by the malignant deposits. Serum *creatinine* should be estimated to rule out back pressure effects on the kidneys, and liver function tests to rule out replacement of liver tissue by metastases.

Bone scan. Nuclear bone imaging is the best technique for detecting bone metastases, which produce 'hot spots' in the areas of the red marrow i.e. the axial skeleton. The false negative rate is only 2%.

If hot spots are shown, they should be examined by *radiography*, which shows osteosclerotic secondaries in the pelvis and lumbar vertebrae if present.

Transrectal ultrasound gives detailed images of prostatic anatomy. However, only one-third of hypoechoic lesions are cancer; at the same time upto 40% of prostatic cancers are isoechoic and therefore missed. The main function of transrectal ultrasound is to *guide a biopsy needle* to a suspicious nodule; secondly, if cancer is found, to perform six spaced biopsies for mapping the extent of the cancer.

Computed tomography. CT scan can show prostatic size and contour, but is not very accurate in assessing extracapsular spread. It is used primarily to *assess enlargement of lymph nodes* and predict nodal metastases. The use of CT for staging prostate cancers has decreased since the availability of prostatic specific antigen.

Magnetic resonance imaging gives better images of the prostate and seminal vesicles than CT and can differentiate malignant nodules, but often understages capsular invasion. The use of endorectal coils may improve its quality in the near future.

Prostatic biopsy. With spring-loaded biopsy guns and ultrasound guidance, transrectal biopsy is now simple and safe, and can be performed on an outpatient basis without anaesthetic.

Treatment. ***For localized disease.*** If the investigations listed above indicate localized disease, the treatment options include observation alone, external beam radiotherapy and radical prostatectomy.

Observation alone. In some cases, the risk of progression of the cancer in the patient's lifetime is so slight that no intervention is warranted. This applies to men over 80 years of age with localized disease and men over 60 with stage A1 disease, i.e. clinically unsuspected tumour found on transurethral resection of the prostate, with 3 or fewer foci in specimen.

External beam radiotherapy. This is an effective treatment for stage A, B and C prostatic cancer. Standard therapy consists of 5000 cGy over 5 weeks to the pelvis with a further prostate boost of 2000 cGy over 2 weeks. Local control is achieved in 80 to 90 per cent of cases. In most European centres this is the primary therapy for localized disease in all men less than 80 years old; in North America only in men between 70 and 80. Complications occur in about 10% of patients and include impotence, strictures, proctitis and small bowel fistula. In patients with positive margins after radical prostatectomy, external beam radiotherapy can reduce local recurrence rates from 30 to 5 per cent, but survival rates are not improved.

Radical prostatectomy. This implies complete surgical removal of the prostate and seminal vesicles. The operation was associated with a very high complication rate in the past. Recently, detailed study of the neuroanatomy of the region has been carried out and the retropubic approach modified to spare the neurovascular bundles responsible for erection. This has improved both the continence and positive margin rates considerably. Survival after surgery for localized disease is as follows: at 5 years, 80%, at 10 years 70%. Ten to fifteen per cent patients encounter local recurrence.

Surgery versus radiation. In patients with localized disease, the results achieved with radical prostatectomy and external beam radiotherapy are similar. The best course to follow is as follows: for patients with an expected life-span of less than 5 years (i.e. those more than 80 years old), observation is advised. In those with a 5 to 10 year expected life span external beam therapy gives results similar to surgery with less morbidity. For patients under 70 with an expected life-span of more than 15 years surgery is best, because radiotherapy is often followed by persistent elevation of prostatic specific antigen.

For metastatic disease. *Hormonal therapy.* About 80% of patients with metastatic prostate cancer have a measurable response to endocrine therapy, with a mean duration of response of 2 to 3 years. Eventual progression of disease is due to growth of androgen independent cell populations.

Orchidectomy. Bilateral orchidectomy is simple and safe, and produces castrate levels within a few hours. The side effects include gynaecomastia, impotence and hot flushes. General, regional or local anaesthesia may be used. If a normal appearing scrotum is important to the patient, the orchidectomy may be carried out by the subcapsular method (preserving the tunica albuginea), or a synthetic testicular prosthesis may be implanted.

Oestrogens. Exogenous oestrogen blocks androgen metabolism at many levels, i.e. the pituitary, the testis, and the tumour. Unfortunately, at doses necessary to produce castrate testosterone levels (3–5 mg/day), diethylstilboestrol is associated with increased cardiovascular complications and deaths. Smaller doses e.g. 1 to 2 mg daily do not produce these side-effects, but then they do not reliably produce castrate levels either. Although diethylstilboestrol has been supplanted by newer drugs, it is the least expensive therapy, and very low doses are being studied in trials of combination therapy.

Luteinizing hormone releasing hormone (LHRH) analogues. Administration of LHRH analogues causes a rise in testosterone levels, but this level drops to castrate levels within two weeks. The clinical effect is equivalent to orchidectomy or stilboestrol. LHRH analogues are available as daily subcutaneous injections, a nasal spray, or a monthly depot injection.

Antiandrogens. Pure antiandrogens such as flutamide block the binding of testosterone and dihydrotestosterone to the androgen receptor. Side effects include gynaecomastia, flushing and diarrhoea.

Total androgen blockade. This consists of a combination of orchidectomy or LHRH analogues with an antiandrogen; patients with low disease burden and good performance status benefit most from this method of treatment.

Other complications of metastastic prostate cancer:

Spinal cord compresssion is well palliated by both radiation and decompressive laminectomy.

Ureteric obstruction. Local extension can impinge on the trigone and produce obstructive uropathy. Antegrade or retrograde stenting is the procedure of choice.

Bone pain. In case of intractable pain, local radiotherapy and/or oral prednisone may be considered.

PROSTATITIS

Acute prostatitis. Acute prostatitis is moderately common. The usual organisms are *Esch. coli* and the pyogenic cocci. The infection may be haematogenous or from the urinary tract. There may be fever with rigors and dysuria. The initial part of urine, on standing, may show threads. Perineal heaviness and pain on defaecation may be felt. The prostate is tender on palpation.

Treatment is by antibiotics, which should be given in adequate doses and for several weeks.

Chronic prostatitis. Chronic prostatitis usually results from inadequate treatment of acute prostatitis. The organisms are the same as in acute prostatitis, along with trichomonas and chlamydia. In improperly treated cases fibrosis occurs and the prostate becomes shrunken in size.

Clinical features. There may be pain in the perineum or in the lower part of the back, extending down the legs. Mild intermittent fever or premature ejaculations may be the presenting symptoms. The gland may feel normal. The prostatic fluid, obtained by prostatic massage, may show pus cells and bacteria. Urethroscopy may show the inflamed prostatic urethra.

Treatment is by antibiotics, after sensitivity testing. If trichomonas is present metronidazole is used.

33 *Urethra and penis*

CONGENITAL ANOMALIES OF THE URETHRA

CONGENITAL URETHRAL VALVES

These occur in the posterior urethra just around the verumontanum. They prevent urine from coming down freely, but do not hinder the passage of a catheter from below upwards. The prostatic urethra and the bladder may be greatly dilated. Untreated, they lead to hydronephrosis and renal failure. They are best demonstrated during *voiding cysto-urethrography,* i.e. when x-rays are taken during attempts to micturate after the bladder has been filled with contrast medium. During *urethroscopy* they may not be seen, as the irrigation fluid presses them flat against the urethral wall. Congenital urethral valves are *treated* by transurethral resection. *Other causes of retention of urine* from which congenital valves have to be distinguished are: *bladder neck obstruction* due to Marion's disease and *neurogenic bladder.* The former is diagnosed by cystoscopy, which shows up the hypertrophied inter-ureteric bar. The latter is detected by a thorough neurological examination.

HYPOSPADIAS

Hypospadias is the most common congenital anomaly of the urethra, occurring once in every 350 male infants. The external meatus is located at some point on the under surface of the penis or in the perineum. It may be found at one of the following sites:

1. Under surface of the glans (glandular hypospadias)
2. Coronal sulcus (coronal hypospadias)
3. Shaft of the penis (penile hypospadias, Fig. 1)
4. Penoscrotal junction (penoscrotal hypospadias)
5. Perineum (perineal hypospadias)

In all except the first variety the penis is curved downwards (chordee) and the urethra and corpus spongiosum are absent distal to the external meatus. The inferior aspect of the prepuce is poorly developed. The patient passes urine without any problem, but during adult life both sexual life and infertility are interfered with, except in glandular hypospadias. If the penis is curved markedly it is impossible to insert it into the vagina. If the urethral meatus is at the root of the penis the sperms are not deposited into the vagina on ejaculation.

Treatment. The aims of treatment in most cases are two: to straighten the penis and to carry the meatal opening to the tip of the penis. Both these aims have to do with proper coitus and placement of sperms in the depth of the vagina, otherwise as just mentioned, as far as micturition is concerned most of these children have no problem. Only rarely is the meatus narrow, when a simple meatotomy suffices.

In the *milder* forms, i.e. glandular and coronal hypospadias, small flaps from the under surface of the penis are adequate; they can be shifted as one-stage operations.

In the *severe* forms of hypospadias, in the past surgical correction used to be carried out in at least two stages. In the first stage the fibrous tissue on the ventral aspect of the penis was excised, allowing the penile shaft to straighten, i.e. correcting the chordee. In the second stage a skin tube was made from the ectopic meatus to the tip of the glans. The first stage was usually carried out at the age of about two, and the second stage at around four years of age.

During recent years there has been a tendency to carry out the whole correction in one stage. The skin around the whole penile shaft is elevated and the fibrous tissue distal to the ectopic meatus excised, thus straightening the penis. The gap between the meatus and the tip of the glans is now filled by making a urethral tube by one of the following two methods:

1. If the gap is moderate in length, a *preputial island flap* is used. A quadrangular flap is marked out of the delicate skin of the inner side of the prepuce. The subcutaneous tissue of the penis, with its contained vessels, is dissected in such a manner as to make a pedicle for the flap. This flap is now swung to the ventral side of the penis, sutured into a tube and used to make the urethra.
2. If the gap is very long, as in peno-scrotal hypospadias, a *bladder mucosal graft* is used. The prevesical space is opened and the bladder muscle incised. A generous area of bladder mucosa is dissected free and removed; it is used as a free graft to make the urethral tube.

During these operations on the penis the infiltration of 1 in 200,000 adrenaline into the subcutaneous tissues greatly reduces bleeding and facilitates the procedures. Hypospadias surgery is extremely delicate work. It should be carried out only if one has the proper training and the temperament, otherwise more harm is done than good.

EPISPADIAS

Epispadias is very rare, the urethral orifice being situated on the dorsum. The operative treatment is similar in principle to that of hypospadias.

RUPTURE OF THE URETHRA

Rupture of the urethra occurs commonly at two sites: the bulbous urethra and the membranous urethra. At either site it may be complete, i.e. a transection, or incomplete, i.e. a partial tear.

Mechanism of injury & clinical features. Rupture of the *bulbous* urethra is the more common accident. Nearly always it occurs due to a fall astride a projecting object, commonly either the cross-bar of a bicycle or a loose manhole cover. Another important cause of such an injury is urethral instrumentation. The patient presents with bleeding from the urethra, a painful haematoma in the perineum, and retention of urine.

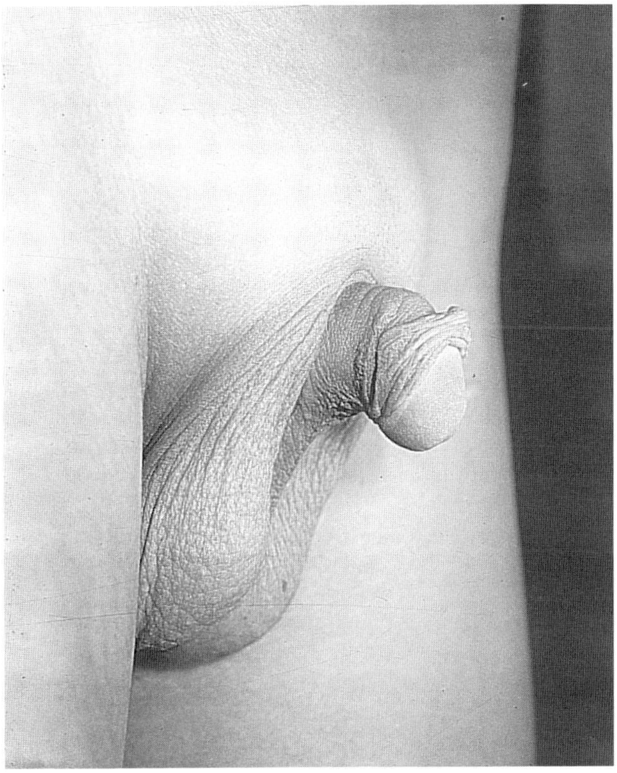

Fig. 1 Penile hypospadias. The shaft of the penis is curved downwards.

Rupture of the *membranous* urethra in males occurs most commonly in association with fracture of the bony pelvis, usually due to a motor vehicle accident. A few cases occur due to falls from heights, industrial crushing injuries, and sporting accidents. The bone disruption produces a shearing force, the prostate and the puboprostatic ligaments being pulled in one direction, the membranous urethra and the urogenital diaphragm in the other. *The injury should be suspected in any patient with a pelvic fracture.* Rectal examination will show the prostate to be in a higher position than normal. This 'high riding prostate' is the result of disruption of the urethra, with the prostate elevated from its normal position by a pelvic haematoma.

Urethrography. When a patient presents in the above manner it is important to find out whether the urethra has been ruptured and if so whether the tear is partial or complete. For this purpose a *retrograde urethrogram* should be carried out. A number 12F Foley catheter is passed into the urethra so that the balloon lies just inside the external meatus. About 1 ml of saline is injected into the balloon to seat it in the fossa navicularis. The patient's pelvis is now rotated to approximately 30° oblique position. About 25 ml of 25% contrast medium is injected into the urethra, and an x-ray taken. The oblique position is best for demonstrating the entire anterior and posterior urethra; in the anteroposterior view the bulbous urethra is foreshortened and the areas of extravasation overlap the urethra, making the interpretation of the x-rays difficult.

The action taken depends upon the findings at urethrography. If the x-ray shows a *normal* urethrogram it means the urethra is not ruptured but merely contused. In such a case the catheter should be advanced into the bladder and cystography performed to rule out a bladder rupture. If the urethrogram shows *extravasation* of the dye but the urethra is *in continuity* and contrast material goes freely into the bladder, there is a partial rupture of the urethra. If *extravasation* is demonstrated and *urethral continuity is lost*, a complete urethral rupture is present.

Treatment. *Urethral contusion.* If the urethrogram is normal and a contusion without rupture is diagnosed, no special treatment is required. The patient is usually able to void normally and his haematoma clears promptly.

Partial rupture. If on urethrography there is *minimal* extravasation and good urethral continuity, the patient may be allowed to void, or a catheter may be placed in the bladder for a few days.

Complete rupture. If the urethrogram shows a complete rupture, whether of the bulbous or the membranous urethra, most surgeons these days place a suprapubic tube into the bladder. This is left in place for about six months, after which staged reconstructive procedures are employed. This time lag allows the extent of the stricture to declare itself and periurethral induration to subside. On the other hand patients dealt with by immediate repair have a much higher incidence of re-stricture, impotence and incontinence.

EXTRAVASATION OF URINE

Extravasation of urine takes place in neglected cases of rupture of the bladder or urethra.

Deep extravasation follows extraperitoneal rupture of the bladder or intrapelvic rupture of the (membranous) urethra. Urine extravasates in the layers of the pelvic fascia and in the retroperitoneal tissues. In these cases it is necessary to drain the prevesical space and to perform suprapubic cystostomy. Later, the treatment is as described above for rupture of the bladder and urethra.

Superficial extravasation takes place after rupture of the bulbous urethra. The membranous layer of superficial fascia (Colles' fascia) is attached to the deep fascia at the midperineal point, ischiopubic rami and just below the inguinal ligament. Therefore, the urine cannot extend down the thighs; it collects in the subcutaneous tissues of the scrotum, penis and abdominal wall. Urgent operation is essential to eliminate spreading cellulitis and the resulting septicaemia. Multiple incisions are made in the skin and superficial fascia, and antibiotics are administered. The subsequent management is by delayed (secondary) repair of the urethra.

URETHRITIS

The most common organism involved in urethritis is the gonococcus, the others being *Chlamydia trachomatis,* staphylococci, streptococci and *Trichomonas vaginalis.*

GONOCOCCAL URETHRITIS

The gonococcus *(Neisseria gonorrhoeae)* is a Gram-negative diplococcus which affects the anterior urethra in the male, and the urethra and cervix in the female. After sexual intercourse with an infected partner symptoms commence after two to ten days. At first there is discomfort on micturition, often progressing to a scalding pain. A urethral discharge appears, being seropurulent at first, then becoming purulent. In chronic cases there may be only a slight morning discharge, or some slight staining of the underclothes. In some cases there may be no symptoms at all. These are the most dangerous cases from the point of view of spread of infection to others, because the patient does not seek treatment and remains infective.

Diagnosis. If urine is collected in two glasses it is hazy in the first glass but clear in the second, because when urine is voided its first part flushes any discharge out of the urethra *(two glass test)*.

Collection of discharge. A specimen of urethral discharge should be obtained from the distal urethra using calcium alginate urethral swabs inserted at least 2 cm into the urethra and rotated gently. The standard cotton-tipped applicators should not be used, because their large size makes insertion uncomfortable. The swabs should be rolled over the slide rather than streaked, otherwise the cellular morphology may be distorted.

Treatment. One of the following regimens is commonly employed for this disease:

Oral. 1. Ampicillin or amoxicillin 3.5 gm (single dose) plus probenecid 1 gm.

2. Tetracycline hydrochloride 500 mg (4 times daily for 7 days).

3. A combination of 1 & 2 above. This is effective against gonorrhoea and coexisting chlamydial infection.

Parenteral. Aqueous procaine penicillin G, 4.8 million units (injected i.m. at two sites), plus probenecid 1 gm by mouth.

For penicillinase-producing N-gonorrhoeae. 1. Cefotaxime 1 gm i.m. (single dose).

2. Intramuscular aqueous procaine *penicillin* accompanied by probenecid: this is a time-honoured and effective regimen. The major advantage is that treatment is given in a single session under the direct supervision of the physician. Thus it is ideal for patients who may not be reliable. The administration of *ampicillin* or amoxicillin in a single oral dose is an effective alternative to parenteral procaine penicillin.

3. The *tetracyclines* are attractive alternatives for the treatment of gonococcal urethritis, because they are also effective against chlamydial infections.

Repeat cultures should be obtained after a minimum of 4 to 5 days following completion of therapy, to ensure that the infection has been eradicated.

NON-GONOCOCCAL URETHRITIS

Patients suffering from non-gonococcal urethritis generally belong to higher socio-economic classes than those with gonococcal urethritis. However, this cannot help in the diagnosis of an individual case. Again, in general symptoms are more severe in gonorrhoea. The most common organisms responsible for non-gonococcal urethritis are chlamydiae, which are small bacteria, but like viruses they are obligatory intracellular parasites. The drug of choice for *Chlamydia trachomatis* is tetracycline hydrochloride. Given in a dose of 500 mg by mouth four times a day for seven days, it is highly effective. If the patient is pregnant erythromycin is preferable. It is given in the same dose and for the same duration as tetracycline.

Trichomonas vaginalis. This is a flagellated protozoan parasite. Its significance as a cause of genitourinary tract disease in men is controversial. It has been associated with urethritis, prostatitis, epididymitis and infertility. Routine tests for trichomoniasis are not indicated for all men with non-gonococcal urethritis. However, there are groups of men with non-gonococcal urethritis who merit investigation for trichomoniasis. These include:

1. Patients whose disease has failed to respond to antibiotics, including tetracyclines.
2. Men with long-standing symptoms.
3. Men whose sexual partners have symptoms or signs suggesting trichomoniasis.

Metronidazole is the drug of choice for the treatment of trichomoniasis, in a dose of 250 mg by mouth, three times daily for seven days; this results in cure rates of about 95%. However, recently *T. vaginalis* organisms resistant to high levels of metronidazole have been isolated.

Complications of urethritis. Urethritis can be followed by one or more serious complications, specially epididymitis and urethral strictures.

EPIDIDYMITIS

This is a fairly common complication of urethritis. Most cases result from retrograde ascent of urethral pathogens via the ejaculatory duct and vas deferens to the epididymis. The testis is also involved by the inflammation, so that most patients really have an epididymo-orchitis. The usual complaint of the patient is painful swelling of the scrotum, commonly accompanied by dysuria or urinary frequency. Urethral discharge is present, but may be mild or absent, specially in patients with chlamydial infection. Below the age of 35 most cases of epididymitis are due to sexually transmitted pathogens i.e. gonococcus, chlamydia etc. Above this age most cases follow infections with coliforms, Pseudomonas, or gram positive cocci. In many cases this infection has been predisposed to by an underlying urological pathology, or by urethral instrumentation. Epididymitis may occur weeks, or rarely months, after urethral instrumentation. It behoves us to take all precautions while passing a catheter or other instrument into the urethra.

URETHRAL STRICTURE

Urethral strictures may arise due to the following:

1. Trauma.
2. Inflammation, e.g. gonorrhoea.
3. Instruments, e.g. indwelling catheters.
4. Operations, e.g. prostatectomy.
5. A few strictures are congenital lesions.

Clinical features. As a stricture develops the stream of urine becomes progressively narrower, so that micturition takes a longer time to be completed. Immediately after micturition dribbling may occur; this is due to urine trickling down from the dilated urethra above the stricture. Increased frequency may be seen. This is due to incomplete evacuation, so that the bladder fills up again quickly. Cystitis resulting from stagnation of urine may also contribute to the frequency. The stricture may be palpable as an induration in the wall of the urethra. The back-pressure effects of urethral stricture produce dilatation of the bladder, the ureters and the kidneys.

Urethroscopy. This allows a very definite and accurate diagnosis. False passages may also be seen, being the result of inexpert use of bougies.

Urethrography. Whereas urethroscopy can show only the lower end of a stricture, urethrography indicates not only the presence of a stricture but also its length, as the dye goes up through it to outline its upper extent. Any urethral diverticulum is also shown up.

Treatment. A urethral stricture is dealt with either by dilatation or operation.

Dilatation. Classically the treatment of a stricture consisted of repeated dilatations for many years, and sometimes for life. For their dilatations these miserable patients sought the indulgence of different surgeons, who got sick of their sight in due course of time. In order to avoid such a fate, a young man would be well-advised to guard his urethra jealously, both from trauma and from gonorrhoea!

Dilatation should be carried out gently, using bougies of gradually increasing size. Force should not be used, because the resulting trauma leads to the formation of even more fibrous tissue and a tighter stricture. Dilatation is usually started using gum-elastic bougies. When the stricture has been stretched by this means to a medium size, metallic bougies are employed for further dilatation.

Operative treatment. If repeated dilatation by bougies fails to provide a sufficiently wide channel, operative treatment has to be undertaken:

1. If the stricture is very short it can be divided through a urethroscope using an *internal urethrotome* under direct vision. A follow-up urethroscopy can be performed at about three months, and the procedure repeated if necessary.
2. If the stricture is a long one it cannot be dealt with endoscopically. In such a case *external urethrotomy* is carried out. In this procedure the strictured urethra, along with a centimetre or so of normal urethra both proximal and distal to it, is laid open. The skin is stitched to mucosa all round and the wound allowed to heal. After about six months, when any fibrous tissue has become soft and supple, the urethral tube is reconstructed.

For making the urethral tube *(urethroplasty)* an incision is made all round the open urethral groove. The skin outlined by the tube is mobilized at its margins and stitched into a tube. Its outer raw surface is covered by mobilizing skin from both sides of the ventral surface of the penis. If this leads to too much tension, this can be released by making a midline incision in the dorsal skin of the penile shaft and allowing skin to slide to the ventral side around the sides of the penis. The dorsal raw area granulates and epithelializes spontaneously; it does not need to be skin-grafted. If it is assured that the buried skin strip is of sufficient width, and that epithelial closure is obtained, the results of such a urethroplasty are good.

PHIMOSIS AND PARAPHIMOSIS

In *phimosis* the preputial orifice is abnormally small. The most common cause of this condition is congenital narrowing of the opening, the other important cause being inflammation of the lining of the prepuce. When the patient passes urine the prepuce balloons out, and a thin stream of urine comes out. Due to difficulty in the passage of urine the bladder empties incompletely, i.e. residual urine results. Due to further back pressure hydroureter and hydronephrosis follows. *Paraphimosis* results when a tight prepuce is retracted but cannot be returned. It acts as a venous tourniquet proximal to the glans, which becomes greatly swollen causing much pain and dysuria.

Treatment. The treatment of phimosis is circumcision. In the case of paraphimosis the urgent requirement is for the relief of the constriction. As the tissues are grossly oedematous the best line of action is simply to divide the constricting band by a short incision on its dorsal aspect. This allows the oedema to subside, and circumcision can be performed at a convenient date a few days later.

CIRCUMCISION

Circumcision has been practised around the world for thousands of years. Among Jews and Muslims it is carried out as a religious ritual, among other communities only if indicated on medical grounds. Muslim barbers have perfected the technique over thousands of years. Millions of circumcisions are carried out by barbers, but rarely does one come across either a stricture or excess or shortage of skin on the penis after a circumcision. If the barbers could adopt aseptic methods this would improve results further. In fact they use fresh ash as a powder on the wound, which is not really such a bad choice.

Anaesthesia. Either general or local anaesthesia can be employed for circumcision; if local anaesthesia is used it is important to inject into the dorsal subcutaneous tissues at the root of the penis, in order to block the dorsal nerve of the penis. Some more drug is then injected around the root of the penis.

Technique. The prepuce is fully retracted and smegma from underneath removed gently. If necessary for retraction, the prepucial opening may be dilated by opening the jaws of a haemostat inside it. The line of the skin incision is now marked around the penis. The prepuce is next held up in two haemostats and a bone forceps applied across it along the marked line, the glans having been retracted backwards to avoid injury to it. The portion of the foreskin distal to the bone forceps is amputated by scalpel. The prepuce is now allowed to retract backwards. Bleeding is controlled by fine haemostats and 4/0 catgut. Sutures of the same material are finally used to approximate the skin with the inner lining of the prepuce. These fine catgut sutures get absorbed and do not require removal.

The cutting of the prepuce can also be carried out by scissors, but the bone forceps gives a more straight cut, and if used carefully is safe. Barbers have used a split fragment of bamboo in place of the bone forceps since time immemorial. The use of the bone forceps introduces the possibility of including the tip of the glans in its jaws. If the prepuce is first mobilized over the underlying glans by

Table 1 Staging of carcinoma of the penis.

Stage I	Confined to glans, prepuce, or both
Stage II	Extending onto shaft of penis
Stage III	With operable inguinal metastases
Stage IV	Involving adjacent structures; inoperable inguinal metastases; distant metastases

removing smegma, and the glands is retracted, such an accident is very rare. The slope of the 'upper' surface of the jaws of the bone forceps also tends to push the glans backwards, out of harm's way. However, care must be exercised.

Particularly in infants, the penis is best left without a dressing, a polymyxin — bacitracin ointment being applied. Any type of dressing gets soiled by urine and creates unhealthy conditions for wound healing. At the same time it becomes adherent to the wound, resulting in pain on its removal. However, a dressing is best for the first few hours, to conceal the wound from the relatives! After 24 hours the patient is encouraged to sit in a basin of warm water twice a day. This irrigates, cleanses and foments the wound, and expedites healing. To the warm water may be added three to four teaspoonfuls of cetavlon for its detergent effect. A certain degree of swelling of the parts always appears, but subsides within a few days.

CARCINOMA OF THE PENIS

Aetiology. Carcinoma of the penis is caused by chronic irritation of the glans and prepuce by smegma. This is proved by its widely varying incidence in different communities, dependent upon their practice regarding circumcision. Thus Jews practice circumcision at birth, and among them carcinoma of the penis is virtually unknown. Muslims circumcise their children during infancy; among them this neoplasm is very rare. Most other communities do not circumcise their boys routinely, and penile carcinoma occurs regularly in their men.

Pathology. Carcinoma of the penis is a squamous cell carcinoma. There are two pathological types of this tumour. The first or *infiltrating* type often commences in an area of leukoplakia. The second type is the *papilliferous* variety; this usually develops in a pre-existing papilloma. The tumour grows slowly. It spreads to the inguinal and then to the iliac lymph nodes. Distant metastases are infrequent. It is classified into four stages as in Table 1.

Clinical features. Although most patients are middle-aged, a fair number are below the age of 40. Mild irritation and discharge of pus may be followed by a blood-stained foul discharge. There is usually no pain. If untreated, the whole glans becomes a fungating, foul-smelling mass. Biopsy should in any case be carried out to confirm the diagnosis.

Treatment. Surgery is the most commonly employed method of treatment of carcinoma of the penis. Any suspicious lesion on the penis should be examined by biopsy. Occasionally a grade I lesion may be cured by circumcision. A local tumour on the glans may be treated locally by radiotherapy, usually employing radioactive iridium. In stage II, radiotherapy may be tried, although local amputation is often necessary. In stage III, radical amputation of the penis is necessary. This includes removal of the corpora cavernosa from the pubic bones. A perineal urethrostomy is then performed. The urethra may require reconstruction by a scrotal flap.

Lymph nodes. If the penile lesion is large, of high grade, or invades the corpora or urethra, bilateral inguinal lymph node dissection is usually performed. In any case, the decision to treat the inguinal lymph nodes should be deferred for a few weeks after treatment of the primary lesion. This is because the lymph nodes may be enlarged not due to secondary cancer but due to infection, in which case the lymphadenitis will settle after amputation of the penis, and obviate the necessity of lymph node dissection.

34 *Testis and scrotum*

THE UNDESCENDED TESTIS

The testis originates on the posterior abdominal wall. It descends into the inguinal canal during the ninth month of foetal life, and should be fully descended in the full term infant. If in the newborn infant the testis cannot be palpated in the scrotum the various possibilities are the following:

1. The testis may be *retractile*. This means that although the testis is normally descended, due to an overactive cremasteric reflex it retracts up into the inguinal area. The child should be examined in a relaxed atmosphere, preferably in the mother's lap, and if the weather is cold the hands should be warmed. An effort should be made to 'milk' the testis down into the scrotum. If the effort is successful it shows that the testis is normally descended and only retracts up from time to time.

Treatment. A retractile testis needs no treatment. The parents should be reassured that no operation is necessary, and that gradually as the weight of the testis increases it will constantly hang low in the scrotum.

2. The testis may be *ectopic*. Such a testis has descended normally through the inguinal canal. However, its further descent into the scrotum is prevented as follows: normally the gubernaculum guides the testis downwards. It has many tails, but the strongest of these is the one which attaches it to the bottom of the scrotum. In the case of an ectopic testis one of the other tails is more thick, and pulls it down in its own direction. Thus it may come to lie at the pubic area, femoral triangle or perineum. Therefore, if the testis is missing from the scrotum and cannot be milked down from above, it should be looked for at these sites.

Treatment. The ectopic testis should be mobilized at operation and placed in the scrotum, where it should be fixed by placing it in a dartos pouch as described below.

3. The testis may be *undescended.* In such a case it cannot be 'milked' down, nor can it be felt at any of the above-named ectopic sites. It is rarely that such a testis is absent. In the vast majority of cases it is incompletely descended, and lies in the inguinal canal or just above the internal inguinal ring. In the majority of cases a hernia sac is also present.

Harmful effects of incomplete descent on testis. 1. Although the testis develops in the abdomen it requires, for its normal growth and function, a temperature a few degrees lower than that prevailing inside the abdominal cavity. Upto the age of six the incompletely descended testis differs little in its microscopic appearance from a normal testis. After that time, due to the higher temperature of its environment, its development becomes retarded. At puberty the incompletely descended testis is quite flabby and small, the eipthelial elements are immature, and by the age of sixteen irreversible changes have occurred in the germinal epithelium. Its power of spermatogenesis is negligible. Its internal secretory activity is also somewhat reduced, but in spite of this the secondary sex characters of the patient develop normally.

2. If an undescended testis is allowed to remain indefinitely in the abdomen, the chances of its developing a *malignancy* during adult life are greatly increased.

If an imperfectly descended testis is brought down satisfactorily before puberty it usually develops and functions normally.

Treatment. An undescended testis should be operated upon and brought down into the scrotum. If the baby presents at birth it is usual to wait for about two years before carrying out orchidopexy, as it sometimes descends spontaneously during this period. If by the age of two years the testis has not descended into the scrotum, it is unlikely to come down at a later date, and operation should be carried out. After the age of 3, the child becomes more and more concerned with his body image. If the undescended testis is left untreated, such children have been found to suffer from psychological symptoms and disorders such as indecision, fear, depression, etc.

Operation. The inguinal canal is opened. Any hernia sac is ligated and excised. The spermatic vessels are gently dissected as they lie retroperitoneally on the posterior abdominal wall, to enable them to lengthen. The inferior epigastric artery and veins are ligated and divided, to allow the spermatic cord and the vas to follow a straight course to the scrotum and thus gain length. These manoeuvres usually allow the testis to be brought down into the scrotum. It is then fixed there by making a pouch for it between the skin and the dartos muscle (dartos pouch), to prevent it from retracting upwards after the operation.

If the testicular vessels are so short that the testis cannot be brought down fully, one of the following courses may be adopted:

1. A two-stage procedure is employed. The testis is brought down as far as possible, and is anchored with a non-absorbable suture. After a year or more, further mobilization is carried out.
2. The testicular vessels are divided, and the testis brought down into the scrotum (Fowler-Stephen procedure). The testis is usually adequately supplied through the arteries of the vas and the cremaster muscle. However, it should be clearly understood by all concerned that *a certain number of testes undergo atrophy after this operation.* To reduce the incidence of such atrophy, the vessels may be divided first, and the orchidopexy carried out after some time.
3. The abnormally short testicular vessels may be divided at the lower pole of the kidney and anastomosed to the origins of the inferior epigastric artery and vein by the use of microvascular techniques, thus gaining very valuable length.
4. If the undescended testis is completely atrophic or the patient has presented after puberty and the other testis is normal, orchidectomy is carried out to prevent the devel-

opment of malignancy, which arises a great deal more commonly in the undescended testis than in the normally placed organ.

Bilateral cryptorichidism. If only one testis is undescended, the cause is likely to be a mechanical block to descent, and has to be treated by operation. It is unlikely to be hormonal deficiency, because if that was the case the other testis would also be undescended. On the other hand if both testis are incompletely descended it is more likely that a deficiency of hormones is responsible. Therefore biweekly injections of chorionic gonadotrophin, extracted from the placenta, are given for six to eight weeks. Longer courses are not employed, otherwise secondary sex characters may develop prematurely. If hormonal treatment fails to bring the testes down, after waiting for a few months they must be brought down by operation, carried out either together or one side after the other.

TORSION OF THE TESTIS

Occasionally a testis undergoes torsion around its longitudinal axis. A painful swelling develops, and if left untreated the testis undergoes infarction followed by atrophy. Torsion does not occur in a normal testis. In cases in which torsion occurs, either the tunica vaginalis extends to a high level so that the testis hangs within the tunica, or the testis is separated from the epididymis and twists around the mesentery joining it to the epididymis.

Clinical features. Torsion commonly occurs between the ages of ten and twenty five years; it is also seen during infancy. There is sudden agonizing pain in the groin with vomiting. If the testis is incompletely descended and lying in the groin the painful swelling may be mistaken for a strangulated inguinal hernia. Torsion of the fully descended testis has to be distinguished from acute epididymo-orchitis. Elevation of the testis usually relieves the pain in epididymitis but increases it in torsion.

Treatment. If the diagnosis is made within an hour of the onset of pain a gentle effort to untwist the testis may be made. However, in most patients it will be unsuccessful and in that case immediate operation should be performed. After detorsion the testis is fixed in position by placing it in a dartos pouch, i.e. between the dartos and the scrotal skin. The opposite testis should also be fixed at the same time, as the anatomical variation responsible for the torsion is likely to be bilateral.

VARICOCELE

In some young adults the veins of the pampiniform plexus become varicose; this condition is called a varicocele. The left side is affected in 95% of cases. Occasionally a varicocele occurs in middle age, due to obstruction of the left testicular vein by the growth of a renal carcinoma along the left renal vein. In such a case the kidneys must be palpated and investigated.

Clinical features. A varicocele may produce no symptoms, but in some cases the patient experiences a dragging pain on the affected side. Due to its increased weight, the scrotum hangs lower than normal and on palpation the dilated, tortuous veins feel like worms in a bag. The testis may be slightly smaller than the opposite side, due to a minor degree of atrophy. When the patient lies down the veins empty. However, a varicocele which is due to a renal carcinoma does not empty on lying down.

Many men suffering from varicocele are subfertile. This is because of the fact that due to venous congestion and the excessive volume of blood in the parts the temperature in the scrotum is raised. The ideal temperature for spermatogenesis is a few degrees lower than that prevailing in the internal organs. This rise in temperature reduces the sperm count and motility and reduces fertility. After a successful operation for this condition both these values improve.

Treatment. The spermatic veins are without any valves, so in the erect posture the pressure of the blood right upto the inferior vena cava is transmitted back to them in the scrotum. Therefore the treatment of choice of a varicocele is ligation of the veins in the inguinal canal or just above the internal inguinal ring so as to abolish this back pressure. After this operation the sperm count and the conception rate both show improvement.

HYDROCELE

A hydrocele is the collection of serous fluid in some part of the processus vaginalis. It may be congenital or acquired:

Congenital. A hydrocele may be a congenital lesion, due to persistence of a part of the processus vaginalis. It presents during the neonatal period or infancy, and may take one of three forms:

1. *Congenital hydrocele.* The processus vaginalis persists in its entirety, its upper end remaining open to the peritoneal cavity (Fig. 1a). In most cases this opening is very small so a hernia does not develop. For the same reason such a hydrocele cannot be emptied by squeezing it. However, when the patient is recumbent while asleep, the hydrocele empties gradually during the night so that it is smaller in the morning. *This is a characteristic clinical feature of a congenital hydrocele.* One should ask the parents whether the size of the swelling is the same on rising as in the evening.

2. *Infantile hydrocele.* Here also the whole of the processus vaginalis persists, but its upper end is closed (Fig. 1b). The size of this type of hydrocele remains constant irrespective of the time of the day.

3. *Encysted hydrocele.* Here the middle portion of the processus vaginalis persists while both the upper and lower portions become obliterated, so that a smooth oval swelling results (Fig. 1c). If gentle traction is applied to the testis the swelling moves downwards and becomes less mobile, confirming the diagnosis. Unlike the first two varieties an encysted hydrocele does not always present soon after birth but may appear later due to collection of fluid in the preexisting sac.

Because the infant skin is quite thin, these hydroceles are usually brilliantly transilluminant.

Acquired. Later in life a hydrocele may be acquired, when it may be either primary (idiopathic) or secondary. As it consists of a collection of fluid in the tunica vaginalis it is called a vaginal hydrocele.

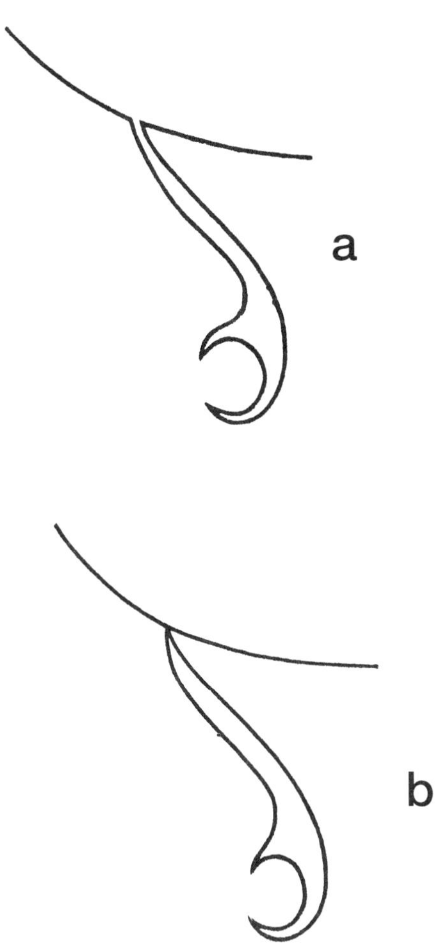

Fig. 1 (a) Congenital, (b) Infantile hydrocele.

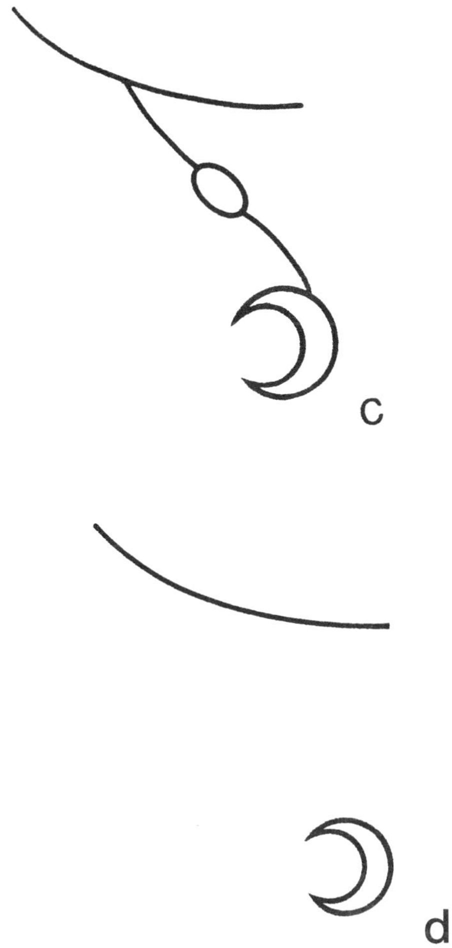

Fig. 1 (c) Encysted hydrocele of cord, (d) Vaginal hydrocele.

1. *Primary vaginal hydrocele.* This is the hydrocele which occurs in adults, and is commonly seen in middle-aged men. Its cause is not known. The only complaint of the patient is the swelling, therefore he sometimes allows it to become very large before seeking relief. On examination the swelling is fluctuant and transilluminant. Unlike an inguinal hernia which comes down into the scrotum from above, in a hydrocele it is possible 'to get above the swelling' at the root of the scrotum (Fig. 1 d). In actual practice this means that if the testis is held in the hand, with the index finger behind the root of the scrotum and the thumb in front of it, the two can be made to meet above the swelling. Unlike the congenital types of hydrocele the primary vaginal variety is always confined to the tunica vaginalis.

2. *Secondary hydrocele.* This is merely an effusion into the tunica vaginalis resulting from certain diseases of the testis, of which the common ones include acute epididymo-orchitis, chronic (usually tuberculous) epididymo-orchitis, and malignant tumours of the testis. Such a hydrocele rarely attains a large size, so the testis and epididymis can usually be palpated through it.

Ultrasound examination. If a clinician uses the relevant clinical methods, i.e. palpation, percussion, fluctuation, and transillumination properly, he does not need the help of an ultrasound examination to find out whether a hydrocele is present or not, and whether it is primary or secondary. However in a doubtful case an ultrasound examination helps elucidate the situation. It is to be hoped that the advent of diagnostic methods like ultrasound will not result in clinicians losing interest in the classical clinical methods, which can provide the same information immediately, without any cost, and anywhere.

Treatment. *Congenital hydrocele.* In congenital and infantile hydroceles the processus vaginalis commonly becomes obliterated over a period of 12 to 18 months. Therefore it is usual not to operate upon a hydrocele during the first two years of life unless a hernia cannot be excluded with certainty. After the age of two, if the hydrocele has not resolved it should be operated upon. The operation of choice for congenital hydroceles is high ligation of the processus vaginalis, as for inguinal hernia. The distal part of the sac is laid open but no attempt is made to remove it. Reaccumulation of fluid in the distal sac is rare.

Primary vaginal hydrocele. If left untreated a hydrocele may continue to enlarge. It may be the seat of haemorrhage or infection, and sometimes calcification occurs in its wall. In the days before surgery became safe, this hydrocele of adults was treated by repeated tapping. The sac used to refill, and over a number of years the wall became thick and less translucent, so that aspirations became more difficult. Today there is little justification for treating a hydrocele by tapping, except in patients with coexisting severe medical conditions.

The treatment of a vaginal hydrocele is by operation, the most popular procedure being *Lord's operation.* An incision is made through the skin and the coverings of the testis including the tunica vaginalis, so that the hydrocele sac is opened. A series of fine catgut sutures are placed radially all round from the cut edge of the tunica to the vicinity of the testis. When these sutures are tied the whole hydrocele sac gets imbricated into a narrow fringe around the testis. The secretory surface is thus greatly reduced. Because very little dissection of tissues is required, only a moderate degree of oedema occurs and the post-operative course is smooth. In any case the patient should be warned that some oedema will result, otherwise he is likely to be alarmed on its appearance.

The treatment of a *secondary hydrocele* is the treatment of the underlying condition responsible for it, e.g. tuberculosis, tumour, etc.

EPIDIDYMO-ORCHITIS

Epididymitis nearly always arises due to spread of infection from the urinary tract. Further, such an infection very commonly spreads to the testis, so that the condition is more accurately termed an epididymo-orchitis.

Acute epididymo-orchitis. Acute epididymo-orchitis follows non-gonorrhoeal urethritis more commonly than gonorrhoea. It can also follow any form of urethral instrumentation, e.g. catheterization, bougienage, cystoscopy, etc. The initial symptoms are those of acute prostatitis. When epididymitis supervenes there is severe pain in the testis and groin, along with fever. The scrotal skin becomes red and oedematous. The swelling of the epididymis may soften and discharge pus. Resolution of the swelling may take many weeks.

Treatment. Strict bed rest is the first essential part of treatment. Urine is sent for culture, and a broad spectrum antibiotic such as a cephalosporin (500 mg 8 hourly) is started while awaiting the results of the culture. More pain is felt in the scrotum if it hangs down; therefore it is supported on a large wad of cotton wool placed between the thighs. Antibiotics are continued for two weeks or more, as necessary. If pus forms drainage must be carried out.

Chronic epididymo-orchitis. Nearly 90% of cases of chronic epididymo-orchitis are due to tuberculosis, which has usually spread to the epididymis from the urinary tract. The onset is nearly always gradual. Commonly a single nodule is noticed in the epididymis. In every case the urine must be examined for tubercle bacilli, if necessary repeatedly. Simple Ziehl-Neelsen staining of the urinary sediment is usually negative; however, Lowenstein-Jensen culture and guinea-pig inoculation are positive in a high percentage of cases; these should therefore be employed. Pyelography and a chest x-ray should also be performed, to rule out pulmonary and renal tuberculosis respectively. Culture of the semen may sometimes help diagnose a case.

Treatment. If a primary lesion is found in the urinary tract or lungs, its treatment should take priority, and the epididymitis will also resolve. If there is no sign of resolution within about four months of antituberculosis treatment, the drug regimen may be changed. However, if there is still no improvement, epididymectomy or orchidectomy should be carried out, but the course of antituberculosis drugs is continued for its full recommended duration.

MALIGNANT NEOPLASMS OF THE TESTIS

About 99% of tumours of the testis are malignant. Of these, the common ones are seminoma and teratoma. These together constitute about 80% of cancers of the testicle. Combined seminoma and teratoma accounts for another 10%. The remaining few neoplasms include interstitial tumours, lymphomas, etc.

Age incidence. A teratoma occurs at a younger age than a seminoma; the peak of its incidence is seen between 20 and 35 years of age, whereas that of seminoma lies between 35 and 45. An imperfectly descended testis is about 10 times more prone to become malignant than a normally placed one.

Pathology. Most testicular tumours arise from the germ cells. They are often characterized by two types of primitive cells, the trophoblast and the yolk-sac cells. When trophoblast is present β-human chorionic gonadotrophin (β-HCG) is produced; when yolk-sac cells are present, alpha-fetoprotein is formed. These two substances act as tumour markers for these neoplasms.

Seminoma. A seminoma arises from the mediastinum of the testis. The testis is firm and smooth, and on section it is homogenous and pink or cream in colour. In rapidly growing seminomas areas of necrosis may be present. Histologically, rounded cells with clear cytoplasm and large rounded nuclei are seen, the cells being arranged in sheets. Infiltration by lymphocytes suggests a good host reaction and better prognosis. Seminomas spread mostly to lymph nodes, blood spread being rare.

Teratoma. These tumours arise in the rete testis from totipotent cells and therefore elements of ectoderm, mesoderm and endoderm are usually represented, although one of these commonly predominates. This tumour may attain a very large size. The cut section is yellowish in colour, and shows cystic spaces containing gelatinous fluid. Cartilaginous nodules may be present.

The *histological* types of teratoma graded in order of increasing malignancy are the *differentiated,* the *intermediate,* the *anaplastic* and the *trophoblastic* varieties. The anaplastic type may show elevated levels of alpha-fetoprotein, while in the trophoblastic type raised levels of human chorionic gonadotrophins may be seen. As the presence of these hormones in the serum helps to indicate the presence of these tumours, they are termed 'tumour markers'.

Although classically testicular tumours have been classified as above, it is becoming clear that different malignant tissues are often present in a single tumour, which is partly seminoma and partly teratoma, and the behaviour of the tumour depends on how much of each type of tissue is present. The presence of yolk sac or trophoblastic tissue in a tumour is associated with a worse prognosis than the presence of differentiated tissue.

The rare *interstitial cell tumours* arise either from the Leydig cells or the Sertoli cells. The former type masculinize the patient, the latter causes feminization.

Clinical features. Commonly, the patient with a testicular tumour complains of a painless swelling, with a sense of heaviness. Unfortunately, upto one-third of testicular tumours are misdiagnosed on the first clinical assessment. *The common errors in diagnosis arise from the presence of pain or hydrocele or a history of trauma.* It should be remembered that pain may result from haemorrhage into the tumour, a hydrocele often accompanies a neoplasm, and the 'trauma' may have merely focussed attention on the tumour. The presenting symptoms may be due only to metastases, e.g. chest pain, dyspnoea and haemoptysis with pulmonary metastases. The rate of growth of tumours of the testis varies greatly. Occasionally a teratoma may have been present for two or three years. On the other hand metastases from a highly malignant tumour may kill the patient within a few weeks (hurricane type of tumour). Similarly, a rapidly growing tumour may be mistaken for a case of epididymo-orchitis.

On examination the testis is enlarged, firm and smooth. Testicular sensation is lost very early. However, the testis should not be squeezed firmly, as this may result in dissemination of cells. A secondary hydrocele is present in a few cases. The cord may be thickened due to hypertrophy of the cremaster, which results from the excessive work this muscle has to do to support the heavy testis. The abdomen should be palpated to detect enlarged para-aortic lymph nodes just above the umbilicus; grossly enlarged para-aortic lymph nodes may be painful. The liver is palpated to find out if it is enlarged. The left supraclavicular region is examined, as spread via the thoracic duct may lead to enlargement of a lymph node at that site.

Staging. Cancers of the testis can be classified into four stages, depending upon the extent of spread:

Stage I: Lesion in testis only.
Stage II: Nodes involved below diaphragm.
Stage III: Nodes involved above diaphragm.
Stage IV: Pulmonary, hepatic or distant metastases.

Note: Stage II is further subdivided into a, b and c depending upon whether the nodes are less than 2 cm, 2 to 5 cm or more than 5 cm in diameter.

Investigations. *Ultrasound* often supports the clinical diagnosis by showing that the mass is solid. An *x-ray chest* shows any metastases in the lungs, which are common in the case of teratomas. Blood should be sent for *tumour markers* (alpha-fetoprotein and β-HCG) both pre- and postoperatively. *Abdominal ultrasound* and *CT scan* demonstrate the spread of a testicular tumour.

Treatment. Successful management of testicular tumours demands careful clinical examination, a high index of suspicion and prompt inguinal exploration if the diagnosis is suggested by the physical findings. The typical testicular tumour feels stony hard and heavy. The primary treatment of choice for tumours of the testis is orchiectomy. This is carried out through a high inguinal incision. Soft clamps are applied over the spermatic cord to prevent venous dissemination of cancer cells, and the testicle is mobilized for inspection and frozen section biopsy, if necessary. If the diagnosis of testicular tumour is confirmed the testis is removed along with the entire spermatic cord.

Further investigations are now carried out:

1. Chest x-ray to exclude pulmonary metastases.
2. Abdominal ultrasound or CT scan to detect metastases in the liver and para-aortic lymph nodes. Further management depends upon the results of the investigations and the histopathology report.

Seminomas. Seminomas are very radio-sensitive tumours. In stages I and II excellent results are obtained by irradiation. In stages III and IV on the other hand, chemotherapy is employed. The commonly used regimen consists of bleomycin, etoposide and cisplatin. These are toxic agents which require close supervision. Gastrointestinal, bone marrow, and skin toxic effects are common. If a seminoma has negative markers and no detectable metastases, orchidectomy should be followed by radiotherapy of 3000 cGy to the retroperitoneal lymph nodes. Survival rate following this is almost 100 percent.

Non-seminomatous tumours. In the recent past the treatment of teratomas used to be by orchidectomy with radiotherapy or retroperitoneal node dissection. The radiotherapy and node dissection have now been replaced by potent chemotherapy. After adequate chemotherapy the patients are re-staged; if persistent bulky disease is present this is resected surgically. The course to be followed after orchidectomy is determined as follows:

In stage I disease. 1. If tumour markers i.e. AFP and HCG are negative, no treatment should be given but a close follow-up instituted.

2. If the markers are positive the patient should be treated with chemotherapy until they become negative.

In stage II, III and IV disease. 1. Four to six cycles of chemotherapy are given.

2. After this if the markers return to normal but a mass persists, surgical excision of the residual disease should be carried out.

Prognosis. *Seminomas.* In cases without metastases as many as 95–100% patients survive five years. If metastases are present the figure drops to 75%.

Teratomas. In stages 1 and 2, 85% survive five years; in stages 3 and 4, only 60%.

Choriocarcinomas. Most patients with choriocarcinomas are dead within 2 years despite intensive therapy.

Section 3

Musculoskeletal system

35 Fractures and dislocations: general principles

A fracture is defined as a break in the continuity of a bone produced by forces that exceed the ultimate strength of the bone. A dislocation consists of a displacement, in relation to each other, of the bone ends taking part in a joint. When a fracture is sustained, a major soft tissue injury usually accompanies it. The surgeon must be familiar with the soft tissues, e.g. nerves and blood vessels, adjacent to a fracture and must look out for damage to them. If the fracture has resulted from violent trauma, the surgeon must examine the patient thoroughly for injuries to other organs. At the same time he should remember that multiple fractures, even when closed, can cause shock from internal haemorrhage.

MECHANISM AND CLASSIFICATION OF FRACTURES

Sufficient force applied to a bone results in a fracture. A single fracture line is called a *simple fracture.* If multiple fracture lines and bone fragments are produced, the fracture is said to be *comminuted.* If a penetrating injury produces a fracture, or fracture fragments protrude through the skin, we call this an *open* or *compound fracture.* When no such wound is present the fracture is classified as *closed. This distinction is very important.* Open fractures are likely to be contaminated with pyogenic bacteria, and this can result in bone infection. Therefore their treatment and prognosis are quite different from those of closed fractures.

Forces applied in different directions result in different types of fractures. A bending force applied to a long bone usually produces a *transverse* or *oblique* fracture line. A direct blow or crushing force often produces a *comminuted* open fracture, along with severe soft tissue injury. A torsion (twisting) force applied to bone produces a *spiral* fracture. The mechanism of a spiral fracture can be demonstrated by twisting a piece of chalk between the two hands; the cut ends have the same shape as the bone suffering a spiral fracture. A compression force applied along the long axis of a bone results in an *impacted* fracture at the junction between the metaphysis and diaphysis; the cortical bone of the diaphysis gets impacted into the cancellous bone of the metaphysis. Finally, violent muscle contraction may produce an *avulsion* of a portion of bone where a tendon is attached.

Fractures in children are often of the *greenstick* type. Just as a green stick bends but does not break, so it is with these fractures; the cortex fractures on the convex side but only bends on the concave side. Again, in children a fracture often passes through an *epiphyseal plate* and results in a disturbance of growth.

If the bone is weakened by some condition it may break after a trivial injury. Such a fracture is called a *pathological fracture.* The most common cause of a pathological fracture is a secondary tumour deposit from a carcinoma. Other causes are senile osteoporosis of the elderly, and metabolic bone-wasting diseases. Finally, healthy bone may fracture with repeated minor trauma. Such fractures are called *stress* or *fatigue fractures.* The most common example is a fracture of the second metatarsal after a long march, where moderate stress repeated thousands of times ultimately breaks the bone.

The signs of a fracture are the following:

There is severe *pain* at the fracture site.

The patient is *unable to use* the part.

The site of the fracture is *tender.*

Within a few hours *swelling* and bruising appear.

If the bone ends are displaced *deformity* is present.

Abnormal movement can be elicited at the fracture site.

Crepitus can also be elicited.This is a grating sensation when the bone ends are moved against each other. However, both crepitus and abnormal movement cause much pain. Therefore they should not be elicited.

ASSOCIATED PROBLEMS

The clinician should not focus his attention only on the break in the bone. He should be aware of the fact that fractures in general, and major and multiple fractures in particular, can be accompanied by widespread effects. Locally, the injury has often damaged different soft tissues. Systemically, compounds released from the injured site can produce serious effects on different organ systems.

Systemic effects of skeletal injuries. Major skeletal injuries may be accompanied by massive bleeding, accumulation of extravascular fluid, and hypovolaemic shock. Fractures of the femur or pelvis result in loss of 500 to 1000 ml of fluid into the tissues. Fat and other substances released from the injured site may result in impaired lung function in the 'fat embolism syndrome'. Unimmobilized fractures continue to bleed and accumulate fluid. They cause pain and generate systemically active mediators that predispose to gut disorders, a sepsis-like state, and multiple organ failure syndromes, with a high mortality rate.

Local effects. Fractures imposing *immobility* increase the risk of deep vein thrombosis, with potential for life-threatening pulmonary embolism and chronic venous insufficiency. Fractures heal slowly, sometimes taking months before full function can be allowed. *Prolonged bed rest* required in major fractures of the axial skeleton results in disuse osteoporosis, joint stiffness, pressure sores, as well as cardiorespiratory deconditioning and psychological stresses. If surgical stabilization can allow at least some use of the injured part, it helps.

Vascular injuries accompanying fractures may cause haemorrhage, ischaemia or both, and the examiner must look for pallor, coldness, empty veins, paraesthesias, paralysis, and pain persisting after fracture immobilization. Arterial injuries threatening ischaemia require immediate repair. This should be followed by distal fasciotomies, because post-ischaemic swelling produces compartment syndromes. Any of the *nerves* passing through the zone of injury may be damaged.

Cases with *multiple injuries* require x-rays of the cervical spine, chest and pelvis; and may need CT scan of the skull, peritoneal lavage or abdominal CT, and bladder catheterization.

Evaluation of the limb must be thorough, with examination for swelling, wounds, deformity, instability and ischaemia. X-rays should be taken as required.

Compartment syndrome. This is one of the most serious complications of trauma to a limb. Muscle groups in the extremities are bound by tough, unyielding fascial envelopes called compartments. If muscle swelling occurs due to fractures, bleeding, surgery or blunt trauma, interstitial fluid pressure rises to a level greater than that of the draining veins. A vicious circle is established, with increasing capillary leakage and increasing pressure. Loss of capillary bed perfusion causes local muscle and nerve ischaemia even though arterial flow is continuing and pulses are palpable. On palpation of the involved compartment tense swelling is obvious. *Volkmann's ischaemic contracture* results, with paralysed and shortened muscles and impaired sensation producing severe disability. Unconscious patients, and those with peripheral nerve injuries, are particularly at risk as they are insensitive to the ischaemic pain.

Whenever a patient has convincing signs of a compartment syndrome, prompt fasciotomy is mandatory. If the diagnosis is in question, intracompartmental pressure can be measured by different methods; this permits observation rather than fasciotomy in doubtful cases. If pressure is higher than 30 to 40 mm Hg below the mean arterial pressure, compartmental perfusion is probably impaired and fasciotomy should be carried out. Any associated fracture is at the same time stabilized with external or internal fixation, and wound closure postponed until swelling has subsided.

Radiography. If a fracture is suspected, the injured part must be x-rayed. While taking the x-rays the following points must be kept in mind:

1. The whole bone must be x-rayed in two planes at right angles to each other. Only thus can one be sure of not missing a fracture.
2. In certain fractures, e.g. of the scaphoid bone, an oblique view must also be taken.
3. In a hairline fracture of the scaphoid the fracture line may not be visible on the first x-ray. Radiographs must be repeated on subsequent occasions, when the fracture sometimes shows up.

STAGES OF HEALING OF A FRACTURE

When a bone breaks, blood vessels are disrupted at the cut surface. The space between the fractured bone ends fills with blood, which clots to form a haematoma. This fracture haematoma is invaded by granulation tissue. Macrophages remove the haematoma and a loose connective tissue is laid down. The osteoblasts of the periosteum and endosteum proliferate and lay down new bone. Histiocytes and osteocytes also probably help in laying down new bone.

About three weeks after the fracture, the cells around the fracture site calcify the matrix and later ossify it. This ossified tissue is called *callus.* It is distributed throughout the area previously occupied by the fracture haematoma. It is visible on x-ray and makes the fracture site increasingly rigid and strong. Thus by about five weeks the bone ends are surrounded by an irregular mass of fibrous tissue and bone.

The callus, which is an unevenly distributed mass of bone, is gradually replaced by bone deposited in *laminae* with a Haversian structure. Over the next few years the mass of bone in the medullary canal and around the fracture site is remodelled so that the anatomy of the bone returns to normal. However, in the adult slight internal and external irregularity persists indefinitely.

If the fracture is *perfectly reduced and rigidly immobilized,* e.g. in internal fixation by a plate or an intramedullary nail, callus formation does not occur. Instead, capillaries invade the bone and grow across it to unite with each other. Cells derived from these capillaries remove dead bone and lay down new bone so that a living cortex is directly remade. This process is called *primary bone healing.* This process is unlike healing by callus. It is not visible radiologically, and it takes months rather than weeks to be completed.

With fracture of a cancellous bone abnormal movement and crepitus are usually absent, because the honeycomb structure is *impacted.* On x-ray the callus does not appear as a bony mass surrounding the fracture but is seen as a zone of increased radiodensity *(sclerosis)* at the fracture site.

The clinical stages of union. Clinically, the process of union of a fracture passes through three stages:

1. *The 'sticky' stage.* The fracture haematoma gradually becomes organized to form fibrous tissue and later spongy bone. Abnormal movement at the fracture site diminishes. However, slight movement can still be elicited, and local tenderness persists. At this stage the fracture is described as 'sticky'.
2. *Union.* By about six weeks healing has progressed further. No abnormal movement can now be detected. There is little tenderness, and stressing the fracture is only slightly painful. Such a fracture is described as 'united'. Bone bridges the fracture, but it is spongy rather than in the form of proper lamellae as seen in normal uninjured bone (the Haversian systems). Therefore it does not look like normal bone on x-ray.
3. *Consolidation.* As the spongy bone becomes replaced by Haversian bone the fracture becomes completely painless. On x-ray the bone around the fracture site starts looking like the rest of the bone. It is no longer more bulky than elsewhere. The bulky callus has been reabsorbed and replaced by the more compact but stronger bone laid out in the Haversian manner. In the beginning the differentiation between the cortex and the medullary cavity is lost. As

consolidation progresses, the medullary cavity becomes visible on the x-ray, while the fracture line can no longer be seen. Such a fracture is described as *consolidated.* At this time the healing process can be regarded as having been completed.

To sum up, then, in the early stages nature arranges for spongy bone to be rapidly formed, in order to quickly stabilize the fracture. Later on at leisure this spongy, bulky, not-too-strong bone is gradually replaced by permanent bone which has great strength, because it has regularly arranged laminae, like the arrangement of steel bars in reinforced cement concrete.

The time taken for union. This depends on the age of the patient, the limb involved, the direction of the fracture line etc.:

1. Fractures in adults take twice as long to unite as fractures in children.
2. Lower limb fractures take twice as long to unite as upper limb fractures.
3. Transverse fractures take longer to unite than oblique or spiral fractures, because in the latter types the fractured surface is greater in area.
4. Open fractures unite very slowly.

A few examples will help elucidate the above points. An oblique fracture of the humerus in a child takes about 3 weeks to unite. The same fracture in an adult takes 6 weeks. A transverse fracture of the tibia in an adult takes 12 weeks, whereas a open fracture of the same bone may take upto 24 weeks.

DISTURBANCES OF NORMAL HEALING IN BONES

Delayed union and non-union. *Delayed union.* The usual periods of time by which fractured bones normally unite are listed above, although they may be exceeded. If a bone is not united by such time, i.e. it displays tenderness and abnormal movement at the fracture site, it is said to display delayed union. The callus may be invisible on x-ray, or may not fully bridge the fracture site. A fracture displaying delayed union may continue to heal until it finally unites.

Non-union. In this condition the healing process stops before union has occurred. Abnormal movement persists, and on x-ray the fracture line remains visible permanently. Such a fracture is said to display non-union. The fracture is bridged by fibrous tissue, the bone ends are sclerotic, and the medullary canal may be obliterated. On x-ray the bone ends are seen to be rounded. This is *fibrous non-union.*

In other cases movement at the fracture site is so persistent that cartilage is laid down between the fractured ends. A cleft develops between the layers of cartilage covering each fracture fragment. Cells at the periphery of the cleft develop into synovial cells, producing a false joint *(pseudarthrosis).*

The causes of delayed union and non-union. A number of factors may interfere with healing of fractured bones:

1. *Excessive movement* at the fracture site may produce delayed union because the callus is being constantly 're-fractured' by the movement occurring in the healing tissue.
2. *Infection* of the fracture haematoma in an open fracture upsets the healing process.
3. *A poor blood supply* at the fracture site delays healing because the invasion of the haematoma by blood vessels is slow or absent. Therefore, osteoblasts are slow to appear in the fracture haematoma. In fracture of the neck of the femur the vessels ascending the neck to the femoral head may be ruptured by the fracture. In such cases union fails to take place, because the blood supply of the head is lost.
4. *Interposition of soft tissues,* e.g. muscle, between the fracture fragments. The soft tissue physically separates the fractured ends, so it is impossible for them to unite.
5. *Systemic disease* e.g. uraemia may interfere with healing generally.

Malunion. A fracture which unites in a position of deformity is said to be malunited. For example a long bone may unite with significant angulation at the fracture site, or with over-riding of the fragments. This occurs due to imperfect reduction and usually results in impaired function. Besides, the deformity is cosmetically unattractive.

Impairment of function after union. 1. *Adhesions.* If adhesions form between the fracture site and the overlying muscles, the latter when stimulated cannot glide over the bone and contract, so that movement at the adjacent joints is limited and the effectiveness and force of the muscles is reduced.

2. *Sudeck's atrophy.* Normally some osteoporosis occurs after a fracture. Occasionally this may be grossly exaggerated, with pain and joint stiffness. This syndrome is called Sudeck's atrophy. It may be due to extreme reluctance of the patient to use the limb after removal of splintage, or from another cause. No specific treatment is available. The patient is encouraged to use the limb under the supervision of a physiotherapist.

Open fractures. Any fracture in which the overlying skin is broken is potentially contaminated with bacteria, from the skin or the environment. The bacteria produce an inflammatory reaction and the fracture becomes infected. *The chances of eradicating infection from the fracture haematoma become fewer with the passage of time.* Therefore the treatment of an open fracture is an urgent matter, and is discussed at length later.

THE TREATMENT OF FRACTURES

The management of a fracture is best considered under two headings: general management of the patient, and local management of the fracture.

GENERAL MANAGEMENT OF THE PATIENT

The general care of the patient with a fracture includes measures to deal with the pain and the blood loss caused by the fracture, the care of any associated injuries, and the emergency splinting of fractures.

Pain. A good deal of pain occurs in most fractures, and must be relieved. This can be done by splinting, and by analgesics such as pethidine and morphine, or if the pain is less severe, paracetamol etc. *If a patient has to travel to a hospital for reduction of his fracture, the doctor who refers him should apply a plaster-of-Paris slab before send-*

ing him. This is the best kind of splint, as it moulds itself to the contours of the body while being applied, and is therefore both more comfortable and more effective than ordinary splints made of wood or Kramer wire.

Blood loss. In all fractures some blood is lost, but mostly it is an insignificant amount. However, in major fractures a good deal may be lost. For example *a patient with a fracture of the femur may lose over a liter of blood into the thigh muscles* without much swelling. Such blood loss produces shock and must be replaced. At the same time, the use of inflatable pneumatic trousers ('military anti-shock trousers' or MAST) for transport may help maintain blood pressure and decrease ongoing blood loss in these cases.

Associated injuries. Fractures of the pelvis can cause injury to the bladder or urethra. These injuries must be looked for, so that they are not missed. Their care is described in the appropriate chapters. Fractures of the long bones may cause injury to neighbouring nerves and vessels. The injured extremity should be evaluated rapidly for neurovascular compromise, soft tissue injuries, and joint instability. Peripheral pulse and capillary refill are evaluated, and motor and sensory examinations carried out to the extent of the patient's ability to cooperate. All findings must be carefully documented for comparison with any later changes.

Emergency splinting of fractures. After the neurovascular examination is completed and soft tissue trauma or wounds evaluated, fractured extremities should be splinted to minimize further injury. Plaster splints, pillows, or air splints can be used to stabilize the extremity. A fracture of the humerus can be splinted with a sling. Femur fractures are best splinted in a Thomas splint with skin traction.

MANAGEMENT OF THE FRACTURE

The aims of treatment of a fracture are three: reduction, immobilization and rehabilitation. The fracture, if displaced, must be reduced as accurately as possible *(reduction).* It must then be held in place for as long as is required for it to unite *(immobilization).* In the meantime the soft tissues, specially the muscles in the area, must be exercised as far as possible, in order to prevent their atrophy through disuse *(rehabilitation).*

REDUCTION

This means restoring the bones to their normal anatomical position. Reduction, when required, can be accomplished by closed manipulation or open operation.

Closed manipulation. This has the great advantage that the skin remains intact and there is no chance of the fracture becoming infected. Therefore, whenever possible, closed reduction is to be preferred.

Anaesthesia. General anaesthesia is commonly used. This not only makes the procedure painless but also relaxes the muscles so that the manipulation becomes easier (manus = hand; manipulation = to move something by the use of the hands). If general anaesthesia cannot be used the fracture haematoma may be infiltrated with a *local* anaesthetic. The local anaesthetic may also be used intravenously distal to a tourniquet (intravenous regional anaesthesia).

Having anaesthetized the patient or the part, the bone ends are manipulated to restore the normal anatomy. The actual movements required for the reduction of common fractures are described in the following chapter. However, in general the surgeon seeks to reverse the mechanical events which caused the fracture.

Open reduction. Open reduction has to be carried out under the following circumstances:

1. If closed reduction fails in bringing the fracture fragments into a satisfactory and acceptable position.
2. In situations where it is common knowledge that closed reduction cannot succeed in its objective. Some examples follow:

i. If soft tissues are interposed between the bone fragments.

ii. If the surgeon cannot obtain any purchase on one of the two fracture fragments, as in a fracture through the anatomical neck of the humerus accompanied by dislocation of the head of the humerus.

iii. In fractures around joints in which there are several small fragments whose accurate replacement is essential for normal joint function. Examples include certain fracture-dislocations around the ankle and depressed fractures of the tibial condyles.

IMMOBILIZATION

The *aims* of immobilization are two:

1. To maintain correct alignment of the bones while healing is taking place.
2. To prevent movement of one fragment over the other. This is extremely important if union is to take place. If movement occurs at the fracture site the delicate granulation tissue or early callus is broken, and healing has to start again from the beginning. In fact if such movement occurs repeatedly, delayed union or even non-union may result.

Methods of immobilization. Immobilization may be provided externally or internally:

External fixation may be provided by:

1. Splints.
2. Traction.
3. External fixators.

Internal fixation is commonly provided by the use of:

1. Intramedullary nails.
2. Bone plates and screws or steel wires.

EXTERNAL FIXATION

1. Splints. i. *Wooden splints.* In a first-aid situation an appropriately sized piece of wood or other stiff material may be used as a temporary splint; it is bandaged to the side of the broken limb.

ii. *Plaster of Paris.* By far the most commonly used splint is a plaster of Paris slab or cast. *Every medical student should be taught to apply a plaster of Paris slab during his work in the emergency department (Fig. 1a).* In case any student has not seen a plaster being applied, the correct method of applying a plaster slab should be demonstrated to each batch of students, and one of them should be asked to repeat it.

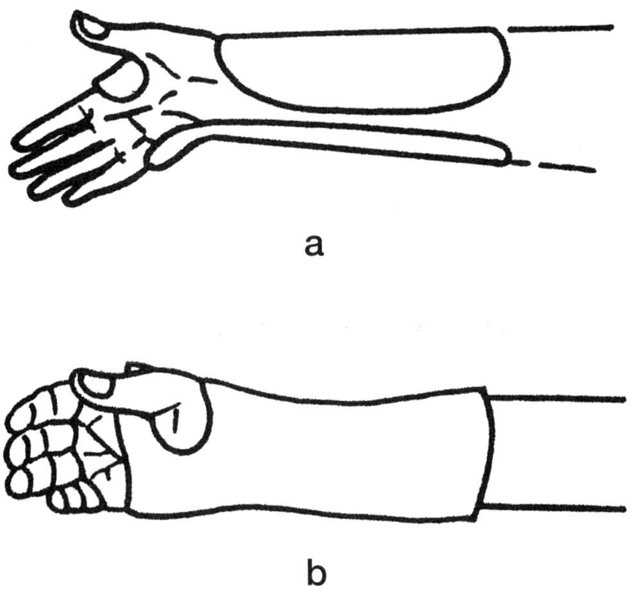

Fig. 1 (a) plaster slab, (b) plaster cast.

While applying a plaster cast (Fig. 1b) the limb is held in the desired position, and is usually enclosed in a layer of cotton wool which serves as padding material. Gauze bandages impregnated in plaster are now soaked in warm water and applied around the limb. The plaster sets in a few minutes to hold the limb in a fixed position.

In order to be effective the plaster cast must generally extend to include *the joint above and the joint below* the fractured bone. In a first-aid situation it is usually best to apply a plaster slab rather than a cast, and to leave the final application of slab or cast till after the fractured limb has been x-rayed in hospital.

The advantages of plaster of Paris. 1. It is cheap and easily available.

2. It is readily applied and quickly sets in the correct position, abolishing movement of bone ends over each other and virtually eliminating pain.

3. It moulds itself to the contours of the limb; therefore, it is comfortable.

4. It is fairly strong.

5. It is radio-translucent, so that x-rays can be taken through it.

The disadvantages of plaster. The necessity of immobilizing the neighbouring joints is one of the most important disadvantages of the use of plaster-of-Paris. It means that sometimes when the plaster is removed these joints are stiff and the muscles weak.

Other disadvantages of plaster are the following:

1. Any wounds which are present cannot easily be treated in plaster.

2. The material is fairly heavy.

3. It is not always easy to maintain the reduction while the plaster bandage is being applied.

However, the most serious hazard of the use of plaster-of-Paris is the one which is described now.

The major hazard of splinting by plaster. After every fracture, swelling occurs at the fracture site. If plaster is applied soon after the fracture, the further swelling which arises results in a rise in pressure, because it cannot expand the rigid plaster cast. The raised pressure obstructs the veins. The venous return is occluded and the part swells further. With increasing swelling and pressure the arteries are occluded. If arterial occlusion persists for more than a few hours the muscles and nerves are infarcted and later replaced by fibrous tissue. If the occlusion is allowed to continue for a longer period gangrene can occur and necessitate amputation of the limb, which is a very major disaster.

Thus if plaster-of-Paris is to be applied to a fresh fracture the following precautions must be observed:

1. The plaster should not completely encircle the limb. This can be achieved by applying a plaster *slab,* leaving a gap on one side of the limb. Alternatively, if the plaster is completely encircling the bone, it can be *split* longitudinally.

2. Any such plaster should be *well padded* inside with cotton-wool so that swelling may occur without compressing the soft tissues.

3. The limb should be *elevated* after applying the plaster, to encourage venous and lymphatic drainage and discourage swelling.

However, in spite of these disadvantages plaster still remains generally the cheapest, most convenient and most widely employed form of splintage.

Clinical features of impaired blood flow. The circulation in the exposed skin distal to the fracture should be carefully examined in the hours following the application of the plaster. If the skin is *pale* or there is *poor capillary filling* in the limb it means that the blood supply is impaired. The other signs of insufficient blood flow include pain, paraesthesias and pulselessness.

Pain at the fracture site is always present but pain in the muscles on active finger movements is an ominous sign. This may manifest itself as inability to move the fingers. *Paraesthesia* results from an impaired supply of blood to the nerves, and is a reliable early sign of reduced blood supply.

Pulselessness may be a late sign and in some cases may not be present, yet the blood supply to the muscles may be interrupted. If this happens, the muscles cannot contract and the fingers will be stiff. If infarction occurs, fibrosis of the muscles and nerves is the result. The fibrous tissue contracts, causing deformity and stiffness. The condition is known as *Volkmann's ischaemic contracture.*

The whole plaster should be split from one end to the other and all padding divided so that the skin is visible throughout the length of the split in the plaster. It is very important to follow this instruction closely. If even a single strand of plaster remains undivided the constriction could continue and have disastrous consequences. If significant swelling occurs there will be increasing discomfort and pain at the fracture and distal to it. In that case also the plaster should be opened. If splitting of the plaster does not improve the circulation the artery should be explored promptly; at the same time fasciotomies should be carried out if required.

2. Traction. In a few situations fractures are immobilized by exerting traction on the involved limb. The common bone injury treated by this method is fracture of the shaft of the femur. This is necessary because the powerful thigh muscles contract and cause overriding of the fragments unless traction is maintained on the limb. The methods of applying traction to the limb are two: skin traction, and skeletal traction.

Skin traction. Adhesive plaster is applied to the whole length of the medial as well as lateral side of the lower limb. The limb is now placed in a Thomas splint. The adhesive strips, or cords attached to them, are pulled firmly and fixed to the foot end of the splint. (Fig. 7, chapter 36). *Every medical student should be taught to apply a Thomas splint as a first-aid measure.*

The advantage of this technique is that unlike skeletal traction there is no pin track passing through the tibia, so that there is no possibility of infecting the bone. However, the disadvantage is that the traction is not very forceful. Therefore it cannot overcome the pull of the strong thigh muscles in an adult. Thus it can be used only in children. In adults it is used only as a temporary measure. If a fracture in an adult is to be managed by traction, skeletal traction is normally used.

Skeletal traction. For this purpose a Steinmann pin is commonly passed through the tibial tubercle and a stirrup is attached to it. The limb is placed on a Bohler-Braun splint. A rope is attached to the stirrup and passed over the pulley, and weights are suspended from it (Fig. 6, chapter 36).

3. External fixators. If a *contaminated open* fracture is treated by internal fixation, infection may result. If fixation is not employed, the fracture remains unstabilized and cannot heal. To resolve this dilemma, external fixators are sometimes employed. In this method a minimum of two pins are passed into the long bone above, and a similar number below the fracture site. The shafts of the pins close to their outer ends are attached to a steel bar. The fracture is now reduced under anaesthesia and the joints between the pins and the bar tightened (Fig. 2a). In this way the bone ends are rigidly and accurately held against each other for the required number of weeks until the bone ends unite .

INTERNAL FIXATION

This is normally provided after exposing the bones at a surgical operation, which may be required for a fracture in the following situations:

1. If reduction is impossible by closed means. This may be due to the fact that:

i. Soft tissues e.g. muscles are interposed between the bone fragments, and need to be extracted at open operation to allow the bone ends to be brought together.

ii. One of the two fracture fragments cannot be manipulated, e.g. in fracture of the neck of the humerus with dislocation of the shoulder.

2. If it is impossible to maintain reduction by external splintage. This is commonly seen in fractures of the neck of the femur.

3. If it is hazardous to the patient to maintain reduction by closed methods. Thus in inter-trochanteric fracture of the femur the fracture can be immobilized by traction.

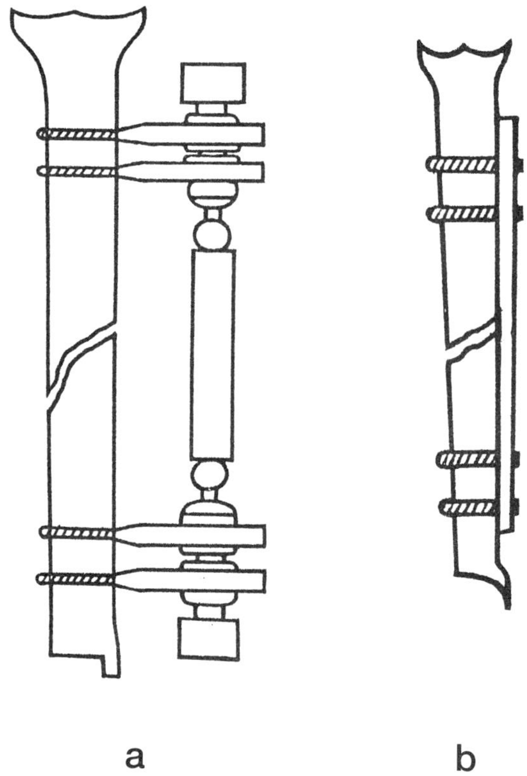

Fig. 2 Treatment of fracture of a long bone by (a) use of external fixator, (b) onlay bone plating.

However, this requires prolonged immobilization in bed. In elderly patients this may produce bedsores, hypostatic pneumonia, or deep vein thrombosis which may lead to pulmonary embolism and death. Therefore this fracture in the elderly is best treated by open reduction and internal fixation.

Common methods of internal fixation. Different methods of internal fixation are employed depending upon the type of fracture:

1. *Intramedullary nailing*. A nail is passed down from one end of the bone along the medullary cavity to the other end.

2. *Onlay bone plate.* This is placed on the bone and fixed in place usually with four to six screws, i.e. two to three screws into either fragment (Fig. 2b).

3. *Pin and plate.* This is used in intertrochanteric fracture of the femur. The pin is passed up the neck of the femur. The bone plate is placed on the shaft of the femur and held in place by screws. The two are joined together. Newer versions include *dynamic hip screw* fixation.

4. *Compression plating.* A special plate is used. It is applied in such a manner that the fracture fragments are compressed together. This greatly expedites fracture union.

USE OF A PROSTHESIS

If the surgeon feels that a fracture fragment cannot survive, (e.g. femoral head in a fracture of the neck of the femur) the fragment should be excised and replaced by a prosthesis made of stainless steel or a plastic material.

Management of soft tissues. Muscles may form adhesions with the fracture site. This interferes with their efficient functioning. *To preserve function and mobility the patient is instructed to move daily, through a full range of movement, all those joints which are not immobilized.* Otherwise the muscles become wasted and adhere to the bone.

When a joint is immobilized the synovial cavity is gradually obliterated with the formation of fibrous tissue. The joint becomes stiff. Therefore the plaster splint should include only those joints which have to be immobilized. At the same time joints which are not immobilized should be actively exercised to prevent stiffness. It has recently been shown that early movement at a joint is essential for its nourishment and function. With this in mind, the tendency is to shorten the period of time for which the plaster of Paris cast extends from a joint above to the joint below. As soon as the fracture gets 'sticky' the cast is shortened to allow early joint movement.

OPEN FRACTURES

An open fracture constitutes an orthopaedic emergency. It is extremely important to prevent infection developing in the wound. Infection in a fracture, once established, can be very difficult to eradicate and markedly increases the risk of nonunion. Therefore, very strict aseptic precautions should be undertaken during the operation.

Open fractures are *classified* into type I, i.e. those with a wound less than 1 cm in length; type II, those with a wound more than 1 cm with moderate soft tissue damage; and type III, those with severe soft tissue injury or loss.

Treatment. This is carried out on the following general lines: the wound is cultured and covered with a sterile bandage and the extremity splinted. Penicillin, a cephalosporin, and an aminoglycoside are administered intravenously.

In a sterile operating room the patient is anaesthetized. The wound is irrigated with several liters of saline, and the extremity painted with an antiseptic. The surgical procedure should be carried out under a good operating light.

1 to 2 mm of the skin edges are excised. All devitalized muscle or debris is excised, the fracture surface curetted to remove all foreign material, and the wound irrigated with more saline. This removal of dead tissue and debris is called *debridement.*

The most important part of the operation is *excision of dead muscle.* The extent of muscle damage can be assessed by the four C's: colour, consistency, contractility and capacity to bleed. Changes in colour of the muscle, loss of contractility on mechanical stimulation and failure to bleed, all demand wide excision of the muscle, specially when contamination by gas gangrene organisms is suspected, because if left behind they would provide a culture medium for bacteria.

Repair of tendons and nerves in an open fracture is rarely indicated. Vessels require repair if the blood supply to the limb is threatened. Finally, the fracture is reduced and the skin loosely approximated, leaving part of the wound open if necessary to avoid tension but covering exposed bone, nerves, vessels and tendons. The fracture is stabilized with plaster or more commonly an external fixator to allow wound access. Antibiotics are continued for a minimum of 10 to 14 days postoperatively. Repeat wound inspections at 24 and 48 hours are advisable, specially for type III injuries. If secondary wound closure to achieve bone coverage is not feasible, skin grafts or muscle flaps can be employed.

In most cases it is safest and best to *leave the wound open* to granulate. If it is closed and becomes septic the tension in the wound rises and further soft tissue damage as well as septicaemia can result. It is legitimate to suture such a wound only if contamination is minimal and one is sure that the patient will be very closely supervised postoperatively. Even in such a case the sutures must be tied very loosely. If fever or excessive pain develop, the sutures should be removed promptly.

Wounds sustained during war are always left open, because a soldier with a wound may have to be evacuated over long distances to the base hospital. During the journey it may be impossible to provide sufficiently close supervision and treatment to the wound. If the wound has been sutured and becomes infected, the pus would not find an exit. The raised pressure in the tissues would drive the septic material into the veins, producing septicaemia which is dangerous and could prove fatal. If on the other hand the wound is left open, any pus which forms drains freely onto the surface, so that there is little risk of septic absorption.

Antibiotics. Although excision of dead tissue and leaving the wound open are of crucial importance in the healing of a compound fracture, appropriate antibiotics help prevent infection if started early. It should, however, be remembered that *antibiotics are no substitute for proper surgical debridement.*

REHABILITATION

It used to be thought that rehabilitation should be started after the fracture has healed. We know now that this is an incorrect approach, because by this time stiffness has already taken place in joints which have not been exercised. Rehabilitation should commence immediately after reduction and immobilization. In fact *psychological rehabilitation* should proceed from the moment the injury is sustained, by means of words of reassurance and explanation.

As far as the *physical* aspects of rehabilitation are concerned, *those joints in the limb which are not immobilized should be put through their full range of movement daily from the beginning* so that they do not stiffen. For example in Colles' fracture which occurs in old people the shoulder and elbow can become stiff very quickly. Therefore the hand should be placed behind the head (full abduction and external rotation at the shoulder) and behind the back (full adduction and internal rotation) at least once every day.

The treatment of nonunion. If there is an obvious cause of nonunion such as infection, the underlying pathology should be treated. Sometimes there is no evident cause of the fibrous nonunion. In that case two measures are usually employed together, namely absolute fixation and the use of a bone graft. Absolute immobilization can be more certainly produced by internal fixation. Thus a common method of dealing with fibrous nonunion is this: an intramedullary nail is passed for rigid internal fixation. At the same time the periosteum around the fracture site is elevated and cancellous bone chips packed under it. The common site for obtaining cancellous bone chips is the patient's iliac crest. The cancellous bone acts as a scaffold on which new bone is formed.

INJURIES TO ARTICULAR CARTILAGE

Adult cartilage cells do not undergo mitosis. Therefore loss of a portion of cartilage is not made good. Because the defect is not repaired, the articular surface remains irregular. This may lead to osteoarthrosis, specially in the weight-bearing joints. Injury to a cartilage in a joint produces no specific signs, but haemarthrosis and swelling of the joint accompany cartilage injury. A loose fragment of cartilage becomes rounded and is called a *loose body*. It may get stuck between the joint surfaces and produce 'locking' of the joint. Blood in a joint eventually clots and organizes into fibrous tissue. It adheres to the cartilage surfaces and synovial membrane, and mechanically limits movement.

INJURIES TO LIGAMENTS

Bony injuries to the limbs are often accompanied by ligamentous injuries. In addition, a ligament injury can occur independently as a primary injury to a joint; these are referred to as sprains. Ligament injuries are graded as follows:

Type I: Stretch, but no disruption of fibres.
Type II: Tear of some ligament fibres.
Type III: Complete discontinuity of the ligament.

Ligaments heal by progressive scar formation and contracture, and recent studies indicate that if gross instability is not present, repair is improved by early motion.

Type I and II injuries are *treated* by immobilization or protected motion. Treatment of type III injuries varies from non-intervention (as in type III acromioclavicular separation) to immediate surgical reconstruction (as for a torn anterior cruciate ligament in a professional athlete).

FRACTURES IN CHILDHOOD

Fractures in children differ from those in adults in many ways:

1. They unite more rapidly.
2. Moderately angulated fractures get corrected by remodelling during growth.
3. Joint stiffness is rare after immobilization.
4. The bone may fracture incompletely (*greenstick fracture*).
5. The fracture may involve the epiphyseal plate. This may interfere with growth, though fortunately rarely.

THE BATTERED BABY SYNDROME

The term battered baby is used for a young child who receives serious, deliberately inflicted injuries at the hands of a parent or other adult. The injuries are unsuspected because the child is unable to give a history. The children are usually under the age of two years. When they are taken to hospital the parents are unable to explain the injuries, or they suggest some minor accident, which does not correlate with the severity of the injury. The common injuries consist of bruises, abrasions, and fractures of long bones, ribs or skull. The 'battered baby syndrome' is a modern disease. It is more common in the advanced countries. It is the external evidence of the frustrations caused by the rat-race of life in our cities, and by broken homes. Such child-abuse is repetitive. Therefore it is important to make the diagnosis and take action appropriately. The child should be admitted to hospital immediately to protect it, while the social worker investigates the case, to arrive at a diagnosis and to suggest measures to prevent repetition of the abuse.

36 *Injuries to the limbs*

Upper limb

The upper limb is a single functional unit, the directly active part being the hand. The arm has no function other than to carry the hand this way and that, so as to place it in the desired position where it can perform its functions of grip etc. If the hand is no more, the arm has no function to perform. The really active parts of the hand are the thumb and fingers. Therefore, injuries to the thumb and fingers have an importance quite out of proportion to their size.

THE PECTORAL GIRDLE

Acromio-clavicular dislocation. This injury commonly occurs from a violent downward blow on the point of the shoulder, commonly in contact sports. Dislocation can occur only if the coracoclavicular ligament is also ruptured. The scapula is pulled downwards by the weight of the arm, and the clavicle upwards by the sternomastoid. The outer end of the clavicle produces a prominence. X-rays are taken both with and without the patient holding a 10-lb weight, which accentuates the subluxation. Partial tears are *treated* with a sling until comfortable, and then progressive exercises. Complete tears can be treated conservatively in less active individuals. If the deformity is accepted and early functional rehabilitation emphasized, the result is usually serviceable in spite of distal clavicular prominence. However, in those concerned with the deformity, surgical reconstruction may be indicated. In patients with persistent pain excision of the distal clavicle gives satisfactory results.

Fracture of the clavicle. Fracture of the clavicle is a common injury. It usually occurs in the middle third of the bone from falls on the outstretched hand. The lateral fragment is displaced downwards by the weight of the limb; the medial fragment is held up by the sternomastoid muscle. The essential *treatment* is to support the weight of the limb by a triangular sling. Nearly always the fracture is clinically united within three weeks and functional recovery is complete within about two months. The figure-of-eight bandage, crossing between the shoulder blades, may be applied to brace back the shoulders, and kept for three weeks. However it should not be used in every case. In the simplest undisplaced fractures a sling is all that is necessary. Again, in the elderly this bandage may prove dangerous by causing pressure on the axillary vessels and nerves. Here also a sling is enough. If the clavicle is broken lateral to the attachment of the coracoclavicular ligament displacement is rare, and an analgesic for pain is all that is required.

Fracture of the body of the scapula. Comminuted stellate fractures occur in the body of the scapula from direct violence as in motor vehicle accidents. Scapular fractures rarely cause symptoms and usually heal uneventfully. The arm should simply be rested in a sling until pain subsides enough to allow mobilization of the shoulder. Fractures of the ribs usually occur at the same time, and should be treated appropriately. If both the scapula and the clavicle are injured, the integrity of the brachial plexus should always be checked.

THE SHOULDER

Dislocation of the shoulder. This is a common injury. The head of the humerus usually dislocates forwards from the shoulder joint so as to lie beneath the coracoid process to produce a subcoracoid anterior dislocation. The injury results from forced extension and external rotation of the abducted arm. The head of the humerus dislocates forwards, either rupturing the capsule or avulsing the labrum from the glenoid. If the labrum is avulsed it rarely heals because it is avascular. The head comes to lie beneath the coracoid and the humerus is locked in this position by spasm of the muscles. Rarely, the humerus dislocates posteriorly, and very uncommonly it subluxates vertically downwards. The *clinical findings* in a subcoracoid dislocation are typical. The outer aspect of the shoulder is flattened, the arm is held in a position of slight abduction and cannot be moved. On x-ray the head of the humerus is seen to be lying below the coracoid. The rare posterior dislocation is less easily diagnosed because the clinical appearance of the shoulder is essentially normal. Also, on x-ray the head of the humerus is not displaced medially to any great extent. Special x-ray views called *axillary views* are required to show up this dislocation.

Treatment. If the patient is given a general anaesthetic relaxing the muscles, reduction of a dislocated shoulder is easy. It can be accomplished simply by pressure in the correct direction over the head of the humerus. If this does not succeed *Kocher's method* is employed. Traction is applied to the humerus which is then externally rotated to the full extent, in order to stretch and abolish the spasm of the subscapularis muscle. Traction is now maintained and the elbow brought across the body to fully adduct the shoulder. The patient's hand is next brought to his opposite shoulder so as to rotate the shoulder internally. During this final rotation reduction is felt to occur and the contour of the shoulder returns to normal. Postreduction anteroposterior and trans-scapular x-rays are essential. The arm is kept in a sling and bandaged to the side of the trunk for three weeks. After this the shoulder is gradually mobilized, but avoiding external rotation in abduction. In the elderly, exercises are started sooner to prevent stiffness.

Recurrent dislocation of the shoulder. After reduction most dislocations of the shoulder heal and cause no further disability. However, occasionally the shoulder becomes unstable and repeatedly dislocates after trivial violence. This causes considerable disability and requires relief. MRI or arthroscopy can help surgical planning by identifying tears of the anterior labrum, which cause persistent disability. Operation is the only satisfactory method of treatment. The shoulder is approached from the front. The rupture in the capsule or glenoidal labrum is repaired. The subscapularis muscle is then overlapped in front of the joint to reinforce the capsule.

Fracture of the neck of the humerus. Fracture of the *surgical neck* is a common injury in adults specially females due to a fall on the outstretched hand, while in children the *anatomical neck* is involved. The patient complains of pain in the shoulder and cannot move the joint. However, in impacted fractures through the surgical neck a limited degree of movement is possible.

Treatment of fracture of the *surgical* neck is simple. The arm is rested in a sling until pain has subsided sufficiently to allow mobilization of the shoulder to be started. Fractures of the *anatomical* neck without dislocation of the shoulder are treated in a similar manner. A certain degree of angulation can be accepted in view of the large range of motion of the shoulder joint. Marked angulation requires percutaneous pinning or open reduction. The treatment of fracture of the anatomical neck combined with dislocation of the shoulder is difficult, and open operation is required. The shoulder becomes stiff after these injuries. This improves over the next few months but some stiffness may remain.

Fracture of the shaft of the humerus. The shaft of the humerus is usually fractured in the middle third, either from an indirect twisting force (which causes a spiral fracture) or from direct violence (resulting in a transverse or comminuted fracture). This fracture occurs in adults. There may be no displacement, or marked angulation or overlapping may result. The proximal half of the humerus is also a common site for pathological fracture from carcinomatous metastases.

Treatment. Reduction of these fractures is often not necessary since gravity acting on the arm exerts steady traction which tends to correct any angulation that may occur. Support of the wrist with a collar and cuff allowing the elbow to hang free may be sufficient. However, in order or minimize the pain a plaster slab is usually applied which runs from the acromion down the lateral side of the arm, below the elbow and up the medial side of the arm. Immobilization is maintained for about 3 weeks, during which period the hand is kept mobile. For the next 3 weeks the arm is removed daily from the sling to exercise the shoulder. If satisfactory reduction cannot be achieved or maintained, surgical treatment with compression plating or intramedullary nailing is appropriate. At the same time, patients with multiple trauma are treated with intramedullary nailing to allow rapid mobilization, so as to prevent pulmonary and other complications.

Radial nerve injury occurs occasionally, usually a neurapraxia or axonotmesis, with an excellent prognosis. If recovery does not take place within 3 months electromyography should be carried out to determine whether subclinical recovery is occurring. Exploration is indicated if

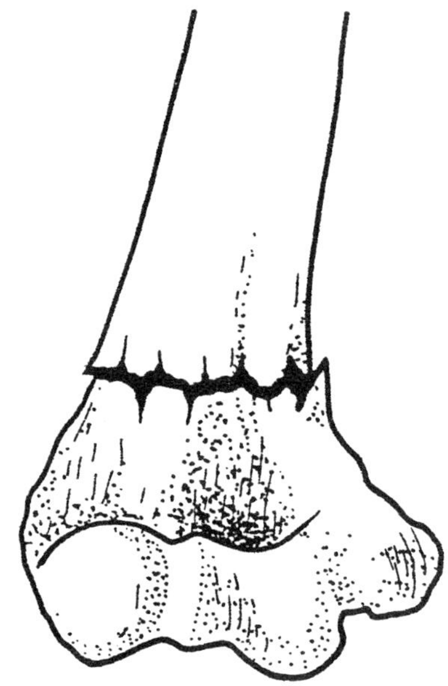

Fig. 1 Supracondylar fracture of humerus.

such recovery is not evident. Patients with radial nerve palsy need wrist and hand splinting and therapy to maintain joint mobility.

THE ELBOW

The elbow very often becomes stiff following an injury. The cause of this stiffness is not known. It is thought to be due to adhesions in and around the joint capsule. Soon after injury the joint should be protected. After 2 or 3 weeks movements are gradually encouraged.

Supracondylar fracture of the humerus (Fig. 1). *This is one of the most common and serious fractures of childhood.* It does not often occur in adults. It should always be regarded as potentially dangerous because of the risk of injury to the brachial artery. The fracture occurs through a fall on the outstretched hand. The deformity is nearly always the same, the lower fragment being displaced backwards and tilted backwards.

Clinical findings. The elbow swells markedly and this obscures the other physical signs. However, the olecranon and the two epicondyles can be palpated. They are found to be normally related to each other. On the other hand in posterior dislocation of the elbow the olecranon lies abnormally posterior to the epicondyles. This distinguishes the two conditions.

The most important point to keep in mind is the possibility of the blood supply to the forearm being interrupted due to this injury. This may happen at the time of the injury if the brachial artery is contused or lacerated by the proximal fragment of the humerus. The radial pulse will not be palpable. More commonly the radial pulse is present at the time of the injury, but is obliterated by swelling and by flexion of the elbow after reduction. Therefore *the radial pulse must be repeatedly palpated* during the first two days after injury.

Treatment. *Undisplaced* fractures can be treated with a posterior splint with 90 degrees of flexion. Further flexion can be hazardous because of swelling, and all patients should be observed closely following immobilization. *Displaced* fractures have classically been treated by closed manipulation and immobilization in as much flexion as tolerated without circulatory embarrassment. Currently, however, percutaneous pinning under fluoroscopic guidance has become the most popular method. This allows the maintenance of more anatomical reduction *without the need for excessive flexion* at the elbow. Postoperatively the limb is kept in a posterior splint with not more than 90 degrees of flexion. If there is evidence of impaired circulation or compartment syndrome, immediate brachial artery exploration and forearm fasciotomies must be carried out to restore the blood supply and tissue perfusion. The pins are removed at 3 to 4 weeks and active exercises started.

Dislocation of the elbow is usually caused by a heavy fall on the outstretched hand with the elbow slightly flexed. The dislocation is nearly always posterior or postero-lateral. This means that the ulna and radius are displaced backward, or backwards and laterally, in relation to the humerus. The patient cannot move the elbow, which lies in a position of slight flexion. The point of the olecranon can be felt to be abnormally posterior to the humeral epicondyles. This distinguishes posterior dislocation of the elbow from supracondylar fracture. AP and lateral x-rays of the elbow show the dislocation (Fig. 2).

Treatment. The dislocation should be reduced as soon as possible. The patient is given a general anaesthetic to relax the muscles. It is then easy to reduce the dislocation by applying traction in the long axis of the slightly flexed ulna, while pressure is applied behind the olecranon. Once reduced the elbow can be put through a full range of movements. The elbow is now rested in a plaster slab in 90 degrees of flexion for three weeks before exercises are begun. A plaster affords the best conditions for healing of the soft tissues. It also allows greater freedom of movement to the shoulder and hand than the collar-and-cuff sling which is sometimes prescribed for this injury.

Fracture-dislocation of the elbow. In severe trauma posterior dislocation of the elbow may be accompanied by fracture of the coronoid process and of the radial head. These are much less stable injuries than simple posterior dislocations. Open reduction may be necessary, with reattachment of the avulsed coronoid fragment. For further stabilization of the elbow prosthetic replacement of the radial head may be required. The silicon radial head can fragment over a period of time. Therefore, once the elbow has stabilized, the prosthetic head is sometimes removed.

Fracture of the olecranon. This is usually caused by a fall onto the point of the elbow. The fracture line runs across the narrow part of the olecranon. If the triceps expansion is intact over the fracture site there is no separation of the fragments and the case may be treated by immobilization for 3 weeks in a padded plaster cylinder, followed by gentle mobilization. If the fragments are separated (Fig. 3), the fracture must be reduced and immobilized by internal fixation. Following sound internal fixation early movement of the elbow should be commenced.

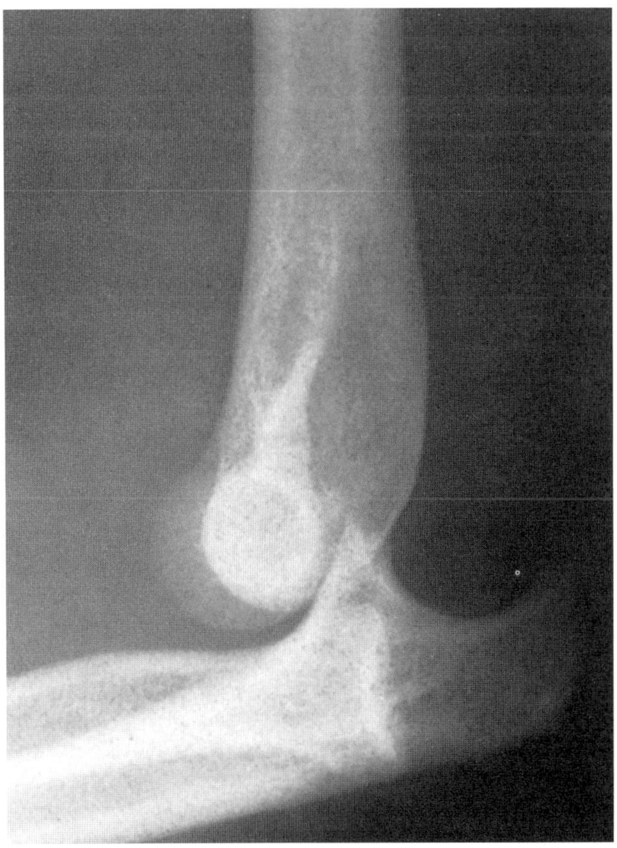

Fig. 2 Posterior dislocation of elbow.

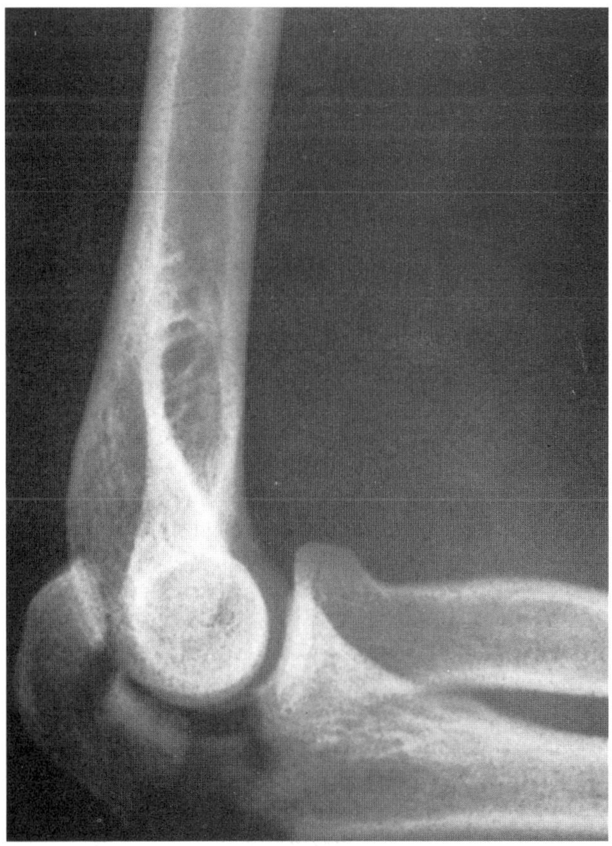

Fig. 3 Fracture of olecranon.

Fracture of the head of the radius. This fracture occurs due to a fall on the outstretched hand. The neck of the bone may be fractured, or alternatively a fragment may be split off from the head. There may be only some painful limitation of movement with tenderness over the head of the radius. The injury is shown on x-ray.

Treatment. If the fracture line runs through the neck of the radius or through the head with little displacement, the elbow should be immobilized for three weeks in a plaster slab. If the fracture involves the articular surface and significant comminution has occurred, the head of the radius must be excised. If this is not done the resulting irregularity of the head limits movement. Also, late osteoarthrosis results. In children the fracture usually involves the neck of the radius. If it is displaced, closed reduction should be tried. However, if this fails, open reduction is carried out. *The head of the radius is not removed in children,* because it results in arrest of growth at the proximal end of the radius. This causes severe shortening of the radius and produces progressive derangement at the elbow and the radioulnar joints.

THE SHAFTS OF THE RADIUS AND ULNA

Fracture of one bone without angulation. This may occur due to a direct blow to the forearm. The fracture requires immobilization in an above-elbow plaster for 6 weeks in an adult, and 3 weeks in a child.

Fractures of both forearm bones. These fractures usually occur at approximately the same level, and are caused by a direct blow. Occasionally the bones may be fractured by torsion of the forearm; in this case the fractures are oblique and are placed at different levels in the two bones. These fractures often produce severe displacement which is very difficult to correct without open operation. Displacement is usually more severe in adults; children often suffer no more than a greenstick fracture with minor angulation. In severe trauma the excessive swelling of muscles within tight fascial compartments may cause muscle ischaemia (compartment syndrome), which may require urgent fasciotomy to release the affected muscle groups. Untreated, this can lead to Volkmann's ischaemic contracture.

Treatment. Accurate reduction is important in these fractures because even slight displacement may interfere with pronation and supination. Perfect reduction is usually impossible by closed manipulation. One attempt may be made at *closed manipulation*, and if successful, a plaster cast should be applied for six weeks. Check x-rays should be taken after 10 and 20 days to detect any redisplacement and correct it. If, as is much more common, the attempt at closed reduction fails, *open reduction* should be performed. Internal fixation is then carried out, usually with dynamic compression plates and screws. These plates have eccentrically placed holes that allow compression together of the fractured ends as the screws are tightened. After operation the internal fixation may be protected by plaster for the first few weeks. However, if the fixation of both bones is mechanically adequate no plaster is required, and the early mobilization helps recovery of function. In a *child* an acceptable reduction can sometimes be obtained by closed manipulation but if not, the fractures are treated by internal fixation using thin intramedullary pins, because such fine pins do not interfere with growth of the bones.

Fracture-dislocations of the forearm bones. These take one of two forms. *The Monteggia fracture-dislocation* consists of a fracture of the ulna and dislocation of the superior radio-ulnar joint. The usual case is due to a blow on the back of the upper forearm; the force breaks the ulna with anterior angulation, and dislocates the head of the radius forwards (anterior Monteggia). Much more rarely the reverse deformity occurs (posterior Monteggia). *The Galleazi fracture-dislocation*, consisting of a fracture of the radius and dislocation of the inferior radioulnar joint, is much less common.

The presence of a displaced fracture of one forearm bone should alert the clinician to the possibility that the superior or inferior radioulnar joint is also dislocated. The general rule that fracture of the shaft of a long bone demands an x-ray not only of the bone itself but also of the proximal and distal joints is nowhere more true than in these fractures.

Treatment. Closed manipulation usually fails. Therefore treatment is commonly by open reduction. After reduction the fractured bone is dealt with by internal fixation, usually by a plate with screws. This may be protected for a few weeks by a plaster extending above the elbow. However, movements of the fingers should be carried out from the beginning to prevent stiffness.

THE DISTAL RADIUS & ULNA

Colles' fracture. This is a fracture of the distal end of the radius produced by a fall onto the palm of the outstretched hand. It rarely occurs below the age of 45. Above this age it is the most common of all fractures specially in females, due to the frequency of osteoporosis in postmenopausal women. The fracture occurs about 2 cm above the wrist joint. The lower fragment is displaced laterally and backwards, and is tilted backwards. Therefore the articular surface, instead of pointing downwards and slightly forwards, is directed downwards and backwards. At the same time the lower fragment is impacted into the upper. Quite often the styloid process of the ulna is detached from its origin by the pull of the medial collateral ligament.

Clinical findings. Just above the wrist there is a prominence at the back caused by the posterior displacement of the lower fragment. This appearance is given the name of *dinner-fork* deformity. The fracture site is tender. The radial styloid no longer lies at a lower level than the ulnar styloid; instead, the two styloid processes are nearly at the same level.

Treatment. The fracture is reduced by manipulation and immobilized with a plaster slab. This is completed after 24 hours to form a plaster cast. The wrist is immobilized in palmar flexion and ulnar deviation. The plaster extends from the distal palmar crease to just below the elbow, but most surgeons apply an above-elbow cast for 3 weeks and replace it with a shorter cast to just below the elbow for another 3 weeks. While the limb is in plaster the patient is encouraged to use the hand freely for everyday activities, and exercises of the fingers, elbow and shoulder are carried out. At the same time the patient is instructed to place her hand behind the head and behind the back at least once daily to prevent stiffness of the elbow. This is necessary because in the age group in which Colles' fracture is common, joint stiffness occurs very commonly after immobilization.

Complications. Most cases have full recovery of function. However, the following complications occur from time to time:

1. *Malunion.* To detect this an x-ray should be carried out 10 days after reduction. If redisplacement has occurred the fragments should be manipulated again into position.
2. *Stiffness* of the fingers or shoulder from disuse: to prevent stiffness, exercises of the fingers and shoulder should be carried out both in the plaster and after removal of the plaster, as explained above.
3. *Carpal tunnel syndrome.* If the diagnosis is confirmed after nerve conduction studies, the flexor retinaculum should be divided.
4. *Sudeck's atrophy* of the bones of the wrist and hand.

Smith's fracture. This is the reverse of Colles' fracture, the distal fragment being displaced anteriorly rather than posteriorly. It is uncommon. After reduction it is immobilized in an above-elbow plaster cast for six weeks in supination and slight dorsiflexion.

THE HAND

THE CARPUS

Any of the wrist bones may be injured but by far the most common injury is fracture of the scaphoid, followed by dislocation of the lunate.

Fracture of the waist of the scaphoid. This injury occurs commonly in young adults from a fall on the outstretched hand. There is pain in the wrist, but function may be nearly normal. There is tenderness over the anatomical snuff-box. Physical signs suggest a sprained wrist. X-rays (which should include a 17-degree oblique view) may sometimes not show the fracture, because no displacement occurs at the fracture site.

Treatment. If a fracture of the scaphoid is seen on x-ray a plaster cast should be applied to include the thumb and extending from the distal palmar crease to just below the elbow. This is kept in place for about eight weeks. Sometimes when a wrist is sprained a fracture of the scaphoid may be present but not visible on x-ray, because of the hair-line nature of the fracture line. In such a case a 'scaphoid' type of plaster, as described above, should be applied. After two weeks the plaster is removed and another x-ray taken. If a fracture was present, by this time some resorption of bone will have taken place at the fracture site so that the injury will be obvious on the x-ray. The plaster should now be reapplied and kept on for eight weeks. *Non-union* may occur in spite of the above management. The reason is that blood supply to the proximal part of the scaphoid enters through the distal pole, and is lost when the bone is fractured across its waist. Avascular necrosis occurs and leads to osteoarthrosis of the wrist. If non-union occurs one can accept the un-united fracture, because it does not cause significant disability. Alternatively, the proximal dead fragment of the scaphoid may be excised.

Dislocation of the lunate. When a person falls on the outstretched hand the lunate may be squeezed out from between the capitate bone and the radius. It comes to lie in front of the wrist bones, with its concave surface forwards, and is best visualized on lateral x-rays. It may compress the median nerve in the carpal tunnel and produce anaesthesia in the lateral three and a half digits and motor paralysis in the distribution of the nerve.

Treatment. Reduction by manipulation is attempted under general anaesthesia. Strong traction is first applied to the hand. The wrist is hyperextended and direct pressure applied over the displaced bone, when it may pop into position. A plaster is applied for four weeks. If unsuccessful, open reduction through a palmar approach is carried out with ligamentous repair and pin fixation. The blood supply of the displaced lunate is greatly reduced because most of its soft-tissue attachments are torn. So in a certain number of cases avascular necrosis occurs, and is followed later by osteoarthrosis. Therefore, if the lunate is avascular it should be excised. If the median nerve is compressed it should be immediately released. At operation the lunate is reduced or excised, and the flexor retinaculum divided to prevent compression of the nerve.

THE METACARPALS

Fractures of the metacarpals. These are produced by the knuckles striking an object, or by a blow on the dorsum of the hand. Fracture of a single shaft is splinted by adjacent metacarpals and is stable. In fractures of the neck some forward angulation occurs, but upto 30 degrees this causes only minimal loss of extension at the metacarpophalangeal joint and is insignificant.

Treatment. An aluminium splint is applied with the finger in the position of function, i.e. the metacarpophalangeal joint in full flexion and the interphalangeal joint in extension, the splint being kept on for three weeks. When pain disappears, mobilization is started. If forward angulation of the neck is excessive or involves the index or middle fingers, percutaneous pinning is necessary to maintain acceptable reduction.

Bennett's fracture. This injury is caused by a blow to the tip of the thumb. It is a fracture-dislocation of the base of the thumb, which is pulled dorsally by the long muscles of the thumb. Minimally displaced fractures can be treated by closed reduction and a plaster cast to include the thumb. Because of the inherent instability of the fracture the most common method of treatment involves closed reduction with percutaneous pinning of the metacarpal to the trapezium.

THE FINGERS

Dislocations of the finger joints. These are easily reduced, and are fairly stable after reduction. They are supported by strapping two fingers together, and movement is allowed immediately. Occasionally the head of the proximal bone 'button-holes' through the capsule. Closed reduction is then impossible and the injury is treated by open operation.

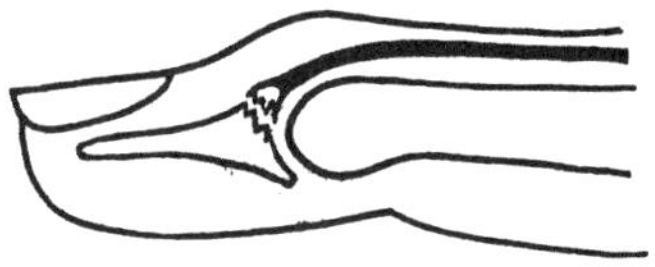

Fig. 4 Mallet finger.

Fractures of the proximal and middle phalanges. *Nondisplaced* phalanx fractures are treated by splinting in a position of function (metacarpophalangeal joints flexed 70 degrees and interphalangeal joints in slight flexion). Malleable aluminium splints with foam padding held in place by adhesive tape are used. *Displaced* fractures require manipulative reduction prior to splinting.

Fracture of the terminal phalanx. The terminal phalanx is commonly fractured by a crushing injury. The pulp is also usually crushed. Often there are associated injuries of the nail and nail bed, which may be more of a problem and are commonly neglected. The skin may be lacerated so that the fracture is open. If the wound does not heal satisfactorily the finger-tip becomes permanently tender. The patient does not use the finger, which gradually becomes stiff.

Treatment. Any wound should be cleansed to prevent infection. If a subungual haematoma is present it is drained by piercing the nail with a red hot paper clip; this gives considerable relief from pain. Nail bed lacerations should be repaired with fine absorbable sutures. The fracture is now splinted with a protective aluminium splint for 3 weeks. Angulated fractures should be reduced and, if unstable, pinned with a K-wire before splinting.

Mallet finger. In this injury the terminal slip of the extensor tendon to the distal phalanx becomes avulsed, usually taking a small fragment of bone with it. It is caused by sudden forced flexion of the terminal phalanx while the extensors of the finger are contracting (Fig. 4). There is localized pain and swelling. The patient is unable to extend the terminal phalanx, which remains in a position of 30 degrees flexion. If a piece of bone has been avulsed it should be sutured back into place. If not, the injury should be treated in a splint holding the terminal phalanx in full extension for three weeks. If the deformity still persists it should be accepted; not only is the disability slight, but suture of the tendon in any case usually stiffens the distal interphalangeal joint.

Lower limb

The function of the lower limb is locomotion and weight bearing, and both legs function together as a single unit. Stiffness of one lower limb produces a limp and interferes with the function of both legs. The foot is not as important as the hand. Even after amputation of a part of the foot e.g. in tarso-metatarsal amputation, or of the whole foot as in Syme's amputation, the function of the lower limb can be carried out to a reasonable extent. Not so in the hand. Amputation of the hand is really equivalent to amputation of the arm.

THE PELVIS

Fractures of the iliac crest. These fractures are of no significance, and should be treated like severe soft tissue injuries. Bed rest is advised for a week or two till pain subsides.

Fractures of the pelvic ring. These occur due to a blow applied directly to the pelvis. Pelvic fractures are classified into the following types:

A. Stable injuries.

B. Vertically stable but rotationally unstable injuries.

C. Vertically and rotationally unstable injuries.

Type A. The pelvis is a rigid ring. If it is broken only in *one* place, as in this type of injury, no significant displacement occurs. Such a fracture can be treated conservatively, with bed rest and subsequent protected weight bearing.

A fracture through *two* places, as in Type B and C injuries, is a far more serious matter because the pelvis becomes unstable and it may be very difficult to reduce the fracture:

Type B. The injury may fracture the pubic rami on both sides leaving a central loose fragment. If the symphysis is separated by more than 3 cm, treatment by a plate or external fixator is required.

Type C. The fractures may pass through the symphysis or rami anteriorly, and the sacroiliac joint posteriorly, when the hip bone can slide vertically upwards. Such an injury requires skeletal traction to draw the hip bone downwards.

Associated injuries. It is very important to note that a fracture of the pelvis may produce considerable internal haemorrhage and injury to the viscera — the male urethra, the bladder, and rarely the rectum and vagina. Blood loss should be replaced. In fractures of the pubic rami rupture of the urethra may be present. If the patient passes urine extravasation will occur in the perineum. Therefore he is asked not to pass urine, and urethrography is carried out under full aseptic precautions. A rectal examination is carried out to exclude the rare perforation of the rectum by a fragment of bone.

Open pelvic fracture. An open pelvic fracture is defined as a pelvic fracture with a direct communication between the fracture site and a vaginal, perineal, rectal or skin laceration. Such fractures used to have a very high mortality rate, e.g. 40%, most deaths resulting from haemorrhage and sepsis. This has been reduced considerably by the following measures:

1. By controlling sepsis.

2. By controlling haemorrhage before massive blood loss leads to coagulopathy, i.e. disseminated intravascular coagulation. Bleeding is controlled by various measures:

i. Direct ligation.

ii. Bilateral ligation of internal iliac arteries, to reduce the blood supply to the pelvic bones and viscera.

iii. Transcatheter embolization of bleeding points.

iv. Application of an external fixator after reduction of the fracture; this reduces blood loss from the cancellous bone.

Further, pneumatic anti-shock trousers (which compress the legs to prevent pooling in these parts) help improve the circulation. Most of the haemorrhage in cases of pelvic injury is from fracture surfaces and venous lesions. For its control, it is best to tamponade the low-pressure retroperitoneal bleeding by splinting the pelvis and to provide blood transfusions, sometimes in massive amounts. If the rectum is injured, not only should the faecal stream be diverted by a sigmoid colostomy, but also the faeces present in the rectum at the time of the operation should be irrigated out.

THE HIP

Dislocation of the hip. This injury is not common because the acetabulum is a deep cavity and the surrounding muscles are strong. It usually occurs when the hip is flexed and adducted, because in this position the head of the femur is covered by capsule rather than bone. Thus a force applied in the long axis of the femur may dislocate the head over the posterior lip of the acetabulum, which may also be fractured. For example, when a front seat passenger in a car is thrown forwards and the knee strikes the dashboard, a posterior dislocation can result. The head of the femur escapes into the sciatic notch where rarely the sciatic nerve may be damaged. The leg is held flexed, adducted and medially rotated. X-ray confirms the dislocation and any associated fracture. If force is applied to an abducted hip an anterior dislocation can result.

Treatment. Reduction is usually accomplished by longitudinal traction, followed by gentle abduction and external rotation. After reduction skin traction is used for 1 to 2 weeks. For the next three weeks walking is allowed on crutches. Full weight-bearing is allowed in six to eight weeks. In a high percentage of cases post-traumatic arthritis develops 10 to 30 years after injury.

Central acetabular fracture-dislocation. This is caused by a blow on the greater trochanter which drives the head of the femur through the floor of the acetabulum. If the superior dome of the acetabulum is intact, the fracture can be treated with skeletal traction for 8 to 12 weeks. In young active patients restoration of an anatomic acetabulum reduces the likelihood of post-traumatic arthritis. Generally, the operation is delayed for about a week until the patient is stabilized, because immediate surgery can be associated with significant blood loss. Postoperative complications include thromboembolic complications, hip stiffness and late osteonecrosis of acetabular fragments or femoral head. Operative treatment of acetabular fractures requires particular skill. If an experienced surgeon is not available, the patient should be transferred to another centre, or non-operative treatment employed.

THE FEMUR

Fractures of the femur are common injuries, and can be classified as follows:

1. Fractures of the proximal femur.
   i. Femoral neck fractures.
   ii. Intertrochanteric and subtrochanteric fractures.
2. Femoral shaft fractures.
3. Supracondylar fractures.

Fractures of the proximal femur are common in persons above the age of 60, in whom generalized osteoporosis makes the bones increasingly fragile. The incidence continues to rise as the number of elderly increases. The causative injury is often slight, usually a fall or stumble. Before the advent of internal fixation for these fractures patients were treated with bed rest and traction, and mortality rates were very high; although modern methods of management have improved the situation significantly, they are still quite high. These fractures occur much less commonly in young adults or children, and then from high-energy trauma such as motor vehicle accidents.

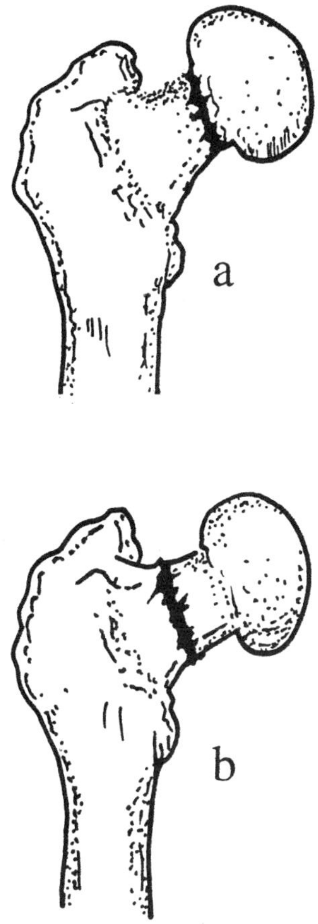

Fig. 5a, b Fractures of neck of femur: a. subcapital, b. midcervical.

Femoral neck fractures (*Fig. 5a,b*). The patient complains of pain in the groin or thigh and is unable to bear weight on the extremity. The leg appears shortened and externally rotated, and any attempt at motion causes severe pain. Ecchymosis may be seen behind the greater trochanter. Undisplaced fractures may be difficult to diagnose and initial x-rays may be negative. Some patients with undisplaced fractures have surprisingly little pain and are even able to bear weight. If a patient has unexplained bone pain and negative x-rays after a fall, MRI or a CT scan readily demonstrates a fracture if present.

Treatment. Because the femoral head is covered all round with cartilage which has no blood vessels, its blood supply comes in mostly through the neck. A fracture of the neck disrupts these blood vessels, so that osteonecrosis and nonunion are common. In *displaced* fractures in the elderly this takes place in as many as 10 to 30% of cases; these are therefore commonly treated by replacing the femoral head by a prosthesis. If the hip is arthritic, total hip replacement

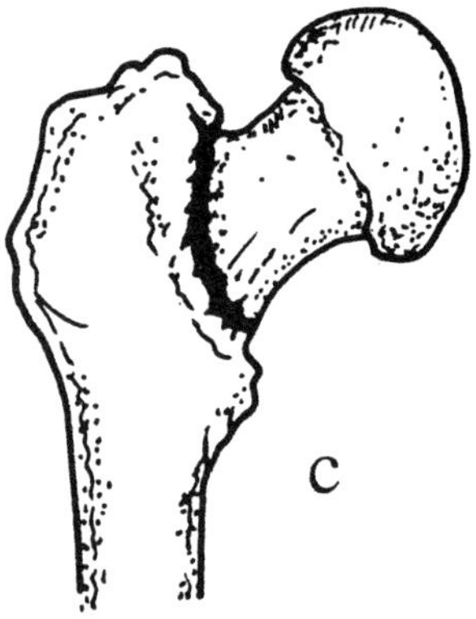

Fig. 5c Intertrochanteric fracture of femur.

arthroplasty is indicated. *Undisplaced* fractures can be treated conservatively. However, the elderly find it difficult to cooperate with protected weight bearing; further, the possibility of later displacement remains. Therefore internal fixation is generally recommended. In demented bedridden patients with other medical problems conservative treatment is usually indicated. However, even medically ill patients can usually tolerate internal fixation, specially if carried out percutaneously with multiple pins under local anaesthesia. Internal fixation should be carried out as early as possible. However, the elderly patient must be medically stabilized first.

Intertrochanteric** (Fig. 5c) **and subtrochanteric fractures. Patients present with inability to bear weight, shortening, external rotation of the leg, and swelling or ecchymosis about the hip. In the elderly, internal fixation with a compression screw and plate allows early mobilization and prevents thromboembolism. In a young patient, or in one with a medical contraindication to surgery, skeletal traction through a tibial pin can be used; however, union requires 4 months or more. In intertrochanteric fractures the blood supply to the femoral head is not disrupted, therefore osteonecrosis and nonunion are uncommon. However, subtrochanteric fractures have a significant incidence of delayed union and nonunion.

Prophylaxis. In the elderly patient with a fracture of the proximal femur, prophylactic measures should be employed before and after operation to avoid thromboembolic disease: low-dose aspirin, antiembolism stockings, and rapid mobilization with sitting in a chair within 24 hours if possible.

Fractures of the shaft of the femur. Fractures of the shaft of the femur occur at any age. They are usually due to severe violence, e.g. from a road accident. The limb is unstable, with pain on motion, rotational deformity and shortening. There is usually marked displacement with angulation and overlap, and muscles may be interposed between the fragments. As is the case of the humerus, the upper half of the femur is a common site for pathological fracture due to secondary tumours.

Damage to the sciatic nerve or femoral artery may be present, therefore neurovascular examination is essential. If signs of distal ischaemia are present arteriography is essential. Considerable blood loss, often more than a liter, may take place into the muscles of the thigh. This blood must be replaced. At the same time, the use of inflatable pneumatic trousers for transport may help maintain blood pressure and decrease blood loss in these cases.

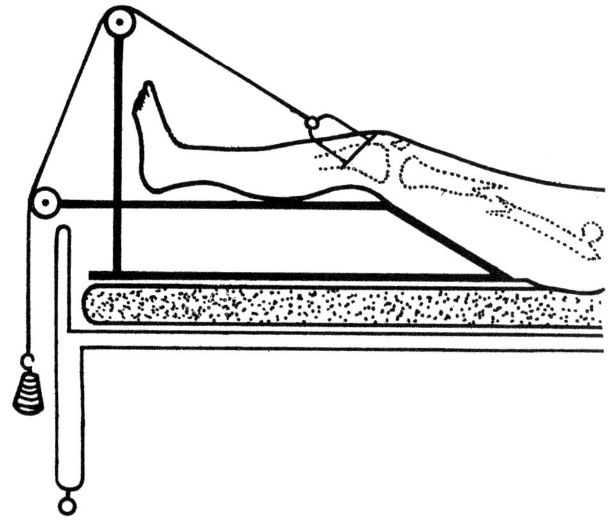

Fig. 6 Bohler-Braun splint.

Treatment. The aims of treatment are three:

1. The alignment of the femur must be restored.

2. The length must be restored. Shortening is produced by the pull of the powerful thigh muscles. This pull must be neutralized. This can be done either by continuous traction on the distal fragment until the fracture unites, or by internal fixation of the fracture by an intramedullary nail or a bone plate and screws. At the same time, upto 1.5 cm of shortening is acceptable, as this amount is concealed by pelvic tilt.

3. Stiffness of the knee must be prevented. This is a common complication of fractures of the femoral shaft due to scarring in the thigh muscles and adhesion formation in the joint.

Conservative treatment (traction). In fractures of other bones it is common practice to overcome shortening by manipulation under anaesthesia, and then to maintain this length simply by encasing the limb in plaster. In fractures of the femoral shaft it is impossible to maintain length in this manner. The reason is that contraction of the very powerful muscles of the thigh causes over-riding of the fragments with considerable shortening. It is therefore essential to apply traction to the distal fragment in order to overcome this constant tendency to produce shortening. There are two methods of applying traction, sliding traction and fixed traction.

Sliding traction. In this method traction is usually applied through bone (skeletal traction). To exert a pull on the femur a Steinmann pin is driven through the upper end of the tibia and a stirrup attached to the pin. A cord leading from the stirrup passes over a pulley, and a weight of upto 6 kg, depending upon the size of the patient, is suspended from the cord. Counter-traction is provided by the weight of the body, by raising the foot end of the bed by 15–20 cm. The limb usually lies on a Bohler-Braun splint (Fig. 6).

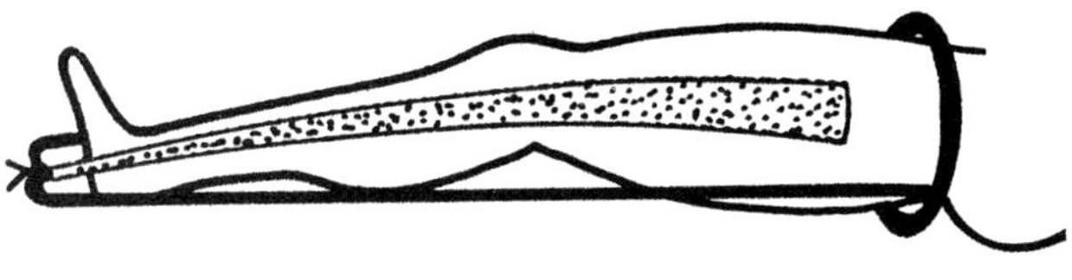

Fig. 7 Thomas splint.

Unlike internal fixation, the patient is not exposed to the risk of an infected fracture. The main danger of the method is that if traction is excessive, bone contact may be lost resulting in delayed union.

Fixed traction. For this a Thomas splint is commonly employed. The ring is passed up around the limb until it rests against the ischial tuberosity. Broad strips of adhesive are attached along the length of the lateral and medial sides of the thigh and leg, and these are further secured in place by a crepe bandage. The fracture is now reduced under general anaesthesia. The adhesive strips are pulled taut. Cords attached to these strips are firmly fixed to the foot end of the splint (Fig. 7). If it is used for an extended period of time, two problems arise with skin traction: the inadequate pull exerted, and pressure sores at the rim of the Thomas splint.

Every medical student should be taught to apply a Thomas splint, because it is the best way to render emergency aid to a patient with a severe injury of the lower limb, before sending him to hospital.

A fracture of the shaft of the femur takes about 12 weeks to unite if treated by traction. During this period the muscles of the lower limb must be exercised. When the fracture is united, traction is removed and the patient allowed to mobilize the leg in bed. If no pain occurs at the fracture site he is allowed up on crutches and gradually returns to full weight-bearing.

A *gallows splint* is useful for children below the age of 3 years. Strips of adhesive plaster are applied to the sides of the legs, which are slung up to an overhead beam so that the pelvis is just lifted off the bed. The child's weight exerts the traction.

Internal fixation. In a fracture of the middle or lower third of the shaft of the femur an intramedullary nail is often passed. Modern interlocking nails allow multiple screws to be driven across the femur and nail both proximally and distally; thus both rotation and lengthening are prevented. Infection rates with internal fixation are low, of the order of 0.5 to 1 percent. Therefore, there is an increasing tendency to treat fractures of the femur by internal fixation. This is of special benefit in the elderly, who do not take to prolonged immobilization kindly. If the fracture occurs in the subtrochanteric part of the shaft, the grip of the nail on the upper fragment is quite insufficient, therefore a nail and plate has to be employed. The nail is passed up the femoral neck, the plate is screwed onto the shaft, and the two are screwed together. Alternatively a one-piece nail-plate is used. *If internal fixation is used, the strictest aseptic routines must be enforced,* as infection can spell disaster.

Supracondylar fracture of the femur. This fracture presents a special problem because the gastrocnemius flexes the distal segment, producing posterior angulation at the fracture site. This is very difficult to control conservatively, and the fracture is best treated by internal fixation using a blade plate.

Fractures of the tibial and femoral condyles. The condyles of the femur and the tibia have a great deal in common. All four condyles are large masses of bone taking part in the formation of the knee joint. If the tibia is abducted on the femur the medial collateral ligament of the knee may be stretched and ruptured. At the same time, one of the lateral condyles, either of the femur or the tibia, may collapse due to compression. As their articular surface is concave, the tibial condyles caves in more commonly than the femorals. Fractures due to direct violence are usually produced by motor-car bumpers hitting pedestrians. The fracture may be comminuted with numerous fragments, or the whole condyle, with an intact articular surface, may be depressed. Tomograms are helpful in assessing the injury.

Treatment. Patients with less than 10 mm joint line depression can be treated conservatively, with immobilization in a cast or brace and protected weight bearing, specially if the patient is over 50 years of age, is not very active, has osteoporosis, or has medical contraindications to operation. Young active patients with more than 10 mm joint line depression are candidates for surgical treatment, which consists of elevation of depressed articular surfaces, bone grafting if necessary, and internal fixation with screws. Ruptured collateral ligaments are also repaired. Postoperatively, continuous passive motion aids in recovery of range of motion, and protected weight bearing is allowed for 8 to 12 weeks in a brace.

THE PATELLA

Fractures of the patella. These may be caused by direct or indirect violence. *Indirect* violence commonly takes place when a person slips on one foot. To save him from falling, the quadriceps muscle on the opposite side contracts violently, resulting in a clean break of the patella into an upper and a lower fragment. If the prepatellar expansion of the quadriceps is *not ruptured* the two fragments of the patella remain undisplaced. Such a fracture is detected as a crack on lateral x-ray of the knee. The patient can extend his knee, but only with pain. Treatment is by immobilization of the knee in a plaster cylinder for 6 weeks combined with quadriceps exercises. This is followed by mobilization of the knee. If the prepatellar quadriceps expansion as well as the patellar retinacula are *ruptured* the fragments are widely separated. The gap is palpable on examination, and obvious on x-ray. The joint fills with blood and clot. Without operation the proximal fragment of the bone remains retracted, the gap fills with scar tissue, and repair takes place with lengthening of the tendon and permanent limitation of active extension. Surgical treatment is therefore required. If the fracture is comminuted, the smaller fragments are excised and the patellar or quadriceps tendon attached to the larger fragment using wires or non-absorbable sutures through drill holes. For transverse fractures the fragments are brought together by tension band wiring, including a figure-of-eight wire. The knee is immobilized in a cylinder cast in extension. If extreme comminution is present, the patella is excised and the retinacula repaired. A *direct* blow on the patella also usually produces a comminuted fracture. It is impossible to restore a perfectly smooth articular surface, so osteoarthrosis results. These fractures should therefore be treated by removal of the patella. After this operation powerful active extension of the knee is possible, but there may be some loss of flexion.

THE KNEE

Injuries to ligaments. Injuries to the ligaments of the knee joint are common among athletes. Clinical examination provides useful clues to diagnosis. X-rays are usually normal, but MRI helps define the extent of the injury.

Collateral ligaments. A blow on the lateral side of the knee while the patient is standing abducts the tibia on the femur and places stress on the *medial collateral ligament.* The classic example of this type of injury is seen when the bumper of a car hits the outer side of a pedestrian's knee. With minor violence only a few fibres of the ligament are torn, but the ligament itself remains intact. If the blow is more severe the ligament is ruptured. An even stronger forced abduction may rupture one or both cruciate ligaments. If the medial collateral and cruciate ligaments are ruptured the tibia becomes completely unstable on the femur. *The lateral collateral ligament* is injured much less often than the medial, because very few blows fall on the knee from the inner side.

Cruciate ligaments. If the front seat passenger of a car is thrown forwards and the front of his tibia hits the dash-board the posterior cruciate ligament may be ruptured. On the other hand if the knee is forcibly hyperextended a rupture of the anterior cruciate ligament may occur. An exact description of the injury helps distinguish one lesion from the other. Gross *swelling* within an hour or two indicates haemarthrosis. Swelling arising slowly over a period of 24 hours means an effusion and points to a less severe injury. Localized *tenderness* may be elicited over an injured collateral ligament. If a ligament has been sprained but not ruptured, stressing the ligament causes pain. If the ligament is ruptured the knee may be too painful to elicit abnormal movement.

The joint should be *examined under anaesthesia.* The tibia in full extension is abducted and then adducted, and any abnormal movement compared with that in the other knee. If excessive movement is present it means that the appropriate *collateral* ligament is ruptured. In order to test the *cruciate ligaments* the knee is flexed to a right angle. The upper end of the tibia is now drawn forwards. Normally the anterior cruciate ligament prevents this movement. If this displacement can take place it means the ligament is ruptured. Similarly, if abnormal backward displacement can occur, it indicates that the posterior cruciate ligament is torn. A stress x-ray of the knee will show up the tilting of the tibia over the femur. MRI shows up the rupture of a cruciate ligament.

Treatment. Collateral ligaments. A minor sprain of the *medial ligament* requires little more than a crepe bandage and a walking stick or crutches for a while. Active sport is forbidden for six months to prevent further stress. An isolated tear of the ligament will heal if the joint is immobilized in plaster for eight weeks. However, if there is gross abnormal movement surgical repair is undertaken, because this means that a cruciate ligament is also torn. *The lateral ligament* is rarely ruptured alone. The fascia lata and the biceps tendon are usually torn at the same time. Sprains require no more than exercises with avoidance of sport. Ruptures require open repair followed by plaster immobilization for eight weeks. In some cases the *lateral popliteal nerve* may also be stretched and bruised. Conservative treatment is advised, because the paralysis will recover. In other cases the nerve may be completely torn. No attempt should be made to repair this nerve, as the intraneural damage is extensive. Instead, the tibialis posterior muscle should be transplanted to the dorsum of the foot to restore active dorsiflexion of the foot.

Cruciate ligaments. These injuries are often missed because the history of the mechanism of injury is not taken in detail, and because physical signs of abnormal movement cannot be elicited in a painful knee. It is essential that such an examination be performed under anaesthesia whenever there is doubt about the diagnosis. MRI shows up these soft tissue injuries to advantage. Minor damage to the cruciate ligaments need not be repaired. However, if the ligament is torn across, repair is necessary. The operation for a ruptured cruciate ligament is quite interesting. The ligament is replaced by the middle 1 cm of the ligamentum patellae. A block of bone, from the femur and the tibia respectively, is taken along at each end of the ligament, so that bone joins up with bone. A tunnel is drilled through the appropriate condyle of each bone in the correct direction. The ligament with a block of bone at either end is passed through the tunnel. Screws are driven in between the bone blocks and the condyles to secure the blocks in position. Fixation of the new ligament in a taut position is thus assured, so that movements can be allowed immediately to prevent any tendency to stiffness or disuse atrophy.

Injuries to the menisci. Injuries to the menisci (semilunar cartilages) are common in men under the age of 45. The medial meniscus is torn much more often than the lateral. A tear is usually caused by a twisting force with the knee semi-flexed. This injury most often takes place while playing football. An early tear starts as a longitudinal split. If this extends throughout the length of the meniscus it becomes a *bucket-handle tear*, in which the fragment remains attached at both ends. This is much the most common type. Its chief effect is that it limits full extension of the knee. The inner two thirds of each meniscus is avascular. Therefore when a meniscus is torn there is no haemarthrosis. Instead there is an effusion of synovial fluid.

Clinical findings. After a twisting injury the patient falls, and has pain and tenderness at the anteromedial aspect of the knee. He cannot straighten the joint fully. The next day the whole joint is swollen. In about two weeks the swelling lessens and he resumes his activities. In some cases, at the time of the injury the torn portion of the meniscus may become interposed between the tibial and femoral condyles and prevent full extension of the knee. Such a mechanical block to flexion or extension is called *locking*. Because of pain and limitation of movement it may not be noticed that the joint is locked. As the effusion settles, the displaced meniscus may itself return to its original position so as to unlock the joint. In other cases it may require manipulative reduction. Many months after a return to apparent normalcy the knee may still be prone to locking and 'giving way'.

There are no specific features on plain *x-ray*, but meniscal tears can be demonstrated by arthrography or arthroscopy. In arthography air is injected into the knee. This separates the meniscus from the tibial and femoral condyles, so that it shows up better. In *arthroscopy* the interior of the knee is examined through an endoscope (arthroscope) introduced through a small incision. However, MRI scans provide accurate diagnosis of all types of internal derangements of the knee, including meniscal tears, osteochondral injuries and cruciate ligament tears.

Treatment. Once a definite diagnosis is made the correct treatment consists of excision of the torn meniscus, as it will not heal spontaneously. This can be carried out through an arthroscopy tube without opening the joint, with minimum morbidity, decreased postoperative pain, and more rapid return to function. The menisci are important stabilizers of the knee, and retention of as much periphery of the meniscus as possible is beneficial. Complete meniscectomy is followed by late degenerative changes in the affected compartment of the knee.

THE TIBIA

Fractures of the tibia may be divided into fractures of the condyles, of the shaft, and of the distal end of tibia (i.e. ankle fractures).

Fractures of the tibial condyles. These have much in common with fractures of the femoral condyles, and have been discussed with them above.

Fractures of the shaft of the tibia and fibula. Most fractures in this region involve both the tibia and fibula, and the following description applies to such injuries. Fractures of either bone alone are considered later.

Mechanism and displacement. Fractures of the tibia and fibula occur from direct or indirect violence. Road accidents are the most common cause of fractures due to *direct violence*. A car bumper hits the leg and breaks both bones. These fractures occur at about the same level in the two bones, are transverse, oblique or comminuted, and are often open from without. *Indirect violence* may be applied to the tibia and fibula in the form of torsion, when the body turns during a fall on the fixed foot, e.g. during sport. The injury may be open from within, through a small wound. As many as a third of tibial shaft fractures are open injuries.

Treatment. Fractures of both bones of the leg can be treated by one of the following methods:

1. *Manipulative reduction* and a long leg plaster cast: this is the method of choice in children under the age of 16, and in those adults in whom stable reduction can be achieved. Conservative treatment is more attractive for these fractures than in the case of the femur, because the patient is usually able to get about well in plaster, he need not remain in hospital, and he may even return to work while the leg is still in plaster. The tibia takes about twelve weeks to unite, but it is rarely fit to take weight without support before twenty weeks.

2. If acceptable alignment cannot be achieved, internal fixation with plating or intramedullary nailing is advisable. This is particularly indicated in multiple trauma patients and in the elderly. It has the advantage that the joints can be mobilized early, but the disadvantage that the fracture may become infected during operation.

3. Open fractures are treated by primary debridement. Enclosing the limb in plaster prevents dressings and makes wound care difficult, while intramedullary nailing opens up tissue planes and can spread the contamination in the wound far and wide. In such cases pins may be passed through the tibia both above and below the fracture and fixed to an external metal frame – an *external fixator*.

Fracture of the shaft of the tibia alone. This fracture occurs commonly due to torsion, causing a spiral fracture. It is usually sufficient to apply an above-knee plaster cast. Delayed union often occurs, because the intact fibula acts as a strut preventing the fragments of the tibia coming into close contact.

Fracture of the shaft of the fibula alone. This fracture occurs usually from a direct blow on the fibula or an eversion injury at the ankle. Treatment need be nothing more than a firm bandage and analgesics for pain. The removal of the major part of the fibular shaft causes so little disability that it is sometimes used as a bone graft. However, the upper and lower ends of the bone are not disposable; they have important roles to play in the knee and ankle joints respectively.

THE ANKLE

FRACTURES OF THE ANKLE

Fractures at the ankle are very common. They are often grouped together loosely under the general title of *Pott's fracture* after the 18th century surgeon who described them.

Mechanism and patterns. Fractures of the ankle may occur from the application of four types of force:

Lateral rotation injury. First the lateral malleolus suffers a spiral fracture. Further force ruptures the inferior tibiofibular ligament. The talus can now rotate in the joint, and as it does so, the deltoid ligament avulses the tip of the medial malleolus. The ankle is now unstable.

Abduction injury. The talus presses the lateral malleolus outwards. The inferior tibiofibular ligament can rupture, rendering the ankle unstable. Alternatively, the shaft of the fibula breaks higher up.

Adduction injury. This may either break the medial malleolus or avulse the lateral ligament.

Vertical compression injury. This occurs due to a fall from a height. The talus is driven up into the distal tibia, which suffers a comminuted fracture.

Treatment. This depends upon the site and extent of the injury:

1. ***Fractures.*** i. Fractures of the lateral malleolus: these need to be immobilized in a short leg plaster for six weeks.

ii. Fractures of the lateral malleolus with tenderness over the medial malleolus, denoting rupture of the deltoid ligament: these require to be immobilized in a long leg plaster for six weeks.

iii. Fractures of both malleoli without disruption of the ankle mortice: these should be treated by open reduction and internal fixation of both fractures.

iv. Fractures of both malleoli with disruption of the ankle mortice (as shown by a wide gap between the malleolus and the talus: here the treatment of choice consists of open reduction and fixation of both fractures, along with the passage of a screw across the fibula into the tibia.

2. ***Injuries to ligaments.*** *Lateral ligament.* A *sprain* of the lateral ligament should be treated by compression bandaging for two weeks using a crepe bandage. The ankle is mobilized within the limits of pain. A *rupture* of the lateral ligament should be protected by a below-knee plaster for not less than six weeks. If it is treated as a simple sprain, with early exercises and activity, the torn ligament may fail to heal and recurrent subluxation of the ankle may occur. Some surgeons prefer to suture the torn capsule and ligaments at operation to ensure that the torn ends of the ligament are correctly apposed. After operation the ankle is protected in plaster for six weeks.

Inferior tibio-fibular ligament. Rupture of this ligament is best treated by internal fixation using a screw passed through the fibula into the tibia. Plaster-of-Paris is applied for six weeks.

THE FOOT

Fracture of the calcaneum. This fracture is caused by a fall from a considerable height onto the heel. Thus both heels may be injured at the same time. In many of the more severe cases there is also a compression fracture of a thoracic or lumbar vertebral body. The whole calcaneum is flattened and widened. The subtalar joint is damaged, causing marked restriction of inversion and eversion. Therefore this injury leaves the foot stiff irrespective of treatment.

Treatment. Classical teaching has taken the view that it is no use trying to restore the anatomy of the bone because this does not improve the function of the foot, and that the best results are achieved by accepting the deformity and concentrating on early non-weight-bearing mobilization. The foot is elevated and a crepe bandage applied over cotton wool in order to control swelling. Weight-bearing is started in about twelve weeks. However, in young active patients open reduction with elevation of the subtalar joint and bone grafting is being increasingly used. For severe late subtalar arthritis fusion of the subtalar joint is appropriate.

Fractures of the talus usually occur through the neck. The usual mechanism is dorsiflexion of the foot, so that the neck strikes the anterior lip of the distal tibia and is broken. The body of the talus is covered on most sides with cartilage and is supplied with blood through the neck. Therefore osteonecrosis of the body is common in these fractures, and leads to non-union and osteoarthrosis of the ankle. If the body is displaced, open reduction is usually necessary and fixation is achieved with two screws. The ankle is immobilized for 6 weeks in a plaster boot. Weight-bearing is avoided for 3 months. If collapse of the body occurs secondary arthritis develops, and ankle arthrodesis is often necessary.

Fractures of the metatarsals. These fractures are caused usually by a heavy weight falling on the dorsum of the foot. Sometimes the soft tissues of the foot are also severely crushed. In such a case the metatarsals unite but the foot remains thickened, stiff and painful. If only *one or two* metatarsals are fractured reduction is usually not required. Early mobilization in a short leg cast with non-weight-bearing exercises is encouraged. Full function is commonly restored in 8 to 12 weeks. If *more than two* metatarsals are broken the foot is unstable and is immobilized in a plaster boot for 4 to 6 weeks. After this period active mobilization is carried out.

Avulsion of the styloid process of the 5th metatarsal is a minor injury. The process is avulsed by the pull of the peroneus brevis contracting during forced inversion of the foot. The foot should not be immobilized. Only adhesive strapping is applied to support the foot and control swelling.

Fractures of the phalanges commonly occur when a phalanx is struck by a dropped object or is struck against an object. Treatment consists of restoring alignment, taping the digit to an adjacent digit, and pain relief.

37 Diseases of bones and joints

Congenital diseases of bones and joints

Congenital diseases of bones and joints include developmental anomalies and dysplasias. In *developmental anomalies* the abnormal growth occurs in utero and is static at birth. Any changes after that time are only secondary. In *dysplasias* abnormal growth occurs both in utero and after birth.

Some congenital diseases are genetic in origin, while others are due to disturbances in the intrauterine environment. For the majority the aetiology is unknown.

DEVELOPMENTAL ANOMALIES

Congenital dislocation of the hip (CDH). Unstable hips occur in about 8 per 1,000 live births.

Pathology. At birth the hip may be dislocated or dislocatable. The bones taking part in the hip are normal but the ligaments are unduly lax. Therefore the femoral head can be dislocated from the acetabulum. During the first few months of life these ligaments shorten to a normal size. If during this period the femoral head is maintained in the acetabulum the hip becomes stable and normal development takes place. On the other hand if the femoral head is allowed to remain out of the acetabulum, the ligaments get shortened, and this makes reduction of the dislocation difficult. If the hip remains dislocated until the child walks, the acetabulum and the head of the femur fail to develop normally. It is then difficult to return the hip to normal by any means, and osteoarthrosis of the joint usually develops in adult life.

The condition runs in families. The factors considered important in the *aetiology* include female sex of the infant, an inherited tendency to lax joints, and breech position of the foetus.

Diagnosis. Congenital dislocation of the hip may be diagnosed at birth, or later.

CDH at birth. CDH should be diagnosed within the first few days of life. *Every doctor and midwife should be aware of the existence of this condition and know how to demonstrate its presence.* The hip is flexed to 90° and adducted. Now the femur is pressed proximally along its long axis. If the sign is positive a 'clunk' is felt as the femoral head slips out of the acetabulum (*Barlow's* sign). The hip is now gently abducted and pressure exerted distally on the femoral shaft by the little finger placed over the greater trochanter. The femoral head can be felt to reduce into the acetabulum with a soft 'clunk' (*Ortolani's* sign). If the signs are positive it means that the hip is unstable. If it is left untreated it develops into a congenital dislocation of the hip.

Treatment. All that is required is to keep the hip in 90° flexion and 50° abduction until the joint becomes clinically stable and normal development is occurring radiologically. When the hip is kept in this position the head of the femur keeps pressing against the acetabulum, which therefore becomes deeper and develops a good upper edge, so that the head cannot dislocate upwards. The standard treatment at the time of birth is the Pavlik harness, which keeps the hip in such a position. Usually within a week the harness can be switched to night use only, when a Von Rosen splint can be used instead. Treatment for three months usually suffices.

CDH at age one year or more. If every newborn is examined as described above, diagnosis in the older infant should not be necessary. If one hip is dislocated, the skin creases at the groin are asymmetrical. Further, whereas the normal hip abducts to the full 90°, the dislocated hip will abduct only to about 45°.

The important *x-ray signs* are the following:

1. The epiphysis of the femoral head is displaced laterally and upwards.
2. *'Shenton's line'* is broken. This is the continuous curve produced by the inferior cortex of the femoral neck and the inferior margin of the superior pubic ramus. If the hip is dislocated the femur moves upwards and this line is broken.
3. The epiphysis of the femoral head is late to develop and so is smaller than on the normal side.

Treatment. The aim of the treatment of congenital dislocation of the hip is to replace the head in the acetabulum and keep it there while normal development takes place. Traction is applied for a few weeks in gradually increasing abduction. Sometimes the head gets reduced during this procedure. If it does not, closed manipulation is tried. If this also fails, open reduction is carried out. After the femoral head is reduced, the hip is kept in abduction so that the head remains in the acetabulum. The continued pressure of the head results in the acetabulum developing normally into a deep cavity, from which the head can no longer dislocate.

CDH in the older child. If congenital dislocation of the hip is diagnosed only when the child is older, the results of treatment are poor. If anything has to be attempted surgically at this stage, it consists of different types of osteotomies, a detailed discussion of which lies outside the scope of this book.

Club foot. Club foot or talipes describes a number of different abnormalities in the shape of the foot. If the foot is plantarflexed and cannot be fully dorsiflexed the deformity is called *equinus* (L. *equus* a horse); the opposite deformity is named *calcaneus*. If the foot is inverted and adducted so that it cannot be everted it is called *varus*; the opposite to this is *valgus*. Nearly always two deformities are combined. The most common deformity is *talipes equinovarus.*

Aetiology. The cause of club foot is unknown. Raised intrauterine pressure deforming the foot, ischaemic contracture of the calf muscles and disordered development of the neck of the talus have all been considered responsible, but there is no agreement in this regard. Treatment never produces a perfectly normal foot. The foot is usually smaller than its fellow. This may be partly due to the time the child has spent in casts.

Pathology. In the common talipes equinovarus the bones of the fore-foot are adducted and externally rotated. All the bones of the foot are plantar-flexed. The ligamentous structures on the medial side of the foot are shortened. The muscles of the calf are hypoplastic. The skin is adaptively shortened on the medial side.

Clinical findings. Cases with moderate or severe deformity are obvious at birth. Mild deformities may be difficult to distinguish from normal. In the normal newborn the foot can be dorsiflexed until the dorsum touches the front of the leg. If this is impossible, a minor degree of talipes equinovarus exists. *Thus examination of a newborn should include putting the foot through a full range of movement.* If the delivery is not supervised by a physician a club foot may not be detected until later. By this time the deformity has become fixed and callosities have developed on the skin of the foot where it bears weight. By adult life secondary degenerative changes develop in the deformed joints.

Treatment. Without treatment the condition is permanent and ambulation difficult. Treatment is started immediately in the newborn period, with stretching exercises and plaster casts changed weekly. Adduction is corrected first, then varus, and finally equinus. Conservative treatment is successful in 50% of cases. If the deformity recurs, manipulation will not suffice for correction and surgical treatment is required. This consists of release of soft tissues on the posteromedial side, and is best carried out between 3 and 6 months of age. In more severe cases the Achilles tendon may need to be lengthened and the tibialis tendon transferred laterally.

Phocomelia (Gr. *phoke* seal + *melos* limb). This is a condition in which the limb may totally or partially fail to develop. Certain drugs, e.g. thalidomide, may interfere with the development of the foetus and produce phocomelia. In minor phocomelia only one or more fingers may be missing. In the 'lobster hand' there is only one finger and the thumb; in this condition function is surprisingly good and no treatment is required.

Syndactyly (Webbed fingers). Syndactyly occurs as a *congenital* anomaly. A bridge of skin connects two or more adjacent fingers. *Acquired* syndactyly occurs after burns. The fingers in either case are separated by operation. When this has been carried out the sides of the fingers are usually lacking in skin cover, and split skin grafts are employed to cover the defects.

DYSPLASIAS

Brittle bones (Osteogenesis imperfecta). In this condition the bones are unduly fragile. Therefore multiple fractures occur after trivial injuries, and result in progressive deformity. With the passage of time the tendency to fracture gets reduced. Diagnosis is helped by the fact that the colour of the sclerae is blue in these cases instead of the normal white. Individual fractures should be treated on their merits. They heal normally.

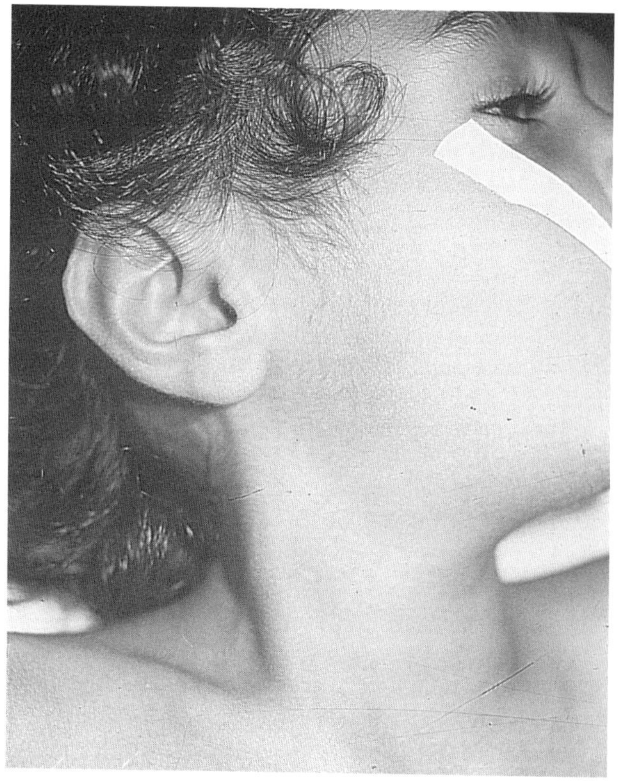

Fig. 1 'Congenital' torticollis with shortening of sternomastoid following after sternomastoid 'tumour' in infancy. The muscle is standing out like a tense cord.

Multiple exostoses (Diaphyseal aclasis). This is a familial disorder which is more common in males. A large number of exostoses develop in the metaphyseal region of the long bones. No treatment is required. However, if an exostosis becomes painful or continues to grow after the period of skeletal growth it raises a suspicion of malignant change. Therefore it should be removed and biopsied.

'Congenital' torticollis. This is not a truly congenital condition. It is almost certainly due to infarction of the central portion of the sternomastoid muscle. Soon after birth this part of the muscle is found to be swollen – a 'sternomastoid tumour'. This lump can be distinguished from other neck swellings in the newborn by demonstrating by palpation that the upper and lower poles of the swelling are continuous with the sternomastoid muscle. After a few weeks the swelling gradually subsides and disappears. However, the matter does not end there. The damaged muscle is replaced by fibrous tissue, which contracts over a period of time. The result is that when the neck grows the sternomastoid fails to grow with it. Due to the shortness of the sternomastoid the head is tilted towards one side. In severe cases the muscle stand out like a cord (Fig. 1). If left untreated it leads to gross asymmetry of the face, which is a serious matter.

Treatment used to consist of stretching exercises. However, these do not correct the deformity and surgical release of the muscle is required. This is carried out through a transverse skin crease incision.

Disorders of the growing skeleton

Disorders which affect the epiphyseal plate or epiphysis are peculiar to the growing skeleton. They may take the form of disturbances of growth and osteochondritis.

DISTURBANCES OF GROWTH

If growth on one side of a limb proceeds faster than on the other, the limb becomes curved, being convex on the side of the more rapid growth. Unequal growth in the leg produces bow-leg or knock-knee. In the spine it probably produces 'idiopathic' scoliosis.

Knock-knee and bow-leg. Normal infants when they start walking may be noticed to have some degree of knock-knee or bow-leg. The parents get worried. Both these conditions occur as part of the normal pattern of growth, and should be regarded as deformities only if severe and progressive. The degree of knock-knee can be measured by noting the distance between the medial malleoli of the ankle when the knees are placed side by side. Bow-leg is measured by noting the distance between the medial femoral condyles when the ankles are placed together.

Treatment. The deformity is usually self-correcting. If significant deformity persists after the age of 7, treatment with long leg braces or corrective osteotomy of the proximal femur or distal tibia may be needed.

Scoliosis. Scoliosis is defined as a lateral curvature of the spine. However, it is always accompanied by a rotational deformity. In the thoracic region, this deformity is transmitted to the ribs and produces asymmetry of the thorax. Scoliosis is classified according to its aetiology.

Idiopathic scoliosis. The cause of this, the most common form of scoliosis, is not known. The primary curve is balanced by secondary curves in the opposite direction above and below it. Therefore in mild curves no abnormality may be visible when the patient is dressed. However, a severe scoliosis is very disfiguring. Not only is there a loss of as much as 15 cm of height but a rib hump develops and gives the patient a hunch back. The rib hump is characteristic of idiopathic scoliosis. It is produced like this: when the dorsal spine curves to one side the vertebrae undergo rotation, and along with them the ribs also rotate. Because of deformity of the ribs and spine, a thoracic scoliosis may limit the vital capacity seriously, and the patient may die of respiratory tract infection.

Idiopathic scoliosis may resolve spontaneously. However a few cases become progressive. The earlier the onset of the scoliosis and the more severe the curve at first presentation, the greater the chances of its progression. Once advanced structural deformity has developed nothing can be done to restore the spine to normal. The deformity may rapidly increase until the patient becomes a dwarfed hunchback.

Treatment. Mild curves i.e. under 20° may be kept under observation. Curves between 20° and 40° are treated conservatively by the Milwaukee brace and by exercises. Curves greater than 50° are treated by operation. However, as far as possible surgery should be postponed until near skeletal maturity. During operation for this condition correction of the curve is first carried out. After this, either the laminae or the vertebral bodies are fused together.

Congenital scoliosis. This occurs due to a hemivertebra, spina bifida etc. Anomalies of the spinal cord and of the kidneys often coexist. An MRI and intravenous pyelogram are therefore carried out if surgery is planned.

Paralytic scoliosis. Post-polio paralysis of vertebral muscles produces muscle imbalance, and may result in scoliosis. A collapsing spine results so that the patient cannot sit up and respiration is embarrassed. In treating this condition the scoliosis is first corrected, and then fusion is carried out to maintain the correction attained. However, as the muscle imbalance remains uncorrected, there is often a recurrence of the deformity.

Postural scoliosis. This affects children of school age. There is a simple curve without rotation of the vertebrae. It is due to bad posture while sitting at school desks. Treatment consists of gymnastics and training in good posture.

Pulmonary scoliosis. Fibrotic disease of one lung or pleura, e.g. empyema, may result in contraction of the chest wall on that side and scoliosis. Treatment consists of removing the thick layer of fibrosed pleura from the surface of the lung (*decortication*). This allows both the lung and the chest wall to expand fully, at the same time correcting the scoliosis.

Perthes' disease. *Pathology.* During the period of growth blood reaches the upper femoral epiphysis only through vessels passing around the periphery of the epiphyseal plate. It seems that some factor interferes with this blood supply and produces avascular necrosis of the ossification centre of the epiphysis.

Clinical findings. The disease affects children between 5 and 10 years of age, mostly boys. Some cases are bilateral. There is pain in the front of the thigh and knee and the child limps. On examination there is restriction of abduction and internal rotation, first due to muscle spasm and later due to flattening and deformity of the femoral head.

X-ray findings. The ossific nucleus of the femoral head is smaller than on the other side. The hip joint space is increased due to effusion. The x-ray findings have been classified into four groups by Catterall as follows: no sequestration, and sequestration involving half, more than half, and the whole of the head. Patients with partial involvement (group I and II) have a much better prognosis than those with more extensive involvement (group III and IV). Osteoarthrosis is the long-term complication of the disease, although it may be delayed for upto 40 years.

Treatment aims at containing the diseased epiphysis within the acetabulum until reossification is complete; this affords the best chance of obtaining a spherical head. It may require the patient to walk with the hip in a position of abduction. For this a walking abduction brace is used for the duration of healing (12 to 18 months). The outcome depends upon the stage of the disease, the final sphericity of the head, and the congruity with the acetabulum. Degenerative arthritis can present in the fourth to sixth decades.

Generalized diseases of bone

Paget's disease. This is a disorder of accelerated regional bone turnover. This disease is rare under the age of 40 but becomes common with advancing age. It occurs slightly more commonly in men. The spine, the skull, the pelvis, the femur and the tibia are most commonly affected. First of all the existing bone, both cortical and cancellous, gets resorbed by osteoclasts. Later, osteoblasts regenerate an abnormal type of bone with sclerosis and thickening of the trabeculae and cortical bone. Because of the disorganized collagen in the woven pagetic bone tensile strength is poor and fractures can occur.

Clinical features. The disease may be discovered incidentally when a patient is examined for some other condition. The patient may complain of thickening of the bone. There may be pain, specially in the weight-bearing bones. The new bone formed is not as strong as normal bone, so it may bend under the body weight and the leg may be bowed. The patient may come to the doctor because of one of the complications of the disease, for example:

1. Osteogenic sarcoma: this occurs in as many as 5% of patients with Paget's disease. Signs of malignant degeneration include progressive pain, a soft tissue mass, and x-ray changes with bone destruction.
2. Pathological fracture of the tibia or femur.
3. Heart failure of the high output type, due to arteriovenous fistulae in the affected highly vascular bone.
4. Deafness due to bony involvement of the middle ear.

X-ray findings. The involved bone is thickened and shows patches of sclerosis. The line of demarcation between cortex and medullary canal is blurred.

Laboratory findings. The serum calcium and phosphorus are normal. Serum alkaline phosphatase is often very high, but this is not specific, because it occurs in most diseases in which osteoclasis is occurring. During bone resorption collagen breakdown is increased, and this results in an increase in the excretion of hydroxyproline in the urine.

Treatment. The pain of Paget's disease can be relieved by treatment with an antiresorptive agent such as etidronate, or with calcitonin. Treatment is continued until biochemical parameters and symptoms improve, usually in about 6 months. In cases of spinal involvement with neurological deficit mithramycin is the drug of choice, rapidly inhibiting pagetic activity. However, it is not suitable for long-term therapy because of hepatic and renal toxicity. Sarcomas must be treated by radical resection and prosthetic limb reconstruction, and if the patient can tolerate the toxicity, chemotherapy.

Osteoporosis. Osteoporosis is defined as abnormal rarefaction of bones. It may be localized or generalized. Osteoporosis may occur in a *localized* form following disuse (e.g. due to paralysis or immobilization), or due to local inflammation.

The *generalized* form of osteoporosis occurs either *primarily,* being a part of the process of getting old, or *secondarily* following endocrine disorders. Osteoblasts have been shown to have oestrogen receptors and respond to oestrogen anabolically, which may explain the accelerated postmenopausal bone loss.

Senile osteoporosis. This becomes manifest in women after the menopause and in men after the age of 65. However, it does not pose a problem until about 15 years later. The main cause of the condition is disuse, due to the generally reduced level of activity in the elderly. In women the change in their hormonal environment at the menopause also plays an important part. In this condition the amount of calcium in the skeleton is reduced.

Investigations. 1. Plain x-rays show the change only when approximately 40% of the skeleton has been lost. However, two radiological methods are now available for accurate measurement of bone density: quantitative CT scans for the spine, and x-ray absorptiometry for any bone.

2. Vitamin D deficiency must be ruled out as the cause. This can be done by a bone biopsy from the iliac crest analyzed by histomorphometric methods. At the same time, accurate serum measurements of vitamin D metabolites and parathormone levels are now available.

There are no symptoms except backache with progressive kyphosis and loss of height. However, the bones are more liable to fracture than normal bones. The injuries which commonly occur are Colles' fracture and fracture of the femoral neck. The fracture should be treated in the usual manner ignoring the osteoporosis, which does not interfere with healing. Acute vertebral fractures are treated with a lightweight brace, analgesics and early mobilization, as bed rest aggravates the osteopenia. Calcium supplementation (1000 to 1500 mg daily) is recommended and can slow down the rate of loss. Physiological doses of vitamin D (400 U daily) help to ensure calcium absorption. In perimenopausal women oestrogen therapy is of proven benefit. The patient must be encouraged to begin a regular program of weight-bearing exercises such as walking, which is important in maintaining bone mass and preventing fractures.

Vitamin D deficiency. Deficiency of vitamin D may arise during childhood, when it produces the condition called rickets. If deficiency arises during adult life it results in osteomalacia.

Rickets. Rickets is defined as the disturbance in normal ossification which is produced by a deficiency of vitamin D. This in turn may arise either due to an insufficient quantity of vitamin D in the diet, or a defect in the absorption of this vitamin because of chronic disease of the small intestine. In rickets uncalcified bone matrix is deposited normally but fails to calcify. This tissue is called osteoid. The disease affects bones which ossify in cartilage as well as those which ossify in membrane. It may present at any time during growth. Characteristic deformities develop in the skeleton. The long bones get bent under the body weight. The costochondral junctions enlarge to produce a row of nodules which is called a *rickety necklace.*

Treatment of nutritional rickets is by supplementation with high doses of vitamin D (3000 U daily, normal daily requirement 400 U). Calcium supplementation enhances the rate of healing. For persistent deformities correction is delayed until the underlying metabolic defect has resolved, at which time osteotomies can be performed.

Osteomalacia. In adults deficiency of vitamin D affects the bones of the pelvis, and they are rendered quite soft. This condition is called osteomalacia (*malacia* = softness). The causes include nutritional deficiency, malabsorption, anticonvulsant therapy, and hepatic and renal disorders. The body weight pushes the sacral promontory downwards. Similarly the femoral heads push the acetabula upwards. This results in a triradiate pelvis and greatly narrows the pelvic outlet. The condition is much more common in females, and usually develops to its full extent during lactation, due to the drain on the calcium stores in the blood. The narrow pelvic outlet may result in obstructed labour.

Treatment. Vitamin D is administered, usually in the form of cod liver oil. Early bone deformities can be dealt with by splintage. Severe deformities may require division of the bone (osteotomy) for correction.

GOUT

Gout is an abnormality of uric acid metabolism that results in the deposition of sodium urate crystals in joints, kidneys and soft tissues. In the joints it produces acute arthritis; in the kidneys, stones; and in the soft tissues, chalky deposits of urates called tophi. The condition is more common in the upper social classes due to the higher intake of meat and wine. There is hyperuricaemia due to overproduction or under-excretion of acid. A high dietary intake of purines can be an additional factor but does not itself produce hyperuricaemia.

Gout is predominantly a disease of men, mostly beginning in middle age. Asymptomatic hyperuricaemia is 10 times more common than gout. The typical acute attack begins suddenly in the early hours of the morning with excruciating pain in the big toe. Attacks may be precipitated by dietary or alcohol excess, starvation, diuretics or a surgical operation. The typical gouty joint is red, warm, swollen and exquisitely tender. The presence of tophi in the ear lobes or around joints may provide a clue, but they occur late when the nature of the problem is obvious. Patients with gout have a higher than expected incidence of vascular disease, hypertension and renal disease.

Investigation. *Synovial fluid examination.* The affected joint is aspirated and the fluid examined under a polarized light microscope. In acute gout, the presence of long, needle-shaped negatively birefringent crystals is diagnostic.

Serum uric acid has a limited value as a test due to a high incidence of false-positive and false-negative results. However, acute gout never occurs with a serum uric acid in the lower half of the normal range. In the first few attacks the uric acid level is often below the upper limit of normal; the level also falls after an acute attack. Thus a normal value does not exclude the diagnosis of gout. However, the test is useful in monitoring treatment.

Management. ***Acute attacks*** are treated with anti-inflammatory drugs. Indomethacine 50 mg thrice daily produces relief within 48 hours, when the dose should be halved. The attack should resolve completely within a few weeks. Intramuscular adrenocorticotrophin (ACTH) is effective in difficult cases. Effusions in large joints should be aspirated and a corticosteroid injected to reduce inflammation.

Long-term therapy. *Prevention.* Measures to reduce uric acid levels include reduction of weight and alcohol intake; avoidance of food and drink containing high levels of purines, such as red meat and wine; and abundant fluid intake.

Drugs. Allopurinol (a xanthine oxidase inhibitor) is the drug of choice, in a dose of 300 mg daily. Side effects are uncommon but include skin rashes. The tophi disappear slowly with reduction in the level of serum urate. In patients allergic to allopurinol, *probenecid* (a uricosuric drug) is used as an alternative. Asymptomatic hyeruricaemia, found on routine screening, does not require treatment. The simple measures outlined above are, however, usually advised.

Diseases of muscles, tendons and fasciae

Tennis elbow. In this condition the patient complains of pain in the elbow specially when he uses the hand and therefore contracts the wrist and finger extensors. The attachment of the extensor muscles of the forearm to the lateral epicondyle is tender. When the extensors of the fingers or the wrist are contracted against resistance, pain is felt at the elbow at their origin. Analgesics or steroid injections usually relieve the pain. If not, the origin of the extensors from the epicondyle may have to be divided.

Supraspinatus tendinitis. In this condition pain is felt in the shoulder, specially on abduction and rotation, and localized tenderness is present over the insertion of the supraspinatus tendon. It should be remembered that *whenever the shoulder is painful from any cause it rapidly becomes stiff* because of disuse. This is probably because the acromion lies very close to the humerus so that adhesions readily form between the two bones which limit movements of the humerus on the scapula. In middle age the blood supply to the supraspinatus tendon often becomes defective, probably because of compression between the acromion and the proximal humerus. Therefore the tendon may degenerate, become painful, and calcify. It may even rupture.

Pain occurs on moving the humerus, specially during the middle of the range of abduction, when the inflamed supraspinatus tendon passes under the acromion. Due to the pain the patient holds the shoulder still. Adhesions therefore form which limit shoulder movements further. After a few months the pain may subside and the range of movement become normal. This sequence of events is called *frozen shoulder.* This is not a specific clinical entity but a response of the shoulder to any painful condition.

Aetiology. Tennis elbow and supraspinatus tendinitis are both examples of *non-articular rheumatism.* This is the name given to a group of conditions which present as pain localized to the aponeurotic attachment of a muscle to bone. The tender area does not regularly show any pathological features. Perhaps the condition is caused by a tear in the collagen fibres attaching the muscle to the bone.

Because the area is repeatedly exposed to stress, it fails to heal satisfactorily.

Treatment. The treatment for supraspinatus tenditinis is conservative. A sling is applied for one to two weeks until relief from pain is complete. Then gentle and gradual exercises are started to increase the range of movements. If this fails, cortisone is injected into the shoulder. The joint may also be manipulated under anaesthesia to break the adhesions and restore movement.

Stenosing teno-vaginitis. In this condition, the cause of which is not known, the sheath of a tendon becomes thick. Pain and limitation of movement result. The condition is seen most often at the common sheath of the abductor pollicis longus and extensor pollicis brevis where it is called *de Quervain's disease.* It is also seen in the fingers, where it results in a '*trigger finger*' which develops in the following manner: the flexor sheath of the tendon thickens and gets narrowed. The tendon develops a constriction under the narrowed part and a bulge distal to it. The finger may lock in flexion, and attempts to passively extend it are painful. *Treatment* is by dividing the retinaculum overlying the tendon. It is interesting to note that the tendons do not subluxate after such an operation.

Carpal tunnel syndrome. The median nerve may be compressed at the site where it passes through the carpal tunnel, which lies between the flexor retinaculum and the wrist bones. The cause may be obvious; for example swelling of flexor tendon sheaths in the tunnel sometimes takes place in rheumatoid arthritis. In most cases, however, there is no obvious swelling. The patient complains of pain in the distribution of the median nerve. The pain may also be felt in the arm, causing confusion with cervical spondylosis. The pain is usually worse at night. There may be wasting of the thenar muscles. *Treatment* consists of simple decompression of the tunnel by longitudinal incision of the flexor retinaculum, which cures the condition.

Dupuytren's contracture. This is a thickening of the palmar, or rarely the plantar, aponeurosis. The fascia thickens, becomes nodular and contracts so that the corresponding finger becomes flexed. The disease usually starts near the base of the little or ring finger. In long-standing cases permanent changes take place in the concerned joints so that the fingers cannot be straightened even after excision of the palmar aponeurosis. The cause is not known, but the condition is familial. Early cases may sometimes be helped by splintage and gentle stretching by the patient. In most cases, however, operation is required, with excision of the contracted fascia.

Ganglion. A ganglion is a localized, tense, cystic swelling containing clear gelatinous fluid (Fig. 2). It usually overlies and communicates with a joint. The origin of ganglia is uncertain. They are mostly seen on the dorsum of the wrist (Plate IV-I). If a ganglion does not resolve spontaneously, excision is carried out.

Chronic bursitis. Chronic bursitis is the result of repeated pressure or injury to various bursae, e.g. prepatellar bursa (housemaid's knee), olecranon bursa etc. A semimembranosus bursa often communicates with the knee joint. In that case it may enlarge when there is effusion in the joint, e.g. in osteoarthrosis. It is then called a *Baker's cyst.*

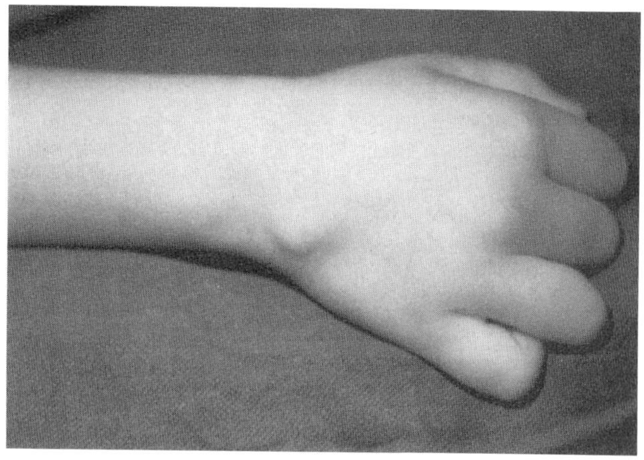

Fig. 2 Ganglion wrist. The site is rather unusual, the common location being on the radial portion of the back of the wrist.

Paralysis of muscles. There are two important results of paralysis:

1. *Loss of function.* This is due to failure of the affected muscles. An important effect is loss of joint stability.
2. *Liability to deformity.* In the *adult* this is not a serious problem. The non-paralysed muscles are liable to develop contracture, but this can be controlled by passive movements and by splintage.

In the *child* the problem is much more serious because growth is disturbed. The non-paralysed muscles become short, so the joints become fixed in the direction of the active muscles. Secondary bony deformities develop, and cause even greater fixation of the joint. It should be remembered that in a totally paralysed limb no deformity develops, because there is no muscle imbalance to distort it.

The management of paralysis. The aims of treatment of a case with paralysis are three:

1. *Elimination of deformity.* In the adult passive movements and splints are able to prevent deformity. In the child this is not enough, and the contracted tendons of the unopposed muscles have also to be divided.
2. *Prevention of recurrent deformity.* For this purpose it is necessary to restore muscle balance across the joint. Either the paralysed muscle group is reinforced, or the non-paralysed muscles are weakened.

The paralysed group is usually reinforced by *tendon transfer.* The tendon of a normally acting muscle is divided and inserted into a new site so that its mode of action is altered. Often it acts in place of its antagonists. The non-paralysed muscle group may be weakened by *tenotomy* or by *lengthening* of its tendon.

3. *Restoration of joint stability and function.* Joint stability may be restored by tendon transfer. If this is impracticable or fails, in the adult *arthrodesis* (fusion of the joint) is usually carried out. In children external splintage is the only solution until they are old enough for arthrodesis.

Poliomyelitis. Poliomyelitis is an acute febrile illness due to a neurotropic virus. It produces irregularly distributed flaccid paralysis by damaging the anterior horn cells. In the advanced countries the disease has been virtually eliminated by mass immunization. Unfortunately, it is still prevalent in some parts of the world. The paralysis and wasting are nearly always asymmetrical, affecting particularly the proximal parts of the lower limbs, and the spine and trunk muscles. There is no sensory loss.

Management. In the early and recovery phases the paralysed limb is splinted to minimize deformity. After 2 years no further recovery can occur and reconstruction can begin. For example in the foot due to paralysis of the dorsiflexors foot-drop occurs. For this the shortened tendo-Achilles is lengthened. Also the tibialis posterior may be transferred anteriorly to produce dorsiflexion.

Infections of bones and joints

ACUTE OSTEOMYELITIS

Before the days of antibiotics acute osteomyelitis used to be a serious and often fatal condition. Nowadays it can be dealt with satisfactorily if detected in time.

Aetiology. The vast majority of cases of acute osteomyelitis are due to bacteria, the infection being bloodborne. In some cases the primary focus may be evident in the form of a boil, but quite often there is no obvious cause. It is thought that lowered general resistance of the patient and local trauma predispose to this condition, but there is no proof of this. The usual organism is *Staphylococcus aureus.* Group A streptococcus and *H. influenzae* are the next most common organisms. Acute osteomyelitis occurs mostly during the period of skeletal growth, the peak incidence being during childhood. Males are affected more often than females.

Pathology. The disease nearly always begins in the metaphysis. During infancy, and again in adult life, there are communications between the blood vessels of the metaphysis and epiphysis. Therefore at both these ages infection can spread to the epiphysis and end up as a septic arthritis. During childhood the epiphyseal cartilage acts as a barrier, so arthritis does not occur as a complication of osteomyelitis.

The infective process moves towards the surface, producing thrombosis of the vessels and leading to avascular necrosis of bone in the process. Finally, the exudate lifts up the periosteum, causing severe pain. The pus under the periosteum is under tension, so the patient rapidly develops signs due to the toxic absorption. The pus tracks around the bone, stripping the periosteum and interrupting the periosteal vessels. Thus progressively larger areas of the cortex lose their blood supply, i.e. become infarcted. Untreated, the pus finally perforates the periosteum and tracks through the muscles to discharge as a sinus on the skin.

The dead piece of bone is called a *sequestrum.* The new bone around it which is laid down by the periosteum is called the *involucrum.* The openings in the involucrum through which pus is discharged are called *cloacae.*

Clinical findings. The onset of acute osteomyelitis is usually sudden, with marked toxicity. The pain rapidly increases in severity. The child keeps the limb motionless. The temperature is often markedly raised. Local tenderness is the essential physical sign. It usually comes on before the swelling. If the maximum tenderness is over the metaphysis of a long bone it should be presumed to be due to acute osteomyelitis until proved otherwise. The adjacent joint may contain an effusion, raising the possibility of suppurative arthritis. However, some movement of the joint is possible in osteomyelitis, whereas in septic arthritis absolutely no movement is possible.

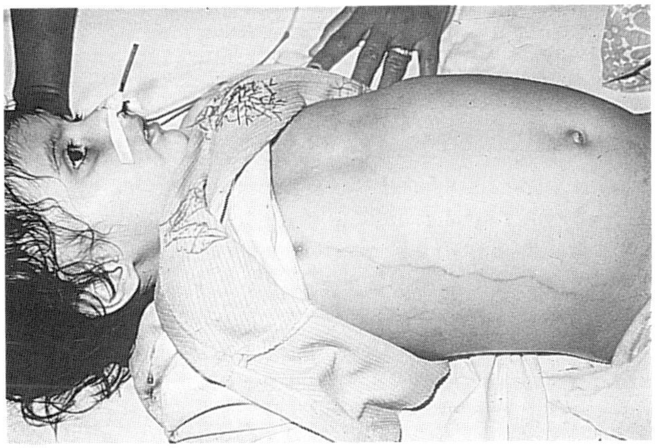

Fig. 3 Septic thrombosis of inferior vena cava showing dilated vein running upwards along side of trunk (see text).

The history must be taken very carefully. A history of trauma may divert attention from osteomyelitis.

Example. A young girl was brought to a hospital with a history of a fall, with pain and tenderness in the thigh. X-ray showed no fracture. A diagnosis of soft tissue injury was made, and a firm crepe bandage applied. Next day the child was brought in severe endotoxic shock, with pyaemia and septic thrombosis of the inferior vena cava, as shown by veins running upwards on the sides of the trunk (Fig. 3).

It was obvious that it had been a case of acute osteomyelitis all along. The history of injury had misled the clinician. Because osteomyelitis was not suspected, she was of course not placed on any antibiotics. To make matters worse, the firm bandaging (meant to give support to the 'soft tissue injury') had forced the pus into the veins and caused pyaemia. In spite of immediate drainage of pus and every possible intensive treatment the child died.

Always remember that if your initial enquiries set you on the wrong diagnostic track, no power on earth can bring you back on the correct path. The consequences can be as tragic as in this case.

Conditions which can mimic osteomyelitis include *Ewing's sarcoma, rheumatic fever* and *leukaemia.*

Exogenous osteomyelitis is most often the result of a *compound fracture.* Symptoms are usually less severe, because some drainage is available via the wound through which the micro-organisms entered.

X-ray. For the first week or more, x-rays of the bone are normal. However, in 2 or 3 weeks new bone can be seen deposited under the elevated periosteum. At this time some rarefaction of bone due to local hyperaemia may also be visible.

Treatment. The child is admitted to hospital and the limb splinted. Toxic patients require intravenous fluids and electrolytes. If the patient is seen within 48 hours of onset, antibiotics are immediately started. However, before they are commenced blood should be taken for culture. If antibiotics are started within 48 hours of onset, the area of disease can be sterilized and complete resolution of infection occurs. If not, the condition becomes chronic and poses a long-term problem.

Antibiotics are administered parenterally. As most cases are due to *Staphylococcus aureus,* cloxacillin is commenced in a dose of 500 mg 6 hourly. In patients allergic to penicillin clindamycin 150 mg b.d. may be used. In infants *Haemophilus influenzae* is often the cause, and ampicillin 250 mg 6 hourly is used. If the case fails to respond, chloramphenicol may be substituted.

If the patient is seen 48 hours or more after the onset, pus may be present requiring drainage. If the temperature settles down to normal within 2 or 3 days and tenderness gradually disappears, antibiotics are sufficient. If, however, the temperature subsides but does not become normal, pus is present or the antibiotic is inappropriate to the sensitivity of the organism. In either case the area must be explored to drain any pus and obtain the organism for culture.

Operation is carried out under general anaesthesia. Incision is made over the tender area and deepened. Pus is usually found deep to the periosteum. The abscess cavity is fully opened and pus taken for culture. A drill hole is made in the bone. If pus flows out from the hole the opening is enlarged until free drainage is achieved. The wound is either left wide open or closed over a suction drain. The limb is splinted and antibiotics continued postoperatively.

Complications. The complications of acute osteomyelitis may be general or local.

General complications. These include septicaemia and pyaemia which may prove fatal or result in metastatic abscesses.

Local complications. These include the following:

1. Suppurative arthritis, if the epiphyseal line is intra-articular.
2. Spontaneous fracture.
3. Chronic osteomyelitis.

CHRONIC OSTEOMYELITIS

Acute osteomyelitis may pass into chronic osteomyelitis if it is not treated early or is treated inadequately, so that infected bone dies to become a sequestrum. It may take one of two forms:

1. Acute haematogenous osteomyelitis leaves behind a large sequestrum.
2. A *Brodie's abscess* may form. In this case the disease is localized, resulting in a chronic abscess within the bone. Pus and granulation tissue are surrounded by sclerotic bone. It may follow a pyogenic septicaemia, leaving a bone abscess which may remain dormant for years; or it may be seen in a patient who in the past had osteomyelitis in a different bone.

Amyloidosis may follow long-standing chronic osteomyelitis.

Clinical findings. Chronic osteomyelitis may remain quiescent for months or years. However, from time to time acute exacerbations occur with fever, local pain and swelling, which may end in discharge of pus. An x-ray may reveal a sequestrum in a cavity. A CT scan can also show up the sequestra. If a sinus is present a sinogram may be carried out to outline the cavity.

A Brodie's abscess is a localized form of chronic osteomyelitis. It becomes painful from time to time. Examination shows tenderness and thickening of the bone. X-ray shows a band of sclerosis around a radiolucent area. The reasons why such a abscess fails to heal are these: firstly, the abscess cannot close by collapse of its walls as happens in the soft tissues. Secondly, infection provokes the formation of dense bone around it, so that white cells, antibodies and antibiotics cannot reach the contents of the cavity.

Treatment. Antibiotics and splintage can help an exacerbation of chronic osteomyelitis to subside, but they cannot cure the condition. For eradication of the disease surgical treatment is required.

The purpose of *surgical treatment* is removal of dead bone and elimination of dead space. A sequestrum may be detected by probing a sinus or by x-ray. At operation the sequestrum is approached by removing the overlying portion of the involucrum. If a cavity is present the overhanging walls are removed with an osteotome until it is *saucerized,* i.e made to look like a saucer, which is a broad and shallow vessel.

A Brodie's abscess should be treated by laying open and curetting the cavity under antibiotic cover.

The best after-care consists of *leaving the wound completely open* i.e. unsutured, and treating it with dressings. This allows the wound to fill with granulations and then finally epithelialize. However, some surgeons prefer to close the wound by suture and irrigate it constantly with antibiotic solutions. If this course is followed, postoperative supervision must be very watchful.

ACUTE SUPPURATIVE ARTHRITIS

Aetiology. Acute suppurative arthritis may occur due to one of the following:

1. A penetrating wound or a compound fracture involving the joint.
2. Blood-borne infection, the common organisms being streptococcus, staphylococcus and pneumococcus.
3. Local extension from a neighbouring focus e.g. osteomyelitis of the neck of the femur, because the femoral neck lies inside the hip joint capsule.

Staphylococcus aureus and haemolytic streptococcus are the two most common organisms that cause pyogenic arthritis, apart from gonococcal and coliform organisms and *Haemophilus influenzae* (in children). Septic arthritis is more common in debilitated patients or those undergoing steroid therapy or immunosuppression.

Clinical findings. There is steadily increasing pain and malaise. The patient tends to avoid movement of the joint, and is severely toxic with a raised temperature and pulse rate. On palpation the joint is hot and tender. Movements are prevented by muscle spasm and are extremely painful. *X-rays* reveal effusion with increased joint space. In more advanced infections erosions and joint space narrowing may be seen. Diagnosis is made by *aspiration* of the joint with culture, Gram staining and analysis of the synovial fluid. The presence of organisms and an elevated white cell count in the fluid may be diagnostic; the count may range from 25,000 to 40,000, with upto 90% of neutrophils.

Treatment. If the white cell count is high antibiotics are started with coverage for *S. aureus* (cephalosporin), streptococci (cephalosporin or a penicillin), and in children *H. influenzae* (ampicillin). When the culture report arrives the antibiotic may have to be changed. For hip infections, which can rapidly be followed by osteonecrosis and are difficult to aspirate, urgent surgical drainage is indicated. Chronic infections with loculation or thick pus also require surgical drainage, and removal of hypertrophic infected synovium can be advantageous. For the knee arthroscopic drainage may be appropriate. Shoulder and ankle infections can be managed by serial aspiration or surgical drainage. In general patients who undergo drainage improve more rapidly and surely. Intravenous antibiotics are indicated for 2 to 4 weeks, but if the joint infection has resulted from an adjacent osteomyelitis, for about 6 weeks. Cases where articular destruction progresses despite treatment should be treated by arthrodesis, resection arthroplasty, or in rare cases, joint replacement arthroplasty.

TUBERCULOUS ARTHRITIS AND OSTEOMYELITIS

Pathology. Tuberculosis of the bones and joints is haematogenous in origin. In countries without mandatory pasteurization of milk the infection enters the body through the gastrointestinal tract due to ingestion of the bovine strain of the bacillus in imperfectly sterilized milk. In countries where tuberculosis has been virtually eliminated due to pasteurization and BCG immunization, the human bacillus is responsible for the few cases that are still seen. However, the disease is common among immigrants from developing countries, patients with HIV infection (AIDS), and patients on chronic immunosuppression therapy.

The most common site in the skeleton is the spine. At the same time the disease may start in any synovial joint, specially a joint with extensive synovial membranes e.g. the hip or knee. Typically, tubercles develop in the synovial membrane which becomes bulky, and an effusion collects in the joint. If the infection can be diagnosed and cured at this stage, full function may be restored to the joint. If, however, the disease progresses, hypertrophic infected synovium (pannus) gradually covers the cartilage surface and erodes the subchondral bone, destroying the cartilage as well. Healing leaves a fibrous ankylosis. Free mobility of a joint depends upon the presence of articular cartilage; when this is destroyed, loss of mobility is bound to occur.

In the spine the diagnosis is rarely made until the bodies of two neighbouring vertebrae are involved. If treatment is delayed an abscess forms and the vertebral bodies collapse. The pus may track long distances; for example pus arising from a lumbar vertebra may track inside the psoas muscle sheath to present in the groin. Vertebral collapse produces a forward angulation of the spine – a kyphosis. Pressure from the pus and from angulation of the spine may damage the spinal cord and produce paraplegia.

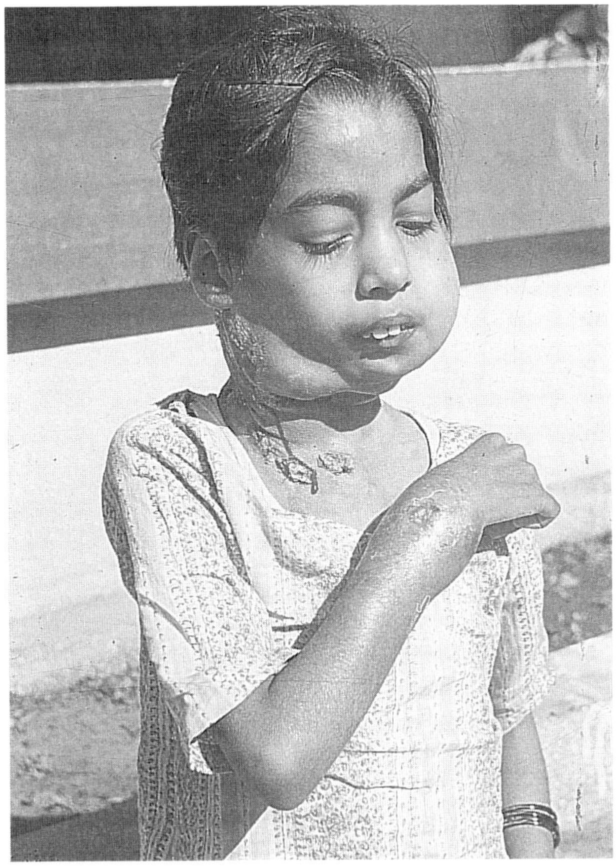

Fig. 4 Young girl with sinuses discharging tuberculous pus from the jaw, neck, wrist, etc.

Clinical findings. ***Symptoms*** arise from the diseased joint and from the systemic effects of the disease. Usually the first symptom is *pain* in the joint which is often more severe at night. The pain gets worse, and increasing stiffness comes on. The stiffness is due to bone destruction and muscle spasm. There is *swelling* of the joint, which is made more prominent by the wasting of the associated muscles. As the bone is destroyed the joint dislocates and the *local deformity* becomes obvious.

In the *spinal column*, because of its deep location, the swelling is not visible until a good deal of pus has collected, and stiffness may be slight and go unnoticed. Therefore a mild ache may be the only symptom of this serious disease. *Systemically* the patient feels unwell, weak and feverish, and may have 'night sweats'.

Signs. In superficial joints the *synovial thickening* and *effusion* may be visible. The muscles acting on the joint are markedly *wasted.* The joint is moderately *tender.* The skin over the joint is not red, only slightly warm.

In the *spine* the only physical sign in early disease is *tenderness* on percussion of the spinous processes. Later, a *kyphus* may be seen and an *abscess* may be visible in the groin.

In really poor patients the infection even today runs riot. Fig. 4 shows a young girl from a village. She is pouring out pus at multiple sites from tuberculosis of various bones and lymph nodes. It is a pity that in this day and age, when man is reaching upto the moon and mars, there should be people suffering misery like this. A fraction of the billions spent on the arms race could eradicate tuberculosis from the whole world.

Laboratory findings. The ESR is raised. The white cell count is high, with a lymphocytosis. The Mantoux test is usually strongly positive.

X-ray findings. The earliest changes are soft tissue swelling and distension of the capsule by effusion. Later, destruction of the articular cartilage causes narrowing of the joint space. Bone destruction is seen as areas of osteolysis. Extensive destruction of joint surfaces causes deformity. As healing takes place, the areas of necrosis are seen to be surrounded by osteosclerosis. The appearance may be that of a cyst surrounded by sclerotic bone. A chest x-ray is always taken and may sometimes show active tuberculosis.

Diagnosis depends on recovery of organisms from the joint. Joint aspiration and/or biopsy is essential, with demonstration of acid-fast bacilli on smears, or positive cultures. If aspiration is not diagnostic open synovial biopsy is necessary.

Differential diagnosis. Tuberculous arthritis must be differentiated from rheumatoid arthritis occurring in a single joint, and from septic arthritis. In the spinal column the differential diagnosis is from pyogenic osteomyelitis, ankylosing spondylitis, prolapsed disc, and tumours.

Treatment consists of antibiotic therapy, symptomatic treatment of the affected joint, and surgical debridement. General supportive measures include rest and proper caloric and protein intake. Patients are started on antituberculosis chemotherapy. The treatment is highly successful if initiated before necrosis and abscess formation has taken place. Triple-drug therapy is employed for 6 to 12 months at daily doses of isoniazid 300 mg, ethambutol 15 mg/kg, and rifampicin 600 mg for 3 months, then 300 mg for 6 to 9 months.

Surgery. Involved joints should be immobilized by traction or splinting. The synovial stage of the disease can be arrested by antibiotics alone, so surgery is not required. However, if the synovial membrane is markedly inflamed and thickened, synovectomy may be helpful. If an abscess has formed it is evacuated after about a month of antibiotic therapy. The bone ends can then be brought into apposition and sound arthrodesis usually takes place. If subchondral bone is involved or the joint fails to respond to the drugs, surgical debridement is indicated. In joints with severe destruction arthrodesis is the treatment of choice. If the disease has been inactive for over 10 years total joint arthroplasty can be considered.

The rheumatic diseases

OSTEOARTHROSIS

Osteoarthrosis is a term used to describe degenerative changes in joints. It is a very common condition in middle age. Usually it is primary. However, sometimes it may be secondary to an injury to the joint during childhood or youth.

Aetiology. Articular cartilage is designed to bear loads and stresses. If the loads applied to the joint increase, or the same loads are applied through unusually small areas because the joint surfaces no longer match each other, this equilibrium is disturbed, because the applied stresses increase in severity. The equilibrium is also disturbed if the disease damages the cartilage so that it is no longer strong and smooth. Thus osteoarthrosis can occur in any joint whose mechanics have been disturbed. When osteoarthrosis develops after a predisposing event it may be called *secondary osteoarthrosis.* The predisposing factors either damage cartilage or reduce the contact area in the joint. Thus:

1. *Injuries to articular cartilage* may render the joint liable to develop osteoarthrosis over the next few years.
2. *Diseases which make the joint surfaces irregular* e.g. Perthe's disease or slipped femoral epiphysis, predispose the patient to the development of osteoarthrosis by reducing the contact area in the joint, so that the pressure on the cartilage is increased and the tissue damaged.
3. Articular cartilage may be damaged by *bacterial or other enzymes*, e.g. in septic arthritis, tuberculous arthritis, or rheumatoid arthritis, and secondary osteoarthrosis may result.

However, the great majority of cases of osteoarthrosis at the hip and knee are idiopathic and are called *primary.* It is felt that these are mostly due to anatomical variations in joint surfaces which produce high local contact pressures.

Pathology. The first change consists of loss of proteoglycans in the territorial matrix of the chondrocytes. Swelling and fragmentation of the collagen network of the cartilage occurs, so that its articular surface becomes rough *(fibrillation).* This process extends deeper until bone is exposed, a condition which is called *ulceration.* Scarring and fibrosis of the capsule occur, with loss of range of motion. At the same time, new bone formation occurs at the periphery of the joint, producing outgrowths which are called *osteophytes.* Where the cartilage is destroyed the subchondral bone and trabeculae become sclerosed. The subchondral bone may degenerate with formation of *cysts.* These cysts may collapse; this deforms the bony articular surfaces, and at the same time loose pieces of bone are separated.

Clinical findings. ***Symptoms.*** The first symptom is *pain* on exercise or at night. It gets more severe as the joint is used, specially in the weight-bearing joints. Pain is also felt when the joint is first moved after a period of immobility. Pain may wake up the patient several times during the night. With the passage of time the joint loses some of its range of movements. In the joints of the lower limb pain and stiffness produce a *limp.* As the disease progresses the *stiffness* becomes increasingly severe until all movement at the joint is lost. The joint may become stiff in a position which is functionally useless. If more than one joint is involved the patient may be crippled and forced to use a wheelchair.

Signs. There may be some *swelling* of the joint due to effusion. *Movement* in certain directions may be restricted. If the hand is placed over the joint as it moves, a sensation of grating may be felt; this is called *crepitus.*

X-ray. The x-ray findings are characteristic. The normal 'joint space' in an x-ray is due to the thickness of two articular cartilages. As this cartilage gets thinner, the joint space diminishes. Bony changes next become evident: sclerosis of subchondral bone, cyst formation and osteophytes. Finally the bone collapses. *The great deal of bone formation distinguishes this condition from rheumatoid arthritis* in which bone loss is the important finding.

Treatment. Therapeutic measures include the following:

1. Modification of activities to avoid excessive strain on the joint.
2. Anti-inflammatory analgesic drugs.
3. Weight loss to reduce the burden on the lower limb joints.
4. Range of motion exercises to minimize contractures.
5. Walking aids such as a stick. Osteoarthrosis tends to be very slowly progressive and symptoms can be satisfactorily managed for many years. However, when symptoms become intolerable surgical intervention may be indicated.

Surgical treatment. Some of the operations used in osteoarthrosis are the following:

1. If one condyle of the tibia is damaged, the knee develops an angular deformity concave in that direction, and weight-bearing becomes malaligned. The alignment can be restored to normal by a *wedge osteotomy.*
2. If it is felt that the damage to the joint has become too extensive for osteotomy to be useful, the joint must be either stiffened (arthrodesis) or replaced by an artificial joint (arthroplasty):

i. *Replacement arthroplasty.* Total hip replacement has been used for primary and secondary osteoarthrosis as well as rheumatoid arthritis. Upto 90% implants survive upwards of 10 years. The major problems consists of loosening of the bone-cement interface and infection. For this reason uncemented porous prosthetic designs have been introduced that allow bony ingrowth to provide permanent stability. With a successful operation pain is abolished and the joint rendered mobile and stable. But if the prosthesis becomes loose or infected the preoperative disability returns and may then be difficult or impossible to relieve. The chances of loosening or infection are greater if the prosthesis has to stay in for a long time. Therefore, although a prosthesis is good treatment for a patient over sixty years of age, its use should be avoided in the young as far as possible, because of their longer expected life span.

ii. *Arthrodesis.* Failure rates of total hip replacement are higher in young active patients. At the same time, because of their longer life expectancy, the risk of long-term failure is also greater. Therefore arthrodesis, i.e. fusion of the femur to the hip bone, is more often employed in those under the age of 40.

RHEUMATOID ARTHRITIS

Pathology. Rheumatoid arthritis is a systemic disease. However, its major manifestations are in the *joints.* The cause of rheumatoid arthritis is unknown. The most popular theory considers the disease to be immune in nature. The disease affects all the supporting structures of the joint, including synovium, tendons, tendon sheaths and bursal tissues. The hypertrophied synovium (pannus) creeps over the articular surface, destroying the cartilage. At the joint margins the inflamed synovium induces osteoclastic bone resorption and creates periarticular erosions. The bone becomes osteoporotic from a combination of hyperaemia, immobility due to pain, and increased osteoclastic activity due to inflammatory cytokines. The ligaments and joint capsule become lax, allowing subluxation of the joint. Ultimately the process in a particular joint can become 'burnt out', with subsidence of the infection and ankylosis of the joint. *Systemic* manifestations of the disease include pericarditis with valvular involvement, granulomas in the lungs, and uveitis.

Clinical findings. ***Symptoms.*** Women are more commonly affected by rheumatoid arthritis than men. The disease may commence any time in adult life, or in childhood. It usually affects more than one joint, and often starts in the small joints of the hands or feet. Later, all the movable joints in the body may be involved together, or one after the other. Each involved joint becomes painful, stiff and swollen. It may remain so far a couple of months, then settle down for many months. The patient feels unwell, and may have low grade fever.

Signs. The inflamed joint shows marked synovial thickening, and typical deformities develop. Limitation of movement, muscle wasting and deformity gradually develop, so as to cripple the patient. The most characteristic deformity in rheumatoid arthritis consists of subluxations at the metacarpophalangeal joints.

X-ray findings include joint space narrowing, periarticular erosions, soft tissue swelling and osteopenia. Gradually, the destruction of bone and stretching of the capsule allows the joint to subluxate and finally dislocate. The active disease may remit, leaving the articular cartilage destroyed. This joint may now progressively develop osteoarthrotic changes, and the x-ray may look like that from a case of osteoarthrosis.

Laboratory findings. The ESR is raised. An abnormal immunoglobulin known as the *rheumatoid factor* may be demonstrated in the blood by the Latex or Rose Waaler tests. However, this factor is found in some healthy individuals and in many chronic infections, and is not always present in rheumatoid arthritis. Therefore, its presence is not diagnostic. It may be mentioned that in osteoarthrosis the blood picture is entirely normal and there is no systemic disturbance.

Treatment involves a team effort of the rheumatologist, orthopaedic surgeon, physical therapist, occupational therapist, and social worker. The aim of treatment is to halt progression of the disease, restore or maintain function, and relieve pain.

Medical treatment. The drugs employed include analgesics (aspirin, codeine), mild anti-inflammatory analgesics (ibuprofen/naproxen), strong anti-inflammatory/analgesics (phenylbutazone/indomethacin), and drugs that modify the immune response (gold salts, penicillamine). Corticosteroids are usually reserved for acute exacerbations or life-threatening situations such as vasculitis.

Orthopaedic management. The aim should be to maintain muscle strength and range of motion of joints, and to avoid deforming forces. Symptomatic joints should be protected with splints or walking aids. If symptoms persist despite medical treatment, surgery may be required and can take one of many forms:

1. *Synovectomy.* Surgical synovectomy slows the progression of the disease. In the knee arthroscopic synovectomy can be undertaken and provides results similar to those obtained by arthrotomy. Radiation synovectomy using intraarticular injection of a short-half-life isotope such as dysprosium-165 ferric hydroxide also produces comparable results. Finally, synovectomy by external beam irradiation has been employed with some success in early cases.
2. *Replacement arthroplasty.* In the hip with disabling pain and stiffness, and the knee with instability due to collateral ligament laxity, total replacement arthroplasty is preferred over synovectomy.
3. In the ankle *arthodesis* gives better results.
4. *Other* operations include release of a carpal tunnel syndrome and silicone replacement arthroplasties to restore mobility to the metacarpophalangeal joints.

ANKYLOSING SPONDYLITIS

Ankylosing spondylitis is one of the group of seronegative spondyloarthropathies. The condition is more common in men. It is a serious illness which makes the patient a cripple. There is calcification and later ossification of the ligaments of joints, which results in complete bony ankylosis of the axial skeleton. The tissue antigen HLA-B_{27} occurs in nearly all patients with ankylosing spondylitis, but only in a small percentage of the normal population. Thus tissue typing can help in diagnosis, but it is not clear how this genetic factor predisposes to the disease. The joints most affected include the sacroiliac and costal joints, and the joints of the hips, the spine (ascending from the lumbar level), and the shoulders. The spine is not only ankylosed but also becomes increasingly concave forwards, so that the patient is bent down and cannot look forwards. Patients in whom the thoracic cage is ankylosed and the spine flexed may die of pulmonary infection, because of stagnation of secretions due to severe reduction in their vital capacity.

Investigations. The ESR is high. *This test should always be carried out in young adults with persistent low backache.* X-rays show obliteration of the sacro-iliac joints and ossification in the spinal ligaments *(bamboo spine).*

Treatment. There is no specific treatment. However, nonsteroidal anti-inflammatory drugs (NSAIDs) help relieve pain. Slow-release indomethacin (75 mg at night) is often the best choice. An exercise programme is essential to maintain movement, relieve symptoms and prevent deformity. Exercises should be carried out at least twice daily. In addition, patients should be encouraged to take part in whatever sport they like. Surgery plays little part, but total hip replacement arthroplasty is occasionally required.

Tumours of bones and joints

Tumours of bones are named after the predominant type of tissue formed by the tumour. Benign tumours take the suffix '-oma', and malignant tumours '-sarcoma'. For example, benign and malignant tumours arising from cartilage are called chondroma and chondrosarcoma respectively, those from fibrous tissue fibroma and fibrosarcoma, and so on.

COMMON FEATURES OF BONE TUMOURS

Bone tumours present with pain, a lump, a tender area, or a pathological fracture. The diagnosis depends upon the clinical features, x-ray appearances and histology. Even then an exact diagnosis can be made only in about 90% of patients.

A *genetic basis* for some bone tumours is suggested by:

1. The increased incidence of bone sarcomas in cases of hereditary multiple exostosis, osteogenesis imperfecta, enchondromas, Paget's disease, familial cancer syndromes, etc.
2. The reports of an increased frequency of osteosarcomas in siblings and cousins of patients with osteosarcoma.

Clinically, a benign tumour presents as a mass; a malignant growth often presents with pain or a pathological fracture. On *x-ray* two features particularly suggest malignancy: an ill-defined osteolytic lesion in the bone, and evidence that the tumour has penetrated the periosteum and invaded the soft tissues.

Before treatment *biopsy* is essential, and open biopsy is preferable. Needle biopsy can be used in tumours of the spine. However, as it yields only a small sample of tissue it is not as reliable as open biopsy.

SPECIFIC BONE TUMOURS

Bone forming tumours. ***Osteoma.*** This small, sessile, benign tumour occurs most often in the skull as an abnormal outgrowth on the surface. It neither causes symptoms nor requires treatment.

Osteoid osteoma. This is a small area of trabeculae of osteoid and bone with a vascular connective tissue ground work. Dense bone forms around it. It is seen most commonly in the second decade, in the long bones.

Osteosarcoma. This is a highly malignant tumour that occurs most commonly in the second and third decades of life in the metaphyseal region of long bones, specially those of the leg. Paget's disease predisposes to a sarcoma, usually an osteosarcoma; these tumours develop in old age because Paget's disease occurs in the elderly. The tumour contains small pleomorphic spindle cells which destroy bone, producing an osteolytic lesion with ill-defined edges on x-ray. It also lays down abnormal bone of irregular structure. Patients present with pain and a mass or swelling. *Spread* occurs via the blood-stream to produce secondary tumours in the lung, and evaluation of the chest by CT is necessary. Bone scan is also carried out to rule out bone metastases, and CT or preferably MRI of the region is performed for surgical planning.

X-ray. If the tumour has lifted the periosteum, neoplastic bone gets deposited as spicules of bone radiating from the shaft to give a 'sun ray' appearance. As the periosteum is lifted above and below the tumour new bone may be formed subperiosteally. On x-ray this bone appears as a triangle *(Codman's triangle).*

Treatment. Osteosarcoma is not particularly sensitive to radiation, but does respond well to combination chemotherapy including methotrexate. Usually, after 6 to 8 weeks of *preoperative chemotherapy*, definitive surgical excision is carried out. This may be in the form of limb preserving excision or limb ablative amputation. If the limb is saved, resected bone can be replaced by prosthesis or allografting. The removed tissue is examined to see if it has responded to chemotherapy. If it has shown a response, the same chemotherapeutic regimen is continued; if not, a different regimen is instituted.

Radiotherapy, whether preoperative or postoperative, has not been found to be of any use. However, it has some effect on secondaries. Results of combination chemotherapy with resection are better than even radical surgical amputation without adjuvant chemotherapy. Preoperative intra-arterial chemotherapy and radiation have also been tried instead of neoadjuvant chemotherapy, and results are comparable.

An interesting mechanism is utilized to make methotrexate fully effective: methotrexate is effective against osteosarcoma cells only in large doses. However, such a dose would result in unacceptable toxicity to normal cells. This is where citrovorum factor comes in. It is an antidote to methotrexate, but only normal cells possess the cell membrane transport system which can enable them to utilize it to save themselves. When large doses of methotrexate are given along with citrovorum factor, the latter protects ('rescues') the normal cells, while the tumour cells are destroyed by the methotrexate. The phenomenon is called citrovorum factor rescue.

Cartilaginous tumours. ***Osteochondroma.*** An osteochondroma almost certainly arises due to localized disturbance of growth of the bone at an epiphysis. A portion of epiphyseal cartilage gets left behind in the periosteum of the metaphysis. The cartilage cap proliferates, endochondral ossification occurs in it, and the osteochondroma grows. As the bone grows, gradually the epiphysis shifts away from the tumour. The growth of an osteochondroma ceases with the completion of bone growth. Excision is curative if all the cartilage is removed.

Chondroma. This tumour is a lobulated mass of cartilage. It occurs most commonly in the metacarpals, phalanges and metatarasals. A chondroma may arise in the medulla *(enchondroma)*. In such cases the bone is thinned by the tumour and pathological fracture may occur. In other cases the tumour may be on the surface of the bone *(ecchondroma)*. The tumours may be solitary or multiple. In multiple tumours malignant change sometimes occurs. The usual treatment is curettage and bone grafting. The most serious concern is the possibility of malignant degeneration, and careful sampling at the time of biopsy is required to exclude the possibility of chondrosarcoma.

Chondrosarcoma. This tumour affects a broad age range (20 to 60). The pelvis, femur, tibia and other long bones are usually involved, and lesions closer to the axial skeleton are more likely to be malignant. The *treatment* of a chondrosarcoma is by excision or amputation, because it is radio-resistant. Commonly it arises in the hip bone or scapula, as mentioned above. In that case it has to be treated by hind-quarter or fore-quarter amputation respectively.

Fibrous lesions. ***Fibroma.*** Small intracortical fibrous lesions are common incidental findings on x-ray in the metaphyses of long bones in children.

Fibrosarcoma. This tumour contains spindle-shaped fibroblasts. It may arise in bone or soft tissue. These tumours metastasize through the blood to the lungs. The 5 year survival rate is about 30%. Fibrosarcoma is treated by early amputation, or in the trunk by wide block resection. The tumour is moderately radiosensitive, and adjuvant chemotherapy can be effective in improving survival rates.

Cystic lesions. ***Solitary bone cyst.*** These lesions occur in children in the metaphyses of long bones, commonly the humerus or femur. They are painless and can present with a pathological fracture as the initial manifestation of the disease. The cysts show on x-rays as osteolytic defects. As the skeleton matures, the cysts tend to gradually disappear. In young children partial or complete healing can be obtained by a series of three intraosseous injections of methylprednisolone. Cysts in older children are best treated by curettage and bone grafting.

Aneurysmal bone cyst. These cysts occur usually in the ends of long bones. They form expanding osteolytic lesions containing bloody fluid. Pathological fracture can occur through the cyst, and callus formation after such a fracture may obliterate it. The tumour is composed of fibrous tissue, vascular spaces, giant cells, and reactive bone. Local resection and bone grafting is the preferred treatment.

Round cell tumours. ***Ewing's sarcoma.*** This is a highly malignant bone tumour of children aged 5 to 15 years, arising usually in the middle of a long bone. X-rays show layers of subperiosteal new bone (*onion-skin appearance.*) A painful hot swelling appears with irregular fever. Therefore the condition has to be distinguished from acute haematogenous osteomyelitis. A soft tissue variant of this neoplasm, primary neuroectodermal tumour (PNET), occurs as well. On immunohistochemical examination it exhibits neural differentiation.

Other tumours. ***Giant cell tumour (Osteoclastoma).*** This tumour is seen most commonly in young adults, in the epiphyseal regions of long bones, specially around the knee. It contains undifferentiated spindle cells and multinucleated giant cells. A giant cell tumour is osteolytic. It expands and thins the bone, sometimes resulting in a pathological fracture. Remnants of the original bone run across the cavity produced by the tumour. Thus it has a *soap-bubble* appearance on x-ray. Although usually benign, a malignant variant sometimes occurs, and even the benign lesions show local aggressive behaviour and a tendency to recur after surgical treatment.

Treatment. Curettage is followed by recurrence in 25 to 50 percent of cases. Therefore wide resection is usually carried out. Alternatively, the cavity left after curetting is filled with methyl methacrylate cement. During polymerization of the cement, heat is generated which kills tissue within several millimeters of the margin in bone. In the long run the cement can cause degeneration in the articular cartilage. It is therefore usually removed after about two years and the cavity filled by bone grafting.

Secondary tumours in bone. The majority of secondary tumours in bone arise from carcinomas of the breast or prostate. A fair number arise from the bronchus, kidney and thyroid. The majority are osteolytic. A few, mostly from the prostate, are osteosclerotic. Treatment consists of a combination of analgesics, radiotherapy, and internal fixation in anticipation of pathological fractures.

Diseases affecting the hand and foot

THE HAND

INFECTIONS

Hand infections occur most often in manual workers and house-wives. The infecting organism is most commonly *Staph. aureus,* besides *Strep. pyogenes* and gram-negative bacilli. Early detection of pus is important. Inflammatory oedema commonly occurs, specially on the dorsum of the hand, because most of the lymphatics travel on the dorsum. The fibrinous exudate is followed by a degree of fibrosis, which is an important cause of stiffness of the hand.

Types of infection. Infections may take place around or under the nail; in the terminal pulp space, web space, or palmar space; or in the synovial sheaths of the flexor tendons.

Acute paronychia. This is the most common infection of the hand. It lies under the skin around the margin of the nail. Antibiotics given early may abort the infection. If pus has formed it must be let out. The eponychium is stripped gently and completely from the base of the nail. If pus has extended under the nail the undermined portion of nail is trimmed away.

Chronic paronychia. The onset of chronic paronychia is slow, and the history dates back many months. The infection may be caused by bacteria or fungi. If the infection is bacterial, antibiotics are ineffective, but freely opening up the infected area helps. If fungi are responsible, anti-fungal remedies e.g. nystatin ointment can be tried.

Apical subungual infection. This infection arises from a prick or splinter under the nail. A small bead of pus forms at the edge of the nail. A V-shaped segment is removed from the free edge of the nail and the pus evacuated.

Infection of the terminal pulp space. This is the second most common infection of the hand. Bacteria usually enter through a prick. The pulp space is closed at its proximal end by a septum of deep fascia. Through the fat of the pulp run the terminal branches of the digital artery. When pus collects in this closed space, its pressure may cause thrombosis of the artery and lead to avascular necrosis of the terminal phalanx.

Clinical findings. Dull pain and swelling are the first symptoms. The pain is worse when the hand is dependent, because the venous engorgement of dependency further raises the interstitial tissue pressure, which is already elevated due to the inflammatory oedema. When pus forms there is throbbing pain. The regional lymph nodes may be enlarged and tender. If the pulp feels hard pus is present.

Treatment. In the very early stage when there is no localization, large doses of antibiotics may cause resolution. Once pus is present immediate drainage is necessary. A short incision is made over the point of maximum tenderness.

Infection of the web space. In this condition the web is swollen and the adjacent fingers separated. Untreated, the pus can track into an adjacent web space, and also along the proximal segments of the adjacent fingers. A transverse incision is made and the pus evacuated.

Deep palmar abscess. This type of abscess lies under the palmar fascia. It is a serious but fortunately rare infection of the hand. The fingers are held flexed, because this position relaxes the palmar fascia. There is gross oedema of the dorsum of the hand because the lymphatics draining the hand lie on the dorsum, and lymphangitis occurs. It is drained by a transverse incision along a flexion crease.

Acute suppurative tenosynovitis. Infection into a flexor tendon sheath is commonly introduced by a needle prick. The whole sheath may be involved rapidly. The organism is *Staph. aureus* or *Strep. haemolyticus*. The classical signs are four:

1. The whole finger is swollen.
2. The finger is flexed, with pain on extension.
3. There is tenderness over the sheath.
4. There is uniform swelling.

Spread. The sheath of the thumb extends up to the forearm as the radial bursa. Again, the little finger sheath joins up with the ulnar bursa, which surrounds the tendons of all the fingers in the palm. Therefore infection from these two digits may extend upto the hand or even forearm.

Treatment. Full doses of cloxacillin are given. The hand and forearm are placed in the position of rest, splinted and elevated. Splinting gives rest to the part, and elevation helps in drainage of the oedema fluid. Unless rapid improvement occurs, incision and drainage is carried out. Transverse incisions are given both at the distal palmar crease and the distal digital crease (i.e. the upper and lower ends of the sheath) to drain pus. Using a fine catheter, the whole length of the sheath is irrigated with antibiotic solution.

Complications of hand infections. *Suppuration* may continue, and require re-exploration.

A stiff digit may result. It should be remembered that in some professions a stiff finger is a very serious disability; in such cases amputation of the useless digit may be preferable. However, one should not be in a hurry to suggest this to the patient; rather one should let him ask for it himself, if he feels it is necessary. In the case of the *thumb* one must save all that is possible even though it may be stiff, because the thumb alone is almost equal to all the fingers due to its very important role in the grip. While holding any object the thumb is normally on one side, while all the fingers combined are on the other.

Principles of treatment of hand infections.

1. *Antibiotic therapy.* This is started immediately. Cloxacillin and ampicillin can be used first. When culture reports are received, the antibiotic may be changed.

If pus has formed one must not depend on antibiotics. Drainage must be carried out at once.

2. After operation the hand is placed in the *position of rest*, which is the one assumed while holding a cricket ball. A light plaster-of-Paris slab, moulded to fit the palm and forearm, is applied. The forearm is suspended in a sling as high as possible to lessen oedema. In all cases rest is

insisted upon. When the acute phase has passed, gentle voluntary movements are encouraged.

3. Adequate *after-treatment* is necessary, with physiotherapy to restore mobility.

INJURIES

Serious injuries of the hand cause a great deal of disability.

Evaluation of the injury. Careful examination of the injured hand is essential in order to find out the extent of damage to arteries, nerves, tendons, bones and joints. Because of the pain and swelling all the clinical methods cannot be easily employed, but the maximum possible information should be obtained. Injuries to the hand cause a great deal of disability. They can be classified into the following types:

1. *Tidy injuries.* These are due to sharp agents, e.g. glass, knives etc. The cuts are clean and incised. Tendons, nerves and blood vessels may be divided.
2. *Untidy injuries.* These injuries are commonly due to industrial accidents. The skin wound is irregular. There may be one or more fractures.
3. *Indeterminate injuries.* e.g. severe crush or burn. It is impossible to know the full extent of the injury immediately. One must wait for a week or two to see what remains. Only then is excision of dead tissue carried out, followed by repair. It is essential to get skin cover after excising all dead tissue. If feasible, the skin is sutured. If not, a free graft or a flap may be used. One should not carry out primary repair of nerves or tendons in these injuries.

Principles of technique in hand surgery. Hand surgery requires meticulous attention to detail:

1. A bloodless field is essential for accurate surgery, so a *tourniquet* is used.
2. As a tourniquet has to be used, the patient is more comfortable under a *general anaesthetic.* If local anaesthesia is used, adrenaline must not be used with the local anaesthetic agent in the fingers, as it may cause spasm of the digital artery and result in avascular necrosis of the digit.
3. Careful wound *toilet* is essential. All dirt and debris must be removed.
4. All *dead tissues* must be excised.
5. Absolute *haemostasis* is essential, because a haematoma may result in infection and spoil an otherwise excellent result.
6. *Antibiotics* and *tetanus* toxoid are employed.
7. In the postoperative period *elevation* and *immobilization* is essential, to give rest and to drain the oedema fluid. The hand is splinted in the *position of function*, in which the metacarpophalangeal joints are flexed, while the interphalangeal joints are extended.
8. In tidy injuries even *digital nerves* may be repaired. This kind of work requires the use of microsurgical techniques, with magnification of the operative field.

THE FOOT

Flat-foot. At birth the foot is flat. The normal arch of the foot is acquired when the infant stands up. It is maintained by the shape of the bones of the foot, by their ligaments, and by the action of the muscles. Flat-foot in adult life may be due to persistence of the infant shape, or to collapse of the arches which had developed. Flat-foot may not be the cause of the pain in the foot. Soldiers with flat feet often do not complain of any pain in their feet.

Idiopathic flat-foot. This is the most common form of flat-foot in the adult. It is seen most often in people who stand for a long time e.g. hairdressers. The medial longitudinal arch collapses, causing pain in the medial part of the sole of the foot. Local tenderness may be found in this area. If these ligaments are stretched by dorsiflexing the foot, pain occurs. At a later stage the foot is painless, but the gait is awkward and inelastic. *Treatment* is required only if there is pain. Rest is prescribed. Arch supports help relieve the pain. In severe cases a change of occupation to a sedentary job is advised in severe cases.

Infantile flat-foot. This is physiological, and self-correcting.

Traumatic flat-foot. This is caused by fractures which abolish the longitudinal arch, e.g. fracture of the calcaneum, or fractures involving the subtalar joints.

Ingrowing toe-nail. An ingrowing toe-nail is commonly seen in the big toe, from encasing the feet in tight shoes and by cutting the toe-nails short and convex. One edge of the nail (usually the lateral edge) curls inwards, and gets buried in the groove in which it lies. Granulations develop and chronic infection persists.

Treatment. Conservative methods succeed in early cases. Tight shoes are avoided, the nail is cut straight, and hot sitz baths help the inflammation to resolve. If these measures fail operation is carried out.

Operation. The part of the nail-bed which lies under the proximal part of the nail is thick and white. This is the area from which growth of the nail takes place, and which must be removed for cure. Only about one-fourth of the germinal matrix on the affected side has to be removed; the remaining three-fourths of the nail continues to grow as before. The operation is carried out under local anaesthesia (Fig. 5). The germinal matrix can also be destroyed chemically by applying a drop of phenol. In resistant cases the

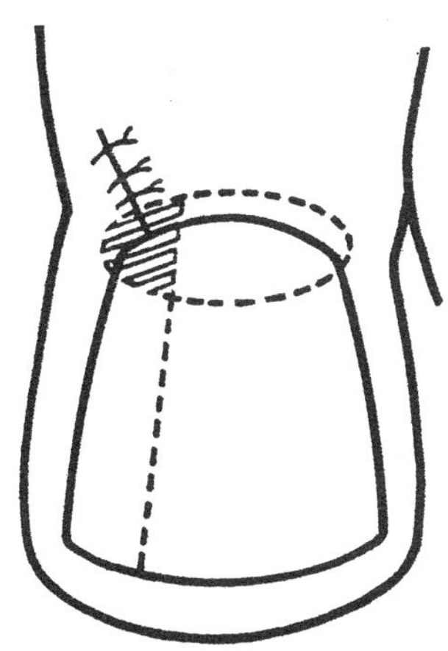

Fig. 5 Operation on ingrowing toe-nail. The shaded part of the growing nail-bed is excised.

whole of the nail and nail bed may have to be removed (*Zadik's operation*).

Madura foot. This is a chronic granulomatous disease found mostly in tropical countries, notably in India and Africa. It is usually caused by a filamentous organism *(Nocardia madurae)* which resembles actinomyces and is found in road dust. The foot is grossly thickened, nodular and hard, with multiple sinuses [PLATE IV-II]. The infection may burrow deeply and numerous cavities develop in bone. Secondary infection usually occurs, with deterioration of the condition.

Treatment. For secondary infection a broad-spectrum antibiotic is used. For the fungus itself dapsone (100 mg. b.d.) is employed. However, many patients come at such an advanced stage that no medical treatment is of any use, and amputation of the foot may have to be considered.

Section 4

Thorax

38 Breast

BENIGN LESIONS OF THE BREAST

Congenital anomalies. The milk line is an ectodermal thickening stretching from the mid-clavicle to the groin in mammals. In some mammals many nipples develop on the milk lines; in women normally only one develops on either side. The most common congenital abnormality of the breast is the presence of additional nipples in the milk line; these are called *supernumerary nipples,* and should be removed by operation not only for cosmetic reasons, but also because any abnormal structure is more liable to undergo malignant change than a normally developed organ.

Extramammary breast tissue is occasionally found, commonly in the axilla (Fig. 1). It usually makes its appearance in adult life, when stimulated by pregnancy or lactation. The treatment of choice is excision of these supernumerary structures.

One or both nipples may rarely be *absent.* Occasionally, a nipple fails to evert following birth, and remains inverted or *retracted* throughout life. A problem arises when the mother tries to breast-feed her baby.

Infantile mastitis. Placental oestrogen may produce a swelling of the breast in the newborn. The condition is called *infantile mastitis.* It is self-limiting, but may occasionally lead to cellulitis.

Precocious puberty. Adrenal cortical and ovarian tumours may produce *precocious puberty and breast hypertrophy*, which may be the earliest signs of the presence of the underlying endocrine disorder.

Gynaecomastia. Gynaecomastia is the development of a female type breast in a male. It is usually unilateral, and occurs in young men (Plate VI-I). *Unilateral* gynaecomastia is not due to hormonal dysfunction, because if such was the case both breasts would have enlarged. Thus it is the target organ, i.e. the breast on the affected side, which is excessively responsive to a normal level of hormones in the blood. On the other hand, in *bilateral* gynaecomastia one must look for a hormonal cause. It is common in hepatic cirrhosis, where there are high levels of circulating oestrogens; also after oestrogen administration for prostatic cancer. Drugs used for cardiovascular diseases like digitalis, spironolactone, methyldopa and calcium channel blockers can all produce gynaecomastia. Other drugs associated with breast development include cimetidine, diazepam and tricyclic antidepressants.

Treatment. It is not normally necessary to be concerned about malignancy in a case of gynaecomastia. However, this mass often produces a good deal of psychological stress in the otherwise healthy young man, and is best removed. If the lump is quite small, subcutaneous mastectomy can be carried out through a circumareolar incision, leaving no residual scar; if it is too large for this approach, a curved submammary incision can be used. In older men the mass is often irregular, and a biopsy is required to rule out a carcinoma.

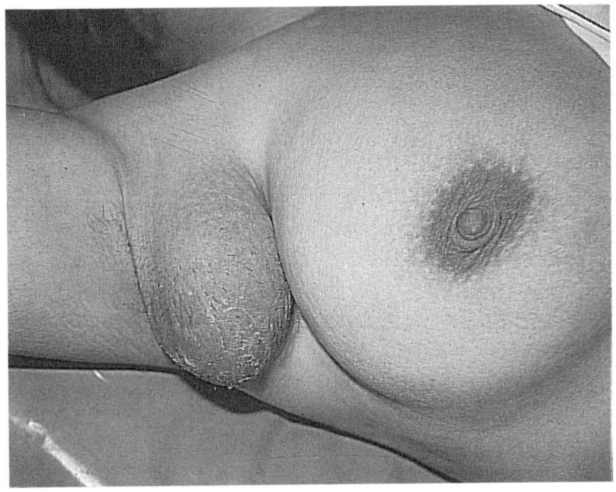

Fig. 1 Accessory breast in axilla.

ABERRATIONS OF NORMAL DEVELOPMENT AND INVOLUTION

Many so-called diseases of the breast are now regarded more correctly as disorders due to aberrations of normal development and involution (ANDI). The term disease is now reserved for disorders of such severity that they are frankly abnormal. Aberrations of development and involution can account for most, if not all, benign breast disorders. For example, most premenopausal women experience breast discomfort and nodularity before menstruation. For most, this is little more than an inconvenience and is regarded as a normal physiological process. In 2 to 3 percent of women the symptoms are more severe and they are referred to a breast clinic with 'cyclical mastalgia'. In the past most such women were described as suffering from 'fibrocystic disease' although often there is little evidence of either fibrosis or cyst formation.

Symptoms of benign breast disease. The following symptoms may be associated with the presence of conditions listed under each symptom. However, this listing does not indicate whether the condition is physiological or pathological, nor is it possible to correlate pathological and x-ray findings with clinical features:

Breast pain (mastalgia)

1. *Cyclical.*
2. *Non-cyclical.* Sclerosing adenosis, musculoskeletal, postoperative, cervical root pain.

Breast lumps. Fibroadenoma, cyclical nodularity, cysts, galactocele, sclerosing adenosis, fat necrosis, lipoma, chronic abscess, normal structures (e.g. prominent rib).

Nipple disorders. Discharge, retraction, sepsis.

Infection. Lactational, non-lactational.

Breast pain. Pain is the most common reason for referral to a breast clinic. The patients fall into two clear-cut groups: those whose symptoms are related to the menstrual cycle (cyclical mastalgia) and those where there is no such correlation (non-cyclical mastalgia).

Cyclical mastalgia. This is much the more common type of pain. The discomfort lasts for a varying period of time prior to menstruation; this is therefore a condition of premenopausal women. The pain is usually bilateral, and is felt in the upper outer quadrants. There are no mammographic or pathological characteristics of cyclical mastalgia. *Symptoms* of this condition correlate with the menstrual cycle, therefore the cause must be hormonal. The following factors have been considered important by different researchers: excess of oestrogens, abnormal prolactin production, and inadequate intake of essential fatty acids.

Most patients require reassurance only, specially to the effect that no neoplasia is present. For the few patients who experience pain in spite of reassurance, drug therapy is required. Excess of oestrogens can be countered by the anti-oestrogen tamoxifen in a dose of 10 mg daily. Danazol (200–400 mg daily) acts as an antigonadotrophin. Abnormal prolactin levels can be lowered by the prolactin lowering agent, bromocriptine (5 mg daily). Each of these drugs, however, is associated with some side effects.

Non-cyclical mastalgia tends to be more chronic, unilateral and located in the medial quadrants of the breasts. Analgesics should be prescribed.

Sclerosing adenosis constitutes one of the causes of non-cyclical mastalgia. Microscopically, proliferation of terminal duct lobules and myoepithelial cells is seen, along with stromal fibrosis. Macroscopically, sclerosing adenosis may have a star-shaped appearance and may calcify; it may thus mimic carcinoma both clinically and radiologically. Other causes of non-cyclical mastalgia include cancer, previous biopsy for benign disease and, in the elderly, referred root pain from cervical spondylosis.

Breast lumps. ***Fibroadenoma.*** Fibroadenoma is a common, well-circumscribed lesion of the breast that tends to occur in young women or girls. The peak incidence is between 21 and 25 years of age. The lump is *movable*, smooth, painless, lobulated, and without any fixation to the overlying skin. The mobility of the mass is a characteristic feature of fibroadenoma; it is so freely movable that it is called a *breast mouse*. Microscopically, fibroadenomas are of two types, intracanalicular and pericanalicular. The former is smaller and firmer, whereas the latter tends to grow to a large size. Fibroadenomas are *treated* by excision and biopsy because of their continued growth and the need to be certain of the diagnosis.

Giant fibroadenoma. A giant fibroadenoma grows rapidly, sometimes to a very large size. The microscopic appearance is the same as in the common fibroadenoma The treatment consists of enucleation through a cosmetic incision.

Phyllodes tumour. These tumours occur in premenopausal women. They have the features of a common fibroadenoma but can grow rapidly to a large size to involve much of the breast. The skin may be stretched over the lesion but is not actually involved by the tumour. Axillary node metastases are rare, and this helps distinguish this tumour from carcinoma. It would be very rare to see a carcinoma totally replacing the breast tissue where both the skin and the axillary glands were not involved; such a situation is seen in a phyllodes tumour. If axillary lymphadenopathy occurs, it indicates an extremely aggressive form of the disease. The neoplasm may outgrow its blood supply and areas of necrosis may occur. Phyllodes tumours should be removed with a 1 cm margin. Very large tumours or those with aggressive histology require wider excision or even mastectomy.

Cyclical nodularity. This condition presents with a lump the size of which varies with the menstrual cycle. Examination shows a diffuse nodular swelling that may be slightly tender. The change usually resolves with the next menstrual cycle. If it does not, aspiration cytology or biopsy is indicated. If malignancy can be excluded, patients with this condition can simply be reassured, but follow-up is essential.

Breast cysts are quite common. They can be regarded as aberrations of normal lobular physiology. They are commonly seen in perimenopausal women. They commonly appear suddenly. Before this, the cyst has existed in a flaccid state; accumulation of an excess of fluid makes it tense and brings it to the patient's notice. The lump possesses some mobility, but not as much as that of a fibroadenoma. *Diagnosis* is straightforward, as the aspiration of the cyst confirms it. Breast cysts are *treated* by aspiration. *However, if the aspirate is blood-stained or the fluid collects again, the cyst should be excised.* Thus it should be remembered that if a cyst is treated by aspiration, it must be followed up properly.

Galactocele. If during lactation a duct gets distended with milk and desquamated epithelial cells, a galactocele is the result. It usually lies under the areola, and can often be emptied by pressure. It should be excised, because it can become infected. Also, it can calcify and be confused with a malignant lesion.

Fat necrosis. If a firm or hard lump has developed in the breast, and has not enlarged since it appeared, it can be an area of fat necrosis. It usually follows trauma, which exposes the fat to calcium, leading to the formation of calcium soaps. It may be impossible to distinguish it from carcinoma on clinical examination or even on mammography. Skin retraction, irregular edges, and fine stippled calcification may all be present. Usually a history of trauma can be obtained. The fat may liquefy to produce a cyst, but the longer-standing cases are scarred and contracted. Excision biopsy is the treatment of choice, so that the diagnosis is beyond any doubt.

Acute mastitis and breast abscess. Breast infections can be divided into two types:

1. *Lactational abscesses.* These are the result of infection by *Staphylococcus aureus,* and develop:

i. At the commencement of breast feeding due to a cracked nipple.

ii. At weaning due to engorgement from incomplete drainage of breast milk.

If seen before frank suppuration, antibiotic treatment alone is sometimes successful. Many cases are due to penicillinase-producing staphylococci; therefore a second-line penicillin or a cephalosporin should be employed. If pus has formed drainage is necessary. The incision should be placed in the dependent part of the abscess to allow drainage of pus under the influence of gravity. The wound is left open and packed loosely with antibiotic-soaked ribbon gauze. However, primary closure under antibiotic cover has also been recommended.

2. *Non-lactational abscesses.* These arise in the periareolar area in cases of duct ectasia, due to stagnation of the contents of a dilated duct. The infecting organisms are a mixture of bacteroides and anaerobic streptococci. Treatment is carried out on lines similar to those employed for lactational abscesses, the antibiotics commonly used being metronidazole and flucloxacillin. Definitive treatment requires excision of the dilated duct when the condition has become quiescent.

Acute mastitis should ideally be *prevented.* During breast-feeding strict nipple hygiene should be adhered to, and any cracks or inflamed areas promptly treated. If some redness develops, an ice-pack gives relief, and a breast pump prevents stasis and intraductal growth of bacteria.

Chronic abscess. A chronic abscess is rare. It can look like a carcinoma, though it is often due to *tuberculosis*. The lesion is not warm and is not tender. Sinuses can develop in old-standing cases. Diagnosis can only be made by biopsy. Treatment requires adequate drainage.

A chronic abscess may also result from *inadequately drained mastitis*. The induration and oedema can make it look like a carcinoma. Wide local drainage with careful biopsy to rule out malignancy is required.

Intraduct papilloma. These benign lesions of the lactiferous ducts occur beneath the areola. The most common symptom is a bloody nipple discharge. They often cannot be palpated, being soft and small; they have to be located by milking the duct in which they lie, so as to express blood from the nipple. If a patient presents with a small palpable mass under the areola and a bloody nipple discharge, there is a 95% chance that she has an intraductal papilloma. When no mass can be felt, a deep-lying carcinoma with invasion of a duct must be looked for.

Intraductal papillomas should be *treated* by excision of the duct as a wedge resection. If a mass can be felt, the area around it should be excised as a wedge. If no mass is palpable, the duct from which blood can be expressed should be probed, and an incision made along the probe until the papilloma is identified. The portion of the duct bearing the papilloma is then removed.

Carcinoma of the breast

Breast carcinoma is the most common form of cancer in women, and is one of the leading causes of death in women above the age of 30. In the Western world one in 14 women can expect to develop breast cancer.

Risk factors. Although the cause of breast cancer remains unknown, certain risk factors can be enumerated:

Sex. Breast cancer is 100 times more common in women than in men. Thus sex is an important risk factor for this cancer, although it is often forgotten as such.

Social class. The greatest mortality rate is seen in the highest socio-economic class. It is thought that dietary factors and obesity affect the solubility of fat-soluble oestrogens.

Age. Breast cancer is almost unknown before puberty and is very rare under the age of twenty. From then onwards the incidence keeps rising till old age.

Age at menarche and menopause. Women whose menarche occurs before the age of 12 are at twice the risk of those starting menstruation after this date. Similarly, women whose menopause comes after the age of 55 run twice the risk of those who stop menstruating before the age of 45.

Family history. If a first-degree relative has suffered from this condition, the risk is increased two-fold; if a second-degree relative, then 1.5 times.

Nulliparity removes a protective effect against breast cancer; thus single and nulliparous women have a 1.5 times higher risk than parous women.

Obesity. Obese women run a nearly 2-fold increased risk.

Previous breast cancer. The relative risk of developing a second breast cancer 20 years after the first is 1.5.

Irradiation. Atomic bomb survivors from Nagasaki and Hiroshima and women who have had multiple chest x-rays for treatment of pulmonary tuberculosis have a higher incidence of breast cancer.

PATHOLOGY

Carcinoma of the breast can arise from the nipple, the ducts, or the lobules.

1. ***Paget's disease*** *(1%).* This is a carcinoma of the ducts of the nipple. It commences as a weeping eczema of the nipple, and may so remain for many years, until ultimately an underlying mass develops. Therefore, any eczematoid lesion of the nipple in a female which persists for more than a few weeks should be biopsied to exclude the possibility of Paget's disease. At the same time, this condition should also be distinguished from a frank tumour that is simply eroding the skin of the nipple. The prognosis is better than for the average carcinoma of the breast if treated by mastectomy and axillary clearance.

2. ***Ductal carcinoma.*** i. *In situ.* (5%) This is a pre-invasive form of breast cancer. It is confined to the duct system and does not invade the basement membrane or the surrounding tissues. Comedo and papillary forms are the most common and both are associated with multicentric disease.

ii. *Invasive.* These tumours can be subdivided into the following types:

(a) *Infiltrating ductal carcinoma with productive fibrosis*, not otherwise specified (NOS), i.e. *scirrhous carcinoma* (65%). This tumour presents typically in a perimenopausal or postmenopausal woman as a solitary, non-tender, firm, ill-defined mass. The tumour possesses a poorly defined border. The cut surface shows a star-shaped tumour

Table 1 TNM system for staging of breast cancer.

T (primary tumour)	
TIS	Carcinoma *in situ.*
TO	No demonstrable tumour in breast.
T1	Tumour 2 cm or less; skin not involved or involved locally in Paget's disease.
T2	Tumour 2 to 5 cm.
T3	Tumour greater than 5 cm.
T4	Tumour of any size with any of the following: skin infiltration, ulceration, peau d'orange, attachment to pectoral muscle or chest wall.
N (regional lymph nodes)	
NO	No palpable axillary nodes.
N1	Palpable, movable, axillary nodes. N1a: metastasis not suspected. N1b: metastasis suspected.
N2	Palpable, fixed, axillary nodes.
N3	Supra or infraclavicular nodes; oedema of arm.
M (distant metastases)	
MO	No distant metastases.
M1	Clinical or x-ray evidence of distant metastases; skin involvement beyond the breast.

with a chalky-white streak, so that is cuts like an unripe pear. The cells are arranged in single rows that occupy irregular cleft spaces between collagen bundles ('Indian filing'). These tumours account for two-thirds of all invasive mammary cancers, and have a relatively poor prognosis. However, factors such as tumour size and axillary node involvement are of more prognostic importance than histological features alone.

(b) *Medullary carcinoma* (6%). These are soft, well-circumscribed, bulky tumours with smooth contours. There is intense infiltration of the stroma with small lymphocytes. They are often large, yet axillary involvement and distant spread are late. This diagnosis indicates a favourable prognosis, the overall 5 year survival rate being as high as 85 to 90%.

(c) *Papillary carcinoma* (2%). These tumours are also well-circumscribed. They demonstrate the formation of papillae, and are associated with a good prognosis.

(d) *Mucinous (mucoid) carcinoma* (2%) consists of masses of jelly-like material, with small clumps of tumour cells lying in a sea of mucoid material. The prognosis is better than for the average carcinoma.

(e) *Inflammatory carcinoma* is a clinical label applied to a very aggressive and lethal form of breast carcinoma which is not related to any specific cell type. The tumour cells are undifferentiated. The lymphatics are blocked with carcinoma, so that the breast is red, hot, swollen and painful. The surface veins and axillary nodes are also full of cancer cells. *This tumour is usually seen postpartum* in younger women with the full breasts of lactation. The prognosis is grave, and treatment is usually unable to control the disease.

Table 2 TNM criteria for actual staging.

Stage	Tumour	Nodes	Metastases
I	T1	NO or N1a	MO
II	TO	N1b	MO
	T1	N1b	
	T2	NO	
		N1a	
		N1b	
III	T3	Any N	MO
	T4	Any N	
	Any T	N2 or N3	
IV	Any T	Any N	M1

3. ***Lobular carcinoma.*** i. *In situ.* This is a preinvasive form of breast cancer, possessing the potential for becoming invasive. It is usually discovered by chance. It has no mammographic features and is usually found on biopsy performed for other reasons.

ii. *Invasive* (10%). This tumour is characterized by the 'Indian filing' of invading malignant cells, and shows a *tendency to occur bilaterally.*

CLINICAL STAGING

By clinical staging the surgeon makes an attempt to identify the extent of the malignant lesion. Not only does clinical staging of cancer provide a reasonably accurate indication of prognosis, but it also *serves as the primary method for comparing different techniques of treatment.*

TNM system of staging. The TNM system of staging has achieved universal acceptance, not only in the case of breast cancer but also in many other types of cancer. It is based on clinical examination for the tumour (T), regional lymph nodes (N), and distant metastasis (M). The TNM system in respect of the breast is shown in Table 1.

The actual staging is carried out as in Table 2. In the case of every patient with breast cancer *a staging sheet* as well as *a diagram* for locating the mass within the breast should be completed and kept as a part of the hospital record. It provides an accurate description for anyone examining the patient on follow-up visits. It also makes it possible to compare one's work with that carried out anywhere else, or to collaborate with an institution anywhere in the world.

DIAGNOSIS

The most common initial evidence of breast cancer is a lump in the breast, usually painless and discovered by the patient herself. A painful breast mass, a nipple discharge and a retracted nipple are all much less common as presenting signs than a painless lump. Other less common accompanying complaints are skin puckering, breast enlargement and arm oedema.

Occasionally systemic metastases to the bones, axilla, supraclavicular area or lungs produce the initial symptoms or signs of disease. Generally, breast cancer tends to spread quite early by both lymphatic and haematogenous routes and with widespread metastases. However, a few cases remain locally invasive for years, without showing evidence of distant spread.

Even when the most experienced clinicians examine a breast and give their opinion about the presence or absence of cancer, they are correct only 70% of the time. Therefore any discrete lump or mass in the breast must be considered as possibly a carcinoma.

About 50% of breast cancers are found in the upper outer quadrant of the breast, the remainder arising in the other quadrants and the areolar region. Tumours do not usually become palpable until they are greater than 1 cm. in diameter. It has been calculated that it takes approximately 5 years for a tumour to reach this size from the single cell stage. *Thus it is easy to understand why distant metastases have so often taken place before the tumour is detected* by the patient or the surgeon.

Mammography. Mammography is an x-ray examination of the breast. It requires special techniques, an x-ray film designed for examining soft tissues, and a radiologist skilled in interpreting the x-ray images of the breast. The classic features of breast cancer on mammography include: tissue asymmetry, mass effect, microcalcification, skin thickening and nipple inversion. A combination of *mass effect and microcalcification* is the most reliable evidence. Mammography is specially useful in the following situations:

1. In screening procedures, specially in high-risk populations, e.g. patients with previous breast cancer or with relatives having breast cancer.
2. When a mass is palpable in the breast but the diagnosis is uncertain: fine calcification, irregular borders, and variable density of the lesion suggest a malignant lesion. However, it should be remembered that only 50% of cancers show calcification on mammography. Therefore, the *absence of calcification does not rule out malignancy.*
3. In a large fatty breast, when the patient has symptoms but no lump is palpated: tumours cannot easily be felt in such breasts, but the mammogram is most accurate in the fatty breast.
4. Preoperative mammography also acts as a baseline for radiological evaluation of the breast in the years after the initial mammogram.

Mammography can detect some tumours which cannot be found in any other way. *The 5 year survival rate for tumours found in this manner may be as high as 90%.*

Thermography. The skin over a malignant tumour of the breast is usually warmer than the surrounding areas. Using heat sensors it is possible to delineate these *hot spots* on the film. Unfortunately the number of false negatives and false positives is high, and the technique has been abandoned. However, research continues to improve the method.

Ultrasonography. Ultrasound clearly differentiates a cystic from a solid mass. However, it is unsatisfactory for diagnosing early breast cancers because of its inability to detect microcalcification, or to discriminate lesions smaller than 5 mm. It may be mentioned that for the diagnosis of a cystic lesion needle aspiration is as effective as an ultrasound examination.

Biopsy. *No patient should be subjected to a mastectomy for cancer until and unless histological proof of the presence of cancer has been obtained.* This can be done only by some form of biopsy:

1. *Fine needle aspiration cytology* has the advantage of being an outpatient procedure and producing immediate results. However, it requires expert and specialized interpretation. At the same time the method has its limitations:
   i. The *false-negative* rate is about 15%, due to missing the tumour at the time of aspiration or from failing to aspirate a particularly hard scirrhous carcinoma.
   ii. The *false-positive* rate is about 2%, due to confusion with an excessively cellular fibroadenoma or the effects of pregnancy, lactation or hormone therapy on normal breast tissue.
   iii. Aspiration cytology cannot differentiate between *in-situ* and invasive cancer.
2. *Core biopsy* using a Trucut type needle can be employed as an outpatient procedure under local anaesthesia. It offers the advantage that it provides a histological rather than a cytological specimen. However it is liable to miss small cirrhotic tumours.
3. *Open surgical biopsy* is required in patients who are clinically suspected to have cancer yet in whom fine needle aspiration cytology or core biopsy fails to demonstrate malignant disease. It is best performed under general anaesthesia, the patient being discharged home the same day. The definitive operation if indicated is carried out a few days later after discussion of the different treatment options with the patient; this delay in operation has no effect on the recurrence or survival rates. Every open biopsy of the breast for a suspected malignancy should include a small piece of skin in the specimen, to see if it is involved. The submitted tumour tissue should also be tested for the presence of hormone receptors.

Lines of tension in the skin of the breast (Langer's lines) are generally concentric with the nipple, and incisions that parallel these lines result in fine scars. At the same time incisions for biopsy should be kept within the boundaries of potential incisions for mastectomy that may be required for definitive treatment. If possible, the skin incision should be placed in the circumareolar position, because it is more cosmetic, the scar being invisible. If the lesion is small total excision is carried out, but in the case of a large lesion an incisional biopsy is taken.

4. *Frozen section* examination of an excised specimen at the time of the definitive operation was very popular at one time. However, it is not as often employed today:
   i. Because of the wider availability of fine needle aspiration cytology.
   ii. Because the patient being anaesthetized is unable to discuss various treatment options with the surgeon in the light of the pathological findings.

Evaluation. Once the diagnosis of breast cancer has been made, the patient should have chest x-ray, haemoglobin, blood count, electrolytes and liver function tests. The value of other more sophisticated tests is open to doubt.

As far as *scintiscans* are concerned: there is a very low incidence (about 1%) of true positive *bone* scans in 'operable' cancer. There is an even lower positive yield with *liver* and *brain* scanning. However, patients with clinical stage III disease and those with symptoms suggesting metastases should undergo further investigation, the bones being scanned by scintigraphy and the liver by ultrasonography.

TREATMENT OF BREAST CANCER

The treatment of breast cancer requires co-operation between surgeons, radiotherapists, medical oncologists and pathologists, along with counsellors and breast care nurses. *A large number, upto 50%, of breast cancers have metastasized before the patient presents for treatment.* Therefore the treatment of breast cancer resolves itself into two parts, the eradication of local disease and the control of distant metastases. For the control of local disease the mainstays of treatment are: firstly, the different operations available for removal of the cancer, and secondly radiotherapy. For metastases the modalities of treatment used include cytotoxic chemotherapy and radiotherapy. Finally, hormonal manipulation can be used both against local and metastatic disease.

SURGICAL TREATMENT

Surgical treatment has to deal with disease both in the axilla and the breast.

The breast. Cancer of the breast is often *multicentric* in origin, and this constitutes a strong argument in favour of complete removal of the breast in all cases.

The axilla. It is very desirable that histological proof be obtained of the presence or absence of *metastatic disease in the axilla.* This is important for two reasons: firstly, it allows accurate staging of the cancer into stage I or II and enables a more definite prognosis to be given. Secondly, it enables the exact number of affected lymph nodes to be determined, which has great significance. If 3 or less than 3 nodes are affected the prognosis is good. On the other hand, if 4 or more nodes contain tumour, the prognosis is much worse. Therefore, dissection of the axilla has long been regarded as an essential part of any complete operation for breast cancer. However, as far as the actual extent of dissection of the axilla is concerned, recently it has been argued that axillary clearance needlessly overtreats the 50% patients with negative axillary nodes. It has been suggested that the axilla should be *sampled*, and adjuvant radiotherapy to the axilla employed if the nodes are found to be positive. But that in any case, if the nodes are large, i.e. greater than 2 cm in diameter, surgical axillary clearance is still preferable.

In the surgical treatment of breast cancer, the breast and the axillary contents are removed wholly or in part. For ease of understanding, the procedures available for the breast and the axilla will be first listed separately. We shall next examine their various combinations, and finally the choice of combinations for different cases.

Operations on the breast. 1. *Total mastectomy.* The whole of the breast is removed, including the areola as well as the skin over the protuberant breast.

2. 'Conservative' operations, namely *segmentectomy* and *quadrantectomy.* Although these terms are somewhat vague, they do imply removal of the tumour with an adequate margin of normal tissue.

Operations on the axilla. 1. *Axillary clearance.* The contents of the axilla i.e. fat and lymph nodes are removed, staying medial to the axillary vein to spare the lymphatics draining the upper limb.

2. *Axillary sampling.* The nodes of the anterior chain are 'sampled'.

3. Axillary lymphangiography, followed by removal of only those nodes found to contain tumour: this is a recent technique to save uninvolved nodes.

The combinations commonly employed include the following:

1. Total mastectomy and axillary sampling.
2. Total mastectomy and axillary clearance, i.e. modified radical mastectomy.

(Note: In the original radical mastectomy the pectoralis major was also removed. This operation is now rarely employed, as its results have been found to be equivalent to those of modified radical mastectomy).

3. Quadrantectomy, Axillary Dissection and Radiation Therapy (QU.A.RT): in this procedure the quadrant of the breast bearing the tumour is excised and axillary dissection carried out. This is followed by irradiation of the breast.

The choice of combination. 1. Tumours larger than 2 cm are best treated by mastectomy and axillary clearance, which should be considered as the 'gold standard' with which all operations for breast cancer should be compared in respect of absence of local recurrence as well as disease-free survival. This method is suitable for *all* operable tumours, but tumours larger than 2 cm should definitely be provided with the benefit of removal of the entire breast.

2. Patients with tumours *smaller than 2 cm* can be treated by partial mastectomy i.e. 'segmentectomy' or 'quadrentectomy' (plus axillary procedure), *provided radiotherapy and follow-up of a high standard are available*, and then *provided the margins of the removed tissue are shown to be free of tumour.* Even so, the following constitute contra-indications to conservative surgery:

i. If the tumour is poorly differentiated.
ii. If the tumour is centrally placed, as it is more difficult to remove by segmentectomy.
iii. If the tumours are bilateral or multifocal.
iv. If the axillary nodes are palpable.
v. If the patient prefers a total mastectomy.

3. Recently, in the case of tumours less than 3 cm in size, quadrantectomy, axillary dissection and radiation therapy to the breast has been tried. The five year survival figures have been reported to be similar to those after modified radical mastectomy. If this work is confirmed, it is possible that for these smaller tumours this procedure may displace modified radical mastectomy.

International trends favour a reduction in radical procedures. *This will be safe only where this is accompanied by high standards of pathological classification, radiotherapy, chemotherapy, and follow-up.*

Technique of modified radical mastectomy (Patey). The breast and axillary contents are dissected *en bloc.* The excised mass consists of:

1. The whole breast.
2. The skin overlying the protuberant breast.
3. The pectoralis minor.

4. All the fat, fascia and lymph nodes of the axilla. While dissecting the axilla, the surgeon remains medial to the axillary vein. Thus he avoids damage to the upper limb lymphatics accompanying the vein, and prevents the development of lymphoedema of the arm.

Suction drainage. Drainage with continuous suction is achieved by using a non-collapsible drain and connecting it with:

i. A glass bottle in which vacuum has been created by evacuating the air with a sucker, or

ii. A collapsible plastic bottle from which air has been evacuated by compression and which, as it springs open, creates a negative pressure.

This step greatly expedites healing by preventing accumulation of exudate under the flaps. Apart from mastectomy, this method can be used wherever the possibility of accumulation of fluid under skin flaps exists. It may be mentioned that a recently suggested alternative approach avoids drainage and actively encourages the collection of serous fluid as a 'seroma'. This exudate gets organized and fibrosed; it is supposed to partly fill the cavity left behind by the mastectomy and provide a fuller contour. Personally, the author would favour suction drainage, as a method less likely to be followed by complications.

If a wide area of skin has been sacrificed, it may not be possible to approximate the skin edges. A deficiency is left which should be treated by immediate split-skin grafting. When the wound has healed, movements of the arm are encouraged to prevent stiffness of the shoulder.

Breast conservation. As mentioned above, in early cases the breast may be conserved by combining local excision with radical radiotherapy to the breast in place of mastectomy. The cases must be selected with great care. Those which are unsuitable for conservation include:

1. Tumours larger than 3 cm.
2. Tumours which are located centrally.
3. Bilateral and multifocal tumours.
4. Poorly differentiated tumours.
5. Breasts showing Paget's disease of the nipple.
6. Cases with palpable axillary nodes.
7. Cases in which the patient prefers to be treated by total mastectomy.

Breast reconstruction. The mutilation produced by mastectomy can be minimized by breast reconstruction, which should be offered specially to premenopausal women. It may be performed at the time of the mastectomy or delayed for 3–6 months after the operation. The advantage of a few months' delay is this: a reconstructed breast generally cannot match the original, and therefore immediate reconstruction results in unfavourable comparison by the patient. With delayed reconstruction the patient will compare favourably the reconstructed breast with the mastectomy. Breast reconstruction may be carried out by:

1. Implanting a *silicone prosthesis* of the breast under the pectoral muscles.

2. Employing a *latissimus dorsi myocutaneous flap*: In this operation the latissimus is divided from its origin and, along with an overlying ellipse of skin, is tunnelled forwards to be spread out and sutured over the pectoral region. The ellipse of skin ensures that there is no shortage of skin after removal of the breast and its overlying skin. The most recent innovation, which gives a better cosmetic result, employs a myocutaneous flap of *rectus abdominis* muscle supplied by the superior epigastric artery and with an overlying ellipse of skin.

Finally, the areola can be constructed by grafting a disc of skin from the upper medial thigh, and the nipple by taking a segment from the opposite nipple.

ADJUNCTIVE THERAPY FOR BREAST CANCER

Fewer than 50% of women treated surgically for apparently curable lesions are alive 10 years later. This liability to early spread made it necessary to look for adjuncts to the treatment of breast cancer in the hope of altering potential metastatic disease. Three types of adjunctive therapy have been developed: radiotherapy, chemotherapy and hormone alteration.

Radiotherapy. Both preoperative and postoperative radiotherapy have failed to alter *survival rates.* However, post operative radiotherapy has had some effect on *local recurrences.*

Adjuvant chemotherapy. *The use of chemotherapy as an adjunct to primary treatment of breast cancer is one of the most important advances in cancer care.* This fact can be properly appreciated only if it is remembered that, until the 1950's, nothing could be done for the distant micrometastases that had taken place before diagnosis in nearly half the patients with breast cancer. Since that time, an increasingly bright picture of the situation has been emerging.

Although chemotherapy was started with one drug, it was soon found that when two or more drugs were used in combination, the therapeutic effects were cumulative but the side effects were not. This was obviously a great advantage of the method of multiple-drug therapy. Today, a *three-drug* combination of methotrexate, cytoxan and 5-fluorouracil (CMF) is commonly used, 6 three-weekly cycles with these drugs being employed. Further, vincristine and prednisolone are often combined with the above three drugs in the form of a *five-drug* regimen, when the results are even better. This kind of combination chemothrerapy is employed in the following groups of patients:

A. In women aged less than 50:

In node-positive patients: in all cases.

In node-negative patients: may be of value.

B. In women aged more than 50:

In receptor-negative patients, due to doubts about the efficacy of tamoxifen.

In women with one to three positive axillary nodes, the 5 year relapse-free survival rate is as high as 88%, compared with 50% in the group where no adjuvant chemotherapy has been used. Unlike tamoxifen, combination chemotherapy is more effective before the age of 50. Before this age, it reduces mortality at the end of 5 years by 34%, after this age by only 18%. Unfortunately, chemotherapy is often accompanied by serious sequelae, e.g. myelosuppression and alopecia.

Comparison between radiotherapy and chemotherapy. For many decades radiotherapy was the standard adjuvant therapy after radical mastectomy if the axillary nodes were found to contain tumour. Recently it has been found that multiple drug chemotherapy given after operation gives superior results; it is therefore used more often.

This superiority of multiple drug therapy over radiotherapy is not entirely unexpected. The only way radiotherapy could possibly affect metastatic disease could be by whole body irradiation; however, this is known to be associated with an extremely high morbidity. Fortunately, because the side effects of the different drugs used in multidrug therapy do not cumulate, multi-drug therapy achieves control of metastases with a significantly lower level of morbidity.

Adjuvant hormonal therapy. The response of breast cancer to hormones is dependent on the presence in the cancer cells of hormone receptors. If these receptors are present it indicates a more differentiated tumour. *Such neoplasms respond to all forms of therapy better than receptor-negative tumours.* If both oestrogen receptors (ER) and progesterone receptors (PR) are present, 80% of tumours will respond to hormonal manipulation. Tumours that are both ER and PR-negative respond in only 10% of cases. It follows therefore that *when a tumour is removed it should be sent not only for histological examination but also for detecting the presence of hormone receptors.*

The different forms of hormonal manipulation include the following:

1. *Antioestrogens.* Tamoxifen is an antioestrogen which acts by blocking oestrogen receptor sites. The oral dose for best results is 20 mg. per day. Tamoxifen is more effective over the age of 50; above this age, it reduces the risk of recurrence at the end of 5 years by 18%, below it by only 4%. Side effects are minimal. *In oestrogen receptor-positive tumours the response rate is similar to that after adrenalectomy.*

2. *Operations.* The operations available are oophorectomy, adrenalectomy and hypophysectomy. These last two have been virtually abandoned due to the success of the various oral agents. However, in the remote areas of underdeveloped countries there is still a place for *oophorectomy* in premenopausal women, because drugs may not be available in constant supply. If the woman is illiterate, the chances of her adhering to a lengthy drug regimen are few. In such women oophorectomy ensures that the benefit of the desired hormonal manipulation is obtained to the fullest extent.

TREATMENT OF RECURRENT CANCER

Recurrent cancer of the breast may take the form of local recurrences or wide dissemination:

1. *For local recurrences.* i. Radiation is a very useful agent. Examples of such local lesions include subcutaneous nodules and bony metastases.

ii. Operation may also be useful for small local lesions, but only if margins clear of tumour can be obtained.

2. *For wide dissemination.* The important problem in recurrent cancer is usually wide dissemination. The treatment of choice here consists of the use of *hormone therapy* and/or *chemotherapy.* The initial choice out of the above two methods depends upon whether or not the tumour is hormonally sensitive. This can be determined by testing for the presence of hormone receptors. As mentioned before, 80% of patients with breast cancers which are both ER and PR-positive respond to hormonal manipulation. Thus if the patient's hormone receptor status is positive, she should be treated by hormonal manipulation; if she is receptor-negative, chemotherapy should be used.

The methods of hormone manipulation. For hormone manipulation, the following methods may be employed:

1. *Ablation* i.e. removal of oestrogen-generating tissue by oophorectomy or adrenalectomy. Both these operations have given way to medical treatment.

2. *Aminoglutethimide.* This drug blocks the conversion of cholesterol to pregnenolone and thus inhibits the production of adrenal steroids. The effect of aminoglutethimide is often referred to as *medical adrenalectomy.* It eliminates the need for, and has therefore supplanted, operative adrenalectomy. If this drug is used, the patient must also receive replacement hydrocortisone.

3. *Antioestrogens,* e.g. tamoxifen, as described above.

Special situations. ***Locally advanced disease (stage III).*** The management of these tumours has given disappointing results because of poor local control and subsequent metastatic disease, resulting in an overall survival rate of only 20%. The different approaches are as follows:

1. *Neo-adjuvant chemotherapy,* to 'downstage' the tumour prior to surgery or irradiation: not only does the tumour shrink and become more amenable to surgery, but also chemotherapy is delivered to potential micrometastases immediately after diagnosis. This method has only recently been introduced, and early results are promising.

2. *Adjuvant chemotherapy.* This improves the disease-free survival rate.

(Note: The classical method has been *radical mastectomy.* This has produced disappointing results, 40% patients developing loco-regional recurrences within 2 years, with low survival rates).

3. *High-dose radiotherapy* has given results similar to those with radical mastectomy. Local recurrences can be reduced by surgically debulking the tumour, or by giving even higher doses of radiation by an interstitial implant.

In the ***elderly,*** tumours are slow-growing, usually oestrogen-receptive positive with a good prognosis, and can be treated with the anti-oestrogen tamoxifen alone. However, as the cosmetic compulsion to retain the breast is less strong at this age, it is best to add mastectomy, tamoxifen alone being reserved for the very frail.

Pregnancy. During the *first trimester,* pregnancy can continue. However, if the disease is locally advanced it requires irradiation and adjuvant chemotherapy; these are contraindicated during pregnancy, which therefore has to be terminated. In the *second trimester* the decision is more difficult, and the patient's wishes regarding pregnancy should prevail. In the *last trimester,* the standard treatment should be given, adjuvant chemotherapy or irradiation being delayed until after delivery.

Lactation. The tumour should be treated on standard lines, lactation being suppressed by bromocriptine.

Ductal carcinoma in situ (DCIS). The best treatment is a mastectomy, both for extensive disease and for the screen-detected smaller tumours, though many prefer conservative surgery for the latter.

METASTATIC BREAST CANCER

Recurrence of breast cancer is of ominous significance. It is incurable with the currently available methods, with a median survival of 15 months. Treatment aims at alleviating symptoms and prolonging survival. Investigations aim at determining the full extent of the disease, and should include examination of the primary and regional nodes, chest x-ray, abdominal ultrasound, and bone scintigraphy. Brain scanning gives a low yield and is not recommended. Similarly, tumour markers do not have a significant role to play. The longer the disease-free interval after diagnosis of the primary tumour the better the prognosis. Again, loco-regional or bony metastases have a better prognosis than liver or brain secondaries.

Treatment. *Endocrine therapy.* Of tumours which are positive for oestrogen receptors, 60% respond to endocrine therapy; of those which are negative, only 10%. Tamoxifen is as effective in this regard as oophorectomy, aminoglutethimide or progestogens, but with fewer side effects. The success of the various oral agents has reduced enthusiasm for surgical endocrine therapy. Adrenalectomy and hypophysectomy are no longer employed; oophorectomy is used only as second-line treatment after a good response to tamoxifen in premenopausal patients.

Prognosis. With the use of adjuvant chemotherapy the prognosis after treatment for breast cancer has greatly improved. 5 year survival rates of 95% in stage I and 80% in Stage II have been reported using modified radical mastectomy. Even with stage III cancers, using surgery plus adjuvant chemotherapy, 5 year survival figures upto 35% can be obtained.

Indicators of prognosis. Apart from an advanced stage of the cancer assessed by the TNM method of staging there are a few other indicators of a poor prognosis, as follows:

i. *Clinical.* Rapid growth rate, young age.

ii. *Histological.* Poor differentiation, lymphatic permeation, blood vessel invasion and infiltration into surrounding soft tissues.

39 Thorax

TESTS OF LUNG FUNCTION

In the pulmonary alveoli the blood and inspired air exchange oxygen and carbon dioxide across the alveolar membrane. Any severe disturbance of this mechanism may lead to changes in the levels of the blood gases. *Blood* O_2, CO_2 and *pH* determinations measure adequacy of lung function. *Chest expansion, vital capacity* and *forced expiratory volume* measure the patient's ability to ventilate.

Lung scanning. The movement of air in the tracheobronchial tree can be measured by lung scanning after *inhaling* radioactive xenon. If the same radioactive xenon is given *intravenously,* lung scanning can measure the flow of blood in the pulmonary vasculature. In this way the relationship between ventilation and perfusion *(ventilation/perfusion ratio)* can be worked out. If an area of lung is ventilated but not perfused, e.g. in pulmonary embolism, a part of the tidal volume is wasted. The larger such an area of lung the more dangerous the situation. If on the other hand a part of the lung is perfused but not ventilated e.g. in collapse of a lobe, the lobe acts as a right-to-left shunt, supplying deoxygenated blood to the arterial system. If the shunt is large cyanosis may result.

Pulmonary angiography. An outline of the pulmonary vessels can be obtained with radiopaque diatrizoate injected into the right ventricle *(pulmonary angiography).* Both pulmonary angiography and lung scanning help in the diagnosis of pulmonary embolism.

CHEST INJURIES

In civilian practice chest injuries consist either of stab and bullet wounds, or are sustained during road accidents. In war they are quite common. There are two main varieties of chest injuries, namely wounds and crush injuries, though both types may be present in the same patient.

PENETRATING CHEST WOUNDS

Stab wounds. Stab wounds are most commonly found on the left side of the front of the chest, the knife being in the assailant's right hand. If the knife penetrates the heart these wounds are associated with a high mortality rate. If it punctures only the lung they are relatively benign, causing only a moderate-sized haemothorax.

Missile wounds. Missile wounds are much more commonly fatal, because they often go through-and-through, and thus can cause damage to a larger number of structures. Most civilian gunshot wounds occur with *low velocity.* Such missiles core out a hole through the body and damage only those tissues with which they come in direct contact. They cause death by damage to vital structures or exsanguinating haemorrhage. Because of its low kinetic energy the path taken by a hand-gun bullet through the body can be deflected by bone or even parenchymal organs such as the liver.

On the other hand wounds due to *high-velocity* rifle bullets and bomb fragments produce extensive tissue damage by cavitation and shock waves. Energy from the bullet is dissipated into the surrounding tissues which are violently accelerated forwards and outwards. For a split-second this creates a large cavity about 30 times the size of the missile. The cavity has a subatmospheric pressure and is open at both entrance and exit holes. It then collapses sucking air, debris and bacteria into the wound and producing a large volume of devitalized and contaminated tissue.

The mediastinal structures, the diaphragm and the abdominal organs may be damaged. A thoracotomy may be required in order to assess the extent of damage and undertake repair. Damage is directly proportional to the density of the tissue. Liver, spleen and muscle are damaged to a greater extent than tissues like lung which mainly consist of air. The destruction is also inversely proportional to the number of elastic fibres present; skin and lung are resistant whereas bone is shattered.

Thoraco-abdominal wounds. A stab or bullet wound of the lower chest may penetrate the diaphragm and damage intra-abdominal organs. The main indications for exploration are signs of persistent bleeding or the likelihood of the perforation of a hollow viscus. The best route for exposure is through the thorax, because it allows correction of the thoracic injuries while providing adequate exposure of the upper abdomen through the diaphragm.

CRUSH INJURIES OF THE CHEST

These are common in road accidents. There may be bruising of the chest wall, rib fractures, a stove-in chest, a flail chest, lung contusion, or rupture of the aorta or myocardium.

Fractures of ribs. Ribs may get broken either from direct violence or when the chest is crushed. When each rib is broken at only one point and the number of broken ribs is small, the problem is usually a simple one, requiring only rest and analgesics, or at most strapping. When some ribs are broken both anteriorly and posteriorly a flail segment of chest wall results which is dangerous because of paradoxical respiration as explained below.

If a *large number of ribs,* e.g. eight or ten, are broken, even if each one is broken at only one point, a critical situation can arise. Firstly, a single rib fracture can result in a blood loss of 150 ml. Multiple fractures may cause substantial blood loss into the chest wall and pleural cavity. Secondly, because of the fractures the chest cannot expand properly, a problem which is made worse by the considerable pain which results. Secretions therefore get retained, further reducing vital capacity and setting the stage for the development of hypostatic pneumonia. This is even more likely in the case of elderly persons with their reduced vital capacity and diminished ability to fight infections.

In a head-on car crash if the driver is not wearing a safety belt the *steering column* and wheel can hit the front of his chest and produce extensive damage. A fracture-dislocation of the upper end of the sternum occurs, with bilateral fractures of the ribs at their anterior ends. This can also cause paradoxical respiration and pose a danger to life.

Stove-in chest. In a stove-in chest a segment of the chest wall is pushed in and kept there by the surrounding ribs coming over it, reducing the volume of the underlying lung.

Flail chest. A flail chest is more dangerous. In this condition a segment of chest wall becomes loose due to fractures of a few ribs both in front of and behind it. When the chest expands during inspiration and a negative pressure is created, this loose segment instead of moving out is sucked in and prevents expansion of the lung, seriously interfering with ventilation.

The function of the other lung is also interfered with. During inspiration, due to expansion of the chest wall on the uninjured side, the lung expands properly and the pressure inside it becomes negative. Normally air from outside would have filled this partial vacuum with inspired air. However, the pressure inside the lung on the injured side does not become negative as explained above. Therefore during inspiration air flows from the injured side to the healthy lung instead of allowing inspired air to come into it. Similarly during expiration this same air flows back into the injured lung due to the pressure inside the normal lung being higher. Thus air in the two lungs keeps moving to-and-fro, preventing air from outside from coming in. Therefore it will be seen that due to the severe physiological disorder produced by it, even a small flail segment of chest wall can produce a dangerous degree of hypoxia. The serious interference with ventilation results in rapid shallow respirations with cyanosis, tachycardia and hypotension. Respiration is noisy from tracheo-bronchial secretions. Cerebral hypoxia produces confusion and restlessness, and this is followed by unconsciousness in severe cases.

Blood and air in the pleural cavity. ***Traumatic haemothorax.*** In most chest injuries some blood collects in the pleural cavity. The source of the bleeding may be the chest wall, the lung, or the heart and great vessels. Due to constant churning of the blood from the respiratory movements, it becomes defibrinated and therefore does not clot. This is fortunate, because it is easier to remove liquid blood from the chest cavity (by aspiration) rather than to evacuate clotted blood. Bleeding is usually moderate, and should be dealt with by daily aspirations. If accumulation is progressive, indicating a persisting source of blood loss, a thoracotomy may be required to control the bleeding.

Aspiration of the pleural cavity (thoracentesis). This is carried out most conveniently using a 3-way stopcock connected with the aspiration needle. When the valve is turned in one direction, fluid can be aspirated into the syringe. The valve is next turned in the other direction, and fluid flows into a tubing which carries it to a kidney-tray. The great advantage of the use of this simple implement lies in the fact that at no time does the system have to be disconnected, so that the chances of infection or of introduction of air into the pleural cavity are minimized.

Traumatic pneumothorax. In many forms of trauma air enters the pleural cavity, usually with blood as well *(haemopneumothorax)*. It may reach the pleural cavity through a wound in the chest wall. More commonly it leaks from the damaged lung.

Tension pneumothorax. If the leak in the lung is valvular a considerable quantity of air accumulates, producing complete collapse of the lung and displacing the mediastinum to the opposite side (tension pneumothorax). This is a very serious condition and threatens life. If, after trauma to the chest, the patient is in respiratory distress with the intercostal spaces bulging on one side of the chest along with a tympanitic note, and the trachea shifted to the opposite side, a tension pneumothorax is present. This condition is readily apparent on clinical examination and one should not wait for x-ray confirmation. The best immediate treatment consists of water-seal drainage. A needle inserted through the chest wall will confirm the diagnosis but is useless therapeutically. A scalpel incision will relieve tension and restore both ventilation and venous return; an intercostal drain can then be inserted with aseptic precautions.

Surgical emphysema. If the parietal pleura is damaged air may leak into the subcutaneous tissues and cause surgical emphysema. If this air is leaking from a peripheral part of the lung it soon becomes absorbed, and is not of much consequence. On the other hand, if a major bronchus has been ruptured, the air leaks under considerable pressure. The emphysema may spread to the whole trunk and neck, and produce asphyxia by compression of the trachea. In such cases tracheostomy helps, by acting as a safety valve and relieving the pressure in the major bronchi. If the benefit produced by tracheostomy is not sufficient, thoracotomy and repair of the bronchus has to be carried out.

Contusion and laceration of the lung. In most cases of moderate and severe chest trauma the lung is injured. Contusion produces consolidation, but usually resolves spontaneously. Laceration permits the leakage of blood and air into the pleural cavity. Major lacerations produce persistent collapse of the lung and leakage of air, and should be repaired at thoracotomy. The damaged lung often becomes secondarily infected. This can be prevented by chemotherapy, bronchial aspiration and physiotherapy.

Examination. The damage must be carefully assessed. The chest wall is examined for paradoxical movement (multiple rib fractures), depression (stove-in chest), or sucking wounds. The position of the trachea and apex beat, along with a tympanitic or dull note over the affected lung, may indicate the presence of a pneumothorax, a haemothorax or massive collapse of the lung. An immediate chest x-ray is essential for accurate diagnosis.

TREATMENT OF CHEST INJURIES

Advances in transportation have provided an opportunity to sustain life in patients who previously would have died. In the advanced countries helicopter retrieval with resuscitation en route by positive pressure ventilation, ex-

Antibiotics. The initial choice of antibiotic has to be made without microbiological guidance; this may be revised on the basis of the clinical response and subsequent laboratory identification. Ampicillin or cefuroxime eliminate the more common organisms and can be combined with metronidazole if infection by anaerobes is suspected. If a staphylococcal infection seems likely, flucoxacillin is an appropriate choice. Antibiotics penetrate the pleural space well and intrapleural instillation is unnecessary. 14 days of treatment is usually adequate, provided the patient has shown a good clinical response and there is no reaccumulation of fluid.

Drainage. *Aspiration* through a wide bore needle should be carried out on alternate days for two to three weeks, and will usually be found to be sufficient.

Intercostal drainage. If aspirations fail to dry up the empyema a large intercostal tube connected to a waterseal bottle should be introduced. This is because the pus has by now become thick and will not flow out through the needle. Positioning of the tube is important, and ultrasound or fluoroscopy are helpful in deciding upon the correct site for insertion, which is *just above the lower limit of the cavity.* Drainage should be continued until the empyema cavity is completely obliterated, which may take up to two months. The tube can be removed once drainage has ceased. If loculations are lysed with streptokinase and debris evacuated from the cavity employing a thoracoscope, the chances of success of the treatment are considerably increased.

Rib resection. In the pre-antibiotic era if intercostal drainage failed the ribs were crowded together due to fibrosis. There was so little space between the ribs that it was impossible to pass a fair-sized tube between them. A short segment of a rib was therefore resected and a stout tube inserted through its bed for free drainage of the thick pus. With earlier diagnosis and better control of infection with the help of antibiotics today, this operation is less often required.

Decortication. Occasionally the sinus refuses to heal. This may be due to underlying lung disease or osteomyelitis of a rib. It may also be due to improper treatment, e.g. incorrect drainage site, premature tube withdrawal, or a retained drainage tube. Finally, the pus may be viscid and loculated collections may prove difficult to drain. In such a case surgical intervention with decortication may be necessary. At thoracotomy the empyema is completely removed with its fibrous tissue walls, leaving the lung and chest wall free to expand. The operation is followed by a rapid convalescence with excellent functional results. It is specially useful for cases where the cause lies in the lungs, e.g. lung abscess, bronchiectasis or carcinoma, because the underlying pathology can be dealt with at the same time. However, it is a major surgical undertaking, and may be contraindicated in the frail and elderly.

DISEASES OF THE BRONCHI

Foreign bodies. Foreign bodies are inhaled quite commonly into the tracheobronchial tree, specially in children. The most common foreign bodies are teeth, bones, peanuts, pins, screws, etc. The changes produced depend upon the size and nature of the foreign body. Small, smooth metallic objects produce little reaction. Larger objects may obstruct a bronchus partially or completely, more commonly on the right side because of the more vertical position of the right bronchus. Organic foreign bodies undergo fermentation or putrefaction, and produce marked inflammatory changes in the bronchial walls.

The initial *symptom* is usually of an irritating cough. If the major bronchus of a lobe is blocked, collapse of that lobe may be followed by suppuration, with symptoms of cough, sputum and fever. If the obstruction is valvular an obstructive emphysema develops on the affected side. There may be no symptoms at all except for a unilateral wheeze, which may lead to an inappropriate diagnosis of asthma and delay the correct diagnosis. Chest x-ray may show up the foreign body if it is radiopaque. It may also show the collapse or emphysema produced by the foreign body.

Treatment. If the patient presents promptly, immediate bronchoscopy should be carried out before oedema of the bronchial wall has developed, and the foreign body should be extracted using a suitable forceps. If removal proves impossible, thoracotomy and bronchotomy will be required. If the foreign body has been present for a long time and has produced bronchiectasis a lobectomy will be necessary.

Bronchiectasis. Bronchiectasis is a condition in which the bronchi are dilated and infected. The lung parenchyma is also often fibrotic. It may arise due to intrinsic or extrinsic bronchial occlusion:

1. *Intrinsic bronchial occlusion* is uncommon. It can occur from an inhaled foreign body or a benign bronchial tumour causing distal obstruction.
2. *Extrinsic bronchial compression* is much the more common cause of bronchiectasis. It occurs in childhood when the hilar lymph nodes enlarge due to measles, whooping cough or primary tuberculosis, and compress a bronchus. Due to control of these diseases in the advanced countries, bronchiectasis has become quite rare in those areas. With increasingly widespread immunization against these childhood infections in the developing countries, it is expected to become less common there as well.

Apart from bronchial occlusion, the condition can arise due to an immune deficit, or to abnormalities in the cilia as in cystic fibrosis.

Pathology. The bronchi are thickened and irregular. Microscopically the normal elements of the bronchial wall are extensively destroyed, the remnants being infiltrated with inflammatory cells. The lung supplied by the affected bronchi may be fibrotic and airless with loss of alveoli, and infiltrated with inflammatory cells.

Clinical features. Symptoms usually begin in childhood with cough and purulent, sometimes blood-stained sputum, and with episodes of fever. A dry form of bronchiectasis also occurs, with repeated haemoptysis. Clubbing of the fingers is common.

Diagnosis. Diagnosis is established by bronchography. The lower lobes, right middle lobe and left lingular segment are most often involved. Bronchoscopy is carried out to exclude the presence of a foreign body or tumour.

Treatment. For *prevention* of bronchiectasis the respiratory complications of measles and whooping cough should be treated with antibiotics, and if collapse occurs bronchoscopy should be carried out promptly.

In severe bronchiectasis major problems result from: the constant discomfort, excessive sputum and bad breath necessitating jobs which avoid personal contact; repeated time off school or work interfering with education and employment opportunities; limitations of sporting and social activities; and an adverse effect on marital prospects. Depression is common.

Medical treatment. In cases of moderate severity the patient can keep the disease under control by postural drainage twice a day, with prophylactic antibiotics during exacerbations of infection. During postural drainage the patient is placed in such a position that the affected lobe is at a higher level than the draining bronchus, so that pus drains from the lobe to the bronchus and out.

Surgical treatment. Most patients today prefer surgical treatment. The main prerequisite for operation is that the disease be well localized and not scattered throughout both lungs. Depending on the extent of the disease the operation chosen may be lobectomy or segmental resection. Careful preoperative preparation is essential, including intensive physiotherapy, postural drainage and antibiotic therapy. The results of resection for bronchiectasis are good, and the patient's symptoms are usually greatly relieved.

TUMOURS OF THE LUNG

BENIGN TUMOURS

These are rare, and account for only 2% of all tumours of the lung. The only type which is seen with a certain regularity is *bronchial adenoma.* It projects into the lumen of the bronchus as a smooth or lobulated mass of red colour, which can be seen at bronchoscopy. As far as symptoms are concerned there may be none. However, the common modes of presentation are either with recurrent haemoptysis, or with symptoms due to bronchial obstruction and the resultant lung infection. In some cases of lung abscess or empyema the cause is a bronchial adenoma, but the tumour is quite unsuspected until bronchoscopy is carried out. Treatment is by surgical resection, and the risk of recurrence is very small.

CARCINOMA OF THE LUNG

At the beginning of this century carcinoma of the lung was an obscure and rare lesion; it has now become one of the leading causes of death from cancer. Smoke, in one form or the other, is responsible for this increased incidence. The most important part in this increase has been played by the widespread habit of *cigarette smoking.* Apart from active smoking, *passive smoking*, i.e. inhaling the smoke-filled air exhaled by a smoker, has been shown to increase the risk of lung cancer. Similarly, the *exhaust fumes* from hundreds of thousands of motor vehicles are increasing the risk for city dwellers. Finally, *asbestosis* has also been shown to be a risk factor. The condition is ten times more common in men than women, and is seen most often during the fifth and sixth decades of life.

Pathology. Tumours of the lung are classified as follows:

Malignant epithelial tumours.
A. Small cell carcinoma.
B. Non-small cell carcinoma:
i. Squamous cell carcinoma.
ii. Adenocarcinoma.

Small cell carcinoma (25%). This tumour, also called oat cell carcinoma, is the most rapidly progressive form of malignant epithelial tumour of the lung. It produces a wide variety of peptide hormones, including those involved in paraneoplastic syndromes (e.g. ACTH, ADH, serotonin, calcitonin). It is composed of small round cells with scanty cytoplasm. Small cell carcinomas occur most commonly in middle-aged and elderly people. They present symptoms at an early stage because of their rapid growth, tendency for early metastases and ectopic hormone production. Cough, weight loss, chest pain and haemoptysis are the most common symptoms of these lesions, which present as large, non-cavitating hilar masses with extensive nodal or mediastinal metastases in most cases. Symptoms indicating infiltration of neighbouring structures, e.g. dysphagia, hoarseness or superior vena cava syndrome, are more common in these tumours than in non-small cell lung cancers.

These tumours should be *staged* employing the TNM system of staging. Although 85% are stage III or IV at presentation, for patients in stage I surgical resection and postoperative adjuvant chemotherapy offers a better prognosis than non-surgical therapy. The mean *survival* time for untreated cases is only 3 months. For most patients with nodal metastases or extensive disease, combination chemotherapy is the mainstay of treatment, 80% cases showing a response (50% show a complete response). The mean survival is around 10 months; 15% survive disease-free beyond 2 years.

Radiation as primary treatment does not compare with combination chemotherapy. However, it provides excellent palliation of metastatic symptoms, particularly for brain metastases. *Surgery* as primary treatment should be reserved for stage I cases. When adjuvant polychemotherapy is added, survival is as much as 55% at 5 years.

Non-small cell carcinoma. *Squamous cell carcinoma* (40%). Microscopically these tumours show one or more of the following signs of differentiation: keratinization, pearl formation and intercellular bridges. About half the cases produce carcinoembryonic antigen (CEA) which is useful for postoperative surveillance.

These tumours arise in older patients, with a peak around 70 years, 75% being found in the larger bronchi. Cavitation is a common finding. Most cases present with cough, haemoptysis, obstructive pneumonitis or positive sputum cytology. Because of their central location about half the cases are detected by sputum cytology or endoscopic biopsy.

The primary treatment of these tumours is surgical. The prognosis depends upon the grade and stage of the tumour. For patients undergoing resection in the pre-clinical phase the survival rate exceeds 80%. Overall survival is about 7% better stage-for-stage than with other lung cancers. Because of the excellent survival rate second primary lung cancers are sometimes seen in these patients; the second cancer is not necessarily a squamous type. For symptomatic metastases radiotherapy is used most commonly.

Adenocarcinoma (30%). These tumours typically arise from the epithelium of the distal bronchi or bronchioles, and range from well-differentiated to poorly-differentiated types. Most cases present incidentally as solitary, non-cavitating nodules on chest x-rays in asymptomatic patients. The only curative therapy is surgical resection. The overall prognosis is not as favourable as in squamous cell carcinoma.

Spread of the tumour occurs directly, by the lymphatics, and through the blood stream:

1. *Direct spread* takes place to the mediastinum, pleura, chest wall and myocardium.
2. Through the *lymphatics* the tumour spreads to the hilar, subcarinal, paratracheal and finally inferior deep cervical lymph nodes. These last-named nodes can be palpated deep to the sternomastoid muscle, and can be removed for microscopy *(scalene node biopsy).*
3. Through the *blood stream* spread occurs to the liver, brain, bones etc.

Clinical features. The important symptoms are cough, sputum, haemoptysis, dyspnoea, pain and wheezing. Any of these symptoms appearing for the first time in a middle-aged person and becoming more severe with time demands early investigation. Partial obstruction of the bronchus may produce symptoms of obstructive emphysema; complete obstruction produces collapse of a lobe. In the collapsed lobe consolidation or abscess formation can occur, with fever and purulent sputum.

If early diagnosis has been missed and the case is already at an *advanced* stage, the initial symptoms may be due to infiltration of the neighbouring structures, e.g. the oesophagus (dysphagia), trachea (dyspnoea or stridor), recurrent laryngeal nerve (hoarseness), or superior vena cava. In some cases non-specific symptoms, e.g. malaise, anorexia or weight loss may direct attention towards the patient's tumour. A few bronchogenic tumours produce *hormones,* with resulting symptoms due to excess of those hormones:

1. A squamous cell carcinoma may produce excess of *parathormone* and cause symptoms of hypercalcaemia, including mental confusion.
2. An oat cell carcinoma may produce ectopic *adrenocorticotrophic hormone* which results in a Cushing-like syndrome.
3. An anaplastic small-cell carcinoma may produce *antidiuretic hormone* and result in water-intoxication with cerebral symptoms.
4. Some tumours produce a defect in neuromuscular coordination, with a myasthenia-like syndrome.

Investigations. ***Chest x-ray.*** The first investigation to be carried out for a lung carcinoma is a chest x-ray. The tumour may give rise to a hilar or peripheral shadow. At the same time obstruction of a bronchus may be responsible for the x-ray appearances of obstructive emphysema, collapse or consolidation.

Bronchoscopy is the next essential diagnostic procedure. A centrally placed tumour can be seen through a bronchoscope, and is biopsied. If a vocal cord is paralysed it means the recurrent laryngeal nerve is infiltrated and the case is inoperable. Again, if the tumour has involved the trachea or a main bronchus at its origin, or if the carina is widened due to underlying involved lymph nodes, this also signifies inoperability. It should be remembered that bronchoscopy does not show up peripherally placed tumours or those in the upper lobe segments. Fibreoptic bronchoscopy remedies some of this deficiency by reaching down to fifth level bronchi.

Other investigations. *Cytological examination* of the sputum reveals malignant cells in a good number of patients. In the case of a peripheral tumour *needle biopsy* under x-ray control may provide a histological diagnosis. An indentation of the *barium swallow* may point to extension of the growth into the mediastinum or enlargement of the mediastinal lymph nodes. *Tomography* may demonstrate enlarged mediastinal nodes, but is used less often since the advent of CT scans. *Liver, bone and brain scanning* may be required if metastases to these organs are suspected. A CT scan indicates the density of a nodule and can thus differentiate inflammatory from neoplastic lesions. At the same time, whole body CT scanning may be employed for the detection of distant metastases. *Supraclavicular node biopsy* is carried out if these nodes are enlarged. *Mediastinoscopy* is carried out at some centres to biopsy paratracheal lymph nodes, which if enlarged contraindicate operation.

Treatment. ***Surgery.*** Surgical removal of the tumour offers the best chance of cure. The aim of operative treatment is to remove the primary tumour and the regional lymph nodes adequately, but to preserve as much lung tissue as possible. For tumour confined to one lobe, *lobectomy* is a better operation than *pneumonectomy* because, although it is as effective in curing the patient as pneumonectomy, it carries a lower operative mortality rate. However, some patients require a pneumonectomy because of the position of the growth and the extent of lymph node involvement. In all cases the paratracheal, subcarinal and para-aortic lymph nodes are removed. If the chest wall, diaphragm or pericardium are invaded they can be resected with the growth. In an elderly patient a localized peripheral tumour may be treated by segmental resection. The mortality rate of pneumonectomy is about 4% and that of lobectomy 2%.

Radiotherapy. Although surgery is the treatment of choice, in about half the patients preoperative investigations show that the case is inoperable, so that only the other half undergo thoracotomy. Even of these, a resection for potential cure is possible in only half the number, i.e. in only 25% of the original number presenting with lung cancer. Therefore the majority, i.e. nearly 75%, are treated by irradiation. Great advances have been made in both the equipment and the technique available for radiotherapy, and have resulted in improved survival. However, the outlook is still not very bright. Even using the maximum possible radiation dose of 5,000 to 7,000 rads, only 62% survive for 1 year, only 14% for 3 years, and only 6% for 5 years.

Patients selected for *primary* radiation include:

1. Inoperable cases.
2. Recurrent carcinoma after previous surgical excision.

3. Patients in whom operation is contraindicated for medical reasons.

4. Patients who refuse surgery.

Postoperative radiation has not given significant benefit in the past. However, recently it has been shown that if the risk of recurrence after surgical treatment is high, postoperative radiotherapy is beneficial.

Palliative radiotherapy can significantly improve the quality of life in patients with haemoptysis, chest pain and paroxysmal coughing. In addition, patients with the superior vena cava syndrome, as well as those with bone and brain metastases, can get good palliation.

Chemotherapy. In squamous cell carcinoma the results of chemotherapy are not impressive. However, in small cell carcinoma of the lung aggressive chemotherapy is the treatment of choice. The combination of chemotherapy and radiation further improves the results.

Laser therapy. In patients with inoperable lesions the YAG laser can help arrest serious haemorrhage from the tumour in the bronchus, and can also relieve bronchial obstruction due to the neoplasm.

Prognosis. In untreated patients a 95% mortality is seen within 1 year. As far as the treated patients are concerned: of each 100 patients with carcinoma of the lung, half are found to be inoperable from the outset. Of the 50% in whom exploratory thoracotomy is performed, half (or 25% of the original group) are found to have such extensive disease that an operation for cure cannot be performed. Thus, only the remaining 25% are candidates for curative resection. Of this group, only about 30% are alive at the end of 5 years. This means that for the series as a whole the 5 year survival rate is only about 10%. The major factor that influences survival is the extent of the tumour at the time of the operation. When metastases to lymph nodes occur, the chances of survival are significantly reduced. The cell type bears little relationship to survival, except for the poor prognosis associated with small cell carcinoma.

LUNG ABSCESS

Aetiology. A lung abscess is a localized area of suppuration and cavitation in the lung. Lung abscesses may be secondary to tuberculosis, bronchiectasis, hydatid cyst or cavitation of a tumour. *However, the majority of lung abscesses occur due to aspiration of infected material into the lung.* Such material can come from infected teeth, tonsils or sinuses. Aspiration usually takes place when the cough reflex is abolished during sleep, anaesthesia or alcoholism. As the patient is usually in the supine position, the most direct route for the airway embolus to travel is via the right main bronchus into the posterior segment of the upper lobe or the apical segment of the lower lobe. Therefore these segments are most often the seat of a lung abscess. In achalasia of the cardia and stricture of the oesophagus regurgitation and aspiration of oesophageal contents can occur. Therefore these conditions can also be followed by the development of a lung abscess.

Pathology. The septic airway embolus produces an area of severe pneumonitis. The most common organisms responsible are anaerobic bacteria, streptococci, staphylococci, and *E. coli.* As the liquefied necrotic material empties through the bronchus a cavity containing pus and air is formed.

Clinical features. There is usually cough, foul-smelling sputum, fever, pleuritic chest pain, weight loss and night sweats.

Further course. Because effective broad-spectrum antibiotics are nowadays available, lung abscesses can often be aborted in the stage of pneumonitis; therefore the incidence of this type of abscess is on the decline.

Patients in whom the *normal defence mechanisms are lacking* present much more difficult clinical problems. Examples of such patients include those at the extremes of life with serious associated diseases like prematurity, malignancy, etc. In such a patient a lung abscess may occur as a complication of a blood dyscrasia, or the prolonged use of corticosteroids, immunosuppressive therapy or radiotherapy. Such conditions often give rise to multiple abscesses, and the majority of these infections are acquired in the hospital.

Because of the urgent need to identify such abscesses in the very sick patient, invasive means for obtaining secretions may sometimes be justified. Recently, *protected brush catheters* have been introduced, which are used through a fibreoptic bronchoscope for obtaining the exudate for culture.

Complications. 1. The disease may *spread* to other parts of the lung by direct extension or bronchial embolism.

2. Persistent fever and pain may be due to the development of an *empyema.*

3. Pyaemic emboli may reach the brain to produce a *cerebral abscess,* which may present with symptoms of fever, headache or convulsions.

4. Occasionally, severe *secondary haemorrhage* may occur and present as haemoptysis.

Diagnosis. The diagnosis is confirmed by chest x-ray which shows a cavity, usually in the apex of the upper or lower lobe. Further investigations include bronchoscopy to exclude a foreign body or tumour, bacteriological examination of the sputum, and examination of the teeth and respiratory tract. The conditions which have to be excluded include tumour, tuberculosis, hydatid cyst, etc.

Treatment. *Medical.* Most lung abscesses resolve on medical treatment, which consists of antibiotics and postural drainage. Antibiotics must be used in high doses and for many weeks, i.e. 4 to 6 weeks. Penicillin G has been the antibiotic of choice, but in foul-smelling lung abscesses, which are due to anaerobes, clindamycin is preferable. When the results of bacteriological examination are received the antibiotic may have to be changed. Postural drainage should be carried out twice a day. Recently, transbronchial drainage by catheterizing the appropriate bronchus under fluoroscopic control has been helpful.

Surgical. Surgery may be required for the following:

1. Massive haemoptysis.
2. Lack of response to antibiotics.
3. A cavity that is thick-walled or large.
4. A suspected malignant lesion.
5. An empyema.

In most cases the lobe containing the abscess is removed i.e. a lobectomy is carried out.

HYDATID DISEASE OF THE LUNG

Pathology. Hydatid disease (echinococcosis) is a parasitic infestation of dogs and sheep, due to the tapeworm *Echinococcus granulosus,* which is transmissible to man. It is uncommon in the advanced countries; it used to be common in sheep-rearing countries like Australia, but has been nearly eliminated by control of dogs and hygienic slaughtering of sheep. However, it is still seen in some parts of the world, specially in certain parts of the Middle East. The adult form of the parasite resides in the intestines of dogs, and eggs are discharged in the faeces. Sheep and man get the infection by swallowing these eggs. The larval form develops into a hydatid cyst in the liver, lungs and various other organs of these animals. The cycle is completed when a dog eats a sheep's liver and ingests the larvae, which develop into adults in the dog's intestine.

Presentation. A lung hydatid may present as follows:

1. On chest x-ray examination carried out for some other condition, as an incidental finding.
2. With dyspnoea or pain in the chest due to the presence of a large cyst.
3. With haemoptysis due to ulceration into a bronchus.
4. With coughing up of watery fluid and *grape skins* due to rupture into the bronchial tree. Anaphylactic shock and urticaria may occur.
5. With cough, sputum and fever due to secondary infection of the cyst.

X-ray. Radiography is usually helpful:

1. A hydatid cyst produces a spherical, sharply defined homogenous opacity.
2. If the cyst opens into a bronchus a crescentic cap of air may overlie the top of the cyst.
3. Rupture of the cyst admits air into it. The laminated membrane collapses and floats on the fluid (*water-lily* appearance).
4. The development of infection, collapse or pleural effusion may modify the x-ray appearance.

Diagnosis. The Casoni intradermal test gives a positive result in 75% of cases. A complement fixation test is more specific. An eosinophilia of over 4% suggests the condition.

Treatment. Treatment consists of removal of the cyst in all cases, due to the great risk of serious or fatal complications. Uncomplicated cysts should be enucleated without rupturing them, as otherwise spillage of scoleces leads to the near-certainty of recurrence. Infected cysts should be treated by lobectomy.

SURGICAL TREATMENT OF PULMONARY TUBERCULOSIS

The treatment of pulmonary tuberculosis is medical, by the use of specific antituberculosis drugs for 6 to 9 months, and most cases are cured by such treatment. Surgical treatment is only rarely required, for dealing with residual lesions which persist after a full course of medical treatment. Resection is the treatment of choice, and is carried out in the following situations:

1. When a lobe has been totally destroyed.
2. If tuberculous bronchiectasis has developed.
3. In a large tuberculoma where an empyema is present as well.

Thoracoplasty. Before the advent of antituberculosis drugs, surgeons tried to avoid operating upon infected lungs. Therefore very few lobectomies were carried out. Instead, an operation was devised by which a tuberculous cavity was allowed to collapse upon itself and close up. In this procedure the ribs overlying a cavity were removed subperiosteally. The chest wall was then pressed down into the cavity, in order to allow its walls to come together and heal. The operation was called a thoracoplasty. The idea was to avoid having to operate upon tuberculous tissues, because this could lead to dissemination of the disease.

Lobectomy. With the control of the tubercular infective process by drugs, there is no longer the same reluctance to operate upon tuberculous lungs, and therefore when operation is carried out these days, lobectomy is commonly employed. Thoracoplasty is carried out less often.

POSTOPERATIVE PULMONARY COMPLICATIONS

After major operations many different types of pulmonary complications can arise and cause serious morbidity and sometimes mortality. However, they can be prevented by good preoperative and postoperative care.

Predisposing factors. 1. ***The patient.*** i. Complications are more frequent in the very young and the very old.

ii. Chronic *bronchitis* is an important predisposing condition. Many more smokers develop such complications than non-smokers, due to the bronchitis from which they suffer.

2. ***The operation.*** i. Operations on the *upper abdomen* and the respiratory tract are more prone to be followed by such complications, due to the fact that pain in the wound discourages deep breathing and effective coughing, so that secretions get retained in the lungs and become infected.

ii. Operations on *septic* conditions are also followed by a higher incidence of pulmonary complications.

iii. During *anaesthesia* trauma to the tracheo-bronchial tree can increase the incidence of pulmonary complications.

iv. Similarly, prolonged *unconsciousness* after anaesthesia is undesirable.

3. ***The postoperative period.*** i. Postoperative *pain* restricts coughing and deep breathing and allows retention of secretions.

ii. *Lack of mobility* in bed results in a sluggish venous circulation, and *dehydration* increases the viscosity of the blood. Both these factors predispose to venous stasis and thrombosis.

iii. Operations on the *gastrointestinal tract* are followed by a temporary paralysis of the intestines (paralytic ileus). During this period secretions accumulate in the gut. The resulting abdominal distension pushes the diaphragm upwards, compressing the lower lobes of the lungs. Thus secretions can be retained in the lower pulmonary segments and become infected, resulting in hypostatic pneumonia.

Complications. The complications which may arise are the following, although they may merge into one another:

1. ***Bronchitis.*** This is the most common, and it often leads to the more serious complications. It may be the exacerbation of a pre-existing bronchitis. The x-ray shows no changes.

2. ***Aspiration pneumonia.*** This usually follows from the above. It takes the form of a bronchopneumonia. There is patchy consolidation with marked systemic effects. The common organisms are *Haemophilus influenzae* and pneumococcus, but hospital organisms like drug-resistant staphylococci and *Pseudomonas pyocyaneus* may also be present. Their presence should be looked for by microscopy and culture of the sputum. Bronchial breathing may be heard over some areas. X-rays show patchy mottling.

3. ***Collapse*** (atelectasis). This also is a sequel to bronchitis, being produced by occlusion of a bronchus by the thick mucus or pus. The air in the lobe or segment gets absorbed, producing collapse. The important factors predisposing to the development of collapse are reduced ventilation and a depressed cough reflex:

i. *Poor ventilation* results from the following:

(a) *Obesity* or a *distended abdomen,* which compresses the lower parts of the lungs and prevents their full expansion.

(b) *Pain*, due to which the patient tends to avoid taking a deep breath, as this causes more pain.

ii. *The cough reflex* becomes depressed either due to excessive sedation or during sleep. *Collapse usually occurs during the night, after heavy sedation.* Secretions accumulate during sleep, and by the time the patient wakes up and can cough they have blocked the bronchus. The patient feels unwell with some fever and dyspnoea. Physical signs on the affected side consist of restricted chest movements, diminished breath sounds and impaired percussion note over the affected lobe. X-ray shows the dense opacity of the collapsed lobe. A diagnostic feature of the opacity is that its margin is concave, and not straight as in the case of a consolidated lobe.

4. ***Lung abscess.*** If bronchopneumonia or collapse does not resolve promptly it may lead to the development of a lung abscess. This is a serious complication, as the organisms are by now resistant to all antibiotics.

5. ***Empyema.*** This may occasionally follow any of the above conditions, and is treated on the usual lines.

Treatment. ***Prevention.*** *Before the operation* smoking should be discontinued, pre-existing bronchitis treated, and the patient given instructions regarding breathing exercises and coughing.

During the operation such anaesthetics should be used which allow early return of consciousness and cough reflex.

After the operation the patient should be persuaded to cough, take deep breaths, roll over from side to side and move his legs. The patient usually tries to avoid coughing, as this causes pain. If a complication arises, it should be treated energetically. *Coughing* up of sputum should be encouraged by every possible method. *Steam* inhalations and non-sedating saline *expectorants* help loosen up the sputum.

Physiotherapy. The help of the physiotherapist may be obtained, for instructing the patient in coughing and breathing exercises, and in postural drainage. However, the attending medical staff should train themselves, or get trained in, chest physiotherapy, instead of relying entirely on the services of the physiotherapy department.

Management. *Bronchoscopy.* If the simpler methods are not effective bronchoscopy should be performed. If this is carried out with a rigid bronchoscope, thick mucus can be sucked out more easily because this kind of instrument has a wide lumen. The procedure should be carried out under local anaesthesia so as not to abolish the cough reflex. If mucus can be efficiently sucked out, bronchoscopy may bring about aeration of a collapsed lobe.

Tracheostomy. If bronchoscopy fails in its objective or repeated bronchoscopies are required, it may be preferable to carry out a tracheostomy, specially if the secretions are very profuse and the patient is breathless. Tracheostomy abolishes the dead space and greatly improves the efficiency of ventilation. At the same time it provides an easy route for repeated aspiration of the tracheobronchial tree. If tracheostomy is carried out the air in the room must be humidified. Otherwise the dry air entering directly into the trachea without the benefit of humidification in the nose and pharynx causes crust formation, and can result in damage to the respiratory epithelium. A 'Swedish nose' has become available recently for the purpose of humidification of the inspired air in cases with a tracheostomy. It consists of a large-bore T-shaped tube containing cotton-wool gauze in its lumen. The tube is attached to the outer end of the tracheostomy tube. The gauze traps the moisture in the expired air, thus producing the same kind of humid tunnel that is normally provided by the nasal passages. The use of this implement has greatly simplified the care of patients with tracheostomies.

PULMONARY EMBOLISM

As many as 2% of all hospital deaths have been found on postmortem examination to occur from pulmonary embolism. The embolus commonly arises from the veins of the calves, thighs or pelvis. Virchow's research during the last century into the pathogenesis of pulmonary embolism is a classic. He found that patients with pulmonary embolism often also had thrombi in the veins of the legs and pelvis; *further, that these thrombi were of the same histological age as those found in the lungs.* When thrombi were injected into the femoral veins of animals they lodged in the lungs. He concluded that thrombi formed in the systemic veins and that thrombosis was caused primarily by three factors: reduced blood flow in the veins, injury to the veins, and a state of hypercoagulability. These factors remain important in the pathogenesis of pulmonary embolism even today, and are known as *Virchow's triad.*

The lesion in the vein may be one of two kinds, thrombophlebitis and phlebothrombosis.

Thrombophlebitis. The thrombosis is secondary to infection, or rarely to trauma. There is a marked inflammatory reaction; the resulting thrombus is firmly adherent to the wall of the vein so that it is rarely dislodged, and embolism is uncommon.

Phlebothrombosis. Clotting takes place due to stasis in the veins, there being no inflammatory reaction in the wall of the vein. The result is that the clot is not firmly attached to the vein wall, and gets easily detached to become an embolus. For this reason phlebothrombosis is much more dangerous than thrombophlebitis.

Clinical features. Pulmonary embolism is the most dangerous, in fact potentially lethal, complication of phlebothrombosis. If a thrombus gets dislodged, a great deal depends upon the size of the embolus.

A *small* embolus may be silent. However, such repeated emboli can result in pulmonary hypertension by blocking the pulmonary vasculature. A *medium-sized* embolus usually gets lodged in one of the branches of the pulmonary artery. It produces pulmonary infarction without any haemodynamic disturbances. The symptoms include pain in the chest, dyspnoea and haemoptysis. There may or may not be tenderness over the calf. Chest x-rays may reveal a triangular infarcted segment. A *large* embolus lodges in the main pulmonary artery or one of the its main branches. It nearly blocks the circulation and can be fatal. If the patient survives, he complains of severe pain and tightness in the chest and marked dyspnoea. The patient is grey and cold, with a rapid feeble pulse, a very low blood pressure, and a raised venous pressure. He can die of this condition. However, the longer he survives the better his chances of recovery.

Diagnosis. The differential diagnosis includes oesophageal perforation, pneumonia, septic shock and myocardial infarction. The diagnosis of pulmonary embolism is mainly by exclusion. On *ECG,* the most common findings associated with pulmonary embolism are nonspecific ST and T wave changes; more specific signs of right ventricular overload are rarely seen. Therefore, the main value of the ECG is to exclude the presence of a myocardial infarction. Changes on *chest x-ray* are similarly non-specific: central venous enlargement and asymmetry of vascular markings. The chest x-ray therefore mainly serves to exclude pneumonia, pneumothorax, oesophageal perforation or congestive heart failure.

Arterial blood gases show hypoxaemia and hypocarbia. The hypoxaemia results in hyperventilation which washes out the carbon dioxide to produce hypocarbia. A low *central venous pressure* virtually excludes pulmonary embolism as the primary cause of hypotension. A normal *lung scan* usually excludes the diagnosis of pulmonary embolism. Finally, *pulmonary arteriography* is the most accurate method of confirming the presence, size and distribution of pulmonary emboli.

Management. *Anticoagulation.* Minor degrees of embolism can usually be managed by anticoagulation alone. Heparin is given intravenously at an initial dose of 5000 to 10000 units followed by constant infusion at a rate sufficient to raise the activated partial thromboplastin time to 1.5 to 2 times the control value, usually 1000 units per hour. The duration of heparin therapy varies, but 5 to 10 days is appropriate, as this is the time required for thrombi to become adherent to the vein wall. An oral anticoagulant is started at the same time.

Thrombolytic therapy has been advocated for pulmonary embolism, using the plasminogen activator streptokinase, and beneficial effects can usually be seen in 12 to 24 hours.

Vena caval filter. In some cases anticoagulants cannot be used because of associated problems, e.g. peptic ulcer, so a mechanical means of protection against recurrent embolism must be employed. A caval umbrella filter (Mobin-Uddin, Greenfield) can be inserted under local anaesthesia through the femoral or jugular vein, and gets fixed to the wall of the inferior vena cava by its hooks, preventing an embolus from proceeding upwards into the right atrium and pulmonary artery. It should be remembered that complications can arise due to migration of, or thrombosis on, the filter.

Pulmonary embolectomy. If a patient sustains a massive embolism, the response must be rapid and coordinated because survival is a matter of minutes. Heparin and inotropic drugs are pushed while diagnosis is made by pulmonary arteriography, because the clinical diagnosis is often in error. Open pulmonary embolectomy carries a mortality rate of about 50%. An alternative approach utilizes local anaesthesia for transvenous removal of emboli. A cup-shaped device attached to the tip of a steerable catheter is inserted into the femoral vein and the cup positioned under fluoroscopy adjacent to the embolus seen on arteriography. Suction is now applied through a syringe to aspirate the embolus into the cup, where it is held by suction vacuum as the catheter and captured embolus are withdrawn. A Greenfield filter may now be placed in position in the inferior vena cava to protect the patient from further emboli. The procedure is associated with an overall survival of 75%.

Prevention. Prevention of pulmonary embolism is better than cure. *Before any operation* it should be ensured that the patient is not dehydrated, otherwise he should be properly hydrated. *During operation,* specially in the case of lengthy operations on debilitated patients, the patient's heels should be raised on small pillows so that the calf muscles are not compressed against the mattress on the operation table and stasis does not develop in the calf veins. Further, the calf muscles can be stimulated by electric current every 2 to 4 seconds. *Both before and after operation* the patient should be mobilized in and out of bed as far as possible, and the lower limbs elevated 15 to 20 cm for gravity drainage of venous return, so that stasis in the veins of the legs is prevented.

Diaphragm

The important clinical conditions in respect of the diaphragm are *hernias* through it, and these may be congenital or acquired.

Congenital hernias occur at certain specific points, and are due to failure of fusion of the various elements which make up the diaphragm (Fig. 1). They have well-defined sacs and adhesions are uncommon. *Acquired* hernias are traumatic or postoperative. They can occur anywhere in the diaphragm, and extensive adhesions with the surrounding structures are common. Symptoms occur if obstruction or strangulation supervene, or if the hernia is large and produces respiratory embarrassment. Surgical repair is recommended in all cases in order to avoid serious complications.

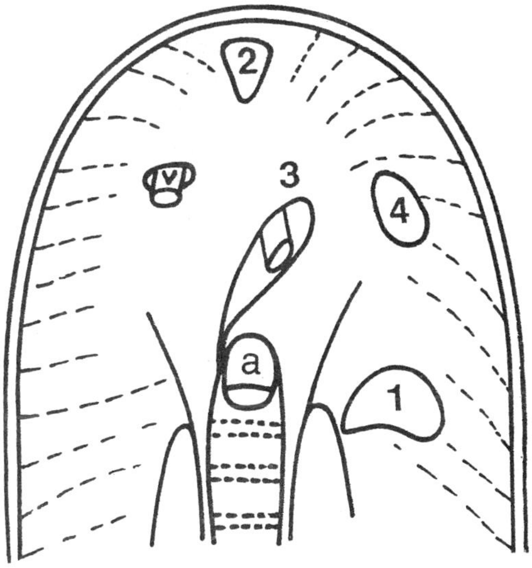

Fig. 1 Sites of diaphragmatic hernias. 1. pleuroperitoneal canal (foramen of Bochdalek) 2. foramen of Morgagni, 3. oesophageal hiatus, 4. dome of diaphragm, a common site for traumatic hernias due to crushing injuries. (a) aorta, (v) inferior vena cava.

The different types of diaphragmatic hernia include the following:

Congenital. ***Eventration.*** In this condition there is defective development of the muscle of the diaphragm, which is replaced by a sheet of fibrous tissue. As this sheet cannot contract like muscle, it gets pushed up by the intra-abdominal pressure and lies immobile. There are usually no symptoms, and the condition is discovered on routine x-ray. If respiratory embarrassment is present the sheet is plicated to strengthen and shorten it.

Hernia through the foramen of Bochdalek (pleuroperitoneal canal). During foetal life the pleural and peritoneal cavities communicate through the pleuroperitoneal canal. Normally this opening closes down. If it persists, at birth a considerable part of the intestines may be lying in the left pleural cavity (the condition is much less common on the right side due to the presence of the liver). The left lung is hypoplastic, and the heart pushed towards the right side, so that the right lung is also compressed. When the baby is born there may be severe dyspnoea, and even cyanosis. The diagnosis is suggested by the presence of bowel sounds over the left chest, and can be confirmed by a chest x-ray which shows air-filled bowel loops in the left chest displacing the heart to the opposite side.

Operation should be carried out urgently through a laparotomy. The gut loops are gently pulled back into the abdomen, and the opening in the diaphragm closed by interrupted sutures of non-absorbable material. The left lung is hypoplastic; it should be allowed to expand gradually, by the use of an intercostal tube leading to a water-seal, which produces a mild degree of negative pressure. It should be remembered that *if dyspnoea or cyanosis is present in a newborn, an immediate chest x-ray is an essential investigation.*

Recently, this congenital diaphragmatic hernia has been diagnosed antenatally by the use of ultrasonography. At the same time, successful repair of such a hernia in the foetus (through a laparotomy on the mother with hysterotomy to expose the foetus) has been achieved. This obviates the high mortality of this condition in the newborn.

Hernia through the foramen of Morgagni. This small foramen lies between the sternal and costal attachments of the diaphragm. It lies anteriorly, and therefore the most common viscus to herniate through it is the transverse colon. Sometimes a hernia through this opening may assume very large dimensions and compress the heart within the pericardium. If it can be reduced immediately and repaired the baby's life is saved.

Acquired. ***Oesophageal hiatus hernia.*** This hernia commonly occurs as an acquired condition in the middle-aged and elderly. It is discussed with the oesophagus in Chapter 19.

Traumatic diaphragmatic hernia. The diaphragm may be perforated by a stab or bullet wound, or ruptured during severe lower thoracic or abdominal compression without an external wound. The defect due to a missile injury may occur anywhere in the diaphragm; that due to a crush injury always lies in the dome. Unlike a congenital hernia a peritoneal sac is not present, and therefore the herniated viscera adhere to the lung. The common symptoms are dyspeptic and obstructive, and strangulation occasionally occurs. Repair of the hernia should always be undertaken.

Postoperative diaphragmatic hernia. After thoraco-abdominal operations the sutured diaphragm may give way resulting in a hernia. Alternatively, herniation may occur through a newly created hiatus e.g. in a colon transplant for the oesphagus. If the condition is suspected operation should be carried out early before any complications develop.

Mediastinal masses

Any lesion producing a mass in the mediastinum requires careful investigation and treatment. *The most important point in the differential diagnosis is the position of the mass in the mediastinum,* which is normally demonstrated by anteroposterior, lateral and oblique x-rays, as well as by CT scan or MRI. The common lesions are the following:

Anterior mediastinal masses
- Retrosternal Goitre.
- Thymic tumours and cysts.
- Persistent thymus.
- Teratoma.
- Pleuropericardial cyst.

Posterior mediastinal masses
- Neurogenic tumours (neurofibroma, ganglioneuroma).
- Foregut cysts.
- Oesophageal hiatus hernia with thoracic stomach.

Masses arising anywhere in the mediastinum
- Lymphadenopathies: tuberculosis, lymphomas (Hodgkin's and non-Hodgkin's), secondary carcinoma, sarcoidosis.
- Lipoma.
- Fibroma.

The majority of benign tumours require removal, in order to avoid the risk of malignant change or compression of the mediastinal structures.

Thymus

Hyperplasia of the thymus. Hyperplasia of the thymus occurs in toxic goitre, acromegaly, some cases of Addison's disease, and in myasthenia gravis. An enlarged thymus in infants may occasionally cause stridor. If the symptoms are persistent, radiotherapy or surgery may be required.

Tumours of the thymus. These tumours are not common. They may be epithelial, lymphoid or teratomatous. They occupy the anterior compartment of the superior mediastinum. Most are discovered on routine x-ray, specially on lateral films. Removal is advised in most cases because of the risk of continued growth and malignant changes.

Myasthenia gravis. In this condition the transmission of motor-nerve impulses at the neuromuscular junctions is blocked by interference with the action of the transmitter acetylcholine on the muscle fibres. The symptoms are profound fatigue after modest exertion and transient paresis of voluntary muscles. Ptosis and diplopia are followed by weakness of the voice and of mastication, dysphagia, and in some cases death from involvement of the muscles of respiration. Diagnosis is confirmed by an injection of neostigmine, which relieves the symptoms within an hour. A lateral x-ray of the superior mediastinum shows a thymic tumour in about 15% of cases.

Treatment. Oral neostigmine relieves symptoms adequately in many cases. In the more severe cases in which it fails to do so, thymectomy is advised.

40 Heart

The heart continues to beat round the clock and round the calendar throughout a person's life span. It pumps blood to the lungs and then to the body both for gas exchange and to facilitate the different processes of metabolism. If this circulation is arrested even for a few minutes life cannot go on. Hence the great importance of the heart both in health and disease.

SPECIAL INVESTIGATIVE PROCEDURES IN CARDIAC SURGERY

Before he can carry out corrective surgery the cardiac surgeon requires all the information he can get, both about the abnormal anatomy of the cardiac chambers and the disordered haemodynamics and physiology of the heart, so that he can arrive at an accurate diagnosis. The available methods of investigation include the following:

1. Plain x-ray chest and fluoroscopy. These examinations give information about the cardiac contours, and show up any chamber of the heart which is enlarged, as it changes the contour in that area.

2. Echocardiography. Ultrasound waves are directed at the heart. Wherever they come across a change of medium they are reflected back. They provide very valuable information about the thickness of the chambers, poor mobility or calcification of the different valves. After myocardial infarction the size of ventricular aneurysms can be assessed, as well as abnormalities in pupillary muscles and the presence of mural thrombi. Estimates can be obtained about muscle mass, velocity of fibre-shortening, ejection fraction, and end-diastolic and end-systolic volumes. Being non-invasive, echocardiography is a very attractive method of investigation for cardiac disorders. At the same time, the information provided by it is sometimes so detailed that it eliminates the need for cardiac catheterization and angiocardiography.

Transoesophageal electrocardiography has made it possible to obtain high quality images during anaesthesia and surgery. In awake patients high quality images of dissection of the thoracic aorta, prosthetic valve dysfunction, intracardiac thrombi and acute mitral valve regurgitation can be obtained. This technique is particularly valuable in chest trauma, where standard echocardiography is inconclusive.

3. Angiocardiography. A radiopaque chemical like Urografin is injected intravenously and numerous x-ray exposures are made at short intervals to follow the passage of the material through the various cardiac chambers and great vessels. This gives very valuable information about the size and shape of the chambers. At the same time it shows the presence of a shunt, or obstruction or incompetence of a valve. The aorta and pulmonary artery and their main branches are outlined. Coronary artery anatomy is also studied. All this is recorded on videotape.

4. Right-heart cardiac catheterization. A catheter is passed through a *vein* and through a vena cava into the right atrium. It is then passed onwards into the right ventricle and pulmonary artery. It gathers a great deal of information. Firstly, radiopaque material can be injected through it and both still and cine pictures can be taken. Secondly, the pressure inside each one of the chambers can be recorded. Thirdly, samples of blood can be taken from each one of the chambers and analyzed for their oxygen and carbon dioxide content. Finally, as far as pressures are concerned: if the catheter has a balloon at its end (*Swan Ganz catheter*) it is advanced further and wedged into a small branch of the pulmonary artery with the balloon inflated. When it is placed in this position, the opening at the tip of the catheter measures the retrograde pressure in the left atrium i.e. in the left side of the heart.

5. Left-heart cardiac catheterization. If a catheter is passed up an *artery*, through the aorta into the left ventricle, it outlines the aorta and the left heart chambers. The arteries commonly used for entry are the femorals and brachials. The coronary arteries can also be outlined, i.e. coronary angiography carried out.

6. Cardiac output measurement. The basic function of the heart is to provide blood to the tissues. Therefore, the ultimate index of function of the heart is the volume of blood pumped by it per minute i.e. the cardiac output. This is not an easy parameter to measure. It requires measurement of the arterial and venous oxygen content, and the tissue oxygen consumption. This is done with a Swan-Ganz catheter as described above under right-heart catheterization. Cardiac output measures the left ventricular function, which affects the risk of operation; therefore the preoperative measurement of cardiac output has considerable clinical significance.

BASIC TECHNIQUES IN CARDIAC SURGERY

Cardiac surgery is different from other types of surgery. The heart is different from other organs. If one wishes to operate upon the bones or the joints, the intestines or the thyroid, one has only to expose that organ and the surgical procedure can commence. The same is not true in the case of the heart.

In order for life to go on, the heart must continue to pump blood to all parts of the body. But if an operation like removal and replacement of a heart valve has to be carried out, the heart obviously has to remain motionless for a considerable period of time. How is life to continue during this period?

The function of the heart is to circulate the blood first through the lungs so that it can be oxygenated, and then through the whole body so that the oxygen can reach all organs, and CO_2 and other waste products can be removed.

The blood is also the most important agent of metabolism. As the blood circulates through all organs constantly an organ requiring an electrolyte, an amino acid, or a hormone, for example can take it up, and another organ secreting a hormone can add it to the blood.

Heart lung machines. If this function of the heart, i.e. to circulate the blood through a 'lung' and then through the body could be taken over for a certain period, for that time interval the heart could be kept motionless and operated upon, without any harmful effects on the body. The heart-lung machines, developed during the last few decades, perform precisely this function. Although different machines vary a lot in their detailed working, the principle underlying them all is the same. Each consists of a pump (the replacement for the heart) and an oxygenator (the 'lung').

Blood returning from the body is withdrawn from the venae cavae, passed through the oxygenator, and pumped into the aorta or femoral artery fully oxygenated. Thus although the blood is diverted from the heart and lungs, it is supplied to the body in a well oxygenated form. Heart-lung machines provide the surgeon with periods for intracardiac surgery of two or three hours with safety, so that even complicated anomalies, e.g. ventricular septal defects, Fallot's tetralogy, and valvular defects can be effectively treated. The temperature of the heart and the body is also reduced, to gain an added margin of safety.

Technique. Most major open cardiac operations e.g. coronary bypass, valve replacements, etc. are performed through a midline sternotomy incision. The pericardium is opened. Both venae cavae and the ascending aorta are surrounded by tapes. The patient is heparinized. A plastic cannula is passed into the aorta through a purse-string suture. Similarly each vena cava or the right atrium is cannulated. The cannulae are connected to the heart-lung machine. Thus during the whole operation the responsibility of oxygenating the blood and supplying it to the body is taken over by the heart-lung machine.

When the operation is completed the cannulae are removed and the heparin counteracted with protamine. During heart-lung bypass the efficiency of the extracorporeal circulation is constantly monitored by measuring the urinary output, and the cerebral activity by measuring the blood gases and blood pressure. Core temperature is also monitored.

Other simpler bypasses. Operations on the thoracic aorta for coarctation or aneurysms do not require a full heart-lung bypass. However, they are facilitated if blood can be taken from a site proximal to the diseased segment of the aorta and pumped into the femoral artery, so that blood supply to the kidneys, other abdominal organs, and the lower limbs is not interrupted. Such a simpler bypass can take one of the following forms:

1. *Left heart bypass.* The left atrium is cannulated and blood delivered by a pump into the femoral artery. The aorta can now be cross-clamped. The left ventricle continues to supply blood to the head and upper limbs, while the bypass keeps the circulation in the lower limbs and the abdominal viscera going.

2. *Femoro-femoral bypass.* If the left atrium is not easily accessible the femoral artery and vein are both cannulated. Blood is withdrawn from the vein and after oxygenation is pumped back into the body via the femoral artery.

Preservation of the myocardium during lengthy operations. During operations on the left heart the surgeon requires a motionless and relaxed heart for a considerable period of time. During this time interval the heart muscle needs to be protected from damage due to anoxia. This can be achieved on the one hand by providing the heart with an uninterrupted blood supply, and on the other by reducing the metabolic needs of the myocardium:

1. *Continuous blood supply.* The coronary arteries are cannulated and perfused with blood during the period of cardiac standstill.

2. *Reducing the metabolic needs of the myocardium.* This can be achieved by one or both of the following two methods:

i. *Hypothermia.* The higher the temperature of the various tissues the greater their metabolic demands. It follows that by cooling the tissues their metabolic needs can be greatly reduced, enabling them to survive short periods of total deprivation of oxygen or longer periods of partial deprivation.

When hypothermia was first used, cooling was carried down only to about 30°C. This gave the surgeon only about 10 minutes of circulatory arrest before endangering the brain, and allowed the performance of simple cardiac operations, e.g. atrial septal defects. The temperature of the tissues could not be lowered much further, because at about 25°C ventricular fibrillation usually occurred.

With the use of cardiopulmonary bypass, ventricular fibrillation is no longer a problem, because with the bypass the heart is stopped anyway. Now therefore, the body temperature can be reduced even down to 15°C, and periods of upto 45 minutes of circulatory arrest can be safely tolerated. Hypothermia is nowadays widely used in the surgery of congenital heart disease in infants.

ii. *Cardioplegic agents* are injected into the coronary arteries to keep the heart still. These drugs serve the dual purpose of providing a motionless heart to the surgeon for his operative procedure, and of reducing its metabolic needs.

Operations without a bypass *(Closed heart operations).* Operations carried out on the main vessels outside the heart or the pericardium (*extracardiac operations*) do not require a bypass. Again, a blind operation where only a finger or instrument is passed to dilate a valve (*a closed intracardiac operation*) does not require a bypass. The only closed procedure which is still employed sometimes is mitral commissurotomy. This was the first operation to be carried out on the heart, and for a decade or more was the only cardiac surgical operation performed routinely.

CONDITIONS AMENABLE TO CARDIAC SURGICAL TREATMENT

These include congenital and acquired conditions affecting the heart.

CONGENITAL HEART DISEASE

A congenital cardiac abnormality occurs about six times in every 1,000 live births. Many anomalies are quite severe, so that they are incompatible with life. Even in babies who survive beyond infancy, life expectancy is greatly reduced, so that surgical correction is desirable in nearly every case.

The anomalies are divided into those with a normal arterial oxygen saturation (*acyanotic* cases) and those with reduced saturation (*cyanotic* cases).

ACYANOTIC CONGENITAL HEART DISEASE

The conditions belonging to this group include patent ductus arteriosus, coarctation of the aorta, and atrial and ventricular septal defects.

Patent ductus arteriosus. This is a common anomaly. The ductus connects the left pulmonary artery with the aorta, and blood flows from the high-pressure aorta into the pulmonary artery. The systolic blood pressure is high and the diastolic low, producing a collapsing or water-hammer pulse. The pulmonary vessels are dilated, and on x-ray screening their pulsations are increased (*hilar dance*). The additional circulation of blood through the lungs and the left heart results in left ventricular hypertrophy.

Many cases with moderate patent ductus arteriosus remain asymtomatic until the second decade of life. Those with a large duct present with cardiac failure during the first year of life. There is dyspnoea on exertion, retardation of growth and repeated chest infections. A typical continuous machinery murmur is audible to the left of the sternum. The important complications of patent ductus arteriosus include cardiac failure and bacterial endocarditis.

Once the diagnosis is made, surgical closure of the duct is indicated. However, a moderate-sized duct sometimes closes spontaneously during the first few months. Therefore, in asymptomatic patients the operation is preferably carried out after the age of 1 year, in order to give spontaneous closure a chance.

Coarctation of the aorta. This malformation consists of a localized severe stenosis of the aortic arch, located just distal to the origin of the left subclavian artery.

Clinical features. The constriction in the aorta produces hypertension above it with headache, irritability, and throbbing and pulsations in the head and neck. Below the constriction there is hypotension, with cold legs and intermittent claudication. Due to the severe hypertension there may be left ventricular failure, intracranial haemorrhage, or even rupture of the aorta. The carotid and subclavian arteries pulsate markedly. Collateral vessels can be seen over the scapular regions. The pulses in the lower limbs are weak or absent. Very few patients survive beyond the age of forty-five, as they die of hypertension.

Diagnosis. On *x-ray* there is left ventricular enlargement, a prominent ascending aorta and notching of the ribs from the enlarged intercostal vessels. *Echocardiography* establishes the diagnosis. *Cardiac catheterization and angiography* delineate the anatomy and measure the size of the isthmus. MRI can demonstrate the precise anatomy.

Treatment. The stenosis can be excised and an end-to-end anastomosis safely performed. The mortality rate is approximately 1 percent. Therefore all children and young adults with coarctation are advised to undergo operation. Relief of symptoms normally occurs after operation.

Atrial septal defect. When the septum between the atria is defective blood flows from the left to the right atrium (L-R shunt), so that the right side of the heart and the lungs are overfilled and the left side receives less blood than usual. Symptoms due to atrial fibrillation always appear by middle age, if not earlier. They are due to overfilling of the right side of the heart and lungs. The pulmonary arteries are actively pulsatile on fluoroscopy (hilar dance), and the increased flow produces a pulmonary systolic murmur. A significant proportion of these defects close spontaneously during the first year of life. Haemodynamically important defects that persist beyond this period are electively closed at a socially convenient time, using a heart-lung bypass.

Ventricular septal defect. This is the most common of congenital cardiac anomalies. It also occurs as part of more complex anomalies *(Fallot's tetralogy and transposition)*. The defect allows the passage of blood from the left to the right ventricle so that the right heart is over-filled, with pulmonary plethora and hypertension. This is a serious lesion if the defect is large. The defect is repaired with the aid of a heart-lung bypass, using either direct suture or inserting a patch of Dacron or pericardium. The operative mortality approaches zero in centres familiar with the operation and the required postoperative care. Risk factors include young age (less than 3 months), multiple defects, and established pulmonary hypertension.

CYANOTIC CONGENITAL HEART DISEASE

In all these anomalies there is central cyanosis due to an intracardiac shunt from right to left.

Fallot's tetralogy. This is the most common of the cyanotic conditions. The pulmonary artery is narrow and there is a ventricular septal defect, so that the aorta overrides both ventricles and some deoxygenated blood passes into it. The patient is undersized with central cyanosis and finger clubbing. There is a systolic thrill and murmur in the pulmonary area. Many of the severe cases die during infancy; the less severe cases may survive into adult life. Before the invention of the heart-lung machine this condition was uniformly fatal. Blalock invented his very ingenious operation to deal with it. He anastomosed the left subclavian artery to the left pulmonary artery, to divert the extra blood in the aorta back into the pulmonary artery. This operation helped a lot, but nowadays Fallot's tetralogy can be corrected completely by using a cardiopulmonary-bypass with hypothermia.

Transposition of the great vessels. In this condition the aorta arises from the right ventricle, and the pulmonary artery from the left. The baby is severely cyanosed. In fact life is only possible because a ventricular septal defect is also present. During infancy an effort is made to increase the shunting between the left and right side of the heart by passing a balloon catheter through the foramen ovale and rupturing the atrial septum. Later, the anomaly is corrected by realigning the arteries.

41 Arteries

Diseases of arteries may take one of three forms: occlusion, dilatation or arteritis. The lumen of the artery may be *occluded* by atheroma, thrombosis, embolism, etc. The artery may be *dilated* due to degeneration of its wall. Finally, the wall of the artery may be the seat of inflammation *(arteritis).*

Arterial occlusion

Arterial occlusion may be partial (i.e. stenosis) or complete. Both types of occlusion are caused most often by atherosclerosis, the other common causes being embolism and trauma. The severity of the symptoms produced by occlusion depends upon whether alternative routes of blood flow, in the form of collaterals, are available.

CLINICAL FEATURES OF ARTERIAL OCCLUSION IN THE LOWER LIMBS

A limb with an occluded artery is usually painful, pale, paralysed and pulseless.

Pain. This may take one of two forms, intermittent claudication and rest pain.

Intermittent claudication. When the patient starts to walk there is no pain. After he has walked a few steps cramping pain appears, most often in the calf but sometimes in the thigh or buttock. If he now stands still the pain is relieved. The distance a patient can walk before pain comes on is called the *claudication distance*. This distance is inversely proportional to the severity of arterial occlusion, i.e. if the distance is short it means the degree of occlusion is severe. *Rest pain* is severe pain felt in the foot even at rest. It is usually worse at night, and is aggravated by elevating the foot.

Pallor. Ischaemic limbs look pale, specially on elevation. When the limb is lowered from the bed it becomes blue; this is due to venous congestion, and indicates sluggishness of any remaining circulation. Bright red spots may also be seen; these are due to extravasation of blood from the capillaries.

Paralysis. Ischaemic limbs are often paralysed and without sensation. These are both bad signs, and indicate a poor prognosis.

Pulselessness. If a main artery is occluded, the arterial pulsations below that level are absent. If good collaterals are present the pulses may be palpable, but are greatly diminished in volume. If a patient has symptoms of arterial disease the following arteries must be palpated for the presence of pulsation: the radials, the carotids, the abdominal aorta, the femorals, the popliteals, and the posterior tibial and dorsalis pedis arteries.

Temperature. Severely ischaemic feet are cold to the touch.

Ulcers and gangrene. In severe arterial insufficiency ulcers may form on or between the toes, or elsewhere on the feet. When gangrene sets in, the affected patch of skin becomes black and dry. If rest pain, cyanosis, oedema and hyperaesthesia are present with or without ulcers, the situation is described as *pregangrene.*

Murmurs. If an artery is narrowed, blood flowing through it produces turbulence, which results in a systolic murmur being audible over the vessel. A complete vascular examination should include auscultation of the following arteries: the subclavians, the carotids, the abdominal aorta, and the femorals. A continuous *machinery murmur* over an artery indicates the presence of an arteriovenous fistula.

Location of atheromatous plaques. Atheromatous narrowing or occlusion are commonly found at the following sites: the aortic bifurcation, the iliac arteries, the femoropopliteal segment, or the distal arteries. Double blocks result in more severe ischaemia.

INVESTIGATIONS FOR ARTERIAL OCCLUSION

Numerous tests need to be carried out on patients suffering from arterial diseases. Most patients suffering from pathological processes affecting the arteries tend to be elderly; *therefore, metabolic and age-related diseases*, e.g. diabetes, hypertension, myocardial ischaemia and bronchitis should be excluded.

Blood tests. Tests to detect abnormalities in the *blood*, e.g. hyperlipidaemia, polycythaemia, and thrombocythaemia, should be carried out, besides the ESR and white cell count.

Plain x-rays show up calcification in arteries.

Blood flow. Three basic parameters are analyzed in the study of peripheral vascular disease: pressure, volume and velocity of the blood flow.

Pressure. Normally, large arteries produce little resistance to blood flow, so that there is almost no pressure gradient between the aorta and the small arteries of the foot. Narrowing due to atheromatous plaques produces increased resistance and a pressure drop across the stenosis. This pressure drop develops even before total flow to the limb is reduced and therefore provides a very sensitive index for assessing the presence of significant arterial disease. A blood pressure cuff is applied to the calf above the ankle. As a stethoscope cannot hear the sounds, a Doppler sensor is used. The normal ankle systolic pressure is about 10 mm Hg higher than the brachial systolic pressure. Thus the *ankle: brachial index* is normally greater than 1.0, and a value below 0.9 indicates the presence of haemodynamically significant arterial disease.

Foot ulcers may be due to ischaemic or neuropathic disease. If an ischaemic aetiology is confirmed by non-invasive tests, the probability of successful healing of the lesion can also be predicted. An ulcer in a patient with an ankle pressure of 30 to 40 mm Hg is not likely to heal unless a vascular bypass can improve the perfusion pressure in the foot. Toe pressure measurements are even more accurate in predicting the probability of successful ulcer healing.

Volume. An *air-filled plethysmograph* is used to measure the changes in volume of the limb during a cardiac cycle.

Velocity. Unlike the above two methods which are indirect studies, *continuous wave Doppler* studies provide direct information about the arterial disease. An ultrasound signal is beamed at an artery. The reflected beam is picked up by a receiver. Its frequency is changed due to its passage through moving blood. The change of frequency is converted into sound, and the loudness of this sound over the concerned artery indicates the volume of blood flowing through it. The Doppler blood flow detector is a very useful instrument. To provide an objective record the signal can be converted into a waveform which is recorded on a strip chart.

Distal bypass grafts may fail for a variety of reasons. Postoperative surveillance allows the failing graft to be identified before occlusion occurs. Duplex scanning provides both B-mode imaging which defines anatomical complications of the graft, and Doppler velocity measurements which identify a low flow state before thrombosis actually occurs. A low flow state exists when the peak systolic flow velocity is less than 45 cm/second. An abnormal B-mode scan or velocity measurement should be followed up with an arteriogram to assess the graft for possible revision.

Transcutaneous oxygen tension measurement. If the oxygen tension in the tissues could be determined, this would be the best proof of the adequacy of the oxygen delivery system. Transcutaneous oxygen tension measurement provides precisely this information. An oxygen-sensing electrode is placed on the skin. The oxygen tension is measured at the foot, the calf and the thigh, with a reference electrode placed over the chest. The normal value in the lower limb is around 55 mm Hg. Values of less than 20 mm Hg are usually obtained in patients with rest pain and ischaemic ulcers. Further, comparing the value at the lower limb with that at the chest yields an index, which should normally be 0.9. The study is valuable in assessing a patient's risk of limb or tissue loss, and in differentiating ischaemic from neuropathic pain. If ischaemic pain is confirmed, the patient is at a high risk for ischaemic loss of tissue or limb, and should be evaluated for vascular bypass procedure.

Ultrasound (B-mode) images provide information about the diameters of the various vessels at different levels, and are very valuable adjuncts of velocity measurements, as explained above.

Arteriography. In this technique a radiopaque dye is injected into an artery and x-rays taken. These show the dye in the vessel and show up any stenosis, occlusion or dilatation. In most cases the dye is placed into some part of the aorta, from where it flows into the different arteries and is photographed. The catheter is introduced usually via the *femoral*, sometimes via the *brachial* arteries. Alternatively, the dye may be injected directly into the aorta by percutaneous puncture through the *translumbar* route. Besides showing up arterial disease, angiography is useful in diseases of organs supplied by the various arteries. For example, different malignant tumours have characteristic arrangements of their feeding vessels, and angiography helps in the diagnosis of such lesions by demonstrating these patterns. The procedure is not without its *complications* including thrombosis, haematoma formation and arterial dissection.

To avoid the hazards of arterial catheters, ***digital subtraction angiography*** has been developed. In this technique first a plain x-ray of the part to be examined is taken. A radiopaque dye is now injected intravenously and further radiographs taken. Using digital techniques employing a computer, the x-ray densities of the first film (due to the non-vascular shadows) are subtracted from the image containing the contrast medium. This greatly enhances the outline of the artery. Reasonably good views of the arteries can be obtained using this method, although the image is inferior to that obtained by conventional arteriography. It is likely that improvement of these images in the future will make invasive arteriography obsolete.

MANAGEMENT OF CHRONIC ARTERIAL OCCLUSION

Most patients suffering from intermittent claudication derive benefit from general advice and medical treatment, others require surgical measures.

General advice. If the patient suffers from *diabetes* or *hypertension* these conditions should be kept under control meticulously. *Smoking* must be given up completely, specially in Buerger's disease, as it makes the patient's condition much worse. *Exercise* should be taken regularly within the limits of pain; this helps in the development of the collateral circulation.

Diet. There are two types of lipoproteins in the serum, those containing cholesterol and those rich in triglycerides. The serum should be tested to see whether the lipoprotein level is raised, and if so which type of lipoproteins are involved in the increase. If the former type are increased, a low cholesterol diet is prescribed; if the latter, weight reduction should be stressed.

Medical treatment. Half a tablet of *aspirin* is prescribed daily, as it has an anti-adhesive effect on the platelets. Rest pain will require relief by *analgesics* such as paracetamol or diclofenac. Oral *vasodilators* may be tried, but are of doubtful value.

Care of the feet. Soft and comfortable socks should be worn. The toe-nails should be trimmed very carefully, avoiding damage to the adjacent skin, specially in diabetic patients, because the sites of such trauma may act as starting points for the development of gangrene.

Buerger's exercises. If the head of the bed is elevated *(Buerger's position)*, the circulation to the feet is increased. The same is the effect of *Buerger's exercises* (raise the limb for 2 minutes, lower it for 2 minutes, repeat the cycle about a dozen times). This routine should be carried out daily for a few weeks.

Sympathectomy. If the above measures fail sympathectomy may be tried. It is of no use in claudication, but it may help some patients with rest pain, because its effect is mainly on the vessels in the skin and subcutaneous tissues. Sympathectomy may be carried out surgically or chemically.

Surgical sympathectomy has largely been abandoned, but may be employed if expertise for chemical sympathectomy is not available. The muscles of the anterolateral abdominal wall are divided or split along the direction of their fibres. The peritoneum is retracted medially. The sympathetic trunk is to be found on the sides of the bodies of the vertebrae. Two or three ganglia with the intervening trunk are removed. In male patients, who constitute the majority, the first lumbar ganglion is not removed, as its loss can be followed by impotence.

Chemical sympathectomy is nowadays more popular. A long lumbar puncture needle is inserted by the side of the erector spinae. It skirts the vertebral column and enters the plane in front of the lumbar fascia which contains the sympathetic trunk. 5 ml of phenol solution in water is injected besides the bodies of the second, third and fourth lumbar vertebrae. The procedure is carried out under x-ray screening control, and the position of the bolus can be assessed by first injecting a small amount of a contrast solution.

ARTERIAL SURGERY FOR OCCLUSION IN THE LOWER LIMB

In atherosclerosis affecting the arteries of the lower limb, surgery has a definite role to play.

Indications for operation. 1. *Rest pain* is an absolute indication for surgery, provided the distal vessels are patent and the patient fit for operation.

2. *Claudication* is a relative indication for operation. If the patient can modify his activity so that claudication is prevented, operation may be avoided.

3. If *ischaemic ulcers* do not respond to treatment, reconstructive surgery may be advised to prevent limb amputation.

4. In arterial occlusion due to an *embolus* urgent embolectomy is indicated to save the limb.

Operations for disease at different sites. *Aorto-iliac artery stenosis.* This condition can be treated by one of the following operations:

1. An *aortofemoral bypass* is the method of choice. A synthetic arterial graft is anastomosed above to the aorta and below to the femoral artery, bypassing the stenosed segment.

2. An *iliac endarterectomy* can also be used, but the long-term results are not so good. In this operation the artery is opened, the atheromatous plaques removed, and the wound in the artery sutured, using a vein patch over the wound to prevent stenosis.

3. If the patient is not fit for major surgery *transluminal balloon angioplasty* may be employed. A balloon catheter is introduced into the femoral artery and passed up to lie across the stenosis. It is inflated with contrast medium to a pressure of 5 to 10 atmospheres, which is maintained for about 15 seconds. Inflation of the balloon produces fissures in the atheromatous plaques, thus dilating the stenosed part. An endothelial lining gradually develops over these fissures, so that the lumen of the artery is enlarged. Restenosis is more common after balloon angioplasty than after reconstructive surgery, but the angioplasty can be repeated if necessary.

Femoral and profunda artery stenosis. This condition responds well to operation provided the vessels above and below the block are normal. A *femoro-popliteal bypass graft* is commonly used. The patient's own long saphenous vein gives the best results. In order to be used successfully, its direction has to be reversed after removal, so that its valves do not obstruct the downward flow of blood. If, along with atherosclerosis in the femoral artery, there is also stenosis at the origin of the profunda femoris, which is otherwise normal, *profundoplasty* is a useful operation to carry out. The incision in the femoral artery is extended along the profunda until normal artery is found. Atheroma is now removed and the opening closed, with a vein patch to prevent narrowing of the vessel.

Arteries below the popliteal. In these vessels direct arterial procedures are unrewarding. The lumen of these vessels is small. Therefore the flow of blood here is poor, and this results in a high rate of graft failure.

Results of operation. When reconstructive surgery is carried out for aorto-iliac disease the results are excellent. However, if femoro-popliteal occlusion develops at a later stage, the outcome may be compromised. Surgery for femoro-popliteal disease is less useful, the success rate at the end of 5 years being only about 50%.

ACUTE ARTERIAL OCCLUSION

Acute occlusion of the arterial supply to a limb represents an emergency. If an extensive collateral circulation is not present, irreversible ischaemic changes begin about 6 hours after the event. Sudden occlusion of an artery may result either from trauma or embolism.

OCCLUSION DUE TO TRAUMA

Blunt trauma to an artery may affect it in one of the following ways:

1. The bruising may cause roughening of the intima so that *thrombosis* occurs, resulting in occlusion.

2. The intima may become detached from the underlying muscle, and the resulting *sub-intimal haematoma* may occlude the artery.

During a long march the muscles in the unyielding *anterior fascial compartment* of the leg may be so swollen as to compress the anterior tibial artery and cause both distal ischaemia and the crush syndrome. The treatment is urgent fasciotomy to release the compression of the artery.

Management. When a limb has been injured its examination must always include palpation of the pulses. If the pulses are absent and the limb is pale and cold, arterial occlusion should be strongly suspected. In such a situation the artery must be immediately exposed. If it is found to be lacerated the affected part may be resected and an end-to-end anastomosis carried out, or a vein graft employed.

If the artery is bruised it may be in spasm. In that case 4% lignocaine solution should be applied locally to overcome the spasm. If the pulse still does not return, the artery should be opened and the thrombosis or subintimal haematoma dealt with, usually by resection of the involved segment of the artery.

EMBOLIC OCCLUSION

An embolus is a body which is foreign to the blood stream and which may get lodged in a vessel and cause obstruction. Emboli may consist of blood clot, air or fat. The most common emboli are made of blood clot. The most frequent site of origin of the blood clot is the roughened intima over necrosed cardiac muscle, in a case of myocardial infarction. Other sites include places where the blood flow is relatively sluggish. Examples include the left atrium in a case of mitral stenosis, and the cavity of a large aneurysm.

Sites of lodgement of emboli. Emboli can get lodged in any organ in the body, producing ischaemia of the part. The most common sites of lodgment of emboli are the *lower limbs,* due to the straightness of the arteries leading to them. There is pain, pallor, pulselessness and paresis. *Cerebral* embolism commonly leads to hemiplegia, and embolism into the *retinal* artery to blindness. In *mesenteric* arterial embolism gangrene of the intestines may follow. Finally, an embolus in the venous system is the most dangerous, and can cause death by lodging in the main pulmonary artery and producing circulatory arrest if the embolus is a large one (*pulmonary embolism).*

Clinical features. In its clinical presentation embolic occlusion differs from the thrombotic occlusion which complicates atherosclerosis. In thrombosis there is a preceding history of claudication, which is lacking in embolism. On the other hand in embolic occlusion a source of the emboli can be found, and paralysis occurs within 4 to 6 hours after the onset of pain; both these features are missing in thrombosis. In a patient who has not had pain in the limb previously, severe pain suddenly develops, and the limb becomes cold with mottled blue and white patches. Movement of the toes and touch sensation are lost. The distal pulses are absent, but the femoral pulse may be more forceful, due to the embolic occlusion immediately distal to it.

Clinical findings suggestive of an embolic cause include cardiac arrhythmia, myocardial ischaemia and valvular disease, and the absence of factors predisposing to atherosclerosis. The presence of normal pulses on the contralateral side is strongly indicative of an embolic source.

Treatment. If a case of embolism is left untreated, stasis of blood occurs both proximal and distal to the embolus, and this results in thrombosis, which spreads in both directions. This extension can be prevented by immediately starting an infusion of 5,000–10,000 units of *heparin* until the embolus can be removed by operation. At the same time, the severe ischaemic pain requires relief by analgesics. The treatment of choice in patients with embolism in a limb artery is urgent *embolectomy* within a few hours. This may be carried out under local or general anaesthesia, depending on the location of the clot. The artery is exposed and held up with tapes. As soon as a longitudinal incision is made into the artery, the thrombus begins to extrude and is removed, together with the embolus. As bleeding occurs arterial clamps are applied. A Fogarty catheter is now passed, in turn upwards and downwards, until it reaches beyond the clot. It is a fine catheter with a balloon at the tip. The balloon is inflated and the catheter withdrawn slowly, bringing out the clot. The process is repeated a few times until brisk bleeding commences, indicating that all clot has been evacuated. The arteriotomy is now closed. Postoperatively, anticoagulant therapy is continued. Prevention of further emboli requires treatment of the cause. If that is not possible, long-term anticoagulant therapy with warfarin is usually started.

Air embolism. If a large volume of air enters the venous circulation it can be very dangerous for the patient. When it reaches the right atrium the air is churned up. The foam enters the right ventricle and causes an air-lock in the pulmonary artery, which may cause right-sided heart failure. Some of the situations in which air may enter the veins are the following:

1. Air may be *sucked* into an open vein. This is most likely to happen during operations on the neck or axilla, where the negative pressure in the thorax helps suck the air into any large vein which may get opened.
2. Air may reach the venous system after *insufflation* into the fallopian tubes, or during illegal abortion.
3. In the days when rigid bottles with *air vents* were used for intravenous infusions, air embolism was more common than with the collapsible bottles in use nowadays. If a rigid bottle has to be used, a spherical plastic float in the drip chamber, which plugs the outlet when the fluid falls to a low level, adds a great measure of safety.

Treatment. The operation table should be tilted so that the head side is low – the Trendelenberg position. This encourages the air to pass into the lower half of the body, where it is relatively harmless. At the same time the patient should be turned onto his left side. In this position the air floats into the apex of the right ventricle, away from the origin of the pulmonary artery. Air may be aspirated from the right ventricle by a needle passed upwards and backwards from below the left costal margin. Alternatively, the heart may be exposed for aspiration under direct vision.

Fat embolism syndrome. The fat embolism syndrome commonly follows extensive and multiple fractures, occurring in up to 5% of patients with combined pelvic and femoral fractures. Fat droplets activate platelet aggregation. The platelets being thus 'consumed,' the patient suffers what is called a consumption coagulopathy. At the same time, fat in globules lodging in the lung is converted by lipase to free fatty acid that causes acute lung injury. Thus the patient presents with dyspnoea, skin petechiae, hypoxaemia, thrombocytopenia, falling haemoglobin and fat globules in the urine. Symptoms arise two or three days after injury and two types are recognized, the cerebral and the pulmonary, depending upon whether the chylomicrons aggregate maximally in the brain or the lung. In the *cerebral* type the patient is drowsy, restless, disoriented, and later comatose. In the *pulmonary* type there is increasing cyanosis with signs of right heart failure. If the condition is suspected *ophthalmoscopy* should be carried out. Emboli in the retinal arteries may cause haemorrhages and 'fluffy' exudate. Petechial haemorrhages are fairly common. The sputum and urine should be examined for the presence of fat globules.

Treatment is supportive and includes vasopressors, inotropes and mechanical ventilation. High-dose corticosteroids probably reduce platelet aggregation. Low molecular weight dextran reduces the viscosity of the blood. Aspirin and heparin carry a significant risk of haemorrhage and are not recommended.

GANGRENE

Definitions. *Gangrene* is defined as death with putrefaction of macroscopic portions of tissue. *Necrosis* indicates the death of individual cells or groups of cells. A *sequestrum* is a dead piece of bone. A *slough* is a piece of dead soft tissue e.g. fascia, tendon or skin.

The classic presentation of gangrene is seen when the condition affects the distal part of a limb. However, certain viscera may be affected by gangrene, notably the appendix, the small intestine, and occasionally the gallbladder.

Causes. Gangrene may result from one of many pathological processes:

1. *Ischaemia.* This may be secondary to one of the following conditions:

i. Atherosclerosis, with thrombosis on an atheromatous plaque.

ii. Embolism, the clot having come from the left atrium in atrial fibrillation, or the left ventricle in coronary thrombosis.

iii. Diabetes, the contributing pathological processes being arteritis and neuropathy.

iv. Thromboangiitis obliterans (Buerger's disease).

v. Raynaud's disease and ergotism, due to repeated arterial spasm.

vi. Inadvertent intra-arterial injection of drugs, specially thiopentone and cytotoxic drugs.

2. *Infections.* The common example consists of gas gangrene.

3. *Trauma.* i. Direct trauma: examples include pressure sores and the constriction groove of strangulated intestine.

ii. Indirect trauma e.g. gangrene of the hand due to compression of the brachial artery by the lower end of a fractured humeral shaft in a supracondylar fracture.

4. *Physical agents.* Examples include burns due to heat, boiling liquids, chemicals, electricity and irradiation.

Clinical appearance. The gangrenous part is cold and motionless. Arterial pulsation, capillary response to pressure and sensation are all absent. The colour changes due to ischaemia take place as follows: at first there is pallor; later, there may be dusky grey or purple discoloration due to the pooling of blood in the part. Finally, the colour changes to a greenish or brownish black, due to the disintegration of haemoglobin and formation of iron sulphide.

Types. Gangrene may be either dry or moist, depending on whether the occlusion of the circulation occurs gradually or suddenly.

Dry gangrene. In atherosclerosis the reduction of blood supply takes place slowly over a period of weeks or months due to gradually increasing narrowing of the arterial lumen by atheromatous plaques. If this happens in an exposed part, e.g. a limb, the parts dry up before the stage of necrosis supervenes. The dryness discourages the growth of bacteria, so that putrefaction does not occur, and there is no foul smell. The part is dry, wrinkled, and black due to the iron sulfide produced by the breakdown of haemoglobin (Plate VIII-II).

Moist gangrene. This results if, at the time when ischaemia occurs, the part is moist. Putrefaction of the tissue proteins takes place and anaerobic infection sets in, producing a foul smell. Examples of this are seen in the following conditions:

1. When an artery is suddenly occluded, as by a ligature or due to an embolus.
2. When *venous* obstruction is present along with arterial occlusion.
3. In *diabetes*, because of the increased likelihood of infection in diabetic tissues.
4. Whenever gangrene occurs in an *internal organ*, e.g. in acute appendicitis and strangulated bowel, because the viscera are always moist.

When seen in a limb, the affected part becomes swollen and discoloured, and the epidermis is raised in blebs. If infection is by gas-producing organisms, crepitus may be felt on palpation.

Natural history. If gangrene remains untreated it may get circumscribed or spread in extent. The outcome depends upon the adequacy of the circulation in the areas adjacent to the gangrenous part. At the distal limit of the living part a layer of granulation tissue develops, which is marked on the surface by a band of hyperaemia. The granulations extend into the dead tissue until those which have penetrated farthest are unable to obtain enough nourishment. At this level the skin and deeper tissues break down, so that an ulcer forms all round the limb. This is the *line of demarcation* between the gangrenous and healthy tissue.

In *dry* gangrene if the blood supply to the living tissues is adequate the line of demarcation develops within a few days, and separation of the gangrenous part takes place with the minimum of infection. When bone is also involved, separation takes longer than when soft tissues alone are affected.

In *moist* gangrene the conditions are more favourable for the growth of bacteria. Therefore, more infection and suppuration takes place, and the line of demarcation develops at a higher level than in dry gangrene, so that more of the limb is lost. Therefore every effort should be made to convert moist gangrene into the dry type.

Spread of gangrene. The moist type of gangrene may spread upwards, either as a whole or in the form of black patches of skin at a higher level than the gangrenous part. Infection may also spread upwards. If a clear line of demarcation does not form, a local amputation runs the risk of leaving gangrenous tissues behind. To avoid this possibility, in the case of the lower limb an above-knee amputation may have to be carried out.

Treatment. As far as possible one should try to save the limb in cases of gangrene. In arterial disease if the blood supply above the gangrenous area is good, or if a poor blood supply can be improved, a conservative excision may be successful and an amputation avoided. Methods of improving the blood supply include direct arterial surgery and interruption of the sympathetic nerve supply. If the limb is badly crushed, or the patient is suffering from gas gangrene or rapidly spreading gangrene, amputation has to be carried out to save his life.

General treatment. In embolic gangrene the patient may need treatment for cardiac failure, atrial fibrillation and anaemia. Diabetes, if present, must be controlled. Pain should be relieved by non-narcotic drugs.

Local treatment. The limb should be kept exposed to encourage dryness, and cool to reduce the metabolic rate and the need of the tissues for oxygen. The pressure areas, e.g. the heel, should be protected by foam pads etc., to prevent the development of fresh patches of gangrene. Where an area of skin becomes hardened, it may need to be lifted, in order to release underlying pus.

SPECIAL VARIETIES OF GANGRENE

Diabetic gangrene. Three factors contribute to the development of diabetic gangrene. Firstly, the peripheral neuritis of diabetes results in trophic changes. Secondly, atheroma of the arteries results in ischaemia. And finally, an excess of sugar in the tissues lowers their resistance to infection.

The *neuropathy* produces a harmful effect in two ways. Impaired sensation results in neglect of minor injuries so that damage to the tissues becomes more widespread. At the same time the muscular involvement leads to deformities in the foot, so that the pressure on the metatarsal heads increases. This leads to the development of callosities, which act as sites of entry for infection. Infections affect the relatively avascular structures like tendons and fasciae to a greater extent than structures which are more richly supplied with blood, such as muscles. Through the tissue planes the infection can rapidly spread upwards.

In diabetic gangrene *major arterial disease* is usually absent, so that the dorsalis pedis and posterior tibial pulses are palpable, and intermittent claudication and rest pain are absent. Any pus is examined, and the blood and urine are tested to detect the presence and severity of diabetes.

Treatment. The diabetic state should be brought under control by diet and drugs. Gangrene is managed along the usual lines. If no major arterial obstruction is present, the effort should be to save as much of the limb as possible. If infection spreads upwards rapidly, free drainage of the area with removal of sloughs must be carried out. If this is done, rapid healing often follows.

Traumatic gangrene. This may be due to direct or indirect trauma.

Direct traumatic gangrene. The most common example of this type of gangrene is a bedsore, besides the ulcers resulting from the pressure of splints or plasters.

Bedsores most commonly develop in a patient who is bedridden, specially if he has suffered injury or disease of the spinal cord. Thus the two most important factors in the development of bedsores are *pressure* and *loss of the trophic influence of nerves*. If the patient is also *anaemic* or *malnourished*, not only is the tendency to develop bedsores increased, but any sores that form tend to spread more rapidly. Again, *moisture* increases the rate of extension of a bedsore. The most common sites for the development of bedsores are over the sacrum, the greater trochanter, and the heels.

While looking after bedridden patients, the *prevention* of bedsores requires extremely vigilant nursing:

1. A foam mattress is employed.
2. The bedsheets must be kept free of all wrinkles.
3. Sweat, urine or faeces must not be allowed to collect over the skin, as these cause maceration of the skin which helps a bedsore spread.
4. The posture must be changed two-hourly.
5. A mattress with a honeycomb of cavities may be employed. Alternate cavities are filled with air and emptied every few minutes by a motorized pump. In this way constant pressure on any area of the skin is prevented. Such a mattress helps considerably in preventing bedsores.

If bedsores actually form, treatment is difficult; hence the very great importance of prevention.

Treatment. All the measures mentioned above under prevention must be continued. As far as the management of the ulcers is concerned: if there is pent up pus, it needs evacuation. Small quantities of slough can be treated by Eusol solution; large sloughs require surgical removal. Oedematous granulations can be made more firm and pink by magnesium sulphate glycerine paste, which withdraws water by its hygroscopic effect. In an otherwise healthy patient excision of dead tissues can be followed up by shifting a skin flap to cover the raw area.

Indirect traumatic gangrene. This occurs due to occlusion of an artery from one of the following causes:

1. *Pressure*, e.g. from a broken bone in a fracture.
2. *Thrombosis*, e.g. following injury.
3. *Ligation* of a main artery.

If the collateral circulation is adequate, gangrene might still not occur after the above incidents.

Treatment. The cause of the arterial occlusion should be dealt with. If the gangrene is dry, a line of demarcation indicates the level above which the tissues are viable, and amputation is carried out above that level. On the other hand moist gangrene spreads rapidly, and amputation is required to save the patient's life.

Frostbite occurs due to exposure to cold. The vessel wall is damaged with oedema, blistering, and finally gangrene. The part should be warmed gradually to body temperature, being wrapped in cotton wool. Warm drinks, analgesics and if necessary paravertebral injection of the sympathetic chain may be employed.

Thiopentone, meant for administration into the basilic vein in the antecubital fossa, may by mistake be injected into the brachial artery. The aspiration of bright red blood, and a cry of agony from the patient during the injection, will indicate to the clinician that a faulty injection has been made. The needle should not be removed, and 5 ml of 1% lignocaine should be injected in order to abolish the vascular spasm, followed by dilute heparin solution. If no improvement occurs, the artery should be exposed and any clots flushed out. Low molecular weight dextran should be given intravenously, to make the blood less viscous.

AMPUTATIONS

Indications. An amputation is indicated when a limb or a part of it is:

1. *Dead* i.e. gangrene is present. This may be due to occlusion of:

i. Major vessels, e.g. from atherosclerosis or embolism.

ii. Peripheral vessels, e.g. in diabetes, Buerger's disease, Raynaud's disease, intra-arterial thiopentone injection, etc.

2. *Dangerous.* This is the situation in both moist gangrene and gas gangrene. The danger to life arises from the absorption of the potent toxins of the clostridia or other anaerobic bacteria. Amputation is required as a life-saving measure. The part may also be a danger to life if it is the seat of a malignant tumour e.g. an osteosarcoma, or an arteriovenous fistula which cannot be dealt with surgically and which has resulted in heart failure.

3. *A total loss.* Some examples of this include the following:

i. When a limb is the seat of multiple severe lacerations and fractures, perhaps with partial amputation, due to a bomb-blast injury or a road accident.

ii. If severe contractures or paralysis, usually after polio, make the limb impossible to use, and interfere rather than help with locomotion.

iii. If, in a patient with an ischaemic foot, severe rest pain makes life miserable. In such a situation amputation improves the quality of life.

It should be remembered that before an amputation is carried out, informed and written consent of the patient must be obtained. This should be a routine before any operation, but specially before an amputation.

AMPUTATIONS AT DIFFERENT LEVELS

Amputations may be classified into minor and major amputations.

Minor (distal) amputations. These are commonly carried out either after injury, e.g. to a finger or toe, or in a patient with small vessel disease (diabetes or Buerger's disease), where gangrene of the toes occurs but the blood supply to the surrounding tissues is good. In such a case a local amputation can be followed by healing.

In *diabetes*, infection plays a major part in the pathological process. Because of the infection the wound has to be left open. At the same time the infection tends to spread up the tendon sheaths. For these reasons the excision of a metatarsal bone ('ray' excision) is often recommended. This opens up the tissue planes, with better drainage of pus.

Trans-metatarsal amputation. This can be utilized in Buerger's disease if more than one toe is affected by gangrene. This operation is carried out employing a long plantar flap, so that the suture line is on the dorsal side, away from the weight-bearing area.

Major amputations. *Above-knee* and *below-knee amputations.* The most common major amputations employed in the lower limb are the *below-knee* and the *above-knee amputations*. The advantages of the one are the disadvantages of the other. In major vessel disease the above-knee amputation provides an absolute guarantee of sound healing of the stump due to the abundant blood supply available from the muscles of the thigh. However, the function of the artificial limb is not as good as in a below-knee amputation. A below-knee amputation provides a lesser certainty of sound healing of the stump. However, should the stump heal the ultimate function of the limb is of a higher quality.

In the past, in cases of major vessel disease, twice as many above-knee amputations were performed as below-knee. However, during recent years this ratio has been reversed, partly because arterial surgery is now available to improve the blood supply to the limb.

Flaps. If muscles, which have a rich blood supply, could be raised as a part of the flap which is to be used to cover the bony stump, the chances of healing of the wound would be increased. In the case of the above-knee amputation because big muscles are present all round the stump, equal anterior and posterior flaps are commonly employed. In the below-knee amputation thick muscles are available only in the calf. Therefore a single long posterior flap is used.

Through-knee amputation. In through-knee amputation a long anterior flap is preferred. The patellar tendon is sutured to the hamstrings so that, acting from below, both the rectus femoris and the hamstrings help in stabilizing the hip joint in the erect posture.

Symes amputation. In a Symes amputation the lower ends of the tibia and fibula are sawn across just above the line of the ankle joint. The stump is covered by a posterior flap consisting of the skin of the heel with its underlying pad of fibrofatty tissue.

Points in technique. The main artery and vein supplying the limb are individually ligated, to avoid the development of an arteriovenous fistula. The nerves are gently drawn down, cut with a sharp knife and allowed to retract upwards, so that the stump neuroma which inevitably forms should be away from pressure. The bone is cut with a saw and any splinters removed, to avoid the formation of spurs. Absolute haemostasis is ensured. However, suction drains are used, to prevent the collection of serum or blood. Muscles are stitched together over the bone, by means of sutures which incorporate the deep fascia.

Postoperative care of an amputation. A gauze and cotton wool *dressing*, held in place by a very carefully applied bandage, is employed. The dressing may be left undisturbed till the time for removal of the stitches, unless excessive pain or fever indicate the development of infection.

An amputation is a demoralizing operation. The modern tendency, therefore is to *fit a prosthesis* not urgently, but in fact *immediately*. In this connection the recently introduced inflatable prostheses are extremely useful. With such a prosthesis a lower limb amputee can get on his feet the day after the operation. This goes a long way in reducing the severity of the acute depression which he is otherwise likely to experience.

Exercises. In the past, exercises of the stump were an important part of rehabilitation, and prepared the stump for the prosthesis. Nowadays, with the prosthesis immediately applied to the stump, mobilization automatically provides exercises for the stump muscles, preventing the development of disuse atrophy and contractures.

Complications. Some of the complications of an amputation, which must be guarded against, are the following: reactionary haemorrhage, haematoma formation, infection, sequestrum formation, wound dehiscence and gangrene of the flaps; and at a later stage, an adherent scar.

Sometimes a patient remarks that he can feel the amputated limb, and that it is painful *(phantom limb).* The surgeon should reassure the patient that these symptoms will spontaneously disappear.

Aneurysms

An aneurysm is a sac formed by the dilatation of the wall of an artery, a vein, or the heart.

Types of aneurysms. An arterial aneurysm may be true or false. A *true* aneurysm contains the three layers of the arterial wall in its sac, and is most often due to atherosclerosis. It may be fusiform or saccular. A *fusiform* aneurysm is spindle-shaped, the stretching process affecting the entire circumference of the artery. In a *saccular* aneurysm only a part of the circumference of the arterial wall is stretched, so that an eccentric localized sac results.

A *false* aneurysm usually arises after a lateral tear in the wall of an artery. The haematoma which collects by the side of the artery gradually develops a cavity which is surrounded by a wall of fibrous tissue and communicates with the lumen of the artery. In its external appearance it resembles a saccular aneurysm. However, unlike the latter its sac contains none of the layers of the arterial wall.

A *dissecting* aneurysm results from haemorrhage which causes longitudinal splitting of the arterial wall, producing a tear in the intima and establishing communication with the lumen. When it affects the thoracic aorta, the dissection may spread down into the abdomen and involve the ostia of the renal arteries. The resulting ischaemia of the kidneys may cause anuria.

Symptoms may be produced by an aneurysm when it:

1. *Expands*, compressing adjacent structures, e.g. the oesophagus, producing dysphagia.
2. *Ruptures*, producing severe haemorrhage.
3. *Gets thrombosed.* For example, if a popliteal aneurysm gets thrombosed, gangrene of the foot can result.
4. *Releases emboli.* For example, emboli from an aortic aneurysm can produce ischaemia of the toes.

Signs. Along the course of an artery is seen a swelling, which exhibits expansile pulsation. A thrill may be palpable, and a bruit heard on auscultation. Proximal pressure causes the pulsation to become less marked; when the pressure is released the force of the pulsation is restored.

Neighbouring structures may be affected by the pressure of the aneurysm. If veins are compressed distal oedema may result; compression of nerves may produce impaired sensation. Similarly the oesophagus or the trachea may be compressed, resulting in dysphagia and dyspnoea respectively.

Differential diagnosis. A *large tumour* lying over the abdominal aorta may pulsate like an aneurysm. However, firstly the pulsation can be shown to be transmitted rather than expansile; secondly, if the patient assumes the knee-elbow position the tumour falls away from the aorta and the pulsation ceases.

If an *abscess* in the axilla or groin is about to be incised, one should make sure that it does not pulsate, i.e. it is not an aneurysm, otherwise incision could be followed by torrential haemorrhage. A highly *vascular tumour* like an osteogenic sarcoma may pulsate and cause confusion.

Investigations. The swelling should be investigated by ultrasound examination, CT scan or MRI to confirm the diagnosis of aneurysm. Finally, arteriography should be carried out to define the runoff bed.

Abdominal aortic aneurysm. An aneurysm of the abdominal aorta may be an incidental finding or may be symptomatic, and its treatment differs accordingly:

1. *Asymptomatic aneurysm.* If an abdominal aortic aneurysm is not producing symptoms, its recommended treatment depends upon its size. If its diameter is greater than 7 cm its chances of rupture are high, and it should be operated upon; if less than 7 cm, it should be treated conservatively.
2. *Symptomatic aneurysm.* Most patients with abdominal aortic aneurysms which are producing symptoms will be dead within one year if left without surgery; most who are operated upon will live. Therefore operation should be carried out in these cases.

Complications of repair. Because of clamping of the abdominal aorta above and below an aneurysm during its repair, the blood supply to the kidney, colon or spinal cord may be jeopardized, resulting in renal failure, ischaemic colitis, or paraplegia respectively.

ARTERIOVENOUS FISTULA (AVF)

An arteriovenous fistula may be a congenital malformation, or it may result from a penetrating wound of an artery and its accompanying vein. These days AV fistulae are also created artificially in the forearms of patients undergoing haemodialysis, so that the catheters in the artery and vein can be connected to the haemodialysis machine.

Effect on the vein. The high pressure arterial blood flowing into the vein makes it dilated, tortuous and thick-walled (arterialized).

Effect on the circulation. In the presence of the fistula the arterial blood, instead of coursing through the capillary bed, follows the easier path and leaks directly into the vein in large quantities, greatly enhancing the venous return. This in turn increases both the cardiac output and the pulse rate. Left ventricular enlargement and cardiac failure follow if the fistula is a large one.

Effect of location of the AV fistula. A congenital fistula in the *distal* part of a limb in a child results in overgrowth of the limb due to the increased circulation. Conversely, a fistula in the *proximal* part of a limb may lead to the formation of non-healing ulcers due to relative ischaemia from short-circuiting of the blood through the fistula.

Clinical features. A pulsatile swelling is seen, over which a thrill can be palpated and a continuous (machinery) murmur auscultated. The veins around the area of the fistula are dilated, as they are helping to carry away the excessive amount of blood. If pressure is applied to the artery proximal to the fistula the swelling diminishes in size, the thrill and the murmur disappear, and the pulse rate and pulse pressure fall to their normal levels (Nicoladoni's sign).

Arteriography confirms the presence of the lesion.

Treatment. Some *congenital* arteriovenous malformations are so small that they require no treatment. Others may be so large and extensive that removal is hazardous. These cases can sometimes be successfully treated by embolization after selective catheterization. A catheter with a bent tip is passed into the parent artery. The tip is introduced into the origin of the artery supplying the AV fistula. Plastic microspheres are injected into the artery; they occlude the lumen of the vessel and result in thrombosis of the vessels constituting the fistula.

Acquired AV fistulae tend to be progressive, and therefore should be operated upon. The vessels are separated. If possible they should be repaired by suture. If this is not feasible, the vein as well as the artery have to be ligated both above and below the lesion (*quadruple ligation*). Alternatively, vascular continuity may be restored by vein or Dacron grafting.

Arteritis

THROMBOANGIITIS OBLITERANS (Buerger's disease)

In this condition inflammatory changes occur in the walls of small and medium-sized arteries and veins, leading to thrombosis and occlusion of the affected vessels. The plantar, tibial, and sometimes the radial arteries are commonly affected, usually in a young male below the age of 30 years. *The patient is nearly always a smoker*; the condition does not occur in women or in non-smokers. The symptoms and signs are those which are commonly seen in occlusive arterial disease. Dry gangrene usually affects the toes, occasionally the fingers. Arteriography may show the occlusions in the distal arteries.

Treatment. The patient *must stop smoking immediately and permanently*; a reduction in the number of cigarettes smoked is not enough to prevent the progression of the disease. Surgery on the affected arteries is not possible due to their small size; however, sympathectomy often results in the healing of ischaemic ulcers and relief of pain.

THORACIC OUTLET OBSTRUCTION

The thoracic outlet is the space through which the subclavian artery, vein and brachial plexus pass from the neck into the upper extremity. It is bounded by the clavicle, the chest wall and the scalene muscles. Occasionally, a rib arises from the seventh cervical vertebra, either on one or both sides. Such a 'cervical' rib is seen in 0.5% of individuals.

Pathology. Obstruction of the subclavian artery and vein, or pressure on the brachial plexus, may occur in the thoracic outlet due to a number of anatomical abnormalities, the most common being cervical rib. This may take the form of a complete rib, articulating anteriorly with the manubrium sterni or the first rib. The anterior part or the whole of the rib may be replaced by a fibrous cord, or the rib may end blindly. In other cases fibrous bands in the insertions of the scalenus anterior or the scalenus medius may be responsible.

At the root of the neck the subclavian artery and the first thoracic nerve pass out through the narrow angle between the upper surface of the first rib and the scalenus anterior muscle. If a cervical rib is present, it further narrows down this angle and forces the artery and nerve to arch over it, both stretching and compressing them. Distal to this constricted segment, a section of the artery gets dilated (post-stenotic dilatation). This dilatation is due to turbulence of the blood flow which causes lateral stresses on the wall of the artery just beyond the stenotic area, eventually leading to the formation of an aneurysm. In the dilated area a thrombus may form, part of which can become detached as an embolus. If showers of small emboli settle in the digital arteries ischaemic episodes occur, which may superficially resemble Raynaud's phenomenon. However, whereas in Raynaud's phenomenon all the fingers of both hands are involved, here only one side is affected, and often only one or two fingers. Again, here the period of ischaemia is longer than in a Raynaud attack.

Clinical features. ***Symptoms*** may be neurological or vascular, and in most cases one or the other type predominates. *Neurological* symptoms and signs result from stretching or compression of the lower roots of the brachial plexus. Pain and paraesthesias in the fingers, hand or arm, and muscular weakness and wasting are common. However, similar symptoms may be produced by compression of the nerves in cases of cervical spondylosis, cervical disc protrusion and carpal tunnel compression. Therefore, evidence of the first two of these conditions must be looked for in the cervical spine x-ray or MRI. Neurological symptoms may be produced not only by a cervical rib but also by a normal first rib, specially in a weak and slim person, and more particularly in middle age due to sagging down of the shoulders. *Vascular* symptoms and signs are due to pressure on the subclavian artery and are strictly unilateral. They may vary from recurrent minor episodes of digital ischaemia to sudden massive ischaemia of the whole limb.

Signs. A cervical rib or other bony abnormality may be visible or palpable just above the clavicle. There may be a palpable thrill and bruit over the artery. The distal pulses may be reduced or absent, and the blood pressure in the affected arm may be lower than on the normal side. Even minor alterations in posture may result in disappearance of the radial pulse.

Investigations. X-rays of the neck, shoulder and thoracic outlet should be taken. MRI is useful, as it can identify the brachial plexus and demonstrate the angulation of the lower trunk of the plexus over a fibrous band. If vascular involvement is suspected aortic arch arteriography should be carried out. Patients presenting with venous obstruction require phlebography. However, clinical assessment remains the most important factor in diagnosis and choice of treatment.

Treatment. If a patient has only *neurological* symptoms he usually derives benefit from correction of faulty posture, with shoulder girdle strengthening exercises. As the scapula rides high, the angulation of the lower trunk of the brachial plexus is reduced, and symptoms are relieved. In the few cases where surgical treatment is required, resection of the cervical rib is the recommended procedure, although in some cases division of the scalenus anterior may be sufficient.

If *vascular* symptoms are present, the need for surgical treatment is urgent. The aims of operation are: to remove the compressing structure, to repair the subclavian artery, and to restore the distal circulation by removing emboli and propagated thrombus. All of these can be achieved through a transverse incision a finger's breadth above the clavicle. Other approaches include the axillary and the infraclavicular routes. A cervical rib which is not causing symptoms should generally be left alone.

RAYNAUD'S SYNDROME

The term Raynaud's syndrome refers to a group of disorders in which intermittent vasopasm occurs in the arterioles of the hands or feet, usually following exposure to cold, so that the fingers become blanched. As the blood flow is greatly reduced, metabolites accumulate in the capillaries. Due to the effect of these metabolites the capillaries dilate and become filled with blood which is rapidly de-oxygenated, the part becoming blue. Finally the arterioles relax, oxygenated blood courses through the parts, and the hands become red, with a burning sensation. Thus the condition is recognized by the change of colour from white, through blue, to red. This symptom-complex may be primary, when no other condition can be identified after appropriate investigation, or it may be secondary to a wide variety of underlying disorders:

Primary

- Raynaud's disease.

Secondary

- Connective tissue disorders, e.g. disseminated lupus erythematosus, rheumatoid arthritis.
- Arteriosclerosis.
- Thromboangiitis obliterans.
- Cold injury (e.g. frostbite).
- Use of vibrating hand tools.
- Polycythaemia vera.
- Ergot poisoning.

In primary Raynaud's syndrome there is an exaggerated vasoconstrictor response to cold by otherwise normal digital arteries. On the other hand in secondary Raynaud's syndrome there is a normal cold-induced vasoconstrictor response acting upon a diseased artery in which there is already reduced blood flow due to narrowing of the lumen.

Primary Raynaud's syndrome (Raynaud's disease) occurs mostly in young women, and affects the upper limb more often than the lower. Many patients with mild to moderate cold sensitivity are not disturbed by their symptoms enough to seek medical advice. It should be remembered that primary Raynaud's syndrome is almost always a *bilateral* condition. If the symptoms are unilateral the cause is much more likely to be an embolus in a digital artery, either from a subclavian artery compressed by a cervical rib, or from an atheromatous plaque in a proximal artery.

Secondary Raynaud's syndrome results in a greater severity of digital ischaemia than the primary form, and patients are more likely to seek medical advice.

Recently the distinction between primary and secondary Raynaud's syndrome has become less well defined, because it has been found that:

1. Patients apparently suffering from primary Raynaud's disease may have low levels of autoantibodies in their serum.
2. Some patients develop collagen disorders a few years after the onset of Raynaud's symptoms.

For these reasons both primary and secondary Raynaud's conditions are now classified under the single banner of Raynaud's syndrome.

Diagnosis. The diagnosis of Raynaud's syndrome depends upon the *history* of colour changes on exposure to cold. Pain in the digits is not a usual feature but may occur, particularly in the secondary variety where there is digital vessel occlusion and a significant amount of tissue damage, leading to ulceration and gangrene. Such ischaemic damage is extremely rare in the primary form of Raynaud's syndrome where the attacks are related solely to vasospasm and there is no obstructive element.

Different *causes* of the secondary disorder must be looked for. History-taking should include enquiry into the use of vibrating tools and ingestion of drugs, specially ergotamine. A history of heavy smoking in a male may suggest thromboangiitis obliterans. During physical examination the clinician must look for painful, swollen joints to rule out rheumatoid arthritis and systemic lupus erythematosus; a subclavian bruit to exclude thoracic outlet obstruction; and absent peripheral pulses to eliminate arteriosclerosis.

Investigations should include x-ray of the thoracic outlet to show the presence of a cervical rib, and x-rays of the hands to show the joint disruption characteristic of rheumatoid arthritis. Blood tests should include ESR, rheumatoid factor, antinuclear factor, anti-DNA antibody, electrophoresis, cryoglobulins, and cold agglutinin assays.

Treatment. *General measures.* No curative treatment is available for Raynaud's syndrome and the aim is palliation by reduction in the frequency and severity of the attacks. Reassurance that the condition is generally benign is important, specially in primary Raynaud's syndrome where progression to digital ischaemia is extremely rare. Most patients can achieve worthwhile improvement by avoidance of cold by the use of thick woollen gloves in cold weather, and by giving up smoking. For the few patients who continue to have frequent or severe attacks, the choice lies between drugs and surgery.

Drugs. *Nifedipine* is a calcium channel blocking agent. It is given by mouth and produces a reduction in vascular tone with vasodilatation. Side effects are common and include headache, flushing, peripheral oedema and blurred vision. *Iloprost* is a prostacyclin analogue. It is given as a 6-hour intravenous infusion daily for 3 days; clinical improvement often lasts for many weeks.

Surgery. The mainstay of surgical treatment in Raynaud's syndrome is sympathectomy, although surgery may be required when the syndrome is secondary to proximal vascular disease, e.g. resection of a cervical rib or band to relieve thoracic outlet obstruction. Good results from sympathectomy can be expected in primary Raynaud's syndrome and in thromboangiitis obliterans, where it should be reserved for patients with recurrent ulceration of the fingertips or severe incapacity from vasospasm in spite of medical treatment. In the connective tissue disorders the results of sympathectomy are uniformly poor.

42 *Veins*

The most important disease processes affecting veins are two: varicosity and thrombosis.

VARICOSE VEINS

A varicose vein is one which is dilated, lengthened and tortuous. The change is commonly brought about by increased pressure in the lumen of the vein, which stretches the vein wall. Stretching in the transverse axis results in dilatation of the vein. When the vein wall stretches in the longitudinal direction its ends remain at the same fixed points, therefore it has to become tortuous in order to accommodate its additional length. Thus the vein becomes both dilated and tortuous.

What causes the increased pressure in the lumen of the vein? The aetiology differs according to the site and underlying pathology. Veins in the submucosa of the lower end of the oesophagus become varicose (oesophageal varices) because of increased pressure in the portal venous system, due to cirrhosis etc. Veins in the lower limbs become varicose when their valves becomes functionless (incompetent). Such an incompetent valve is commonly located at the termination of the long saphenous vein, sometimes at a site lower down the limb.

VARICOSE VEINS IN THE LOWER LIMBS

In European and American communities varicose veins of the legs are an extremely common condition. Not so in the Eastern countries, where this condition is uncommon. The most likely explanation is that the inhabitants of the latter regions have better veins.

Aetiology. The most common lesion leading to the development of varicose veins in the legs is an incompetent (functionless) valve. Such cases are referred to as *primary* varicose veins, and constitute the vast majority of cases. *Secondary* varicose veins are predisposed to by any cause of venous obstruction, e.g. tumour or pregnancy, and by thrombosis of the deep veins. Finally, varicose veins occurring in children and adolescents may be due to a *congenital* arteriovenous fistula or an extensive cavernous haemangioma.

Pathology of primary varicose veins. In the upright position in the normal limb, with each muscle contraction blood is pumped upwards and prevented from returning by the valves in the veins. When this happens, the pressure in the deep veins is reduced. This allows blood in the superficial veins to empty into the deep veins, ready to be pumped upwards with the next muscular contraction. The valves in the superficial veins ensure that only a short segment between each pair of valves can empty through the corresponding perforating veins and widespread transfer of blood from superficial to deep veins is prevented. However, if there is extensive incompetence in the superficial valves, it is possible for blood to spill over from deep veins at a high level, down the superficial veins, and finally to enter the deep veins at a low level every time these veins fall slack after muscle contraction. This is how primary varicose veins develop.

With such a retrograde circuit based on an incompetent long or short saphenous vein, its upper end provides the source, its main stem and branches form the pathway of incompetence, and one or more perforating veins are the re-entry points. This state is usually curable by removal of the source and the pathway of incompetence, but enlarged re-entry points (the perforators) that allow back flow may also need to be closed off.

The main valves affected are located at the following sites:

1. The termination of the long saphenous into the femoral vein.
2. The termination of the short saphenous into the popliteal vein.
3. The mid-thigh.
4. On either side of the tibia and fibula where there are communications *(perforators)* passing through openings in the deep fascia above the ankle.

Symptoms. The most common complaint is of a tired and aching sensation in the leg, specially the calf, towards the evening. There may be itching of the skin over the varices.

Examination. The varicosities are most commonly distributed along the course of the long saphenous vein (Fig. 1); less often, the short saphenous vein is affected.

Identifying the location of the incompetent valve. It is very important to identify the exact location of the incompetent valve or valves, because only then can effective treatment be given by ligation at those sites, to abolish the retrograde flow of blood into the veins below the valves. The best example of such an examination is the Trendelenberg test.

Selective occlusion (Trendelenberg) test. The patient lies down on the examination couch, and the limb is elevated to empty the veins. The suspected pathway of incompetence is *selectively* occluded by compression with fingertips (not with a tourniquet). The patient now stands up and the varicose veins are observed. After a few seconds the compression is removed. If the vein fills promptly only at this stage, this shows that the varicose vein selected for occlusion, fills by down flow and therefore its valves must be incompetent, i.e. the test is positive. This test is of great diagnostic value and when positive it accurately identifies simple (primary) varicose veins. However, no great reliance can be placed on a negative test, as the real source of incompetence (say, short saphenous) may have been overlooked.

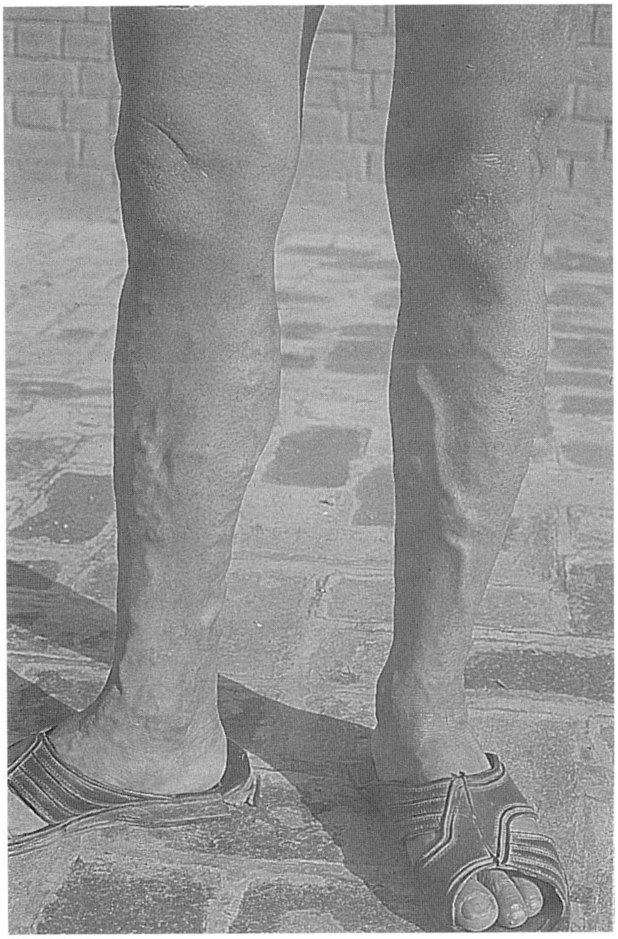

Fig. 1 Varicose long saphenous veins.

Testing for patency of the deep venous system. Before any surgical treatment is planned for a patient suffering from varicose veins, it is important to know whether or not the deep venous system is patent. If there is no history of deep vein thrombosis the deep venous system is usually patent. However, the Selective Perthe's test can be employed to make sure.

Selective Perthes' test. The patient stands up so that the veins are well filled. The suspected pathway of incompetence is now compressed with fingertips and the patient asked to rise on his toes three times. If the veins become visibly less prominent and soft to touch, the test is positive. The compression is now released, when full prominence and firmness of the veins return promptly. The test confirms that the deep vein pumping mechanism is functioning satisfactorily, and the fault lies in the superficial vein under test; it fills the varicosities as fast as the deep veins empty them. If the above tests are inconclusive, confirmation can be provided by use of the directional Doppler flowmeter.

Directional Doppler flowmetry. The probe is placed over the saphenous vein in the lower thigh or upper calf and the response to coughing noted; a burst of downflow should follow each coughing action. The pathway of incompetence is now occluded by finger pressure well above the probe and the test repeated. It will be found that the downflow has been eliminated.

Photoplethysmography. The calf veins are emptied by five contractions of the calf muscles. The plethysmograph now determines the time taken for refilling of the veins. If the valves in the veins are incompetent, the veins refill very quickly, i.e. the 'venous refilling time' is considerably shortened.

Ultrasonography is particularly useful in short saphenous incompetence, where it can give positive confirmation of downflow in an incompetent vein.

Treatment. ***Varicose veins without venotensive changes.*** Here the treatment may be cosmetic, symptomatic or definitive. *Cosmetically,* varicose veins may be disguised by appropriate make-up or elastic support stockings. *Symptomatically,* heaviness or tiredness can be relieved by elastic stockings and elevation of the limbs whenever possible. However, stockings are tedious, specially in hot weather. The most effective *definitive* method is the elimination of superficial vein incompetence by sclerotherapy or by surgery.

Compression sclerotherapy. If there are only a few minor varicosities these can be dealt with by injecting a sclerosing agent in solution, which causes thrombosis in the concerned segment of the vein. The resultant fibrosis causes the vein to shrink down in size, or even get obliterated. A suitable chemical is 3% sodium tetradecylsulphate.

Technique. The injection must be given into an empty vein, so that the walls of the vein adhere to each other without intervening blood clot. After the injection cotton balls are placed over the injection sites and a double layer of crepe bandages applied firmly, the patient being encouraged to walk about normally. The bandages are removed after about a week, elastic stockings being worn for another few weeks. It should *be remembered that compression by elastic bandages and stockings is an essential part of the injection treatment of varicose veins*; without this the veins open up, their valves get destroyed, and they get thrombosed, so that their situation is made worse. If varicosities are extensive, the disadvantages of injection treatment outweigh their advantages and surgical treatment is to be preferred.

Surgical treatment. Surgery constitutes the most important method of treatment of varicose veins of the lower limbs. In this connection it is first necessary to know the sites of the incompetent superficial valves. At the same time one must know whether the deep veins are patent or not:

1. If the deep veins are patent and the valves in the deep veins and perforators are competent the results of surgery for varicose veins are very good.
2. If the deep veins are patent and deep valves competent but the perforators are incompetent the results are reasonable.
3. If deep venous obstruction is present, superficial ligation and stripping should not be carried out, because a marked worsening of the situation usually occurs.

The basic principle of the operative treatment of varicose veins is the ligation and division of those veins into which the high-pressure leak from the deep venous system has primarily occurred:

1. Incompetence at the *sapheno-femoral* junction is treated by ligation at this site. The ligature is applied to the

long saphenous vein flush with its termination, and the tributaries joining the last few centimetres of the vein are ligated and divided, so as to prevent the blood flowing back along them and causing a recurrence of the varices.

2. *Saphenopopliteal* ligation is carried out on the same lines for varicosity of the short saphenous venous system.

3. *Incompetent perforating veins* are individually located by tourniquet tests and marked; they are next isolated by dissection and ligated.

Care must be taken not to damage or destroy normal competent saphenous veins, because they may be needed for coronary bypass operations for coronary occlusion in the future.

Stripping. Apart from ligation of the incompetent valve at the sapheno-femoral (or sapheno-poplileal) junction, the varicose vein may by excised *(stripped)*. In this procedure the long saphenous vein is exposed-below the knee. Its distal end is ligated. The stripper which essentially consists of a flexible steel wire is passed proximally up the vein. At the groin the stripper is anchored to the saphenous vein with ligatures. Firm traction is now applied to the stripper at the knee, and it brings the vein out with it. Simultaneously, a firm crepe bandage is wrapped around the limb over cotton pads. Haemorrhage can occur into the subcutaneous tissues from the torn ends of the tributaries of the avulsed vein, but immediate firm bandaging effectively prevents it.

Complications of varicose veins include the following:

Thrombophlebitis of a vein, which is red and tender. Elastic bandages are applied over foam rubber pads, and the patient allowed to go about.

Eczema may occur because the patient scratches the skin which itches. An ointment containing hydrocortisone, or one containing zinc oxide and coal tar, is used.

Haemorrhage. A varicose vein may rupture and bleed furiously. The patient may not be aware of the simple fact that blood will continue to flow under pressure if he remains standing, or sitting with the leg hanging from a chair. He must be told to lie down at once. The bleeding point is pressed upon and the haemorrhage will promptly stop. A bandage should now be applied over a sterile gauze pad. To aid haemostasis further, the leg should be elevated over one or two pillows.

To elevate a leg with a bleeding varicose vein without compressing the bleeding point can be dangerous; air can enter the vein, and if in a large enough quantity, can cause air embolism. Therefore, compression-bandaging of the bleeding point must be carried out before elevation of the leg.

Venous ulcer (Gravitational ulcer, Varicose ulcer). These ulcers are chronic, tend to recur, and cause considerable disability. They follow either varicose veins or deep vein thrombosis. The cause in either case is venous stasis, which results in local anoxia and oedema. Signs of venous insufficiency are usually present along with dermatitis, with brown discoloration, thickening of skin and oedema. The site of occurrence of a venous ulcer is quite constant; it nearly always lies on the anteromedial surface of the tibia just above the medial malleolus. In this condition syphilis must be excluded by serological tests, and atherosclerotic ischaemia by checking the peripheral pulses. If these cannot be felt because of oedema, the Doppler ultrasound may be employed. Malignant change may occur in a long-standing ulcer (Marjolin's ulcer).

The pathophysiology is not fully understood. In the normal person during walking, the contractions of the calf muscles pump blood in a cephalad direction in the deep system. In a patient with incompetent perforator valves, the high venous pressure in the deep veins is transmitted to the superficial venous system, and causes extravasation of plasma and blood cells. In time the subcutaneous tissue becomes firm, with a leathery feel.

Venous ulcers resulting from varicose veins heal promptly after ambulatory treatment or ligation operations. On the other hand post-thrombotic ulcers tend to be refractory to treatment, and require bed-rest and skin grafting.

The *Bisgaard method* of treatment of venous ulcers is very useful. The limb is elevated. Massage, along with passive and active movements, is now carried out. A firm elastic bandage is next applied from the base of the toes to the knee and the patient encouraged to walk. Movements in walking alternatively stretch and relax the bandage and produce a venous pumping effect.

For the treatment of incompetent perforators, *subfascial ligation,* i.e. ligation under the deep fascia, appears to be a theoretically sound procedure. It is employed by some, but has been abandoned by others.

THROMBOSIS

Apart from varicosities, the most important pathological change affecting veins is thrombosis. The main factors responsible for producing thrombosis are three (Virchow's triad):

1. Change in the *vessel wall*, usually damage to the endothelium, as in injury or inflammation.
2. Diminished rate of *blood flow*, as after operations.
3. Increased *coagulability* of blood, as in infections and after haemorrhage.

The *pathological effects* of thrombosis include the following:

1. *Locally*, the clot may get dissolved and the vein get recanalized. Alternatively, the clot may organize into fibrous tissue. Specially if the thrombus is infected an abscess may form, or pyaemia may occur due to systemic spread of the infection. In the pelvic veins a clot sometimes calcifies, leaving behind a small circular radiopaque shadow, which to the beginner may look like a stone in the lower end of the ureter.
2. *Distally*. If the vein remains blocked a collateral circulation soon opens up, as shown by the appearance of tortuous superficial veins.
3. *Proximally*, the clot may extend into the larger veins, where a portion of the thrombus may become detached, get lodged in a branch of the pulmonary artery, and produce pulmonary infarction. If an infected thrombus, e.g. from septic thrombosed haemorrhoids, gets lodged in the portal vein it may result in the formation of abscesses in the liver (pylephlebitis).

Thrombosis in the superficial veins is commonly accompanied by inflammation (thrombophlebitis), while in the deep veins it usually occurs without it (phlebothrombosis).

Superficial venous thrombosis. *(Thrombophlebitis).* This can occur in one of the following situations:

1. In a grossly varicose vein.
2. In occult malignant neoplasms.
3. In local trauma.
4. In a vein cannulated for infusion.
5. In polycythaemia and thromboangiitis obliterans.

At the site of the vein a painful, red and tender cord is found. When thrombophlebitis occurs below the knee it is usually self-limiting. The risk of thromboembolism is minimal and anticoagulation is not needed. When thrombophlebitis extends above the knee embolization may occur; such patients should be closely observed for cephalad progression of thrombus. Treatment consists of bed rest and a crepe bandage. Aspirin relieves pain, and also helps by reducing the coagulability of the blood. If an abscess forms it must be drained, along with proximal and distal ligation of the vein. Anticoagulation to prevent pulmonary embolism is indicated if the response to conservative management is poor.

Deep vein thrombosis. *(Phlebothrombosis).* Deep vein thrombosis is a dangerous condition because the thrombus is much more likely to embolize to the lungs. Half the patients who develop embolism have no symptoms of deep venous disease. Deep vein thrombosis follows any condition where the intima of the vein is damaged (e.g. in trauma), the circulation of the blood is sluggish, (e.g. major operation or debilitating illness), or the blood is rendered more coagulable (e.g. operation). If more than one factor is at work, the chances of thrombosis are greatly increased. Postoperative thrombosis is common in middle-aged and elderly persons, in the obese, and after operations on the hip and those carried out for malignancies.

The thrombosis often starts in a tributary of a main vein, where the circulation is sluggish. When it extends proximally to reach the main vein the faster bloodstream may break off a portion, which lodges in the pulmonary vasculature as a pulmonary embolus. The most common deep veins affected by phlebothrombosis are the pelvic and calf veins.

'White leg' and 'blue leg'. If a length of deep femoral vein gets thrombosed, oedema and painful venous congestion in the lower limb results. If the lymphatics are also inflamed, a more pronounced and persistent swelling results (phlegmasia alba dolens — 'white leg'). If extensive thrombosis of the iliac and pelvic veins occurs, infarction may affect parts of the lower limb (phlegmasia caerulea dolens — 'blue leg').

Diagnosis. ***Clinical.*** Phlebothrombosis may cause no symptoms, except for some pain in the affected calf. A slight fever may raise suspicion. *After extensive major operations the calves should be examined every day for tenderness.* If the foot is passively dorsiflexed, pain in the calf may be complained of – *Homan's sign*. However, this manoeuvre itself can result in a clot getting dislodged and causing pulmonary embolism.

Diagnostic tests. *Venography.* The most specific test for the diagnosis of deep venous thrombosis is venography, in which contrast medium is injected into a vein on the dorsum of the foot to demonstrate the venous drainage through the popliteal, femoral and iliac veins. A normal result nearly always excludes the presence of venous thrombosis. However, venography may itself be complicated by venous thrombosis. At the same time, extravasation of contrast medium may produce cellulitis and skin ulceration. Therefore, patients are often initially screened by a non-invasive technique and undergo venography if the diagnosis remains in doubt.

Doppler. This technique is a practical, non-invasive method of assessment of blood flow in veins. However, it is less accurate in demonstrating thrombotic disease in the calf. When a Doppler (ultrasound) probe is placed over the normal femoral vein in the groin a venous hum is heard due to the flow of blood. If the patient now contracts his calf muscles a roaring sound is heard due to increased flow of blood. If the deep veins are thrombosed between the calf and the groin, the roar does not occur.

Plethysmography is another useful non-invasive technique. A calf plethysmograph measures volume changes and may detect the oedematous changes associated with thrombus formation.

Radioactive fibrinogen is injected intravenously. It gets incorporated into any developing thrombus. The legs are now scanned by a gamma camera to detect the radioactivity. This is a useful non-invasive test for thrombosis in the calf; in the thighs the high background radioactivity from the pelvic bones and urinary bladder makes the test inaccurate. Scanning of the lower limbs shows deep vein thrombosis in as many as half the patients following prostatectomy or surgery for fractured hip, and about a quarter of general surgical patients after the age of 40.

Magnetic resonance imaging is a reliable method of diagnosing venous thrombosis and can demonstrate thrombi in the pelvic veins.

Management of deep vein thrombosis. ***Prevention.*** In susceptible persons precautions against thrombosis must be taken before, during and after surgery.

Before operation. Women taking oral contraceptives are more prone to develop venous thrombosis after operation. Before elective operations these should be stopped a month earlier. If a patient is grossly over-weight it would be best if he reduced his weight. If an elderly patient has been in hospital for lengthy investigations and has become immobile, he should be sent home for a few days for mobilization before readmission for surgery. Heparin in low doses (5,000 i.u. subcutaneously 2 hours before operation, and twice daily for a few days) helps in reducing the incidence of venous thrombosis. However, anticoagulants should be avoided in operations where a raw bleeding area is likely to be left behind.

During operation. Specially during lengthy operations, the pressure of the table on the calf muscles can occlude the deep veins and render the flow of blood sluggish. To prevent this, the heels should be elevated on foam-rubber pads; at the end of the operation the legs should be elevated and massaged.

After operation. If the legs remain immobile after operation or the patient is dehydrated, the incidence of deep vein thrombosis is high. Massage and active leg movements should be prescribed and supervised, and dehydration corrected. The patient should get onto his feet as early as possible. Low dose heparin as described above is also useful. In highly susceptible individuals Dextran may be used due to its property of inhibiting platelet adhesion. 500 ml is given intravenously during the operation and 500 ml during the following 24 hours.

Treatment. If deep vein thrombosis has developed the whole limb should be *bandaged* using crepe bandages, and *bed rest* advised until the local signs subside.

Anticoagulants should be used in full doses, heparin in combination with phenindione being commonly employed. Anticoagulation prevents the propagation of the original thrombus and the development of new thrombi, while the existing thrombus is lysed by naturally occurring fibrinolysis. Intravenous heparin acts rapidly and its effects can be reversed promptly with protamine sulphate to minimize the possibility of bleeding complications.

Although anticoagulation is the treatment of choice, fibrinolytics such as streptokinase and recombinant tissue plasminogen activator have been evaluated. They can lyse upto 70% of thrombi, a feature that anticoagulants lack. However, complications are significant and the routine use of fibrinolytics has been prohibited by bleeding complications, specially in the postoperative setting.

Pulmonary embolism may be prevented by placing a Greenfield or similar filter in the inferior vena cava introduced under x-ray control down the internal jugular vein. This prevents any dislodged thrombus from getting into the right ventricle and pulmonary artery, and yet allows the flow of blood upwards through its interstices.

VENOUS HAEMORRHAGE

If major veins are damaged by trauma or at operation in the neck, groin and specially the pelvis, bleeding can be torrential, and unless skillfully managed can kill the patient by exsanguination. Tight packing is the best immediate measure. With the packing in place the anaesthetist obtains and transfuses sufficient blood for adequate volume replacement. The surgeon exposes veins both above and below the site of injury for control by vascular clamps, the simplest form of which consists of the commonly available small bull-dog clamps. Even if enough room is available for instituting such control, blood may still continue to flow furiously through myriad anastomosing channels, and often requires all the ingenuity that the surgeon can command for a successful outcome.

43 Lymphatics and lymph nodes

Acute lymphangitis. Acute lymphangitis is said to be present when lymphatic vessels are inflamed. This occurs when, from a focus of infection, bacteria spread proximally along these vessels. It is seen as red streaks in the skin along the course of the lymphatics. Treatment consists of bed rest, elevation of the affected limb, and the use of cloxacillin. Rapid resolution normally occurs. However, if pus forms it has to be drained.

LYMPHOEDEMA

Lymphoedema is defined as the excessive accumulation of interstitial fluid as a result of defective lymphatic drainage. The condition is subdivided into primary and secondary lymphoedema, the latter being much the more common. The different types of lymphoedema are listed in Table 1.

Primary. ***Hypoplastic*** cases constitute 92 percent of these patients. Cases with *distal* hypoplasia are mild and non-progressive. They are seen in young women after puberty. Those with *proximal* hypoplasia have more extensive lymphoedema involving the whole extremity, occurring equally among males and females. *Proximal plus distal* hypoplasia is also progressive.

Hyperplastic cases are uncommon (8 percent). Lymphography shows dilated lymphatics, and in the megalymphatic group there are no valves.

Secondary lymphoedema is most often due to *malignant* disease metastatic to lymph nodes. Surgical *removal* of nodes, specially when combined with radiation, is another common cause.

Filariasis. In parts of Africa, South America and India, filariasis is the most common cause of lymphoedema. The worm enters the lymphatics and lodges in the lymph nodes where a severe fibrotic reaction causes obstruction to the lymphatic pathways which are grossly dilated. This results in severe swelling of the lower limbs called 'elephantiasis'. The diagnosis is confirmed by finding microfilariae. As these enter the blood in large numbers at night, the blood sample should be taken at midnight. A strongly positive complement fixation test suggests active or past filariasis. Treatment with diethylcarbamazine destroys the microfilariae but cannot reverse established lymphoedema; progression of the disease may, however, be slowed or prevented. Established lymphoedema is treated by the same methods as primary lymphoedema.

Table 1 The different types of lymphoedema.

1. Primary lymphoedema
   i. Hypoplasia
      (a). Distal
      (b). Proximal
      (c). Proximal and distal
   ii. Hyperplasia
      (a). Bilateral
      (b). Megalymphatic
2. Secondary lymphoedema: due to
   Malignancy, radiation
   Trauma or excision
   Inflammation, filariasis
   Paralysis.

Investigations. ***Lymphangiography.*** *Isotope lymphangiography.* This is today the primary diagnostic technique. Rhenium sulphur colloid is specifically taken up by lymphatics and allows the presence of lymphoedema to be confirmed as an outpatient procedure. Normally, 0.6 percent of the dose arrives at the groin within 1 hour. Gamma camera pictures provide information that the isotope is reaching the groin lymph nodes; later images may show a failure of progression, indicating proximal obstruction. This should be confirmed by contrast lymphangiography. *Contrast lymphangiography* is the definitive investigative technique for lymphoedema. It is required to confirm the diagnosis and determine the type of lymphatic abnormality present. It provides information on the presence of hypoplasia, megalymphatics and obstruction. It helps guide therapy and assess prognosis.

Ultrasound, CT and *MRI* can all show enlarged lymph nodes, and guided *biopsies* of nodes can be taken if malignancy is suspected. Needle or Tru-cut biopsies are probably preferable, since removal of large fibrotic nodes may worsen pre-existing lymphoedema. To rule out renal and hepatic causes, serum creatinine level and liver function tests should be obtained in all cases.

Treatment. Young women with distal hypoplasia can be managed by limb elevation, massage and elastic compression stockings. Stockings are poorly tolerated in warm climates and women tend to be conscious of their appearance. Antibiotics should be used for cellulitis, as well as prophylactically in low doses if the patient is troubled by repeated attacks.

Surgery. Surgical treatment is appropriate for whole limb lymphoedema that interferes with mobility or results in severe deformity. The lymphatic obstruction may be bypassed or the oedematous subcutaneous tissues excised.

Reduction operations are employed in most cases. The most popular is the Charles operation. All diseased skin and waterlogged subcutaneous tissue down to and including the deep fascia are excised from the ankle to the knee, and split skin grafts, taken from the normal opposite thigh and other sites, are used to cover the muscle.

Lymphatic bypass. In a few patients in whom lymphangiography shows proximal lymphatic obstruction with normal distal lymphatics, the ingenious operation of *mesenteric bridge bypass* has shown the best results. About 5 cm of terminal ileum is isolated on its mesenteric pedicle, reanastomosing the small bowel behind the pedicle. The gut segment is opened along its antimesenteric border and the mucosa stripped off the submucosa. The isolated segment is brought down to the first normal group of lymph nodes below the level of the obstruction and sutured over them after they have been bivalved. Connections develop between the divided nodes and the submucosal plexus and lymph drains up the pedicle into the mesenteric lymph nodes. The operation has produced good results in more than half the patients operated upon.

LYMPHANGIOMA

A cavernous lymphangioma (cystic hygroma) is seen in newborns as collections of lymphatic cysts in the neck or axilla. It is described in the chapter 47 dealing with conditions of the neck.

LYMPHADENITIS

Acute lymphadenitis results when a lymph node draining any area of infection becomes acutely inflamed. The node may suppurate and discharge pus. Treatment is on the usual lines for acute pyogenic infection, including incision and drainage where indicated.

CHRONIC LYMPHADENITIS

Chronic lymphadenitis may be simple (pyogenic) or specific. The common type of specific lymphadenitis arises due to tuberculosis.

Chronic pyogenic lymphadenitis occurs if a persistent focus of infection is present in the area of drainage of the lymph node, e.g. recurrent tonsillitis, or multiple boils in the scalp or over the legs. Treatment requires eradication of the primary septic focus, when the lymph node enlargement subsides.

TUBERCULOUS LYMPHADENITIS

Tuberculous lymphadenitis is by far the most common form of chronic lymphadenitis. Although uncommon in the developed countries due to universal pasteurization of milk, it is still a major health problem in some parts of the world. It is common among children in regions where BCG inoculation is not universal. Lymph nodes of the neck are the most common site of this infection, the reason being that the orifices affording inlet to both the respiratory and alimentary tracts are located in this area, and a large number of lymph nodes guard these portals of entry. The infection is acquired either by contact with cases of open human tuberculosis, or by drinking infected milk.

Evidence of past disease may be seen in the mediastinal and mesenteric lymph nodes in the form of specks of calcification on routine x-rays of the chest and abdomen respectively. Tubercle bacilli reach the node via lymphatics, therefore most of the early tubercles are seen in the cortex. Microscopically lymphocytes, monocytes and giant cells are seen.

If the disease spreads, many lymph nodes are affected. *When infection spreads out through the capsule, adjacent nodes may get matted together,* and this feature helps distinguish tuberculosis from Hodgkin's lymphoma and other causes of lymph node enlargement. The inflamed nodes may break down to form caseous tuberculous pus, which may perforate the deep fascia and present as a fluctuant swelling on the surface. Finally, the skin may break down resulting in a sinus. When healing occurs, a good deal of scarring is produced; in cases with caseation calcification may also be seen.

Investigations. These fall into two categories, the general and the specific.

General. These are helpful but *not diagnostic*. The *differential leucocyte count* may show a lymphocytosis. The erythrocyte sedimentation rate *(ESR)* helps in following up the course of the disease. The *Mantoux* reaction is a test of delayed hypersensitivity to tuberculin. Induration over an area of 10 mm or more across is taken as a positive Mantoux test, and is seen in nearly 80% of the cases. A chest x-ray helps in detecting healed pulmonary tuberculosis (fibrosis or calcification), or coexisting active pulmonary tuberculosis.

Specific. These are *diagnostic* of tuberculous lymphadenitis.

1. *Bacteriological examination.* Slides are made from pus or lymph node imprints and stained with Ziehl Neelsen stains. The tubercle bacilli appear red. The only confirmatory proof of tuberculosis is the isolation of Mycobacterium tuberculosis from the pus or lymph node. Mycobacteria are cultured on Lowenstein-Jensen medium and examined weekly for 8 weeks. Colonies usually appear in 3 to 4 weeks' time. By using a new medium, Middlebrook 7H12, mycobacteria can be isolated within 9 days.
2. *Histopathological examination.* This includes histopathology of the lymph nodes and of the walls of any cold abscess. Histopathology is diagnostic in 98% of cases. A granuloma characterized by epithelioid cells and giant cells of the Langhan's type, with central caseation and a peripheral rim of lymphocytes along with fibroblasts, is characteristic of tuberculosis.
3. *Guinea pig inoculation.*
4. *Biochemical tests* for different mycobacteria.
5. *Serological tests:*
   i. Elisa.
   ii. Radioimmunoassay.
   iii. Flourescent antibody test.

Fine needle aspiration is a useful tool for getting material for the diagnosis of tuberculous lymphadenitis. The diagnostic accuracy rate is 96%.

Treatment. General measures like good nutrition, hygienic living conditions and fresh air are helpful, but the mainstay of treatment is drug therapy. Surgery has a limited role to play in the treatment of this condition.

Drug therapy. As in the case of tuberculosis anywhere else in the body, lymph node tuberculosis is treated by multiple drug therapy. The commonly used drugs are the following:

1. Rifampicin: this is a bactericidal drug used in a dose of 10 mg/kg/day as a single dose. The usual adult dose is 600 mg/day. The main adverse effect is hepatitis.

2. Isoniazid (INH): this is a bactericidal drug given in a dose of 5 mg/kg/day. The usual adult dose is 300 mg/day. There is a risk of peripheral neuropathy with this drug; to prevent this, pyridoxin 25 mg/day is used.

3. Ethambutol: this is a bacteriostatic agent. The usual dose is 15 to 20 mg/kg/day. The main side effect is optic neuritis, and vision should be checked at frequent intervals.

4. Pyrazinamide (PZA): pyrazinamide is a bactericidal drug. The dose is 20 to 30 mg/kg/day, the adult dose being 1.2–2 G/day.

5. Streptomycin: streptomycin is an aminoglycoside which is available in injectable form. The dosage is 10 to 15 mg/kg/day, the usual adult dose being 0.75 to 1 G/day i.m. The main side effects are nephrotoxicity and ototoxicity.

Different combinations of drugs have been used in different regimens. This has reduced the duration of treatment from 2 years to 6 months. The regimens commonly employed at present are the following:

1. Rifampicin + INH + streptomycin + PZA daily for two months, then rifampicin and INH for four months.

2. Rifampicin + INH + ethambutol + PZA for 4 months, then rifampicin + INH for 4 months

Response to treatment is assessed by examining the size of the lymph nodes and by determination of ESR.

Surgery. With the introduction of effective antituberculosis therapy, the role of surgery has become quite limited. Nowadays, surgery is most often needed for *excisional biopsy of lymph nodes* for diagnosis. The other indications for surgery include the following:

1. *Failure to respond* to medical treatment: the involved groups of lymph nodes are removed.

2. Persistent discharging *sinus:* the sinus tracts with the underlying diseased lymph nodes are excised en bloc.

3. *Cold abscesses.* Large cold abscesses not responding to drug treatment should be managed by one of the following methods:

i. Repeated aspirations with injections of streptomycin into the abscess cavity.

ii. Opening the abscess cavity, curettage of all granulation tissue, and closure of the cavity without drainage: this differs from incision-drainage of 'hot' abscesses, in which the abscess cavity after drainage is left open or drained. If that course is followed here, the incidence of secondary infection with pyogenic organisms is high.

Before any of the surgical procedures is undertaken, antituberculosis drugs are administered for at least a week or two to minimize bacteraemia during and after the operation.

Post-BCG lymphadenitis. Occasionally the bacilli in a batch of BCG vaccine are not sufficiently attenuated, and a large number of infants develop lymphadenitis. When the inoculation is given over the deltoid, as is the common practice, one of the lymph nodes in the anterior (pectoral) group of lymph nodes enlarges. The node sometimes liquefies. The baby commonly remains well. If the node is small it can be observed. If large, and specially if it has liquefied, single-drug therapy with isoniazid is considered legitimate. However, in the odd case in which spreading infection develops, multiple-drug therapy is required. Some workers have had better success with removal of the lymph node involved.

LYMPHOMAS

Lymphomas arise from the different types of stem cells (B cell, T cell or histiocyte). In common with other neoplasms, the less histologically differentiated they are, the more rapidly they grow. They can be divided into Hodgkin's lymphoma (Hodgkin's disease) and non-Hodgkin's lymphomas.

HODGKIN'S LYMPHOMA

Hodgkin's disease is the most common type of lymphoma, and can occur wherever there is lymphoid tissue. On section the nodes are pinkish grey in colour and rubbery in consistency. Unlike tubercular lymph nodes they remain discrete. The only exceptions to this rule are seen in some anaplastic forms of Hodgkin's disease. The spleen gets diffusely enlarged. Bone deposits occur in the bones with red marrow, specially the vertebral column and pelvis.

The histological appearance varies, but a constant feature is cellular pleomorphism. Four pathological sub-types of Hodgkin's disease are described: lymphocyte predominance, nodular sclerosis, mixed cellularity and lymphocytic depletion. The first two sub-types are associated with the best prognosis, the last sub-type with the worst outcome. The nature of Hodgkin's lymphoma is disputed. The Reed-Sternberg cells (with mirror-image double nuclei) which are so typical of Hodgkin's disease are also seen in other conditions, notably glandular fever. It is thought that the condition represents an immunological reaction. A few cases may be due to Epstein-Barr virus as the incidence is increased 10 to 20 years after an attack of infectious mononucleosis, and the virus is sometimes found in the malignant cells.

Clinical features. Hodgkin's disease is more common in males. Two peaks of incidence occur, one in young adults and the other which becomes slowly more common with increasing age. A painless and progressive enlargement of the lymph nodes commences in the neck usually without, but sometimes with, constitutional symptoms e.g. malaise, fever and weight loss. Enlarged mediastinal nodes may obstruct the superior vena cava and produce marked congestion in the neck veins. A vertebra may collapse due to bony metastases and result in bone pain.

As stated above the lymph nodes are discrete, except in late or anaplastic cases. The spleen and liver may be enlarged. Later, irregular fever often develops. When the disease becomes disseminated, anaemia and pancytopenia may occur. The disease usually progresses quite slowly, but occasionally follows a rapid course.

Clinical staging. Clinical staging of Hodgkin's lymphoma helps greatly in deciding upon the correct line of treatment. The condition is divided into four stages as shown in Table 2.

Investigations. When the disease is suspected a chest x-ray is ordered to exclude mediastinal node enlargement, and an abdominal ultrasound to detect involvement of the para-aortic lymph nodes, spleen and liver. A CT scan can be used for the same purpose. Excision-biopsy of a lymph node is now carried out to establish the diagnosis, and for accurate histological grading.

Table 2 The stages of Hodgkin's disease.

I	Confined to one lymph node group
II	Affecting two or more lymph node areas, but restricted to one side of the diaphragm
III	Involving lymph nodes both above and below the diaphragm (the spleen is considered a lymph node)
IV	Spread beyond the lymph nodes, e.g. to bone marrow, liver

(Each stage is further subdivided into subgroups A and B according to the absence or presence of associated generalized symptoms such as weight loss, fever, pruritus, anaemia and bone pain.)

Other investigations include mediastinal scanning with Gallium 67 to demonstrate involved mediastinal nodes, and intravenous pyelography to show compression of the renal calyces by retroperitoneal lymph nodes. Lower limb lymphangiograms to demonstrate pelvic and retroperitoneal lymph nodes, and laparotomy for the purpose of staging Hodgkin's disease (staging laparotomy), are required less often since the advent of ultrasound and CT scans, because most of the information is provided by these modern investigative methods.

Treatment. Both radiotherapy and chemotherapy are available for the treatment of Hodgkin's disease. Since both methods can cause bone marrow depression and other toxic side effects, treatment must be very carefully planned, with regular blood counts.

Radiotherapy is the treatment of choice in stages I, II and III-A, combination chemotherapy in stages III-B and IV. Supradiaphragmatic disease is treated by radiotherapy to cervical, axillary and mediastinal nodes, infradiaphragmatic disease by irradiation of the para-aortic and iliac nodes.

Chemotherapeutic agents are given in combination, as their clinical effects are summated but side effects are not. Repeated courses of cytotoxic drugs plus steroids are employed. A popular combination consists of nitrogen mustard, vinblastine (Oncovin), procarbazine and prednisone (called MOPP for short).

In the latest regimen doxorubicin, bleomycin, vinblastine and dacarbazine are also added, in a combination which alternates with MOPP, the side-effects of treatment being further reduced. This technique is referred to as a 'HYBRID' programme. Treatment can usually be given on an outpatient basis and most people are able to lead a normal life.

With the development of highly effective chemotherapy and radiotherapy, there is a limited role for ***surgery*** in lymphomas. *Biopsy* examination is necessary for diagnosis and histological typing. *Splenectomy* in children carries the risk of overwhelming sepsis, most often due to encapsulated cocci (*Streptococcus pneumoniae, Haemophilus infuenzae*). If splenectomy is employed, long-term prophylactic antibiotics and pneumococcal vaccination should be given to these patients.

Interestingly, while 'staging laparotomy' is being used less often, a 'restaging laparotomy' has been proposed, to accurately document residual or recurrent disease, because negative findings would spare the patient further toxic therapy, without compromising his chances of survival.

Results. In early cases a 5 year survival rate of 80% can be achieved by radiotherapy. Even in stage III cases which require the addition of chemotherapy, 50% of cases can survive 5 years. This is a far better situation from that which prevailed a couple of decades earlier.

NON-HODGKIN'S LYMPHOMAS

Non-Hodgkin's lymphomas (NHL) consist of a group of primary malignancies of lymphoreticular tissue. Most of them are monoclonal B-cell tumours. Their clinical course is more variable than that of Hodgkin's disease, the pattern of spread is irregular, and more patients have leukaemic features. They are classified into nodular (favourable) and diffuse (unfavourable) types.

Clinical features. Non-Hodgkin's lymphomas generally affect persons older than those suffering from Hodgkin's disease, the median age of onset being 50 years. In contrast to Hodgkin's disease only about two thirds of patients with NHL have asymptomatic *lymphadenopathy* ; in the rest of the patients the onset of NHL occurs at a site other than a lymph node, commonly as an abdominal mass or a hepatic or splenic enlargement. *Constitutional symptoms* such as fever, night sweats and weight loss are often present. Occasionally, the patient first presents as an *emergency* with superior vena caval syndrome, spinal cord compression, or ureteral obstruction from retroperitoneal node involvement.

Spread. In non-Hodgkin's lymphoma the mode of spread is generally more unpredictable than in Hodgkin's disease, and most patients have disseminated disease when they present, because NHL can rapidly spread to distal nodal and extranodal sites through the bloodstream. This extranodal spread of NHL is comparable with the pattern of metastasis seen in carcinomas.

Treatment. As with Hodgkin's disease, chemotherapy and/or radiotherapy are the mainstays of treatment. Because most patients with NHL have disseminated disease at the time of presentation, chemotherapy has a greater role to play than radiotherapy. The prognosis is more favourable for the nodular than for the diffuse forms of NHL.

Section 6

Head and neck, endocrines, etc.

44 *Brain*

Head injuries

Head injuries are responsible for a great deal of morbidity and mortality. Among children between the ages of 1 and 15 they constitute the most common cause of death. At the same time, many survivors of head injuries are severely handicapped. Although they may appear normal, the loss of some of the higher intellectual abilities responsible for tact and judgement make them difficult to live with.

Patients with head injuries are at many places looked after by general surgeons rather than neurosurgeons, therefore the general surgeon should have a knowledge of the principles and practice in this field. Most patients do not require any neurosurgery but only medical and nursing measures. However, the surgeon must know when specialized investigations at a neurosurgical centre are required. At the same time, CT scan facilities are becoming available at increasing numbers of hospitals. The surgeon should be in a position to decide that an extradural haematoma disclosed by the scan will not brook the delay involved in transfer to a neurosurgical unit, and should be able to evacuate it.

INJURIES TO THE BRAIN

Pathology. All degrees of brain injury result from displacement and distortion of the brain *at the time of impact.* At that moment a diffuse injury to the nerve cells occurs, which causes the immediate clinical picture of brain injury. The *secondary changes* include *oedema* and *intracranial haemorrhage*, and these take time to develop. The rise in pressure resulting from the secondary changes produces a deterioration in the level of the patient's consciousness a few hours after injury. On the other hand the clinical picture in the early stages results from the neuronal lesion alone. The important factors determining the severity of brain injury are the following:

1. *Distortion of the brain.* The brain has some mobility inside the skull because of the presence of cerebrospinal fluid around it. The severe distortion which results may produce widespread damage to neurones, nerve fibres and blood vessels. This distortion causes sudden loss of consciousness. If it produces significant damage to nerve cells, persisting loss of consciousness and possibly focal neurological deficit may occur. The distortion may also damage the midbrain, the cells of which are responsible for normal consciousness by activating the cortex. Thus there may be prolonged unconsciousness without any evidence of injury to the skull.

2. *Deceleration and acceleration.* In most traffic accidents the moving head strikes a stationary object, e.g. the road. There is rapid deceleration of the skull. The brain continues to move and suffers distortion. On the other hand in cases of assault the stationary skull is struck by a moving object and rapidly accelerates.

The extent of damage. In cerebral ***concussion*** the damage is slight. There is only a brief physiological paralysis without structural damage. Transient unconsciousness occurs, followed by complete recovery.

Post-traumatic amnesia. The essential feature of concussion is amnesia for the blow; the patient who can clearly recollect the blow has no concussion. The length of time the patient is amnesic after the blow is called post-traumatic amnesia, and this is the best indicator of the severity of the concussion. Post-traumatic amnesia extends until the patient has continuous memory for who he is, what time it is, and where he is, i.e. 'for person, time and place'. Post-traumatic amnesia is constant and does not recede with time, unlike retrograde amnesia.

'Post-concussional syndrome'. Many patients suffer from this condition, consisting of headache, irritability, depression and vertigo. It is more common after minor concussion, probably because patients return to work too soon. A concussive blow must by definition be followed by full recovery. More severe injuries can cause severe concussion which merges with permanent brain damage.

In cerebral ***contusion*** there is more severe damage, including bruising of grey matter, oedema, damage to nerve cells and fibres, and haemorrhage. In cerebral ***laceration***, in addition to the above changes the brain surface is torn, with haemorrhage into the cerebrospinal fluid.

ACUTE INTRACRANIAL HAEMATOMAS

As a result of the head injury, blood may collect outside the dura, underneath the dura, in the subarachnoid space, or in the brain substance.

Acute extradural haematoma. Extradural haemorrhage commonly follows injury to the anterior branch of the middle meningeal artery, which occurs when a blow on the side of the head results in a fracture of the temporal bone. *If such a fracture is seen on x-ray the patient must be admitted for observation.* Blood passing outwards through the fracture line produces a swelling deep to the temporal muscle. If such a swelling is present, even a conscious patient must be admitted for observation.

Clinical features. A moderate blow to the side of the head produces a short period of concussion, and then the patient regains consciousness – the *lucid interval.* During this time blood is collecting inside the skull and also under the temporalis muscle. After a period of consciousness the patient becomes confused and irritable. Drowsiness follows confusion. The clot presses on the motor cortex producing first twitching and later paralysis of the face, the arm, and then the leg on the opposite side of the body, as the clot spreads upwards. The temporal lobe is pushed inwards and compresses the third nerve. This causes constriction followed by dilatation of the pupil on the same side. The brain stem gets displaced and the opposite crus is pushed against the rim of the tentorium producing hemiplegia, this time on the side of the haemorrhage. *It should be remembered that the level of consciousness deteriorates only late, and then rapidly.*

Finally, increasing pressure inside the skull forces the midbrain downwards, and impaction of a midbrain cone causes decerebrate rigidity and fixed dilatation of both pupils, when it is probably too late to do anything. It should also be remembered that the 'lucid interval' does not always occur. If an extradural haematoma forms in a patient already unconscious from cerebral contusion, there is no lucid interval.

Acute subdural haematoma. If the skull is struck on the front or the back and the brain moves inside the skull the superior cerebral veins, which end in the superior sagittal sinus, may be ruptured where they cross the subdural space and produce a subdural haematoma. The *clinical features* of subdural haematoma resemble those of extradural haematoma. However, there are differences. In the former, there is usually severe brain damage and persisting loss of consciousness without a lucid interval. In the elderly an acute subdural haematoma may follow a trivial injury. A CT scan is required for accurate diagnosis and surgery.

Acute intracerebral haematoma. This is uncommon. Usually cerebral laceration, contusion, oedema and necrosis occur at the same time, compression being due to all these combined.

SECONDARY PATHOLOGICAL CHANGES

Apart from the trauma inflicted on the brain at the moment of impact, certain secondary pathological changes take place later, which may result in a further deterioration in the patient's condition. These changes include brain oedema and respiratory failure.

Brain oedema. The brain swells in response to any insult. The factors producing brain oedema include the following:

1. Hypotension or hypoxia can produce ischaemia, resulting in cell death and consequent cytotoxic oedema.
2. Contamination of CSF with blood can disrupt CSF absorption and lead to hydrocephalus.
3. Inappropriate secretion of antidiuretic hormone or the development of diabetic insipidus can alter fluid and electrolyte balance and aggravate cerebral oedema.

The above changes separately or in combination can result in elevation of intracranial pressure.

Now, the cerebral perfusion pressure is the difference between mean arterial blood pressure and intracranial pressure. Thus, if the blood pressure remains unchanged, any rise in the intracranial pressure decreases the cerebral perfusion pressure; when the latter falls below 50 mm Hg, cerebral perfusion is compromised. The resultant ischaemia produces further brain oedema. Thus a vicious circle is produced leading to increasing intracranial pressure, a deteriorating level of consciousness, and finally, irreversible damage to the brain.

If pressure in the supratentorial compartment continues to rise, the medial side of the temporal lobe herniates down through the tentorial opening and presses on the third cranial nerve. Also, it displaces the midbrain to the contralateral side, so that the opposite cerebral peduncle is indented by the free edge of the tentorium. Compression of the midbrain also blocks the flow of cerebrospinal fluid in the aqueduct which further raises the intracranial pressure. Thus the level of consciousness deteriorates, and on the same side as the compressing mass the pupil dilates and hemiparesis sets in.

Injury to the brain may occur either on the side of the blow to the head (coup), or on the opposite side (contrecoup).

Respiratory failure. Damage to the brain (and specially the brain stem) due to contusion, laceration, haematoma, or the resultant oedema, may produce respiratory failure. This in turn causes more brain oedema leading to irreversible changes. However, hyperventilation should not be employed, because this washes out CO_2, and a low pCO_2 reduces cerebral blood flow and produces ischaemic damage.

Measures to minimize damage. These include the following:

1. Because the brain is at risk from ischaemic damage following injury, a normal *cardiac output* must be maintained.
2. *Hypotonic* fluids should be avoided, because they may be drawn into the cerebral tissue and brain swelling increased.
3. A rise in body *temperature* increases the metabolic demands of tissues and causes a deterioration in the neurological state. In certain cases hypothermia may have to be employed to protect the brain from damage.

MANAGEMENT

Initial management. The attending doctor has four duties when faced with a case of head injury. These are known as the ABCD of head injuries: The **A**irway should be maintained. **B**aseline observations should be made. **C**omplications should be anticipated, and future action should be **D**etermined.

Airway. The most urgent and immediate duty is to clear and maintain the airway. Loose teeth, blood and vomit must be removed and the airway maintained by laying the patient semiprone, with the foot of the bed raised and an airway inserted. If the cough reflex is absent a cuffed endotracheal tube is required to prevent aspiration of saliva.

Baseline observations must be made as soon as possible, so that any change of intracranial pressure can be appreciated. A careful *history* should be taken to ensure that conditions such as diabetic coma, subarachnoid haemorrhage or epilepsy have not caused the patient to fall, the head injury being a secondary event. *The level of consciousness* must be determined by the response of the patient to various stimuli defined by the Glasgow Coma Scale (Table 1). These parameters should be employed rather than ill-defined levels of consciousness which mean different things to different people. If the patient is conscious, the length of amnesia before and after the accident must be assessed, as its duration is proportional to the severity of

Table 1 Glasgow Coma Scale.
The following parameters are recorded at regular intervals:

	Score
Eye opening	
Spontaneous	4
To speech	3
To pain	2
None	1
Verbal response	
Orientated	5
Confused	4
Inappropriate words	3
Incomprehensible sounds	2
None	1
Motor response	
Obeys command	6
Localizes pain	5
Withdraws to pain	4
Flexes to pain	3
Extension to pain	2
None	1
Total score	
Normal	15
Impaired consciousness	9–14
Coma	3–8
The Coma Score is the sum total of the sectional scores	

Author's comment. The Glasgow Coma Scale is extremely valuable. However, it would be better if the numbering was in the reverse direction, i.e. if the numbers increased with increasing unconsciousness. In that case one would not have to list them as 4, 3, 2, 1 but as 1 to 4, which would be more convenient.

the head injury. The *pulse, blood pressure, respiratory rate, temperature,* and size and reaction of the *pupils* should be measured half-hourly.

Complications must be anticipated.

Future action must now be ***determined***, about whether x-rays or CT scans are required, whether the patient needs to be admitted, and whether a neurosurgical consultation is called for.

Skull x-rays are required in the following situations:

1. Loss of consciousness, or amnesia.
2. Suspected fracture.
3. CSF or blood from ear or nose.
4. Neurological symptoms and signs.
5. Difficulty in assessing the patient, e.g. if he is very young or drunk.

Anteroposterior and lateral x-rays of the skull are taken to show the site of a fissured or depressed fracture or lateral displacement of a calcified pineal gland. A lateral x-ray of the cervical spine is also essential. If the patient needs immediate intensive care, x-rays may be postponed.

Admission is recommended in the following circumstances:

1. Confusion or impaired level of consciousness.
2. Skull fracture.
3. Neurological symptoms and signs, e.g. headache, vomiting, seizures etc.
4. Difficulty in assessing the patient.
5. Difficult social or medical circumstances, e.g. no responsible adult with the patient.

In most cases overnight admission for observation is sufficient.

CT scan and *neurosurgical consultation* are indicated in cases with:

1. Skull fracture with confusion, focal neurological signs, or seizures.
2. Depressed skull fracture.
3. Penetrating fracture with leakage of CSF.
4. Persistent confusion without skull fracture.
5. Deterioration of level of consciousness.

The *most common cause of deterioration*, shown by a declining level of consciousness, is raised intracranial pressure due to an intracranial haematoma, brain oedema, or airway obstruction (which itself leads to brain oedema). Other causes include epilepsy, fever and blood loss from other injuries.

The further course of action depends upon whether a CT scan is available or not.

A. *CT scan is available.* 1. If the CT scan is *normal* and physical examination shows no neurological deficit, the patient may be kept overnight or discharged. If he is allowed home, an accompanying person should be instructed to awaken the patient frequently over the next 24 hours to be certain that he remains arousable. Any deterioration in the level of consciousness should prompt re-evaluation.

2. If the CT scan shows an *extradural* haematoma, urgent craniotomy is indicated. The journey to the neurosurgical center can be hazardous, and the surgeon could decide to evacuate the haematoma before shifting the patient.

Evacuation of haematoma. If such a course is adopted, the appropriate side of the scalp is shaved. No local anaesthetic is usually necessary. A 5 cm incision is made over the clot as shown by the CT scan; this is usually in the temporal region just above the zygomatic arch. The incision is made right down to bone. A mastoid retractor is now placed in position and will stop the scalp bleeding. The skull is just perforated using a perforator. This creates a conical hole and dark blood will ooze out. The hole is enlarged using a burr, when the hole becomes cylindrical and blood clot immediately bulges out. The clot is sucked away by a sucker which should, however, not be inserted into the cavity, as this can cause more bleeding as well as damage the brain. The patient can now be transferred to the neurosurgical service.

B. *CT scan is not available.* Here the decision about the best course of action will be more difficult. A feasible method would be to describe the findings of the history and physical examination to the neurosurgeon on the phone and seek his guidance according to the circumstances. The side of the haematoma may be decided by the shift of a calcified pineal gland on anteroposterior x-ray, and the side of the first pupil to dilate. The position of an exploratory burr hole is decided according to the site of the external injury and the site of the skull fracture.

Postoperative management. After removal of any traumatic intracranial mass, the aim of management is to normalize the cerebral perfusion pressure and prevent secondary injury to the damaged brain. Intracranial pressure (ICP) monitoring may be indicated, specially in patients with marked depression or deterioration in neurological function. Because frequent examinations are not possible under general anaesthesia, comatose patients who require emergency abdominal, thoracic or orthopaedic surgery should also have ICP monitoring. The following steps are also helpful:

1. Head elevation facilitates venous drainage and reduces the intracranial pressure.
2. Sedation reduces combative activity which elevates intracranial pressure.
3. Prophylactic use of anticonvulsants prevents cerebral injury from seizures.
4. Mild dehydration protects the brain from insult due to fluid overload.
5. Prevention of hypotension reduces the extension of ischaemic injury. On the other hand aggressive treatment of hypertensive episodes reduces cerebral blood volume and further disruption of the blood-brain barrier.
6. Treatment of hyperthermia avoids an increase in metabolic demands.

If intracranial pressure remains high despite these measures, *mannitol* (0.5 to 1.0 g/kg) can be used to reduce it. Mannitol is an osmotic diuretic which reduces brain swelling by drawing fluid from the extravascular spaces of the brain into the blood due to increase in the osmolality of the plasma. The kidney function must be good. If diuresis does not occur, further administration is delayed. *Furosemide* (0.1 mg/kg) can be used to supplement the action of mannitol; alone it is less effective.

Deep sedation with *narcotics* may be useful. Finally, there is no evidence that *corticosteroids* improve the outlook in severe head injury.

Nursing care. The nursing care of an unconscious patient is very detailed. Every physiological function of the body has to be supervised and aided. The eyes remain open, so they must be protected by bland ointments. A condom catheter obviates the necessity of passing a catheter into the bladder, yet the patient can be kept dry. Nasogastric tube feeding or intravenous infusions are necessary. Constipation develops, due to the small amount of residue which can be given to an unconscious patient in his diet; this requires management with enemas. The limb joints are put through their full range of movements daily, to prevent stiffness and contractures. If a tracheostomy has been performed, it requires to be taken care of; however, it is not often carried out, because an endotracheal tube may be used for upto a week.

FRACTURES OF THE SKULL

These are produced by two types of violence:

1. Compression of the whole skull when it is distorted by hitting a hard, flat surface. This is the most common type of skull fracture.
2. Local indentation, i.e. a depressed fracture.

Depressed fractures. A depressed fracture may result after a blow from two types of objects:

1. *A large round object.* A closed depression results. The brain is bruised but not penetrated. When the injury to the brain heals, the fibrous tissue in the scar may irritate the underlying brain and result in epilepsy. However, with this type of blow the chances of inciting epilepsy are low, being only about 4%.
2. *A small round object.* A compound depressed fracture results. The scalp is torn. The fractured bone lacerates the dura and brain. Infection may result. Epilepsy occurs in as many as 25% of these cases.

A haematoma in the scalp may simulate a depressed fracture, because clotted blood at the margin of the haematoma may feel like the edge of a depressed area. An x-ray may be required for differentiation.

Treatment of a depressed fracture. Operation is required if the fracture overlies the speech or motor areas, or if bone fragments have penetrated the dura mater. A flap of skull and overlying muscle is raised. The depressed bone is raised into position. The dura is opened. Bone fragments are carefully picked out. Removal of pulped brain is best carried out by irrigation with a stream of normal saline from a nozzle.

Pond shaped depressions may occur in the *newborn* due to prolonged pressure of the head against the sacral promontory. Spontaneous elevation occurs within a few weeks; otherwise the fracture is elevated by making a small hole in the skull and hooking it up with an aneurysm needle introduced through the opening.

Compound fractures of the vault. These may be very severe, with escape of brain substance, and are commonly sustained as a result of high-speed motorcycle accidents. Crash helmets have helped reduce their incidence. Only skull x-rays give accurate information; probing of scalp wounds is dangerous.

Fractures of the base of the skull. These are produced by compression of the skull with fissures radiating down from the vault. They become compound by opening into the middle ear, cribriform plate, or the different air sinuses.

Clinical features. The cranial contents i.e. cerebrospinal fluid or blood may escape from the ear or nose, and the cranial nerves may be damaged. *Paralysis* of nerves may occur immediately. If the paralysis recovers within a few weeks it suggests that it was due to compression from blood clot. If it does not recover, the cause was probably laceration of the nerve. If paralysis appears a few weeks after the injury, it means it has resulted from a scar or callus, and will not recover.

Epistaxis indicates the presence of a fracture of the cribriform plate. If the fracture extends into the roof of the orbit a *subconjunctival haemorrhage* results, the patch being wedge-shaped with the apex in front. Such a haemorrhage has to be distinguished from a 'black eye' resulting from a direct blow on the eye. In the case of a subconjunctival haemorrhage resulting from a fracture of the base of the skull, as the blood comes forwards from inside the orbit, the posterior limit of the haematoma cannot be seen (Plate V-I); in the case of a black eye there is an area of white sclera behind it. Blood from the *ear* clots. If it does not, it is probable that it is mixed with cerebrospinal fluid, i.e. that a fracture into the roof of the middle ear is present.

LATE EFFECTS OF HEAD INJURY

Chronic subdural 'haematoma'. Chronic subdural haematoma usually develops after a blow to the front or back of the head. Due to displacement of the brain inside the skull, veins passing from the cerebral hemispheres to the superior sagittal sinus may rupture at the point where they cross the subdural space. A haematoma collects in this space. The fluid gradually becomes thinner and lighter in colour, and resembles cerebrospinal fluid (CSF). Recently it has been suggested that the fluid is CSF from the start, and that it collects in the subdural space due to a tear in the arachnoid matter and not a vein, i.e. that it is a subdural hygroma and not a haematoma.

Clinical features. Even a slight blow to the front or back of the skull may produce this lesion, so the patient may not have become unconscious at all, and this is a point which should be kept in mind. There is mental apathy going on to slowness of response to questions, and finally stupor. The stupor comes and goes, because the volume of the brain varies from time to time. The patient is inaccessible at times, but rouses to answer questions correctly though very slowly. Early diagnosis is important, because when stupor sets in the operative mortality rises sharply, to 30%.

There may be no physical *signs*, specially in older patients, because by that age the brain shrinks in size, so that there is more room for the fluid to collect. There may be only an extensor plantar response on one or both sides. Changes in the size of the pupil occur late, when pressure-cone formation is about to occur. X-ray of the skull for the position of a calcified pineal, along with CT scan or exploratory burr holes, must be carried out if there is a reasonable suspicion of the presence of a subdural collection.

Treatment. Burr holes are made in the posterior parietal areas on both sides under local anaesthesia. The dura is incised and brownish fluid gushes out. This is allowed to flow out, aided by lowering the head. The dura is left unsutured.

Post-traumatic epilepsy. Epilepsy occurring *soon* after injury does not indicate an intracranial haematoma. It is due to primary brain damage which may be slight and from which total recovery occurs. On the other hand *late* post-traumatic epilepsy indicates scarring in the cerebral cortex. In those patients who have suffered early epilepsy, and in major compound fractures with tears in the dura or intracranial haematomas, it is advisable to use anticonvulsant drugs prophylactically for upto 3 years.

The **outcome** after head injury depends on many factors. Predictors of a bad prognosis include increasing age, pre-existing illness, penetrating injuries, delay in treatment and multiple trauma.

INTRACRANIAL ABSCESSES

An intracranial abscess may be extradural, subdural or intracerebral.

Extradural abscess. If infection takes place in the middle ear or the frontal sinus, osteomyelitis of the skull may result. If the pus bursts through the bone it may collect outside the dura as an extradural abscess. The abscess results in acute localized headache, tenderness on percussion of the skull and localized pitting oedema of the scalp. These signs collectively form *Pott's puffy tumour*. The CSF often has a markedly elevated protein level with mild pleocytosis. An MRI defines the extent of the extradural mass. The most common organisms are *Staphylococcus aureus* and the streptococci. Treatment should be immediate, beginning with broad antibiotic coverage until the offending agent is identified. Specific antibiotic therapy should be continued for upto 6 weeks. Surgical drainage is necessary if neurological deficits persist in spite of aggressive medical therapy. Corticosteroids are beneficial in reducing localized oedema, although prolonged use can reduce the host immune response to infection. Recovery of neurological function is directly related to the duration and severity of impairment before treatment.

Subdural abscess. Infections of the frontal sinus or accessory air cells may result in septic thrombophlebitis of the superior sagittal sinus. From here, pus may reach the subdural space through the superior cerebral veins, resulting in a subdural abscess. In other cases open contamination of the subdural space takes place at operation or after trauma. Staphylococci, streptococci, and anaerobic cocci are commonly responsible. Once the subdural space is entered, infection can spread over the whole surface of the brain.

Intracerebral abscess. This may result from one of the following:

1. *Implantation* from penetrating wounds: this is normally associated with a low mortality rate, because the organisms are usually derived from the skin and are not very virulent.
2. *Metastases* from intrathoracic sepsis, specially subacute bacterial endocarditis, lung abscess, bronchiectasis or empyema: in these cases the septic embolus is lodged deep in the white matter close to the ventricle. Fatal septic ventriculitis can occur within a matter of days.
3. *Local extension* due to septic thrombosis spreading from septic foci in the ear or frontal sinuses, or from a penetrating wound.
4. Among patients with *compromised immunity*, either from an underlying illness such as HIV infection, or during pharmacological immunosuppression such as for organ transplantation.

Diagnosis. Clinical diagnosis is based on the following:

1. Evidence of *infection*, e.g. chronic suppurative otitis media or recent mastoidectomy (in the case of a temporal or cerebellar abscess) or frontal sinusitis (in the case of a frontal abscess). Fever and tachycardia are often absent. The white blood count may be high. The ESR is raised in most patients.
2. Clinical features of *raised intracranial pressure.* The symptoms produced by an abscess in the cranial cavity include headache, vomiting, failing vision and deterioration of level of consciousness, while papilloedema, a slowing pulse, and a rising blood pressure constitute the important physical signs.

3. *Focal neurological symptoms.* These depend on the site of the lesion. A temporal lobe abscess may produce dysphasia, along with hemiparesis on the opposite side. A cerebellar abscess may cause nystagmus and incoordination. A subdural abscess can produce epilepsy.

Localization. In the past ventriculography and carotid arteriography have been employed for delineating the site of an intracranial abscess. However, with the availability of *CT scan* and *MRI* the older tests are not required. Both contrast CT scan and MRI are highly accurate in detecting brain abscess and should be carried out before CSF is sampled.

Management. The treatment for cerebral abscess is the same as that for a collection of pus anywhere in the body. The inflammation is treated by antibiotics. Penicillin (20 mu i.v./day) and metronidazole (400 mg thrice daily) are reasonable choices until the culture and sensitivity report comes in. Removal of pus is best achieved by burr hole aspiration. This should be repeated daily until no more pus is obtained. Repeat CT scans are desirable to confirm that there is no recurrence of pus. If aspiration fails because the capsule is too thick, craniotomy and excision of the abscess is necessary. The cause of the infection also requires treatment; this is often frontal sinus disease, middle ear infection, or congenital heart disease.

INTRACRANIAL TUMOURS

General aspects. Intracranial tumours constitute a major component of a neurosurgeon's work.

Primary intracranial tumours include a wide variety of neoplasms. Gliomas are by far the most common growths, accounting for over half the total number of cases. Meningiomas and pituitary adenomas form the next most common groups, constituting about a fifth and one eighth of the total respectively. The other tumours which are seen relatively often include neurinomas, craniopharyngiomas and tumours of blood vessels. *Secondary* carcinoma deposits come most commonly from the lung, but can originate from any organ in the body.

Intracranial tumours can be classified into: (a) extracerebral, (b) intracerebral, and (c) other space-occupying lesions (Table 2).

Table 2 Classification of intracranial tumours.

A. *Extracerebral tumours* (arising from the extracerebral structures)
Meningiomas
Neuromas
Haemangioblastomas
Pituitary tumours
Bone tumours, metastatic

B. *Intracerebral tumours* (only the common tumours are enumerated)
Gliomas–astrocytomas, medulloblastomas, etc.
Metastatic tumours
Lymphomas

C. *Non-neoplastic space-occupying lesions*
Abscesses
Cysts: congenital and parasitic
Granulomas: tuberculomas, syphilitic gummas
Vascular lesions: haematomas, aneurysms, arteriovenous malformations

Clinical features. 1. Every tumour has an initial silent period. If it is near a 'silent' area it will produce no symptoms until the intracranial pressure rises and headache and vomiting starts.

2. Intracranial tumours exert both local and generalized effects by their presence within a closed bony structure:

i. *Local* effects of a tumour are either irritative or destructive. Irritation of adjacent cortex results in focal seizures, while compression of nearby brain tissue produces a focal neurological deficit.

ii. *Generalized* effects are produced by the *raised intracranial pressure* (ICP) due to the presence of the mass. The raised ICP may provide the only evidence of the presence of a tumour, or it may occur along with focal symptoms. In frontal lobe tumours pressure symptoms occur late. Temporal and parietal lobe tumours obstruct the outflow from the corresponding ventricle, so symptoms may occur earlier. Similarly, posterior fossa tumours obstruct the flow of fluid from both ventricles, so that pressure symptoms arise very early. There is headache, vomiting, papilloedema, bradycardia and retarded cerebration. The vomiting of raised intracranial pressure is not preceded by nausea, and occurs without warning.

A few patients present only when *cone formation* is imminent. When the intracranial pressure inside a supratentorial compartment rises, the inner border of a cerebral hemisphere may be forced under the falx cerebri. The temporal lobe may be forced down into the tentorial opening. Further, the cerebellar tonsils may be pushed down into the foramen magnum. The pathways for cerebrospinal fluid absorption being blocked, the pressure rises abruptly. Signs of a threatened cone include violent paroxsymal headache, drowsiness, slow pulse and neck stiffness. Dilatation of one pupil is an urgent sign. *Lumbar puncture must be avoided at this stage.*

3. *Meningeal irritation* may arise due to bleeding in, or malignant infiltration of, the subarachnoid space.

4. *Other* signs may be present, e.g. a primary tumour elsewhere (lung or breast), or an endocrine disorder due to a pituitary tumour.

Investigations. History-taking, general examination in search of primary disease, and neurological examination must be carried out most precisely and thoroughly.

X-rays. X-rays of the skull and chest, and ESR, are essential investigations in every case. The chest x-ray may show an unsuspected bronchial carcinoma as the primary tumour. On x-ray of the skull:

1. Due to the *raised intracranial pressure*, the posterior clinoid processes may be eroded. At the same time, the pressure of tight convolutions on the inner table of the skull may produce a beaten-silver appearance.

2. A bulky tumour in one supratentorial compartment may have caused lateral displacement of a calcified *pineal* body.

3. Astrocytomas, angiomas, meningiomas, etc. may show characteristic *calcification*.

Arteriography. A radiopaque dye is injected into the common carotid artery and x-rays taken. The site of a tumour is shown by the displacement of the cerebral vessels by the neoplasm. Meningiomas, glioblastomas, and haemangiomas show characteristic arrangements of blood vessels in the tumour, the pattern being different for each neoplasm ('tumour circulation').

Ventriculography was employed in the past, air being introduced into the ventricles via catheters passed through burr holes. However, this investigation could be dangerous, allowing the brain in another compartment to push through the tentorial opening and cause cone formation, and is not often employed.

CT scan and *MRI* clearly shows up a tumour when present. Meningiomas appear densely white. Gliomas are less dense. Astrocytoma cysts show as dark areas. Secondary tumours appear as multiple shadows. CT scan and MRI have almost completely displaced carotid angiography and ventriculography.

General management. The surgeon has to manage the tumour itself, its vascularity, its effects on other structures, and the intracranial pressure if it is raised.

Intracranial pressure. If the raised intracranial pressure is not urgently relieved, the outcome may be rapidly fatal. Severe headache and a deteriorating level of consciousness are ominous signs. Intracranial pressure may be lowered by the following measures:

1. *Mannitol* may be administered. Being an osmotic diuretic, it causes dehydration and thus extracts fluid from the CSF.

2. *Dexamethasone* is most useful in those malignant gliomas and secondary tumours which have undergone necrosis. In these cases reduction of oedema may restore a comatose patient to consciousness and eliminate the signs of paralysis. Regular administration of dexamethasone may prolong life. Dexamethasone also reduces the oedema occurring during deep x-ray therapy.

3. In the case of posterior fossa tumours the ventricles may be *tapped*. With supratentorial cysts or abscesses, the cavity of the cyst or abscess itself may be tapped.

4. A supratentorial tumour may be *partially removed*.

Surgery on the tumour itself can only be performed safely if the pressure is normal. To guard against postoperative epileptic fits, anticonvulsant therapy is started two days prior to surgery. At the same time, because of the risk of epileptic seizures the patient should not drive a vehicle for a period of one year after surgery for a supratentorial tumour.

Individual tumours. ***Gliomas.*** These account for over 50% of central nervous system tumours in adults, and most are supratentorial. They are divided into 4 histological grades. Grade 4 gliomas (glioblastoma multiforme) present with a history of a few weeks. They show a good initial response to steroids but carry a poor prognosis. Treatment usually involves a combination of surgery and radiotherapy. In very large tumours surgical reduction of tumour mass is performed as a precursor to radiotherapy, which may take the form of external beam irradiation (5000 cGy over 5 weeks), stereotactic focal irradiation using a linear accelerator, gamma knife or proton beam. Chemotherapy has limited application.

Meningiomas are relatively benign, and are best treated by total excision, including the dura at the site of attachment of the tumour. Careful preoperative preparation, microsurgical dissection and specialized postoperative care produce a very low operative mortality and morbidity. In patients with large vascular tumours, preoperative embolization of the middle meningeal artery (through the external carotid) helps reduce the blood supply and facilitates dissection. In any case, very large meningiomas are best removed in stages.

Medulloblastomas are treated by complete surgical excision followed by craniospinal irradiation after staging by myelography or MRI. Combination chemotherapy provides a valuable adjunct. Despite aggressive surgery, radiotherapy and chemotherapy, patients treated for medulloblastoma have a survival rate of 65% at 5 years, falling to 40% at 10 years.

A ***metastatic*** tumour, if single and in an accessible site, can be excised with excellent symptomatic relief. Radiotherapy (3000 cGy over 14 days) is used after such an excision, as well as for multiple metastases .

TUMOURS OF THE PITUITARY BODY

Tumours of the pituitary arise from one of the types of cells present in the organ. Thus they comprise three varieties of adenoma: chromophobe, acidophil and basophil. Apart from these, congenital tumours derived from Rathke's pouch are seen from time to time.

Chromophobe adenoma. This tumour commonly occurs in females between twenty and fifty years of age. It grows slowly over many years. It compresses the acidophil and basophil cells of the anterior pituitary, affecting the production of thyrotrophic and gonadotrophic hormones. The patient becomes fat and sluggish, and amenorrhoea sets in. Pressure by the enlarging tumour on the diaphragma sellae causes severe headache. The tumour then breaks through the diaphragm and presses on the decussating fibres of the optic chiasma causing bitemporal hemianopia. Finally, massive extension with raised intracranial pressure or epilepsy occurs.

Acidophil adenoma. This tumour is small in size. In children it causes gigantism, in adults acromegaly.

Basophil adenomas. These tumour are also small and produce Cushing's syndrome.

Diagnosis. The presence of most pituitary adenomas can be ascertained by MRI scanning. At the same time, tumours can be identified by an increase in the serum levels of the hormones produced by them, e.g. growth hormone, cortisol, and prolactin.

Differential diagnosis. Other lesions that may enlarge the pituitary fossa include craniopharyngiomas, meningiomas and metastatic tumours. All these lesions can produce hypopituitarism and visual loss, and the diagnosis is usually confirmed only at operation.

Treatment. Most pituitary tumours can be successfully managed by the trans-sphenoidal route. The surgeon incises the septal mucosa in the nasal vestibule and approaches the sella turcica by a submucosal route along the nasal septum, reaching the pituitary fossa via the sphenoidal sinus. Even large tumours can be almost totally removed. Medical management is possible for prolactinomas with bromocriptine, which inhibits prolactin secretion and reduces tumour size. Very ill patients with Cushing's syndrome who are not fit for surgery may be treated by agents that suppress cortisol synthesis, such as ketaconazole. However, the drug is not always well tolerated and is not the first line therapy for the ordinary patient with Cushing's disease.

HYDROCEPHALUS

Hydrocephalus is defined as the abnormal accumulation of fluid in the cranial vault. It may be congenital or acquired. If the ventricles are sealed off at some point the hydrocephalus is described as non-communicating. If they communicate freely with the subarachnoid space the hydrocephalus is communicating.

Congenital hydrocephalus. Congenital hydrocephalus usually occurs along with spina bifida or meningomyelocele. The most common cause is failure of development of arachnoid villi. A few cases are due to obstruction of the CSF pathway. This may be due to the Arnold-Chiari malformation, in which the roof of the fourth ventricle lies below the foramen magnum and there is obstruction of the exit foramina; or it may be due to congenital stenosis of the aqueduct of Sylvius.

Clinical features. The head may be enlarged before birth and produce obstructed labour. After birth rapid enlargement occurs. The fontanelles widen. The forehead bulges forward. The ventricles dilate enormously. The cortex is reduced to a mere shell, but there are no motor symptoms. Intelligence may be preserved in spite of the enormous size of the head.

Acquired hydrocephalus. *Non-communicating* hydrocephalus occurs due to obstruction of the ventricles by tumour or inflammation. *Communicating* hydrocephalus usually follows inflammation and complicates meningitis, or is due to blockage of the cisterns by organizing subarachnoid haemorrhage.

Diagnosis. To diagnose hydrocephalus some degree of ventricular enlargement must be demonstrated. During infancy, while the fontanelle is open, cranial ultrasound is useful for the detection of ventricular enlargement; in older patients CT or MRI are employed for the purpose. The cause may be evident from the history, or from the presence of subarachnoid haemorrhage or meningitis. Further imaging may be required to identify a tumour.

Treatment. If a tumour is the cause of the hydrocephalus it is removed if possible. For the other types of hydrocephalus different *shunting* procedures are useful:

1. A lateral ventricle may be connected to the cisterna magna by a polythene catheter, for treating obstruction of the aqueduct of Sylvius.

2. The proximal end of a fine catheter is placed in the dilated lateral ventricle through a small drill hole in the skull. It is passed beneath the scalp, where it connects with a valve (*Holter valve*). A further tube is then passed under the skin and into the peritoneal cavity, which is entered through a small incision over the anterior abdomen *(ventriculoperitoneal shunt)*. Less commonly, the catheter is led via the neck veins into the right atrium *(ventriculoatrial shunt)*. The valve allows flow of the fluid in only one direction, i.e. away from the ventricles. These tubes are foreign bodies and liable to become infected and blocked. However, the ventriculoperitoneal and ventriculoatrial shunts are satisfactory treatment for hydrocephalus irrespective of its cause.

INTRACRANIAL ANEURYSMS

These may be subclinoid or supraclinoid.

Subclinoid aneursyms. These aneurysms arise from the internal carotid artery within the cavernous sinus. They are below the level of the dura so they do not cause subarachnoid haemorrhage. They produce symptoms by pressing on the third to the sixth cranial nerves in the lateral wall of the cavernous sinus.

Treatment. Ligation of the internal carotid artery might cause hemiplegia, so ligation of the common carotid is preferred, as it allows some collateral circulation.

Supraclinoid aneurysms. These are more important than subclinoid aneurysms. They arise due to a weakness in the media of the internal carotid, middle cerebral or anterior communicating arteries. When such an aneurysm ruptures, subarachnoid haemorrhage occurs into the basal cisterns. This is most common between the ages of 50 and 55. An aneurysm is the cause of nearly half the cases of subarachnoid haemorrhage.

Clinical features. The onset of symptoms is always sudden:

1. Sudden severe headache.
2. Sudden loss of consciousness.
3. Focal neurological deficit, e.g. hemiplegia, dysphasia, ptosis, dilated pupil.
4. Neck stiffness and vomiting, due to irritation of the meninges by the blood.

If the patient survives, the consciousness level improves. However, a second fatal haemorrhage occurs in approximately 40% of patients within six weeks.

Differential diagnosis. Other causes of subarachnoid haemorrhage include hypertension, arteriovenous malformation, blood dyscrasias and anticoagulant drugs.

Investigations. A CT scan should be carried out in all patients. In the rare event that it does not demonstrate subarachnoid bleeding, lumbar puncture can be carried out to confirm the diagnosis. CT scan also documents the presence of complications like cerebral infarction and hydrocephalus. Finally, bilateral carotid and vertebral arteriography is performed. It demonstrates the aneurysm, its neck, and its relationship with parent and branch vessels. It also shows up multiple aneurysms if present. MRI can help in identifying the site of haemorrhage, demonstrating mural thrombus and depicting the relationship of the aneurysm to cerebral structures.

Treatment. The ideal treatment is exposure of the neck of the aneurysm, preservation of adjacent and parent arteries, and obliteration of the aneurysm by applying a metal clip. Experienced teams produce good or excellent results in 80 percent of patients undergoing early surgery, with a 10 percent mortality rate. If the patient is medically unfit or the aneurysm is considered inoperable, endovascular treatment with intraluminal obliteration may be used. However it is still too early for a final evaluation of this method.

45 Vertebral column, spinal cord and nerves

Vertebral column

There are two main reasons for the importance of injuries to the vertebral column. Firstly, this is a very important part of the skeleton, and deformity in this part has deleterious consequences for the patient. Secondly, injuries to the vertebral column are often associated with damage to the spinal cord, with paralysis of the limbs and/or the bladder.

DISLOCATIONS

True dislocations of the vertebral column are most common in the cervical region, where the surfaces of the articular processes lie nearly horizontally. In the dorsal and lumbar regions the vertical direction of the articular processes results in their being fractured.

During *hanging*, the atlas dislocates forwards over the axis. Either the odontoid process gets fractured or the transverse ligament of the atlas is ruptured, allowing forward displacement of the atlas. In this way the space in the vertebral canal is greatly reduced, the brain stem gets crushed, and death results from paralysis of the respiratory muscles.

During a *head injury* the base of the odontoid process may be cracked, and yet displacement may only occur after several days. If occipital pain persists after a head injury, x-ray of the odontoid process should be taken through the open mouth.

Dislocations of the *cervical vertebrae* commonly occur by falls on the head from a motorcycle or diving into shallow water, and affect the lower cervical spine due to its greater mobility. The inferior articular process of the upper vertebra is forced forwards over the upper margin of the superior process of the lower vertebra. If a facet on one side is dislocated forwards, a lateral x-ray shows a forward movement of nearly a quarter of the diameter of the vertebral body; if facets on both sides are dislocated, then over half the diameter. In the latter situation the narrowing of the vertebral canal causes serious neurological effects. Pain is felt in the neck and may be referred along a local nerve root due to pressure. Neck movements are restricted. Posterior tenderness is due to rupture of the interspinous ligament.

Treatment. If cervical spine injury is suspected, the neck should be protected by pillows on either side until x-rays have been taken. If dislocation is present, it should be reduced as soon as possible, but *if there is evidence of cord involvement the situation constitutes an emergency.* Traction should be applied to the skull under anaesthesia, using skull tongs or a halo apparatus. The weights are increased under x-ray control upto 16 kg. When the facets disengage, weights are reduced to about 4 kg. If this fails, closed manipulation or open reduction will be required.

FRACTURES

Fractures and dislocations of the spine follow major trauma such as motor vehicle accidents or falls from a height. Seen from the standpoint of stability, the vertebral column is considered to be composed of three columns. The anterior column consists of the vertebral bodies, discs and longitudinal ligaments. The intermediate column contains the facet joints and their ligaments, while the posterior column consists of the spinous processes and interspinous ligaments. If all three columns are disrupted, the situation is extremely unstable. If on the other hand only one column is interrupted the spine may be regarded as stable.

Stable fractures. These do not interfere with the continuity of the spinal column. Examples include:

1. Fractures of the *spinous and transverse processes,* which usually occur due to direct violence. Fractures of the transverse processes occur commonly in the lumbar region, where the corresponding kidney may also be injured.
2. *Compression* fractures of the vertebral bodies. These usually occur due to a fall on the buttocks.
3. Fractures of the *laminae* or *pedicles*. These may be accompanied by traumatic intraspinal haemorrhage. The bleeding may occur in the cord itself and cause flaccid paralysis by destroying the anterior horn cells; or it may occur outside the cord and cause root irritation.

Unstable fractures. ***Fracture-dislocations.*** These produce complete disruption of the vertebral column. There is rupture of the interspinous ligament, fracture or dislocation of the facet joints, and a fracture through the vertebral body. These injuries occur commonly at the dorsolumbar region, and only rarely in the neck. Damage to the spinal cord or cauda equina is seen in many cases. In most cases the injury occurs between T 12 and L1, and classically from a flexion and rotation force, as in a motorcyclist thrown into the air and landing on one shoulder. The diagnosis is made on the basis of the history of flexion-rotation injury, the displacement, and the palpable gap between the spinous processes. *X-rays* usually show a horizontal 'slice' fracture passing through the upper part of the vertebral body with forward displacement of the upper vertebra on the lower, along with increased space between the spinous processes at the affected level.

Treatment. Most unstable injuries in this region are accompanied by damage to the spinal cord and nerve roots. The T12/L1 interspace is level with the first sacral segment of the cord, so injury at this level can affect the cord only from the first segment downwards. However, the lumbar nerve roots can also be damaged as they pass the lesion, so classically injury at this level consists of a lower motor neurone lesion of the lumbar segments along with an upper motor neurone lesion of the sacral segments.

Most of the damage is inflicted at the moment of injury. Therefore laminectomy for the purpose of general decompression is of no value; in fact, because it increases the instability of the spine, it is contraindicated. Prompt reduction of the dislocation is more effective in relieving pressure. Spinal fusion is unnecessary since the fracture of the vertebral body will unite spontaneously. If the displacement is minimal, alignment may be preserved by simple recumbency; if it is significant, open reduction with internal fixation is preferred. Plates may be bolted to the spinous processes, or rods secured to the laminae by wires going round both.

PROLAPSE OF INTERVERTEBRAL DISC

Each intervertebral disc consists of a central portion of spongy material, the nucleus pulposus, and a tough fibrous ring, the annulus fibrosus. During normal flexion of the spine the disc is deformed and bulges backwards slightly into the neural canal. If a strong flexion force occurs it ruptures the annulus. Portions of the annulus and nucleus escape into the spinal canal and compress the nerve roots. In four-fifths of cases the protrusion follows upon trauma due to a severe strain; in one-fifth it is degenerative.

Protrusions occur commonly in the most mobile portions of the spine. 80% occur in the lumbar region at L4/5 and L5/S1 levels. 19% occur in the cervical region at C5/6 and C6/7 levels. Only 1% occur in the immobile dorsal spine. Most disc herniations are posterolateral because of the presence of the posterior longitudinal ligament in the midline, and consequently the symptoms are usually unilateral. They are uncommon in old people, probably because of age-dependent loss of water content and disc volume.

Lumbar disc protrusion. At first there is low back pain due to injury to the disc. Later, when nerve roots are compressed the pain radiates to the leg. There is root pain, increased on coughing, in the distribution of the affected nerve. Paraesthesias, tenderness in muscles, with sensory loss and motor weakness also occur. The most common roots involved are L5 and S1. Therefore the pain is usually in the back and side of the leg radiating to the sole of the foot, and is called *sciatica*. Sensory loss occurs on the sole and outer side of the foot. The ankle jerk is lost. Attempts at passively raising the straight leg are painful. The more severe the condition, the smaller the angle through which the straight leg can be raised without causing pain *(Straight leg raising test).*

Other causes of sciatica include nerve root compression by tumour, abscess or osteophyte; and peripheral nerve compression within the pelvis or gluteal area by tumour, abscess or haematoma.

Investigations. *Plain x-rays* of the lumbosacral spine centred on L5 are taken in the anteroposterior and lateral views. In cases with a major protrusion of a disc the relevant disc space is seen on x-ray to be narrowed.

Myelography used to be the standard procedure for outlining a prolapsed disc, as it shows the indentation in the column of radiopaque material in the spinal theca. *CT scan* and *MRI* have nearly displaced myelography, as they provide the same information without the need for an invasive procedure. However, in the poorer communities myelography may be the only method of investigation available.

Treatment consists of confinement to bed along with analgesics until symptoms subside, which usually takes two to four weeks. 80 to 90% of cases are relieved by this management. Avoidance of heavy lifting and bending helps prevent recurrence. Operation is indicated if symptoms persist, if severe pain occurs, or if motor weakness is developing. Hemilaminectomy is performed, removing the adjacent margins of two laminae. Through the exposure thus obtained the degenerated disc is removed, relieving the pressure on the nerve root. Alternatively, the disc can be *digested* by percutaneous injection with chymopapain or collagenase. Finally, *microdiscectomy* and *percutaneous suction discectomy* have been introduced as less invasive alternatives, but require further evaluation.

Cervical disc protrusions. These are relatively uncommon. In many cases the diagnosis is mistakenly made in cases of cervical spondylosis or referred pain from a cervical strain.

CERVICAL SPONDYLOSIS

In old age the neck is not as supple and flexible as during youth. The difference is due to the presence of cervical spondylosis in the old person's spine. In this condition the intervertebral discs are degenerate. Also, osteophytes form at the postero-lateral corners of the vertebral bodies and project backwards into the intervertebral foramina. The condition may be symptomless or may cause neurological manifestations. Sudden strain on the spine may cause referred pain and muscle spasm in the occipital or post-auricular regions, along the trapezius, and between the scapulae.

Investigations. Because spondylosis as seen on x-rays is common and often asymptomatic, no investigation can substitute for a careful history and examination. Plain lateral x-rays, taken in flexion and extension, help in excluding other diseases as well as allowing assessment of the size of the vertebral canal and range of movement of cervical spine and intervertebral joints.

Treatment. Symptoms are relieved by wearing a collar, because it restricts movement. If they persist in a severe form, anterior cervical fusion is occasionally required. Compression of nerve roots may be caused by osteophytes in the intervertebral foramina. This may require excision of the back of these foramina by removal of the anterior half of the concerned articular facets *(hemifacetectomy).*

SPONDYLOLISTHESIS

In this condition the body of the fifth (or occasionally fourth) lumbar vertebra gets separated from the laminae and spine due to a defect in the pedicles, remaining attached merely by thick fibrous tissue. The body slips forwards and carries with it the whole of the upper portion of the spine. The spinal canal is not narrowed, but root pressure can cause sciatica. There is long-standing low back pain. Rest and analgesics are required. A stiff corset may be needed in some patients. Surgical treatment is reserved for patients who fail conservative measures, have disabling back pain, have slips greater than 50 percent, and have multiple risk factors. The most commonly used procedure is bilateral posterolateral fusion *in situ*, i.e. without attempting reduction of the slip.

TUMOURS OF THE VERTEBRAL COLUMN

Both benign tumours and primary malignant neoplasms are quite rare. *Secondary deposits* are much more common. Most come from carcinoma of the breast or prostate. A neuroblastoma of the sympathetic chain may protrude through an intervertebral foramen and compress the spinal cord. Severe local pain results. It later becomes girdle in type when the nerves get involved. The next stage is vertebral collapse and paraplegia, but deep x-ray therapy at the early stage may prevent it. Secondaries from the prostate respond promptly to stilboesterol. Those from the breast regress with hormones or aminoglutethimide.

The spinal cord

SPINAL CORD INJURY

Traumatic injury to the spinal cord may result from vertebral fracture, fracture/subluxation, and penetrating injuries such as gunshot or stab wounds. The spinal cord gets injured due to one of the following types of lesion:

1. Long axis stretch causing concussion or rupture of nerve fibres and vessels within the cord, as seen in acute flexion injuries with severe compression fractures.
2. The cord getting nipped between the lamina of the upper vertebra and the body of the lower, as commonly encountered in fracture-dislocations.

The spinal cord ends at the lower border of the body of the first lumbar vertebra, so injuries below this level damage only the cauda equina.

Injuries at different levels. The effects produced by injuries at the various levels differ from each other:

1. Injuries to the *neck* commonly cause dislocation. Here the neural canal is spacious, so cord injury may be slight or absent.
2. The *dorsal spine* is strong and relatively immobile and can be broken only by major forces such as collapse of a roof. Displacement is marked and the space is limited, so cord injury usually results, and is severe.
3. The *lumbar spine* is strong and has vertical articular processes. Therefore only major forces are able to break it and produce fracture-dislocations. The lumbar theca is spacious, so nerve injury may be absent or limited to a few roots of the cauda equina.

Different degrees of damage to the spinal cord. During injuries to the vertebral column the spinal cord may suffer concussion or partial or complete contusion.

Spinal concussion. When the vertebral column is acutely flexed the spinal cord gets stretched. This displaces the neurones and synapses so that synaptic conduction is disturbed. So all those functions which depend upon synaptic activity are lost below the level of the lesion:

1. Each anterior horn cell receives hundreds of synapses. Stimuli passing through these maintain the central excitatory state which keeps the cell ready to respond for *voluntary movement, muscle tone and reflex activity.* Therefore, loss of the central excitatory state causes complete loss of all these three functions below the lesion, producing a flaccid paralysis and retention of urine.
2. *Pain and temperature* sensation cross a synapse in the inferior sensory decussation and therefore are lost.
3. *Joint position sense* ascends the posterior columns without a synapse, and is therefore preserved.

Recovery. If the injury is merely spinal concussion, voluntary power and sensation return within one or two days. If concussion is superimposed on an underlying partial or complete cord injury, the stage of spinal shock is likely to be prolonged; the longer this stage, the less likely is recovery to occur. If a mass reflex appears, usually at three to six weeks, it indicates that no recovery is likely.

Partial or complete contusion of the cord. This results from the cord being crushed between the lamina of the vertebra above and the body of the vertebra below. It produces a transverse zone of contusion and bruising. Oedema may cause a rise in the level of paralysis. Any damage inflicted on the cord is permanent.

Clinical features. Spinal fracture and cord injury should be suspected in patients with head injuries and multiple injuries. It is best to assume that the spine is unstable and immobilize the patient on a backboard with a hard cervical collar until careful examination has been made.

Clinical findings of spinal cord injury include spinal tenderness, weakness of the limbs, numbness or paraesthesia, respiratory embarrassment, and hypotension. Spinal root involvement produces sensory and motor impairment in the corresponding dermatome and myotome. A complete lesion produces absence of reflexes, flaccidity, anaesthesia, and autonomic paralysis below the level of the lesion. If the transection is above T5, hypotension occurs due to the loss of sympathetic vascular tone.

Spinal shock results immediately from a long axis stretch of the spinal cord. There is flaccid paralysis below the lesion and retention of urine. In the early stages cord contusion can be diagnosed:

1. If there is complete loss of all sensation below the lesion.
2. If the level of sensory loss and paralysis rises after the injury.
3. If the stage of spinal shock persists for more than forty-eight hours.

In cord contusion the *clinical course* falls into three stages:

1. The stage of spinal shock.
2. The stage of reflex activity.
3. The stage of septic complications, including urinary tract infections and bedsores.

THE MANAGEMENT OF SPINAL CORD INJURIES

PREVENTION

Injury to the cervical spine is most common in contact sports such as rugby, football and wrestling, besides some non-contact sports like gymnastics, diving and horse-riding. In athletes, high-risk manoeuvres such as spear-headed tackling should be avoided. Strict adherence to rules prohibiting such dangerous moves reduce the incidence of quadruplegia by more than 70 percent. At the same time, helmets providing for protection of the head as well as the cervical spine should be used.

TREATMENT

The *objectives* of treatment are to correct spinal alignment, protect undamaged tissues, restore function to reversibly damaged neural tissues, and achieve permanent spinal stability. To achieve these, reduction and immobilization of a fracture/dislocation must receive top priority.

A: THE STAGE OF SPINAL SHOCK

In the stage of spinal shock care is taken to avoid unnecessary movement or examination which might increase the cord damage.

First aid treatment. Cervical injuries are transported lying on the back with the head supported between pillows without flexion. Dorsal and lumbar fractures are transported with the patient face down. *The patient should be turned onto a stretcher by at least three persons* controlling the head, trunk and pelvis, without torsion of the spine. Sedation should be given to relieve pain and anxiety.

Examination. At the hospital the sensory level to pinprick on the trunk is tested, in order to define the segmental level of the lesion, and to test whether the patient can recognize movement of the foot or knee. If he can, the case is one of concussion. *If all sensations are lost, the outlook is grave.* A lateral x-ray of the corresponding level of the vertebral column is taken without disturbing the patient. The utmost gentleness is necessary to prevent further injury to a partially damaged cord.

Reduction and immobilization. *Cervical region.* Cervical spine injuries are managed as described under dislocations, in the preceding section.

Dorsal spine. Simple wedge compression fractures are very stable. Symptomatic treatment is given and early mobilization carried out. In fracture-dislocations the cord is often transected. The fracture is stable due partly to the support of the rib cage, and surgery is almost never indicated. Treatment is that of the paraplegia itself.

Lumbar spine. If severe displacement is present open reduction is required. The spine is next stabilized by plates bolted to the spinous processes. If there is only minimal displacement, postural nursing is enough. If paraplegia is present plaster is avoided, as it results in pressure sores. If there is no paraplegia the patient can be mobilized in a plaster jacket.

Indications for early operation in patients with spinal cord injury include the following:

1. A penetrating injury with or without a CSF leak.
2. Inability to reduce the fracture/dislocation satisfactorily by closed methods.
3. Severe compression of the spinal cord by an intraspinal mass shown by MRI.
4. Neurological deterioration in a patient with an incomplete cord lesion initially.

It should be remembered that even after surgical reduction and/or fixation, *external immobilization* is required, usually for about 3 months.

Nursing. To prevent bedsores the skin is dried and powdered. The patient is turned every two hours to prevent local pressure. Laxatives or enemas are given to empty the bowels. Breathing exercises are instituted, because hypostatic pneumonia is a danger, specially if accessory muscles of respiration e.g. abdominal muscles are paralysed. Muscle contracture is prevented by frequent passive movements of the limb.

Diet. A high-protein diet should be given to make good the loss of serum proteins from bedsores.

Bladder. In every case of cord injury retention of the urine is present in the initial stages. This may last from a few days to a few months in recoverable lesions. It is permanent in complete lesions. *Most deaths after spinal injury are due to ascending infection from catheterization.*

B: THE RETURN OF REFLEX ACTIVITY

If spinal shock does not recover even partly after 48 hours, partial or complete cord contusion is present. When spinal shock passes off, lower motor neurone paralysis persists in a few muscles corresponding to the level of the lesion, owing to crushing of the anterior horns at this level.

Partial cord lesions. These show spastic paralysis in extension with exaggerated reflexes and extensor plantar responses, and sometimes with uninhibited flexor spasms. Retention of urine may persist for upto one year.

Complete cord lesions. These are followed by spastic paralysis in flexion with gross flexor spasms and mass flexor reflexes of spinal automatism, which indicate complete lack of inhibition of spinal flexor reflex arcs. The slightest touch on the foot produces flexion of the ankle, knee and hip with evacuation of the bladder and rectum. The patient may misinterpret this as return of function. Actually it indicates that function will never recover.

Regional considerations. ***Cervical & thoracic spine.*** In high cervical lesions all respiratory muscles are paralysed. If the fifth segment is injured the patient breathes only with the diaphragm, which is supplied mainly from the C4 segment. In lesions of C6 elbow flexion is present. Lesions at T1 produce paralysis of the small muscles of the hand and Horner's syndrome. At lower levels a band of hyperaesthesia encircles the trunk one segment above the site of injury.

Lumbar spine. The centre for the control of the *bladder* lies opposite the 12th dorsal and first lumbar vertebrae.

In *complete cord lesions above T10 segment* the bladder centre is intact and uninhibited; therefore, an automatic bladder develops. When the intravesical pressure rises, evacuation occurs. The patient has to wear a receptacle for urine in order to remain dry.

Complete lesions involving the bladder centre produce paralysis of the detrusor supplied by the third and fourth sacral nerves. This results in permanent retention with overflow incontinence. However, since the upper abdominal muscles can be contracted voluntarily by the 7th to 10th dorsal segments, the patient can be taught to empty the bladder by straining, and by pressing his hands suprapubically, during the day. He must wear a receptacle at night. The care of the bladder is also discussed in Chapter 31.

The *centre for defaecation* is located in the 1st and 2nd lumbar segments. Damage produces a patulous anus and incontinence.

Cauda equina. In cauda equina lesions the disabilities correspond to the nerves injured. Usually the sacral nerve roots are involved, resulting in anaesthesia in the perineum and urinary retention.

Rehabilitation. The patient is confined to bed for 2 to 3 months until the spine stabilizes by bony healing. A great deal of progress in the care of paraplegics has been achieved due to work at the various paraplegic centres. The aims of treatment are the following:

1. To keep the patient in the best possible physical condition by preventing the development of bedsores and urinary infections.
2. To over-develop the muscles above the site of injury, so that these may move the pelvis.
3. To move the splinted legs by movements of the pelvis.

Rehabilitation of muscle activities. Contractures are relieved by physiotherapy, tenotomy etc. If necessary the lower part of the completely isolated cord is destroyed by intrathecal alcohol to abolish mass reflexes and flexor spasm which would prevent walking.

Rope climbing develops the muscles of the shoulder girdle. On parallel bars the patient learns to move his pelvis. Light aluminum splints are now fitted to the legs. Using sticks, the patient moves the pelvis from his shoulder. The splinted legs move with the pelvis. Thus the patient can walk slowly for short distances to a wheelchair, in which he may move about. He can participate in occupations involving fine handicraft.

In the treatment of a paraplegic, meticulous care of the bladder has a high priority. At the same time nursing of an extremely high standard is required, in order to prevent bedsores from developing. If the above steps are not taken, most paraplegics die within a few years from ascending urinary infections, or due to septicaemia from spreading bedsores.

Prognosis. If any cord function survives the initial injury, additional function usually returns if the cord and spine are protected from further injury. Patients with complete injury rarely recover function below the level of the lesion. Rehabilitation aims at self-care and readjustment of vocation. Life expectancy is reduced in paraplegics, and more specially in quadriplegics.

Causes of death. Paraplegics do not live very long; if they do, it implies excellent nursing and general management. The causes of death in paraplegics include spinal shock, respiratory failure from ascending oedema if the lesion is near C5, hypostatic pneumonia, ascending urinary infections, and septicaemia from unhealed bedsores.

SPINA BIFIDA

Embryology. During the second week of intrauterine life a longitudinal groove appears on the dorsum of the embryo. Its margins unite to form a tube from which the nervous system is developed. This tube of epiblast becomes separated from the surface by mesoblast. In each segment bars of cartilage appear on each side and fuse with each other to form the vertebral arches. If these arches fail to fuse spina bifida results. Its incidence is 0.1%.

The different types of spina bifida include the following:

1. Spina bifida occulta. The vertebral arches fail to fuse but the membranes do not protrude backwards. A patch of hair, a lipoma or a depression in the skin in the lumbosacral region are the only external evidence, and suggest that a spina bifida occulta exists. A fibrous band sometimes connects the skin to the membranes to produce a tethered cord. As the body grows, the spinal cord grows at a slower pace. This causes the band to pull on the membranes and nerve roots causing foot-drop, bed-wetting at night, bowel changes, or backache. A tethered spinal cord can present at any age with these changes. If the condition is suspected, an x-ray shows the gap between the laminae. Further evaluation should be carried out with MRI or myelography and CT scan.

The presence of a subcutaneous lipoma etc. is often noted before symptoms appear. Even if neurological symptoms are absent, surgery to prevent deterioration is indicated in children if tethering of the cord is demonstrated. Any patient with symptoms requires urgent evaluation and treatment. If appropriately repaired, patients with occult spinal dysraphism show entirely normal development and function.

2. Meningocele. This is the most *common* form of spina bifida. A fluctuant and transilluminant swelling is seen in the midline of the back in the newborn. It is due to a protrusion of the meninges through the ununited vertebral laminae and soft tissues. It contains cerebrospinal fluid, and is in communication with the spinal theca (Fig. 1a).

3. Meningomyelocele. The cord or cauda equina lie in the sac. They may be adherent to the posterior aspect, and on transillumination are seen as dark shadows in the midline. Interference with the spinal cord or nerves may occur, with bilateral talipes and trophic changes in the skin of the feet (Fig. 1b).

4. Syringomyelocele. Syringomyelocele is rare; here the central canal of the cord is dilated (Fig. 1c).

5. Myelocele. In this, the most severe form of spina bifida, the neural groove lies open, and at its upper end the central canal discharges cerebrospinal fluid (Fig. 1d). Most cases are stillborn, or death occurs within a few days from meningitis.

Some cases of spina bifida develop hydrocephalus due to associated anomalies at a higher level.

Treatment. Operation for meningocele and meningomyelocele is advised within a few days of birth, as the sac may enlarge and ulcerate. The sac is opened and redundant membrane excised. Membranes are repaired and muscles approximated over the defect. Cases with gross paralysis require care as those with traumatic paraplegia. The expenditure on each patient during a lifetime is exorbitant. It is

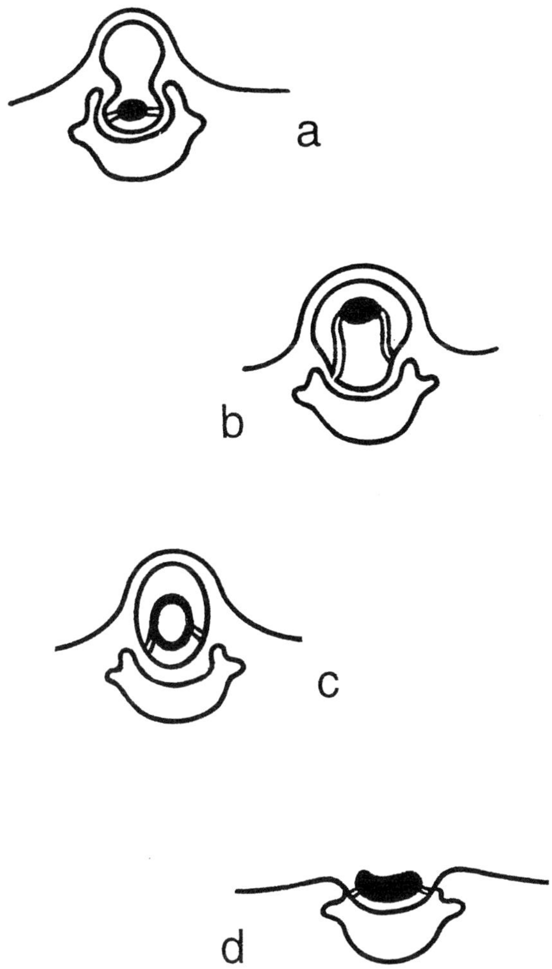

Fig. 1 Different types of spina bifida. (a) Meningocele, (b) Meningomyelocele, (c) Syringomyelocele, (d) Myelocele.

difficult to decide whether this money would not be better used in saving thousands of patients from curable ailments.

TUMOURS OF THE SPINAL CORD AND MEMBRANES

Spinal cord tumours can be divided into the following categories:

1. *Extradural*, e.g. meningioma and neurofibroma.
2. *Intradural*. These can be further subdivided into the following types:

i. Extramedullary tumours, e.g. meningioma and neurofibroma.

ii. Intramedullary tumours: these consist of ependymomas which can be excised, and gliomas which cannot easily be removed.

Clinical features. If the posterior nerve roots are involved, root pain and local sensory loss are the result. If the anterior horns are affected, wasting and loss of reflexes are found. Involvement of the sensory tracts leads to loss of sensations below the tumour. If the pyramidal tracts are destroyed, upper motor neurone paralysis is seen. Involvement of both pyramidal tracts leads to disturbed bladder function.

In *extramedullary* tumours root pain may be present for years before cord compression occurs. If the pain is referred to the shoulder and arms, it may be regarded as due to arthritis or neuritis. In the chest it may be labelled as angina pectoris. In the abdomen it may be thought to arise from the gallbladder or appendix, or from the pelvic organs. A spinal origin should be suspected if the pain is *increased on coughing*. Finally, spastic paralysis sets in with a transverse level of sensory loss below the level of the tumour.

Intramedullary tumours extend over a length of spinal cord, so they cause a wide belt of sensory loss and lower motor neurone paralysis. Root pain occurs late.

Tumours of the *cauda equina* produce root pain, sensory loss and lower motor neurone paralysis in the distribution of the sacral nerve roots.

Investigations. *X-ray spine* may show absorption of a pedicle or enlargement of an intervertebral foramen.

Lumbar puncture may show obstruction to the circulation of cerebrospinal fluid (CSF) by Queckenstedt's test: on compressing the internal jugular veins the pressure of the lumbar CSF does not rise.

Examination of the CSF. The fluid below a block becomes yellow and contains increased amounts of proteins.

Cisternal myelography. A needle is passed into the cisterna magna at the level of the 2nd cervical spine. 3 ml of a radiopaque dye e.g. Myodil is injected. This gravitates down till it is arrested by the tumour, and x-rays are taken.

CT scan and MRI. Both these investigations show up the presence of a spinal tumour to good advantage. They also help greatly in its differential diagnosis from other conditions. They have to a considerable extent supplanted the older methods of investigations. However, in regions without CT scan or MRI, the previously employed methods still have relevance.

Treatment. The treatment of spinal tumours consists of exposing the concerned area of the spinal cord by laminectomy and excising the tumour.

Indications for laminectomy. Laminectomy is indicated for the following conditions:

1. Spinal tumours.
2. Trauma.
3. Paraplegia due to Pott's disease.
4. Chronic pain from malignant lymph nodes in the upper neck, the posterior nerve roots being divided.
5. The pain of an irremovable new growth, the spinothalamic tracts being sectioned.

Nerves

CRANIAL NERVES

The **first** (olfactory) nerve may be injured by fractures of the cribriform plate causing partial or complete loss of smell on the affected side.

The **second** (optic) nerve may be damaged by fractures involving the optic foramen, or by tumours or aneurysms. Primary optic atrophy with partial or complete blindness can occur. However the pupil contracts if the opposite retina is stimulated.

The **third** nerve is involved by tumours, trauma or aneurysm in the skull, sphenoidal fissure or orbit. Pressure on the nerve above the tentorium occurs when a midbrain pressure cone forms. A partial lesion merely causes dilatation of the pupil. In a complete lesion there is also ptosis from paralysis of levator palpabrae superioris, and proptosis from paralysis of the majority of the ocular muscles. A lateral and downward squint occurs due to unopposed action of the external rectus and superior oblique muscles.

The **fourth** nerve supplies the superior oblique, and is rarely involved alone.

The **fifth** nerve. *Trigeminal neuralgia.* In this condition sudden severe pain occurs in one or two divisions of the trigeminal nerve, commonly in a middle-aged or elderly person. The pain may be precipitated by exposure to cold, touch, eating, talking etc. Normally no cause can be found. Treatment is started with drugs. Carbamazepine is the most effective. If this fails treatment is by surgery. The trigeminal ganglion is approached subtemporally. The lateral two thirds of the sensory root are sectioned. Thus the ophthalmic division is spared, avoiding the complication of exposure keratitis due to anaesthesia of the cornea.

The **sixth** nerve has a long intracranial course. It may be affected by fractures of the base of the skull or, along with other nerves, by lesions in the cavernous sinus, sphenoidal fissure or orbit. Internal squint results from paralysis of the external rectus.

The **seventh** nerve may be involved at different sites:

1. ***Intracranial.*** Lesions within the brain are supranuclear, nuclear or infranuclear. In *supranuclear* lesions the upper part of the face escapes, because those muscles have a bilateral innervation. In *nuclear* lesions the whole face, the sixth nerve on the same side, and the opposite arm and leg are affected. In *infranuclear* lesions the auditory nerve is also commonly involved.

2. ***Cranial.*** The intraosseous part of the facial nerve is affected by fracture of the base of the skull or middle ear disease. Paralysis may occur:

i. Immediately after fracture, due to direct injury.

ii. Within a few days due to haemorrhage within the nerve sheath; in this case recovery is possible.

iii. After some weeks due to the pressure of callus; this is unlikely to recover.

3. ***Extracranial.*** i. *Bell's palsy* is a herpetic neuritis of the facial nerve, and follows exposure to cold. The swelling of the nerve extends into the bony canal and compresses the nerve; it usually subsides before permanent damage has occurred, but in a few cases partial or complete paralysis persists.

ii. The branches of the facial nerve may be injured by broken windscreens or badly placed operation incisions.

The paralysed face is flat and expressionless. The eye cannot be closed. Corneal ulceration may follow due to exposure. Epiphora occurs due to drooping of the lower eyelid. The patient cannot whistle, and food collects between the gums and cheek.

Treatment is directed towards the cause. The angle of the mouth may be supported by small strips of adhesive strapping applied under tension. Faradic stimulation and massage are prescribed. If recovery does not occur, the hypoglossal nerve may be anastomosed to the branches of the facial nerve.

The **eighth** nerve may be involved by middle fossa fractures or tumours.

The **ninth** nerve may be injured in a fractured base of skull, with dysphagia due to paresis of the constrictor muscle.

The **tenth** nerve may be damaged in a fractured base of skull. The recurrent laryngeal nerve may be damaged during thyroidectomy, and compressed due to infiltration by a carcinoma of the thyroid. Partial involvement affects the more sensitive abductor muscles only, so that if it is bilateral, asphyxia results and tracheostomy may be required. Complete involvement causes paralysis of both abductors and adductors, so the cord is held in the midway or *cadaveric* position. The opposite vocal cord increases its mobility, reaches across the midline and closes the glottis. The voice is adequate but monotonous.

The **eleventh** nerve is commonly injured during removal of tuberculous lymph nodes in the neck. If the injury is recognized at operation, primary suture should be performed.

The **twelfth** nerve may be injured during removal of the submandibular salivary gland. Hemiatrophy occurs in the tongue, which is pushed towards the paralysed side on protrusion.

SPINAL NERVES

Injuries. Injuries of the nerves are classified into neurapraxia, axonotmesis and neurotmesis.

Neurapraxia. This is the equivalent of concussion. Conduction in the intact nerve fibres is interrupted temporarily due to stretch or distortion, and without organic rupture. It is produced by minor stretch injuries. There is sensory loss, paraesthesiae and paresis for a few days. Fibres remain intact. The axons do not degenerate. When conduction returns, all functions return together within a few hours. Recovery is complete. Treatment consists of splinting the limb in the position of relaxation of the paralysed muscle until recovery.

Axonotmesis. Traction produces rupture of nerve fibres within intact sheaths. This may occur during birth, or by clutching for support while falling. Compression by tourniquets, splints, or by incorrect posture on the operating table may have the same effect. Wallerian degeneration occurs in the distal portions of the broken axons, leaving empty tubules. Slow recovery occurs by the downgrowth of axons into the distal tubules. Some nerve fibres are lost due to fibrosis in the tubules. However, there is little maldistribution of fibres because the sheaths are intact. After a delay of nearly 10 days, axons proceed distally at the rate of approximately 1 mm a day. When they reach their endings it takes three weeks for the end organs to become activated. As such muscles and skin areas farthest from the site of division are reinnervated last.

Clinical features. There is an initial picture of concussion with loss of sensation, tone, power, and reflex activity in the limb. This is followed by incomplete recovery. Numbness and paralysis persist only in those areas where fibres have actually ruptured.

Secondary changes. Disuse results in impaired circulation, and the part becomes blue and cold. The nails are brittle and trophic changes occur due to minor unrecognized trauma. The paralysed muscles are overstretched by the unopposed action of antagonists. Periarticular adhesions fix the immobile joints in a contracted position.

Treatment is aimed at maintaining the nerves and joints in good working order while awaiting the arrival of downgrowing axons. The part is protected by warm padding and splinted in the position of relaxation of paralysed groups. Muscle movement is maintained by regular galvanic stimulation of paralysed muscles. All joints are put through their full range of movements daily to prevent contractures. Moral support and encouragement is provided during the slow process of recovery. If recovery fails to occur the nerve should be explored, when a perineural scar or an intraneural fibroma is usually found, and requires removal.

Neurotmesis. This is commonly produced by penetrating wounds. It results in partial or complete division of nerve sheaths and fibres. In the proximal portions of the divided axons retrograde degeneration occurs as high as the first node of Ranvier. The axons now subdivide to produce numerous end bulbs which grow downwards. But the gap between the nerve ends has by now been filled with organizing blood clot which acts as a barrier. Cells of the distal sheaths of Schwann sprout and grow proximally towards the proximal axons. In this way a very few axons find their way into distal tubules.

Even after accurate nerve suture the quality of regeneration is less perfect than in cases of axonotmesis, due to wastage and maldistribution of axons. The density of scar tissue is increased by local sepsis and inflammation, and by tension at the suture line. Maldistribution is greatest in the case of mixed motor and sensory nerves, e.g. the median and ulnar nerves at the wrist. The quality of recovery is best in purely motor nerves supplying large muscle groups e.g. the radial nerve.

Treatment consists of fine and accurate suture in the absence of sepsis and tension, and placing the nerve in a suitable bed. If there is much loss of skin, plastic surgical operations to replace full-thickness skin must precede repair of nerve. In clean incised wounds immediate primary suture is best. In untidy contaminated wounds suture is postponed for about three weeks, because primary suture would require enlargement of the incision and this would spread infection. Secondly, in three weeks the nerve sheath becomes thick and easier to stitch.

Nerve suture. The two ends of the nerve are identified. The incision is prolonged to expose the nerve well above and below the seat of injury. The ends of the nerve are 'freshened' by a scalpel. Slices are removed until projecting fibres are seen and blood oozes from the cut surface. If necessary the ends are approximated by mobilization and posture. Sutures are inserted through the nerve sheath. Magnification is employed, and 7/0 to 9/0 polypropylene sutures are used, as they cause the least reaction.

If nerve suture is impossible due to loss of tissue, recourse may be had to nerve anastomosis, nerve grafting, tendon transplantation, arthrodesis or amputation (the last-named for persistent ulcers on the foot).

INDIVIDUAL SPINAL NERVES

Injuries of the *cervical plexus* are uncommon and insignificant.

The *phrenic nerve* (C3, 4, 5) used to be crushed to cause temporary paralysis of the diaphragm in order to reduce the size of the pleural cavity in tuberculosis.

NERVES OF THE UPPER LIMB

Brachial plexus lesions. Complete lesions of the brachial plexus are rare, because the severity of the trauma usually proves fatal. Incomplete lesions may be due to stabs or cuts. The main muscle groups are as follows:

C V	Deltoid, biceps and supinator
C VI	Remaining muscles of shoulder, triceps and pronators.
C VII	Extensors of fingers
C VIII	Flexors of wrist and fingers
D I	Small muscles of hand

Upper brachial plexus lesion (Erb's paralysis). This lesion occurs due to excessive depression of the shoulder in infants during a difficult delivery, and in adults after a fall on the shoulder. C5 & C6 are affected. The limb is internally rotated by the unopposed subscapularis. It hangs by the side, with the hand pronated. Function of the hand is preserved, therefore arthrodesis of the shoulder and elbow is useful.

Lower brachial plexus lesion (Klumpke's paralysis). The lower nerve trunk or medial cord are injured by an unreduced dislocation of the humerus. When a falling person clutches at an object the nerve roots may be avulsed from the spinal cord. The first dorsal root is affected. The small muscles of the hand are wasted. Anaesthesia affects the medial side of the hand. Treatment consists of splinting the limb to relax the paralysed muscles. Physiotherapy should be continued for two years before recovery is assessed.

The circumflex nerve winds around the uppermost part of the shaft of the humerus. It may be injured in fractures of the humerus. The deltoid is paralysed and wastes rapidly. Recovery commences in a few weeks if the cause of the compression is removed and the arm supported in right-angled abduction.

The nerve to the serratus anterior is injured by a blow or an operation on the breast or chest wall. 'Winging' of the scapula results. Overhead abduction of the shoulder is not possible.

The radial nerve may be injured in the *axilla* in a dislocation of the shoulder or after the use of crutches. The patient cannot extend the elbow, the wrist, or the fingers, and wrist drop occurs. Anaesthesia is seen over the dorsum of the forearm and hand.

Injury in the *spiral groove* of the humerus may occur due to pressure of the arm on the edge of the operating table, prolonged application of a tourniquet, fracture of the shaft of the humerus, or 'intramuscular' injection of a drug into the radial nerve. Wrist drop results, with inability to extend the fingers. Anaesthesia is found over the ball of the thumb.

The median nerve may be injured at the *elbow* due to fracture at the lower end of the humerus. The index finger cannot be flexed – the *pointing index* – but the other fingers can be flexed by the portion of flexor digitorum profundus which is supplied by the ulnar nerve. The thenar muscles are wasted. Sensation is lost over the lateral three and a half digits in front. Trophic changes occur, specially in the index finger.

Injuries at the *wrist* are common due to cuts etc. The thenar muscles are paralysed and wasted. No part of the hand is completely anaesthetic.

The ulnar nerve may be injured at the *elbow* from:

1. Fracture of the medial condyle.
2. Cubitus valgus due to old injury of the humerus, with increase of the carrying angle. The small muscles of the hand are paralysed, except the thenar muscles and lateral two lumbricals. The patient cannot abduct or adduct the fingers, and cannot grip a piece of paper between the fingers. Wasting is obvious in the interosseous spaces and along the inner border of the hand. Sensations are lost over the medial one and a half fingers.

Injury at the wrist occurs due to cuts. Paralysis and wasting of the small muscles of the hand occurs. Sensation is lost only over the front of the medial one and a half fingers.

NERVES OF THE LOWER LIMB

Injury to the ilioinguinal nerve may occur on the right side during appendicectomy, and on the left side during iliac colostomy. The conjoint tendon becomes weak, predisposing to an inguinal hernia.

The sciatic nerve is injured by wounds, fractures or intramuscular injections. The flexors of the knee are paralysed, but some flexion is possible due to the action of the sartorius and gracilis muscles. There is complete sensory loss below the knee, except for a strip along the inner side of the leg and foot supplied by the saphenous nerve. Trophic ulcers form on the sole of the foot.

The lateral popliteal nerve is injured by fractures of, or during excision of, the upper end of the fibula, and by pressure from plasters or splints. There is complete paralysis of the extensors and peroneal muscles, with talipes equinovarus and sensory loss over the outer side of the leg and dorsal aspects of the toes. Trophic changes also occur in this area.

The *medial popliteal nerve* is rarely injured.

46 Face and mouth

The face develops from five processes around the primitive mouth. At the cephalic side lies the frontonasal process, and on each side a maxillary and a mandibular process. Mesoderm grows medially from each maxillary process to join in the midline and form the palate.

CLEFT LIP AND PALATE

Failure of fusion between the above-mentioned development processes results in a cleft involving the following structures:

1. Lip alone.
2. Lip and alveolus.
3. Lip, alveolus and palate.
4. Palate alone.

During the first two months of pregnancy exposure to x-rays, vitamin deficiency and certain virus infections, e.g. rubella, is associated with an increased incidence of these abnormalities. In 12% cases the condition is familial.

Effects. A cleft lip can ruin the symmetry and appearance of an otherwise extremely beautiful face (Fig. 1).

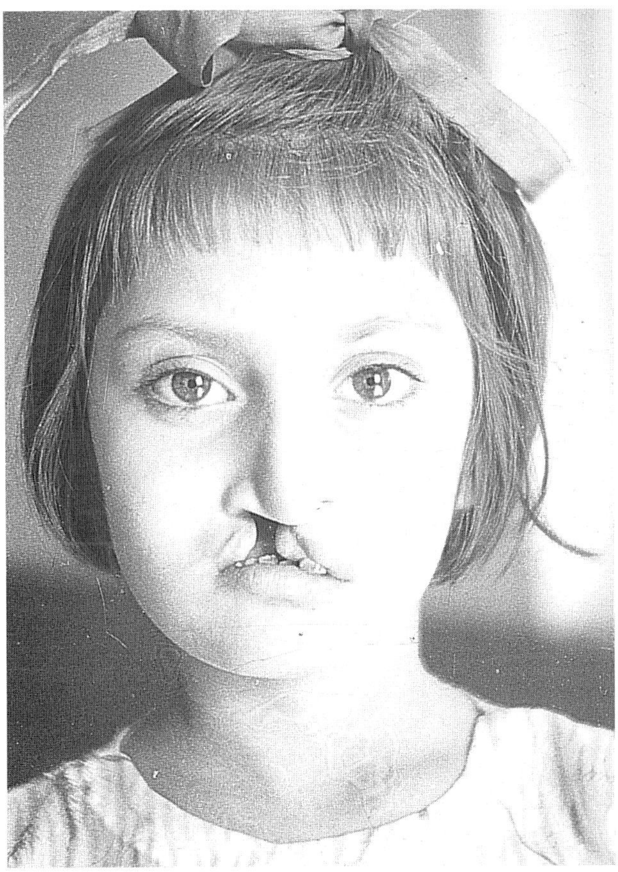

Fig. 1 Cleft lip in a young girl, destroying the symmetry of an otherwise very beautiful face.

A cleft in the palate interferes with numerous important functions:

Sucking. With cleft palate the infant may be unable to suck, as negative pressure cannot be established. Most cases can be dealt with by enlarging the hole in the teat of the feeding bottle; for this purpose a red hot sewing needle may be passed through the opening.

Speech. Because air escapes into the nose the patient with cleft palate cannot make consonants (e.g. B, D and T), and has a nasal speech.

Hearing. There is a slight loss of hearing because regurgitated food causes inflammation of the pharynx and eustachian tubes. At the same time middle ear infections are more common in cases of cleft palate, the reason being as follows: in the normal person, acting from below the tensors and levators palati open out the inner ends of the eustachian tubes during swallowing, allowing air to enter and equalize the pressure inside and outside the tympanic membrane. In cleft palate, as these muscles are severed in the midline they are put out of action. The middle ear remains closed, air gets absorbed, the tympanic membrane caves in and may rupture. Early closure of the cleft in the palate removes this source of ear infections.

The *teeth* are out of line and require orthodontic management.

Treatment. ***Cleft lip.*** The aim is to improve the appearance. Operation is performed at the age of about three months, when the baby is putting on weight. The most popular operation is by Millard, in which the deficiency of tissue on the medial side of the defect is made good by an advancement flap from the lateral side. Further, the curved suture line lies in the position of, and looks like, the missing philtrum column, producing a very good result (Fig. 2). Fine sutures of monofilament polypropylene (size 6/0) result in a scar without stitch marks (Fig. 3).

When there is a bilateral cleft lip with unfused premaxilla, both sides are operated upon together, the better to repair the orbicularis oris across the midline. The constant pull exerted by the reconstructed orbicularis oris ensures that the protruding premaxilla moves back to its normal position. The short columella results in a depressed tip of the nose, which generally requires correction later.

Cleft palate. The aim is adequate speech and dentition, swallowing without nasal regurgitation, and no loss of hearing. Operation is undertaken at the age of 12 to 18 months. The mucosa of the palate is mobilized in the form of flaps. The mucosa on the nasal aspect of the palate is also mobilized. Both layers are sutured. The muscle of the soft palate is stitched carefully. Before operation the parents must be told that in a small number of cases the cleft palate repair can break down, due to the fact that it is a thin, moist membrane, which is subject to very high pressures during the act of swallowing.

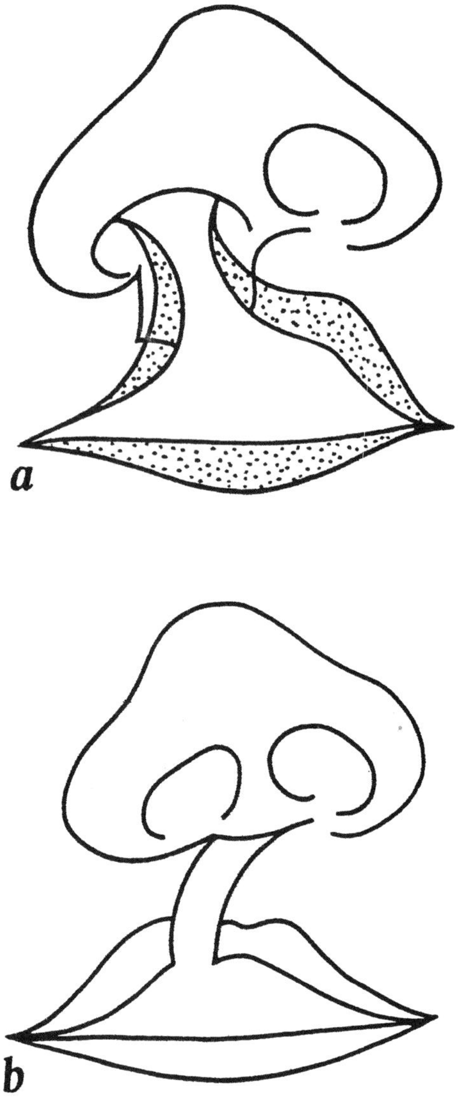

Fig. 2a,b Millard operation for unilateral cleft lip. a. Flaps outlined. b. Incisions made.

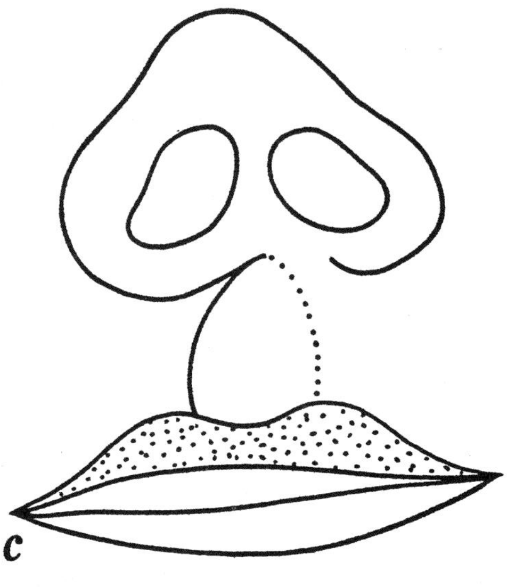

Fig. 2c Millard operation. Final position.

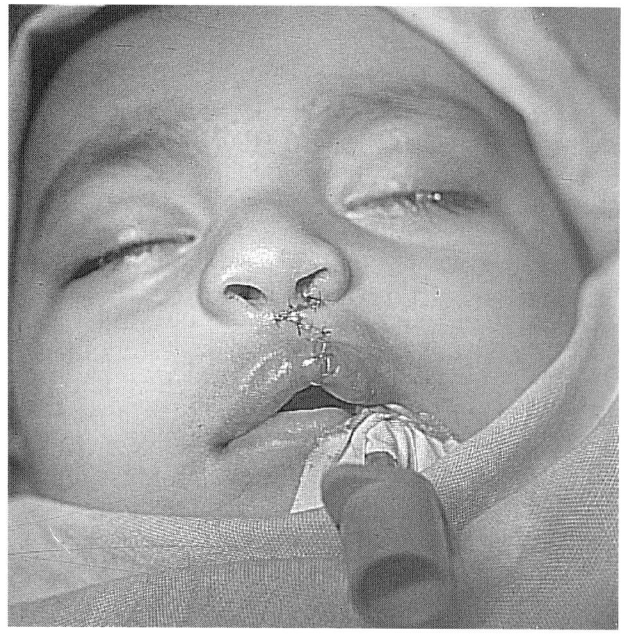

Fig. 3 Before removal of sutures after a Millard operation for unilateral cleft lip.

Even after operation, a gap may remain behind the repaired palate due to its shortness, allowing some air to escape via the nose and interfering with proper speech. Cineradiography in the lateral position helps clarify the situation. If speech therapy fails to deal with the matter, a flap from the posterior wall of the pharynx may have to be raised and its free edge attached to the posterior margin of the soft palate, to remedy the situation ('pharyngoplasty').

The care of an infant with cleft palate should consist of a team effort between a surgeon, an orthodontist, an otorhinolaryngologist, and a speech therapist.

Micrognathia. In this condition the horizontal ramus of the mandible is poorly developed and short. Usually a cleft palate is also present, when the condition is called Pierre Robin syndrome. The pharyngeal airway is narrow, resulting in attacks of dyspnoea and cyanosis.

The baby should be nursed in the prone position so that the tongue cannot fall back and obstruct the pharynx. If this is done, there is no need of the 'tongue stitch' of the past. To hold the chin off the bed in the prone position, a 'cap' of tubinette gauze is worn, which is suspended from an overhead frame. If, however, a sufficient number of nurses or helpers are available, the baby may be carried prone on the hand round the clock. In about six weeks the mandible grows sufficiently, so that symptoms of respiratory difficulty disappear. In adult life the ramus can be lengthened by bone-grafting. However, in many cases, it grows adequately so that recourse to such a procedure is not required.

Preauricular sinus. Six tubercles join to form the external ear. Imperfect fusion results in a preauricular sinus, the opening of which lies in front of the tragus. If the opening closes, a cyst may form. If it becomes infected and bursts an ulcer may result. The only curative treatment is complete excision of the sinus.

Congenital short fraenum of upper lip. If this occurs, a gap between the medial incisors may result, which is cosmetically unattractive. It should be incised transversely and sutured longitudinally. However, sometimes the medial incisors come together in spite of the presence between them of a thick, fleshy fraenum. This suggests that the fraenum does not always stand in their way.

A swelling on the palate may be a tumour of the palatal mucosa or bone, an ectopic salivary tumour, a carcinoma of the maxillary antrum, or an alveolar abscess.

NEOPLASMS OF THE LIP

Lymphangioma and cavernous haemangioma occur from time to time.

Carcinoma of the lip. This tumour is common in men between sixty and seventy years of age, specially fair-skinned individuals who have followed an outdoor occupation, as excessive exposure to sunlight predisposes to this condition. The lower lip is affected in 95 percent cases. It is a squamous-celled carcinoma, and presents as an ulcer, usually with the typical everted edge. Any ulcer on the lip which does not heal readily should be viewed with suspicion and biopsied.

Treatment. Carcinomas of the lip are usually slow-growing and can be cured by surgery or radiotherapy. Early (T1) tumours can be managed by wedge resection, including at least 0.5 cm of normal tissue. More advanced lesions require combined surgery and radiotherapy. The five-year survival rate is 70%. If a tumour is advanced or recurs after radiotherapy, surgical excision leaves behind a large defect, which has to be repaired by rotating a flap from the nasolabial area.

Involvement of submental or deep cervical nodes occurs late. If they are mobile, a neck dissection is performed. In tumours arising in the lip, the recent tendency is to remove the lymph nodes only in the supraomohyoid region of the neck. If the nodes are fixed or the patient is elderly or weak, radiotherapy is used instead. Careful follow-up of all cases is essential.

FACIAL INJURIES

These are very common. Minor injuries e.g. black-eye and small lacerations are due to accidents, sports or fights. In traffic accidents the victims are usually motor car passengers who are thrown forwards against the windscreen or dashboard. The wearing of safety belts reduces the incidence of such trauma.

First aid. The airway may be obstructed by blood, or by the tongue falling back in a bilateral fracture of the mandible. The patient should be placed on his side or semi-prone. A complete examination can be carried out in the operation theatre under anaesthesia. The blood supply to the face is good, so wounds in this area heal well. They can be treated by primary suture even if 24 hours have elapsed since the injury. Dirt and pieces of glass must be removed. 4/0 chromic catgut is used for mucosa and muscles, 5/0 or 6/0 polypropylene for skin. Sutures are removed in 2 to 4 days to avoid stitch marks.

Fractures of the face. ***The nasal bones.*** The injury may be lateral, causing impaction of one nasal bone under the other; or frontal, which compresses the nasal structures backwards. Under general anaesthesia the bones are gripped in special forceps, disimpacted and manipulated into position. They are protected by a plaster of Paris cast.

The malar bone. The malar bone may be fractured and depressed by a direct blow. There may be diplopia and inability to open the mouth. A notch can be palpated on the infraorbital margin. The bone is elevated by a bone lever introduced through an incision in the temple behind the hair margin. It is fixed by wiring it to the frontal bone and maxilla.

The maxilla. These fractures are classified according to *Le Fort*. In Le Fort I fracture the alveolus is separated from the maxilla. In Le Fort II the maxilla is separated from the rest of the skull. In Le Fort III the maxilla, nasal bones, ethmoids and palatal bones are separated from the base of the skull. The patient may be unable to close the jaws.

In Le Fort II & III there may be diplopia due to displacement of the floor of the orbit. In Le Fort III the cribriform plate may be injured and cerebrospinal fluid rhinorrhoea may result.

Treatment. A tracheostomy may be necessary. The displaced maxilla is freed by rocking with bone forceps, restored to its normal position, and held in place by one of the following methods:

1. By internal wire sutures between maxilla and malar bone.
2. By wiring a pliable metal bar to the teeth and fixing this by a system of extra-oral rods to a steel frame around the skull.

At the same time the upper and lower jaws may be wired together.

The mandible. The mandible may be fractured at the following sites:

1. *The neck of the condyle.* The neck is pulled forwards by the external pterygoid muscle.
2. *The ascending ramus*, usually near the angle of the jaw: little displacement occurs. The only symptom is persistent pain.
3. *The body of the jaw* is fractured most often, usually by a direct blow. The fracture commonly occurs at the site of the canine tooth, the long root of which weakens the bone. If the fracture is bilateral the central portion of the jaw is displaced downwards by the anterior bellies of the digastric muscles etc. The fracture is nearly always open due to the firm attachment of the mucoperiosteum to the bone. Diagnosis is obvious, as speech and swallowing are impaired. Blood-stained saliva trickles from the mouth. The line of the teeth is irregular. Fractures of the body of the mandible are rated as favourable or unfavourable according to the direction of the fracture line. Fractures that run downwards and forwards are favourable. The posterior fragment is pulled upwards by the masseter, the anterior fragment downwards by the mylohyoid and digastric; thus the fragments are brought together. The reverse is true if the fracture line runs downwards and backwards.

Treatment. Compression plates produce maximum contact and stabilization of the fractures; the need for intermaxillary fixation is eliminated, so that motion at the temporomandibular joint is allowed. If plating systems are not available, open exposure of the fracture and direct wiring with intermaxillary fixation for 6 weeks is required, fluids being taken through a tube. Warm antiseptic mouthwashes reduce the chances of infection in this compound fracture. Antibiotic cover is required. Complications include necrosis of bone, delayed union and aspiration pneumonia.

Boils and pimples. Boils in the 'mask' area of the face should never be squeezed, as the infection can reach the cavernous sinus by venous connections and cause cavernous sinus thrombosis.

THE TEETH

Impacted wisdom tooth. This tooth is the third lower molar. An adjacent tooth prevents it from eruption. It is overhung by a flap of gum, known as an operculum, where food collects causing infection which may spread to the cheek. If an abscess is present it is drained. When the acute symptoms have subsided the impacted tooth is extracted. If the molar tooth anterior to it is carious, extraction of the carious tooth may afford room for the impacted molar to erupt.

Haemorrhage after extraction. There may be an open artery or a spicule of bone which prevents firm clotting within the socket. The patient may be a haemophiliac. The cavity is mopped with pledgets of cotton wool. Any loose bone spicules are removed. Firm pressure with a pledget for a few minutes may stop the bleeding. Snake venom and absorbable gauze may be used. Persistent bleeding from the gum margin can be arrested by a stitch.

DENTAL CARIES

The incidence of dental caries is highest among affluent people whose diet includes carbohydrates in highly refined form e.g. white bread, and sweets eaten between meals. Carbohydrates are broken down by bacterial enzymes to lactic acid, which can dissolve enamel. Proteolytic enzymes from other bacteria then disintegrate the dentine.

The stages of dental decay. Stages I (erosion of enamel) and II (disintegration of dentine) are painless and symptomless. When stage II caries has reached near the pulp, hot or cold fluids and sweets may cause toothache.

Stage III: Part of the crown collapses.

Stage IV: Acute pulpitis. Pain is throbbing. Untreated it causes an alveolar abscess.

Surgical significance of caries. A mouth full of broken teeth increases morbidity from operations. Stomatitis may result. If there is dehydration, acute suppurative parotitis may occur. Bacteraemia from infected roots may hamper recovery from operation. Therefore in non-emergency cases dental extraction may be considered and operation delayed for a few weeks till the gums are soundly healed. During anaesthesia one should guard against breaking of a tooth, which may be inhaled and cause collapse of a lobe of the lung and lung abscess. If a tooth is inhaled or is missing, a chest x-ray and bronchoscopy should be carried out.

Alveolar abscess. Alveolar abscesses occur most often in childhood and early adult life. In acute pulpitis the putrefying pulp generates gases that exert pressure through the root canal into osseous tissue around the apex of the tooth. The abscess almost always points towards the lateral aspect. If it is not resolved early by antibiotics or drained promptly, osteomyelitis of the jaw results. There is constant dull pain, redness and swelling of the gum and cheek. The regional lymph nodes are enlarged and tender and there is fever with rigors. The cause of the alveolar abscess must be looked for on the x-ray: caries, an impacted 'wisdom' tooth, retained roots, or a dead tooth.

Treatment. Surgical principles must be followed. An abscess must be drained. Antibiotics must not be used in place of a drainage operation. They can be used before pus forms, and later in support of the drainage operation.

Root abscess. An alveolar abscess is acute; a root abscess is nearly always chronic. It arises when infection extends from the pulp through the apical canal. Usually there are no signs, and it is revealed only by a dental x-ray. The absence of pain and of sensory response to hot or cold stimuli means a dead tooth. Treatment is usually by extraction of the tooth.

THE GUMS

Gingivitis and pyorrhoea. In gingivitis the gums recede and there is an excessive deposit of tartar. Food particles accumulate between gums and teeth. The gums are swollen and spongy, and bleed. In pyorrhoea pus can be expressed from gingival pockets. There is a foul smell. The teeth become loose and fall out. Early cases require regular scaling, daily massage of gums with fingers and an astringent mouthwash. If this is unsuccessful gingivectomy is advised. In pyorrhoea cure is unlikely without extracting the teeth implicated.

Tumours of the alveolus (Epulides). There are four varieties of epulides:

1. *Granulomatous epulis*, i.e. a mass of granulation tissue, usually around a carious tooth. The tooth should be extracted and the granulations scraped.
2. *Fibrous epulis*, i.e. a fibroma arising from the periodontal membrane. The adjacent tooth and a wedge of bone (including the portion of the gum containing the growth) must be removed.
3. *Giant-celled epulis*, i.e. osteoclastoma. Ulceration and haemorrhage can occur. X-rays show bone destruction. Small tumours are curetted, larger ones radically excised.
4. *Carcinomatous epulis*, i.e. an epithelioma of the gum, which can ulcerate, invade the bone and spread to the cervical lymph nodes.

THE JAWS

Swellings of the jaw may be classified into the following types:

1. *Inflammatory.* Alveolar abscess, osteomyelitis, actinomycosis.
2. *Odontomes.* Dental cysts, dentigerous cysts, adamantinoma.
3. *Bone tumours:*

i. Benign: (a) Fibro-osseous.
(b) Osteoclastoma and reparative cell granuloma.

ii. Malignant: (a) Osteosarcoma.
(b) Carcinoma of maxillary antrum.

Osteomyelitis of the jaws. In infants this condition may complicate measles or scarlet fever.

Subacute osteomyelitis occurs from an apical dental infection, an alveolar abscess or a compound fracture of the jaw. The mandible is affected more often because it is supplied by a single artery, thrombosis of which causes bone necrosis. X-ray evidence of necrosis appears only after three weeks. In the initial stages antibiotics may abort the infection. If x-rays show bone necrosis operation is performed, to relieve tension and remove dead bone.

Chronic osteomyelitis. The causes of chronic osteomyelitis are similar to the above; in fact this condition usually develops in cases where acute or subacute osteomyelitis fails to heal. The infected area requires to be deroofed. A shallow groove is chiselled in the bone, any sequestrum removed, and the wound left open to granulate. Appropriate antibiotics are given.

Cervico-facial actinomycosis. Actinomycosis is a localized inflammatory condition of the jaw that spreads by multiple fistulae and abscesses into the face and neck. The underlying bone can also become infected, as well as the apex of the lung. The infection is caused by anaerobic filamentous bacilli belonging to the Actinomycetes family. These were once believed to be fungi, because they grow slowly as branched filaments and chains. Diagnosis is dependent upon the presence of characteristic sulphur granules in the pus on microscopy. Special stains should be carried out to exclude fungal infection. Penicillin and sulphonamides are effective against these infections. Abscesses and areas of chronic scarring may require surgery.

THE ODONTOMES

These are cysts, tooth malformations or tumours arising from the epithelial or mesothelial elements of the teeth. Only epithelial odontomes are important, namely dental cyst, dentigerous cyst and adamantinoma.

Dental cyst. This occurs at the root of a normally erupted but chronically infected pulpless tooth. Epithelial cells from the enamel organ form the lining. Usually the fluid is clear and uninfected and the condition is painless.

Dentigerous cyst. This cyst contains an unerupted permanent tooth, usually a third molar.

Treatment of both the above-mentioned cysts is excision of the whole epithelial lining of the cyst.

Adamantinoma. An adamantinoma is an epithelial tumour probably arising from enamel-forming cells. It looks histologically and behaves like a basal cell carcinoma, being locally invasive. It is solid, but with areas of cystic degeneration. An x-ray shows large and small loculi. It recurs after enucleation, so the treatment is resection of the affected portion of the jaw with a margin of healthy tissue. The defect in the jaw is bridged by a bone graft.

BENIGN SWELLINGS OF THE JAWS

The fibro-osseous group. These are probably disorders of ossification in membrane bones. They contain fibrous tissue and bone. Examples are monostotic or polyostotic fibrous dysplasia and ivory osteoma.

Giant-celled reparative granuloma probably results from a haemorrhage within the jaw. It occurs between 10 and 25 years of age, i.e. at an earlier age than osteoclastoma. Its treatment is by thorough curettage.

TUMOURS OF THE JAW

Osteoclastomas occur from time to time in both mandible and maxilla.

Mandible. A primary or secondary cancer is rare in the mandible. However, the mandible may be involved by the spread of a carcinoma of the lip, tongue or floor of mouth. Irradiation causes bone necrosis; therefore, the affected area of mandible must be resected.

Maxilla. Osteogenic sarcoma and squamous-cell carcinoma from the hard palate or gum are seen occasionally.

Columnar-celled carcinoma from the *maxillary antrum* produces a foul blood-stained discharge from the nose. It may grow medially to cause nasal obstruction, upwards to produce diplopia, forwards to produce a facial swelling and downwards to bulge out from the palate. All nasal polyps should be biopsied to avoid missing a malignancy; fragments of the tumour may be washed out by antral lavage and examined microscopically. High-voltage irradiation is given. If some malignant tissue persists, as shown at antrostomy a few weeks later, radium tubes are placed in the antrum. If lymph nodes are palpable a neck dissection is performed.

THE MOUTH

Stomatitis. This is a general term applied to inflammatory, erosive and ulcerative conditions widely affecting the oral mucosa. *Gingivitis* refers to similar conditions confined to the gums. If they spread to other parts of the oral mucosa the term *gingivostomatitis* is used.

Infecting organisms. The mouth contains many organisms. Most of them are harmless under normal circumstances. Their ability to cause damage is reduced by the regular desquamation of surface cells, constant washing of the mouth by saliva, and the integrity of the epithelium. Some organisms take advantage of any weakness in the defences of the oral mucosa to produce an infection (facultative pathogens). Others produce specific infections (true pathogens). An oral ulcer is soon colonized by facultative pathogens e.g. streptococci, staphylococci and Vincent's organisms. A non-specific acute inflammation results. This secondary infection can be treated by 0.2% solution of chlorhexidine as a mouthwash.

Predisposing factors. Deficiency of iron, vitamin B_{12}, folic acid and other B vitamins causes atrophy of the epithelium. The patient may present with a red, burning tongue and angular cheilitis due to secondary infection by *Candida albicans*. Severe protein deficiency produces a similar condition. Cytotoxic drugs, agranulocytosis, aplastic anaemia and hypogammaglobulinaemia reduce the ability to deal with secondary infection. Chronic lead poisoning leads to a blue line at the gum margin, and excessive intake of iodides results in a sore mouth and salivation.

Aphthous stomatitis (Gr. *aphtha* small ulcer). Minor aphthae appear in crops on a cyclical basis. The ulcers are 0.5 cm across, with a yellow base and red margin, and are painful. They heal within a fortnight. Major aphthae are larger and deeper, and heal with scarring. A mouthwash of 0.2% chlorhexidine or of tetracycline helps healing.

Herpes simplex infections. The infection may be subclinical or may result in stomatitis. Vesicles appear and break down to form ulcers. There is fever and lymphadenitis. An analgesic elixir and 0.2% chlorhexidine mouthwash are prescribed. Healing takes place in 10 to 14 days.

Herpes labialis. This consists of a reactivation of the herpes virus on exposure to cold winds, bright sunlight etc. It is infectious, so doctors and nurses should take due precautions.

Vincent's gingivostomatitis. This occurs due to symbiosis between *Borrelia vincenti* and *Bacteroides fusiformis*, both anaerobic and gram negative organisms. It produces a deep ulcer crater covered with greenish grey necrotic tissue which bleeds readily and has a characteristic smell. There is fever, ache in the part and salivation. Both organisms are sensitive to penicillin and metronidazole. However, local factors also need treatment by a dentist.

Cancrum oris. This is a severe form of stomatitis affecting poorly nourished children as a complication of measles etc. During states of toxaemia and dehydration, thrombosis of branches of the facial arteries develops, and results in necrosis of the tissues. Ulceration starts from the gums and spreads into the jaws. It also spreads to the lips and cheeks producing full-thickness tissue loss. Treatment should be prompt, with systemic penicillin and metronidazole, local irrigation and a high-protein, vitamin-rich diet through a nasogastric tube. Defects of the lips can be filled by nasolabial flaps. More extensive cheek defects may require repair by tubed pedicle flaps.

Monilial stomatitis. Candida albicans infection occurs in the form of thrush. This affects debilitated infants and persons with diminished resistance, e.g. the chronically ill, the elderly, and during treatment with steroids and cytotoxic agents. Small soft white plaques form, looking like milk curds. When these are wiped off, bleeding erosions are revealed. Acute candidiasis also occurs after treatment with broad spectrum antibiotics. The lateral part of the tongue is smooth and red with a burning sensation. 1% aqueous gentian violet is used in infants, and amphotericin B lozenges in older patients.

Angular stomatitis. This condition is seen in infants who suck a thumb, and in the elderly, due to leakage of saliva. There are moist cracks at the angles of the mouth, with infection by candida and staphylococci. Treatment is by nystatin cream and fucidate ointment.

The single oral ulcer. The most common cause of this condition is acute or chronic trauma, e.g. from a toothbrush or a denture. If an ulcer persists for weeks or months the possibility of malignancy must be ruled out by biopsy.

Mucous cysts. These may occur on the lips and cheeks. They arise due to retention in, or extravasation from, minor salivary glands. They are small soft round swellings (Plate VIII–I). The treatment is excision.

Ranula. This arises due to extravasation of saliva from a sublingual gland. A translucent bluish swelling forms in the floor of the mouth. There is a delicate fibrous capsule lined by a layer of macrophages. The entire mass of gland and extravasation should be removed by gentle dissection.

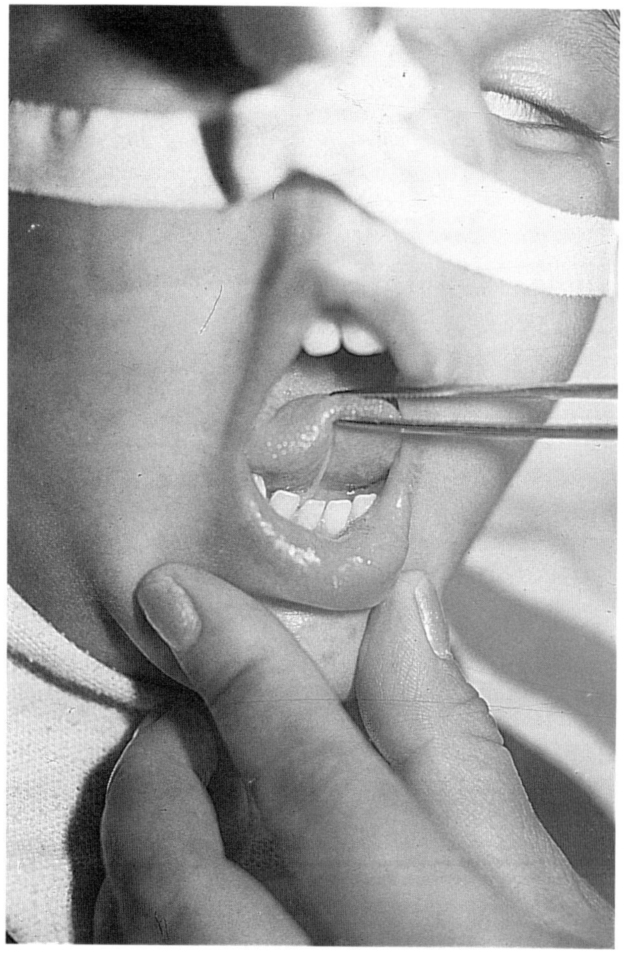

Fig. 4 Tongue-tie.

Sublingual dermoid. This condition arises due to inclusion of skin during fusion in the ventral midline. This produces an opaque swelling. It is lined by stratified squamous epithelium and filled with paste-like keratin. It commonly presents in the midline of the floor of the mouth.

Carcinoma of the cheek. Most of these are squamous cell carcinomas. The incidence is increased by smoking, drinking alcohol and chewing betel leaf. Radiotherapy is the treatment of choice, using external beams or ^{192}*Iridium wires*. Surgery is required for residual or recurrent tumour, or if radiotherapy is not available. If a full-thickness defect results, this is repaired by tubed pedicle flaps from the deltopectoral area. Enlarged neck nodes are treated by neck dissection.

THE TONGUE

Tongue-tie. Tongue-tie and ankyloglossia are terms applied to a short lingual fraenum (Fig. 4).

Attempts to protrude the tongue result in heaping up of the mid-portion of the tongue. The condition can result in considerable speech impediment. It is not commonly realized that stretch on the short fraenum can irritate the neighbouring opening of the duct of the submandibular salivary gland, and occasionally result in excessive salivation. Characteristically, the patient complains that when he wakes up in the morning his mouth is full of saliva. It is only after he has spat it out that he can talk to anyone. The short fraenum should be divided across. The wound takes on a linear shape in the vertical direction, and should be closed with a few fine absorbable sutures.

Lingual thyroid. The thyroid descends from the foramen caecum to its final position in the neck. If it does not do so, it may be seen as a midline swelling at the junction of the middle and posterior thirds of the tongue, i.e. at the foramen caecum. If large, it may cause difficulty in breathing and swallowing. However, before it is removed, a radioiodine uptake scan should be carried out, to ensure that there is some thyroid tissue at its normal site in the neck; if not, the removed lingual thyroid should be sliced, and some of the slices implanted among the muscles of the neck.

CARCINOMA OF THE TONGUE

Carcinomas of the tongue constitute about half of all oral cancers. 97 percent are squamous cell in type, the remainder being salivary and connective tissue tumours. Squamous cell carcinoma predominantly occurs in older men. However, it has also been seen in younger individuals and should therefore not be overlooked in this population. Poor oral hygiene and the use of tobacco and alcohol are considered to be important in its causation. When tobacco and alcohol are used together over a period of time, the risk is greatly increased. Tumours arising from the ventral surface of the tongue extend directly to the floor of the mouth, and it is difficult to distinguish them from tumours arising primarily at this site.

Clinical features. ***Symptoms.*** Tumours of the *anterior two-thirds* present most often as painful ulcers or visible swellings. Dysphagia, or the presence of a lump in the neck, are uncommon features.

Carcinomas of the *posterior third* of the tongue are very different from those of the anterior two thirds; they behave like tumours of the oropharynx, many of them being non-Hodgkin lymphomas. They commonly present either with local pain or dysphagia. A lump of lymph nodes in the neck is also a fairly frequent occurrence.

If there is any fixation of the tongue, difficulty will be experienced in propelling food backwards from the mouth into the pharynx. A lesion near the alveolus may result in toothache or in difficulty in wearing dentures. If a tooth is extracted, its socket may not heal. Generally speaking, the more anterior the lesion the earlier the patient seeks advice. Extensive lesions of the tongue may extend posteriorly to involve the larynx. Even if the larynx is not infiltrated, involvement or resection of the base of the tongue may predispose the patient to aspiration pneumonia and ultimate respiratory failure.

Examination. *Inspection* will show whether the lesion is exophytic (Plate VII-II) or ulcerative. The patient should be asked to move the tongue from side to side; this allows the degree of fixation to be assessed. *Palpation* is an essential part of the examination of any lesion in the oral cavity. Tongue ulcers are like icebergs; while a small part of the tumour may be visible, there may be many times the volume in the deeper tissues of the tongue. This can be assessed only by palpation. *Staging* is based on size and this should be recorded. The extent of induration is also included in this estimate of size.

Nerve involvement is difficult to assess. Anaesthesia means infiltration of the lingual nerve, and since this lies deep, its involvement means extensive spread of the tumour. In the hard palate anaesthesia means infiltration of the greater palatine nerve, and such patients are incurable. *Mandibular* involvement is best assessed on x-ray, but any fixation to bone must be noted clinically. Finally the neck should be palpated for metastatic *nodes*. These usually lie in the submandibular area or the deep jugular chain, but the tongue also has direct drainage to the jugulo-omohyoid node in the lower part of the neck. Lesions in the posterior part of the tongue may spread to the retropharyngeal nodes, and pressure from these on the sympathetic chain may result in Horner's syndrome.

Lymph node metastases constitute the *most important factor in prognosis.* In their absence as many as 80 percent patients survive for 5 years or more; in their presence only 40 percent.

Investigations. If spread to the mandible is suspected, *x-rays* should be taken. They also show the state of the teeth and the presence of any root abscesses; these facts have an important bearing on the use of radiotherapy. If spread to the retropharyngeal area is suspected, *CT scan* is useful. *Biopsy* should be carried out under general anaesthesia; local anaesthesia causes a rise in the tissue pressure, which may result in spread of the tumour. A representative part of the tumour should be chosen for biopsy, not the necrotic centre.

Treatment. Carcinoma of the *anterior two-thirds* of the tongue can be treated by radiotherapy, either using an external beam or by interstitial implantation of tubes into which radium needles or iridium 192 can be placed. External radiation in doses of 6500 rads is useful, but interstitial radiation can deliver doses over 10,000 rads over a small area with greater effect. In general, *surgical* treatment is required for tumours that:

1. Are large.
2. Involve the mandible.
3. Have recurred after radiotherapy.
4. Are accompanied by palpable neck glands.

Surgical therapy consists of resection of the tumour with a margin of normal tissue and block dissection of the regional lymph nodes. Hemiglossectomy is generally carried out for any lesion of the lateral tongue. Due to uncertainty about the ability to obtain clear margins, surgery is often followed by adjuvant radiotherapy.

Carcinomas of the *posterior third* of the tongue are more radiosensitive, so that 2-year local control rates of 75% for T1 lesions and 67% for T2 lesions have been obtained. However, advanced disease at the primary site or disease with cervical metastases requires surgery. If the lesion is lateral enough, partial glossectomy may suffice, otherwise total glossectomy with or without laryngectomy is required. The 3 year survival rate after total glossectomy is around

50 percent, and 90% of patients can maintain adequate nutrition by the oral route. If the larynx is preserved, 80% have intelligible speech.

If *neck glands* are palpable a neck dissection should be carried out. Fixed glands are not necessarily a contraindication to radical neck dissection, as the structure to which they are fixed can often be removed.

Radiotherapy. If preoperative radiotherapy is employed followed by surgery, the cure rate is increased but complications like infection, wound breakdown and bone necrosis are also more frequent. If a tumour recurs after surgery, radiotherapy seldom rescues the patient; on the other hand where radiotherapy has failed, surgery succeeds in about one-third of the cases. Radiotherapy tends to cause periodontal disease, which results in marginal caries. Thus if a patient with intact teeth is irradiated he should undergo a 6 monthly dental check-up for the rest of his life. If he fails to do this and caries starts, pulpitis and apical abscess formation quickly follow, and in the irradiated case the mandible may be lost due to osteoradionecrosis. It is therefore wiser to extract all teeth before radiating an oral cavity. This usually does not meet with any resistance, because patients with a carcinoma of the tongue often have badly diseased teeth.

Reconstruction. Resection of cancers of the tongue or floor of the mouth can leave large defects in the latter. If more than half the tongue is removed or less than 1 cm of the floor of the mouth remains, replacement of soft tissues by a flap is required. A popular flap is the pectoralis major myocutaneous flap. It consists of a pedicle of pectoralis major muscle carrying the pectoral branch of the acromiothoracic artery on its deep surface and an ellipse of skin on its superficial aspect. It is elevated upto the clavicle, tunnelled underneath the skin of the neck and passed through the defect in the floor of the mouth. It is sutured in such a manner that the skin island lies in the mouth and the muscle pedicle lies over and protects the carotid sheath.

In cases where laryngectomy is also required, the resulting gap between the pharynx and the trachea is bridged by a free graft of the jejunum. Using microvascular techniques, the supplying artery of the graft is anastomosed to the superior thyroid artery, the vein (end-to-side) to the internal jugular vein.

A number of carcinomas of the tongue are incurable on presentation due to distant metastases, very advanced local disease, bilateral neck glands or poor general condition.

SALIVARY GLANDS

Investigations. *Sialography.* A radiopaque liquid such as sodium diatrizoate is injected into the parotid duct using a fine catheter, and antero-posterior and lateral x-rays taken. They outline dilatations or constrictions of the duct, as well as any displacements of the ducts due to an expanding lesion.

In the evaluation of patients whose salivary problems are related to underlying conditions such as Sjogren's syndrome, lymphoma, arthritis or other collagen or autoimmune diseases, *immunological* studies and analysis of blood *chemistry* are valuable.

INFLAMMATIONS

Acute parotitis. The two common causes of acute parotitis are *mumps* and *postoperative suppurative parotitis.*

Mumps. Mumps arises due to infection by a virus. High fever is accompanied by painful swelling of both parotid glands, often along with acute orchitis; this is occasionally followed by atrophy of the testes.

Suppurative parotitis. Suppurative parotitis is commonly seen in patients who are severely toxaemic, and where marked dehydration occurs in the postoperative period. *Staphylococcus aureus* is the usual infecting organism. A hard, tender and painful swelling is seen in the parotid region. An abscess often forms and requires drainage.

Prevention. For prevention of acute suppurative parotitis, adequate hydration must be ensured during the postoperative period. Regular mouthwashes help maintain a proper standard of oral hygiene, so that bacteria cannot multiply.

Treatment. Antibiotics and analgesics are administered. The patient's state of hydration and his general condition are improved. Oral hygiene should be attended to, including the use of toothpaste applied with a soft toothbrush. If the general condition does not improve and an abscess forms, it should be incised and drained.

Chronic sialadenitis. The most common cause of recurrent or chronic sialadenitis is obstruction of the duct of the gland due to a calculus.

Salivary calculus. The secretions of the *submandibular glands* are thick in consistency. Therefore, salivary calculi are seen most commonly in these glands. A submandibular salivary calculus can be palpated in the floor of the mouth. It is shown up by x-rays, because it is radiopaque due to its calcium content. For its removal, an incision is made in the floor of the mouth over the duct.

TUMOURS OF THE SALIVARY GLANDS

BENIGN TUMOURS

Pleomorphic adenoma (mixed salivary tumour). A mixed salivary tumour is by far the most common neoplasm of the salivary glands. The sex distribution is equal and the peak age incidence is in the fifth decade. It is a *very slow-growing* tumour, and forms a smooth, firm lump, usually over the lower pole of the parotid. When the tumour attains a large size it becomes lobulated (Fig. 5). It is usually symptomless, apart from the lump. Pain and facial paralysis should raise the suspicion of malignancy.

On *microscopic examination* the tumour shows a mixed appearance. Epithelial cells appear in strands, while others take on a duct-like arrangement. In parts of the tumour a mucoid material is produced between the cells, resulting in an appearance resembling cartilage. The tumour is classified as benign, but strands of tumour cells penetrate the capsule of the gland. Therefore simple enucleation is not advised, as it can leave behind residual tumour and lead to a recurrence. Occasionally, a long-standing pleomorphic adenoma may change to a carcinoma.

Investigations. In suspected neoplastic disease of the parotid, *MRI or CT* scanning should be carried out. *Fine*

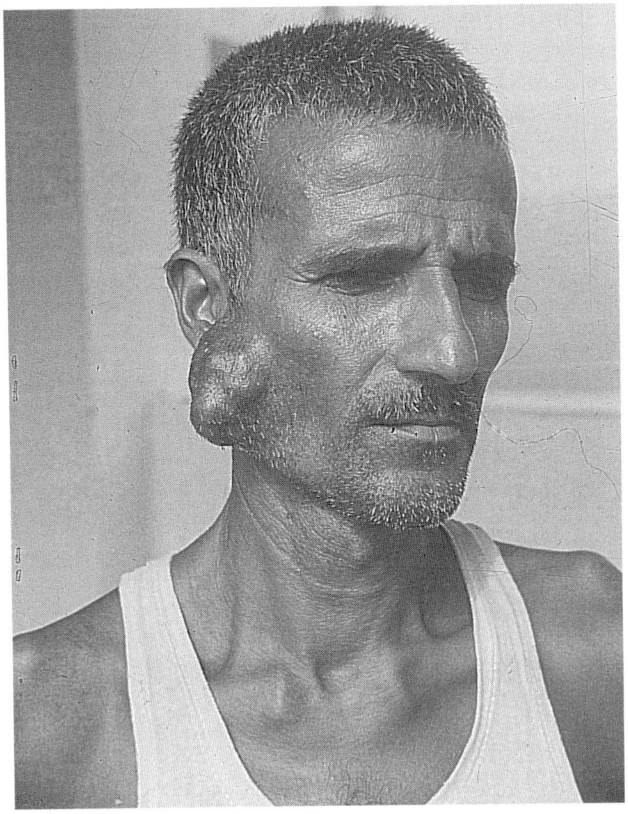

Fig. 5 Mixed parotid tumour of many years' duration; the tumour has become lobulated.

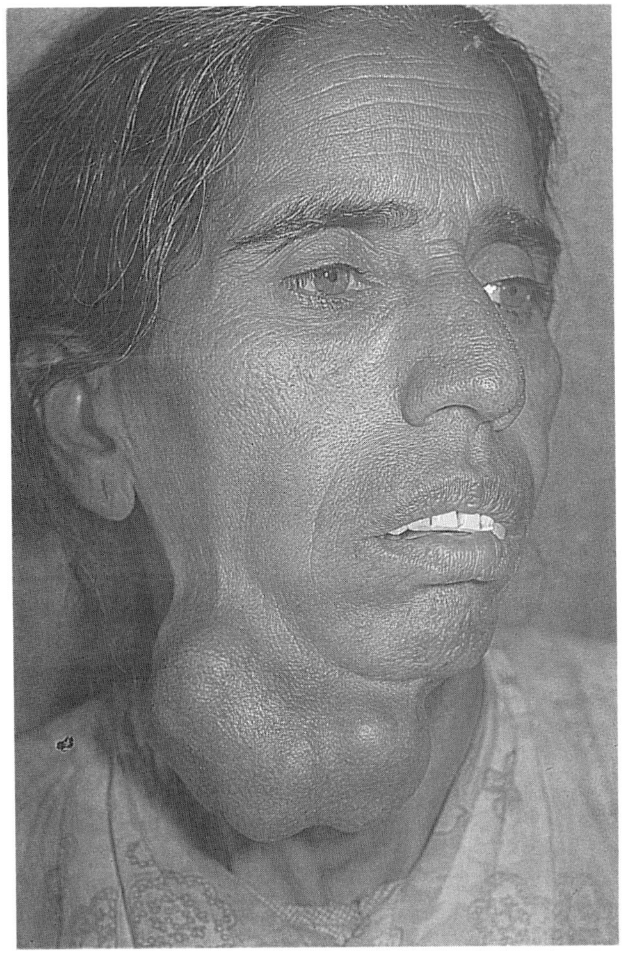

Fig. 6 Mixed tumour of submandibular salivary gland.

needle aspiration biopsy should be used routinely in the assessment of suspected neoplastic disease of the salivary glands. *Open* incisional or excisional biopsies may be required if a granulomatous or autoimmune condition is suspected. However, such biopsies should be undertaken only after careful consideration, since they carry the risk of dissemination of mixed tumours or malignancy.

Treatment. The superficial lobe of the *parotid* gland should be removed, with preservation of the branches of the facial nerve. The main trunk of the nerve is identified outside the stylomastoid foramen, and each branch traced forwards.

In the case of the *submandibular salivary gland* (Fig. 6), the entire gland is removed through a submandibular incision, avoiding the mandibular branch of the facial nerve, which supplies muscles at the angle of the mouth.

Adenolymphoma (Warthin's tumour). This tumour presents a slowly enlarging soft swelling. It is much more common in males, the peak age incidence being in the seventh decade. Bilateral tumours are sometimes encountered. Unlike other salivary tumours, an adenolymphoma produces a 'hot' spot in a ^{99}Tcm scan, so a firm preoperative diagnosis is possible without biopsy.

MALIGNANT TUMOURS

Carcinomas of the salivary glands. The histological types of carcinomas include adenocarcinoma, epidermoid carcinoma, and undifferentiated carcinomas. The adenocarcinomas contain the various cell types found in the salivary glands. The epidermoid and undifferentiated carcinomas resemble those seen at other sites. All these neoplasms tend to produce signs of malignancy at an early stage. These are fixation, resorption of adjacent bone, pain, anaesthesia, and paralysis of muscles.

An *adenoid cystic carcinoma* is the most common malignant tumour of the salivary glands. It is associated with a poor prognosis, because it infiltrates over long distances in the perineural tissues of adjacent nerves, and in the medullary cavity of neighbouring bones, before causing bone resorption. Thus, the tumour is always more extensive than the physical signs or radiological appearances suggest. The most common presenting feature is pain, and the growth may be present for some years before diagnosis. During this period the patient may consult different specialists for facial pain.

Treatment. Carcinoma of a salivary gland should be treated by radical excision of the gland. In the case of the *parotid,* the facial nerve should be resected if its preservation is likely to result in incomplete resection of the tumour. Restoration of continuity of the nerve will require primary nerve grafting.

In the case of the *submandibular gland* radical excision with, if necessary, removal of the adjacent tongue, presents no difficulty.

In mucoepidermoid and squamous cell carcinoma of the parotid and submaxillary glands, metastases to regional lymph nodes occur in about 40 percent of the patients. Therefore in these cases regional node dissection should be carried out. If lymph nodes are palpable neck dissection should be carried out in all cases.

Surgery may be contraindicated if the disease is extensive or the patient severely debilitated; radiotherapy or chemotherapy can then be employed. Postoperative radiotherapy is indicated if surgical margins are close or positive for tumour cells, and in high grade mucoepidermoid carcinoma that shows a propensity for early metastasis.

5-year survival rates vary from 40 percent for high-grade tumours to 90 percent in low-grade neoplasms.

Common features of tumours of the head and neck. Most malignant tumours developing in the anatomic area above the clavicles are squamous cell carcinomas originating from the respiratory and stratified epithelium of the upper aerodigestive tract. The change from normal to malignant epithelium passes through the stages of hyperplasia and hyperkeratosis (grouped together as leukoplakia) and *erythroplakia* or red patch, the last-named of which is premalignant. In the past, *leukoplakia* was also considered a precursor of malignancy, and removal of all leukoplakic areas of mucosa was advised. However, recent thinking suggests that this change is not in itself premalignant but simply evidence of chronic irritation; therefore surveillance rather than removal is recommended.

Malignant tumours of the head and neck cause more disruption of local function than tumours at other sites. The two main vegetative functions of the human body, namely alimentation and respiration, are dependent on the harmonious function of the bone, nerve, muscle and mucosa-lined cavities that constitute the head and neck. Invasive carcinoma disrupts these functions with resultant malnutrition, upper airway obstruction and recurrent aspiration pneumonia. Thus, unlike tumours in other parts of the body, where the fatal event is most often disseminated malignancy, as many as 60% of patients dying with head and neck malignancy have no clinical evidence of metastasis beyond the loco-regional disease.

As with most solid tumours, the best prognosticator of head and neck cancer is the presence or absence of lymph node metastases. Further, in cases with cervical metastases, extracapsular spread of tumour is a bad prognostic sign. It should be remembered that the incidence of extracapsular spread increases with the size of the lymph node.

Flaps for repairing skin and soft tissue defects in the head and neck. While removing advanced cancers in the head and neck considerable areas of the skin and soft tissues often have to be removed. If a simple split skin graft is used to resurface the area, a marked defect of contour may remain. For this reason a variety of skin flaps are employed:

1. ***Random flaps***, e.g. advancement, transposition, and rotation flaps, and Z-plasties as explained in chapter 4.

2. ***Axial flaps***. An axial flap is based on an artery running down its long axis. Therefore it can be a good deal longer than broad, i.e. it can be designed without regard to the length to width ratio. Some examples follow:

i. *Median forehead* flap based on the supratrochlear vessels, for replacement of loss of the tip of the nose or an ala.

ii. *Scalping* flap based on the superficial temporal artery, for loss of the whole nose (Fig. 9, Chapter 4).

iii. *Deltopectoral* flap from the upper chest: this is supplied by the perforating branches of the internal mammary artery. It may be used to supply skin cover, as well as lining in the mouth.

3. ***Myocutanous flaps.*** This type of flap is required where skin as well as underlying soft tissue has been lost. It consists of a large-sized muscle vascularized by a defined artery and vein. A part of the skin covering the muscle, usually in the shape of an ellipse, is left attached to its surface. The muscle is detached from its origin or insertion, or from both. It is tunnelled under the skin lying between the donor and recipient sites. At its destination the skin is sutured into the epithelial defect, while the muscle fills any soft tissue gap, besides acting as a vascularized pedicle for the skin patch.

Resection of cancer of the floor of the mouth may leave a defect in place of the excised portions of the tongue, the floor of the mouth, and the mandible. A suitable flap for reconstruction is the *pectoralis major myocutaneous flap*. The muscle is detached from its origin and insertion but is left attached to an overlying ellipse of skin and its supplying thoracoacromial vessels. It is tunnelled under the skin of the neck and into the mouth. The patch of skin is inset into the mucosal and tongue defect. If a radical neck dissection has been done, then on its way up the neck the muscle also provides cover to the carotid artery, which has been laid bare by the removal of the sternomastoid muscle.

4. ***Free microvascular flaps.*** Unlike the above-mentioned flaps, a microvascular flap is completely divided from its donor site, i.e. it is a free graft. Its supplying artery is anastomosed to an equal-sized artery at the recipient site. As these arteries are small, microvascular techniques have to be employed, using an operating microscope and extremely fine instruments and sutures. The whole operation takes many hours, but can transfer composite grafts over long distances for a very good cosmetic effect.

47 *Neck*

BRANCHIAL CYST

On the side of the neck in the foetus four bars appear; these are the branchial arches, which are separated by the branchial clefts. The first cleft persists as the external auditory meatus. The second arch grows over the third and fourth arches to fuse with the fifth. The enclosed epithelium disappears. If it persists, a branchial cyst results. If the second arch fails to fuse with the fifth, the opening persists as a branchial fistula. A branchial cyst is lined by squamous epithelium and its contents are normally like white paste. It lies under the anterior border of the upper third of the sternomastoid as a fluctuant swelling. If it is infected, it may be confused with lymphadenitis. It should be removed through an incision parallel to the skin creases of the neck.

BRANCHIAL FISTULA

A branchial fistula represents a persistent second branchial cleft. The external orifice of the fistula is located at the anterior border of the sternomastoid muscle, at the junction of its middle and lower thirds. The tract proceeds superiorly and passes inwards through the bifurcation of the carotid artery. The internal orifice lies close to the tonsil, or the track may end blindly outside the lateral pharyngeal wall. The discharge of the fistula consists of mucus or mucopus.

Treatment. In order to get rid of the troublesome discharge of mucus as well as the possibility of repeated infections, branchial fistulae should be excised. Dissection of the tract is facilitated by passing a fine probe into the orifice and utilizing it as a guide for dissection. It is also useful to inject methylene blue dye into the opening. As the tract is followed up in the neck, a series of two or three small transverse incisions in a stepladder pattern are preferable to a long oblique incision, which is cosmetically undesirable.

CYSTIC HYGROMA

In the early embryo primitive lymph sacs develop, one on either side of the neck. Normally they disappear. However, if one of them becomes sequestrated and persists, a cystic hygroma results. It consists of a collection of cysts, like a mass of soap bubbles. A cystic hygroma is usually present at birth; it may occasionally be so large as to obstruct labour. Occasionally, if it is very large, it may compress the trachea and produce respiratory difficulty. It usually lies in the lower part of the posterior triangle of the neck. The swelling is soft and cystic. It is *brilliantly transilluminant,* and this characteristic distinguishes it from all other swellings in the neck.

Treatment. Excision of all the cysts at an early age is the treatment of choice; if left untreated, the hygroma can be subject to repeated infections in its cysts. However, radical ablative surgery is not advised in this benign lesion. Conservative unroofing of remaining cysts is advised, preserving all adjacent crucial structures. Postoperative wound drainage is desirable and is best accomplished by the suction technique.

INFLAMMATORY CONDITIONS

Ludwig's angina. In this condition there is an indurated inflamed area in the submandibular region and the floor of the mouth. The cause is a virulent, usually streptococcal, infection of these parts. If the condition remains untreated, it may assume dangerous proportions. The swollen tongue is pushed towards the palate and forwards through the open mouth. Ludwig's angina is an infection of a closed space, and untreated the inflammation passes to the submucosa of the glottis, so that the patient's life is in danger from oedema of the glottis.

Treatment. If the condition is diagnosed very early, antibiotics may abort the infection. If the swelling does not subside with such treatment, a curved incision is made below the jaw and the mylohyoid muscles divided. This decompresses the closed fascial space.

CERVICAL LYMPHADENITIS

Nearly half the lymph nodes in the body lie in the neck; they guard the portals of entry into the respiratory and gastrointestinal tracts. Bacteria entering these tracts often pass through the mucosa of the throat and reach these nodes; therefore inflammation of the lymph nodes of the neck is very common, and occurs from the oral and nasal cavities, the ear, the scalp, and the face.

Acute lymphadenitis. The affected nodes are enlarged and tender, and there is usually a degree of pyrexia. If the patient comes early, antibiotics and fomentation may help in resolving the infection. If an abscess forms, incision and drainage is required.

Tuberculous lymphadenitis. This condition is described in detail in Chapter 43 dealing with lymphatics and lymph nodes. In the neck, usually the upper jugular chain of nodes is first affected. If widespread lymphadenitis is present, periadenitis often occurs, as shown by matting together of the nodes. If the patient's natural resistance is good, or he receives appropriate treatment, fibrosis or calcification may occur. If not, the caseating material liquefies and a *cold abscess* forms. If the pus erodes the overlying deep fascia and flows into the subcutaneous tissues, it is called a *collar-stud abscess.* If left untreated, the skin over it becomes reddened, and soon a discharging sinus forms, through which secondary infection can occur.

CAROTID BODY TUMOUR

The carotid body, which lies at the bifurcation of the carotid artery, contains chemoreceptors sensitive to changes in the pH of the blood. A tumour arising in this structure is usually very slow-growing; only occasionally does it metastasize to the lymph nodes. This tumour is common in middle age. As it is attached to the carotid artery *it can be moved from side to side but not vertically.* Expansion of the tumour can lead to paresis of the 7th, 9th 10th, 11th and 12th cranial nerves, with symptoms such as dysphagia, choking or hoarseness.

Diagnosis. The possibility of a carotid body tumour should be kept in mind in a patient who presents with a lump in the region of the carotid bifurcation. A misdiagnosis of lymph node enlargement with attempt at excision biopsy can result in excessive blood loss and a great deal of embarrassment. Ultrasound confirms the relationship with the carotid bifurcation and demonstrates the splaying of the carotid arteries by the tumour. Angiography shows splaying of the carotid bifurcation and a tumour blush, and often allows the feeding vessels of the tumour to be identified. MRI, specially with enhancement by gadolinium, provides greater soft tissue contrast. This allows the detection of tumours down to 5 mm in diameter, as well as better assessment of the extent of invasion by a large tumour.

Treatment. If the tumour is asymptomatic and growing slowly and the patient is elderly, removal is probably not required. However, it is easier and safer to remove the tumour before extensive local invasion, and so in most patients excision while the tumour is small is advocated. With tumours greater than 3 cm in diameter it may be an advantage to shrink them preoperatively by embolization. If excision is to be carried out, the surgeon must be prepared to replace the artery with a length of saphenous vein. During the grafting procedure the circulation to the brain should be continued by diverting the blood from the common to the internal carotid artery through a silicone tubing. This shunt also devascularizes the tumour by excluding the external carotid artery from the circulation. Operative mortality used to be high but should now be virtually zero because of the above-mentioned refinements.

SECONDARY CARCINOMA IN THE NECK

Secondary carcinoma is quite commonly seen in the lymph nodes of the neck. In such a case a search must be made for the primary, by examining the possible sites in the region, including the thyroid, the tongue, the larynx, the pharynx, the jaws, the paranasal sinuses, as well as distant sites, such as the breast, the bronchus, the stomach and the testis.

Management. This varies with the situation:

1. If the primary tumour is being treated by surgery and the cervical nodes are palpable, they may be excised en bloc with the primary.
2. If lymph nodes become palpable some time after successful treatment of the primary, a neck dissection should be carried out.
3. If radiotherapy results in resolution of the primary but the metastatic nodes persist, they can be dealt with by a neck dissection.

Neck dissection. For many decades now, cervical lymph nodes have been removed in cases of head and neck malignancies in order to eradicate disease in the primary lymphatic field. However, the extent of dissection recommended has undergone a reduction with the passage of time:

1. In the *classical radical neck dissection* described by Crile, the cervical lymph nodes were removed en bloc along with those structures intimately associated with them, such as the internal jugular vein, the sternomastoid muscle, the accessory nerve and the submandibular gland.
2. A major factor in the morbidity of classical neck dissection is paralysis of the trapezius muscle by resection of the *accessory nerve*, and preservation of this nerve was recommended many years ago.
3. Other surgeons have demonstrated techniques where the *jugular vein* and *sternomastoid* can also be left intact. These methods are particularly useful in *prophylactic* (elective) neck dissections where the lymph nodes are not enlarged.
4. Finally, it has been suggested that only those lymph nodes at risk should be resected. The concept of *selective neck dissection,* customized to the site of the primary disease, has gained support. Thus, for example, for carcinoma of the lip, anterior tongue and floor of the mouth, *supra-omohyoid* neck dissection might be used; in thyroid disease an *anterior compartment* neck dissection may be appropriate; while for a nasopharyngeal lesion a *posterolateral* neck dissection may be employed.

48 *Thyroid*

METHODS OF INVESTIGATION

Assessment of thyroid function by a carefully elicited history and observation of clinical signs is of fundamental importance. Symptoms and signs can be quantitated by using a diagnostic index of thyroid disease. There are separate diagnostic indices for hypo- and hyperthyroidism, (Tables 1 & 2).

Tests of circulating thyroid hormone levels.

Serum thyroxine (T_4) (normal 55–150 nmol/l). This measures the total protein-bound thyroxine and offers a good basic test for thyroid function specially when *myxoedema* is suspected, provided the patient is not on any drug or in a condition which might affect the serum levels of binding proteins.

Serum tri-iodothyronine (T_3) (normal 1.2–3.1 nmol/l). This test is most useful in the confirmation of *hyperthyroidism*, specially when the clinical picture strongly suggests thyrotoxicosis but the levels of serum T_4 are normal.

Free thyroxine (normal 8–26 pmol/l). Since the introduction of a radioimmunoassay in kit form, it is possible to measure the biologically active unbound circulating T_4 with precision and at relatively low cost.

Free tri-iodothyronine (normal 3–9 pmol/l). The free T_3 iminoradioimmunoassay has the same merit as the free T_4 assay, and is the best test in the assessment of *hyperthyroidism*.

Tests of hypothalamic-pituitary function. *Thyroid stimulating hormone* (normal 0.5–5.0 mu/l). When thyroid function is grossly deficient, the negative feedback effect is at a very low level, so that the TSH level rises. Values above 40 mu/l are seen in hypothyroidism, and this test is invaluable in detecting mild degrees of hypothyroidism. Conversely, in hyperthyroidism the level of serum TSH is low. Routine TSH assays cannot identify patients who may have subclinical hypothyroidism and might benefit from replacement therapy. New sensitive immunoradiometric assays (IRMAs) represent the best confirmatory test for

Table 1 Hypothyroidism — diagnostic index.

CLINICAL FEATURES: SYMPTOMS	Present	Absent
Diminished sweating	+6	−2
Dry skin	+3	−6
Cold intolerance	+4	−5
Weight increase	+1	−1
Constipation	+2	−1
Hoarseness of voice	+5	−6
Paraesthesiae	+5	−4
Deafness	+2	0
SIGNS		
Slow movements	+11	−3
Coarse skin	+7	−7
Cold skin	+3	−2
Periorbital puffiness	+4	−6
Slow pulse rate	+4	−4
Slowing of ankle jerk	+15	−6
Totals of positive and negative =		
Final Score =		

−25 or less:	Euthyroid
−24 to +19:	Doubtful
+20 or over:	Hypothyroid

Table 2 Hyperthyroidism — diagnostic index.

CLINICAL FEATURES: SYMPTOMS		Present	Absent
Dyspnoea on effort		+1	0
Palpitations		+2	0
Tiredness		+2	0
Preference for heat		0	−5
Preference for cold		+5	0
Sweating		+3	0
Nervousness		+2	0
Weight	Increase	0	−3
	Decrease	+3	0
Appetite	Increase	+3	0
	Decrease	0	−3
SIGNS			
Palpable thyroid		+3	−3
Thyroid bruit		+2	−3
Exophthalmos		+2	0
Lid retraction		+2	0
Lid lag		+1	0
Hyperkinesis		+4	−2
Finger tremors		+1	0
Hands	Hot	+2	−2
	Moist	+1	−1
Pulse rate			
Less than 80		0	−3
80–90		0	0
More than 90		+3	0
Atrial fibrillation		+4	0
Totals of positive and negative points =			
Final Score =			

Less than 11:	Euthyroid
11–19:	Equivocal
Greater than 19:	Hyperthyroid

both hypothyroidism when levels of TSH are high, and hyperthyroidism when levels are low.

Thyrotrophin releasing hormone test. Thyrotrophin is administered intravenously and TSH levels are measured. An exaggerated response to this test is seen in hypothyroidism, and little or no response in hyperthyroid patients. However, the test is being superseded by the immunoradiometric assay for TSH where this is available.

Tests of thyroid function. *Radioactive iodine uptake test.* The thyroid treats radioactive tracers of iodine (^{123}I) exactly as it treats inorganic iodine. When a tracer dose e.g. 5 microcuries is given, it is rapidly absorbed from the small bowel into the blood. In hyperthyroidism the thyroid uptake is rapid. Ultimately the isotope – now incorporated into the T_3 and T_4 – passes back into the serum and can be measured as protein bound ^{123}I. A rapid uptake of ^{123}I (high counting rate at 4 hours) and a rapid turnover (high serum ^{123}I at 24 hours) are typical of hyperthyroidism. Because the radio-active dose is low it can be used in children, in pregnancy, and for serial tests. ^{131}I was the time-honoured isotope utilized, but it has been replaced by ^{123}I or ^{99m}TC (technetium pertechnetate), because either of these isotopes results in a much lower dose of irradiation to the thyroid.

Isotope scanning provides graphic information about the size and extent of the gland, and about radioactivity in its different parts:

1. When the thyroid is scanned after administration of a tracer dose of ^{123}I the functioning ('hot') parts of the gland, and the non-functioning ('cold') parts can be shown up. Most carcinomas are 'cold', while an autonomous toxic nodule is 'hot'.
2. The scintillation scan may be of value in determining the presence of *abnormally positioned* thyroid tissue, such as substernal or lingual thyroid.
3. After total thyroidectomy, whole body scanning after a tracer dose of ^{123}I can demonstrate *metastases*. However, if the thyroidectomy was partial the metastases are not shown up because they cannot compete with the remaining normal thyroid tissue in the uptake of iodine. This is an important reason why total thyroidectomy is preferred in the treatment of thyroid malignancies.

Basal metabolic rate, ECG, serum cholesterol level, and the T_3 suppression test, are not of much use as tests of thyroid function.

Ultrasonography. Ultrasound examination indicates whether a nodule is solid or cystic. Solid nodules are most likely to be neoplastic, whereas cysts are most often benign lesions.

Biopsy. Biopsy of the thyroid is particularly helpful in two situations: in establishing a diagnosis of thyroiditis, and in differentiating between benign and malignant thyroid nodules. A core biopsy may be obtained with a ***Trucut*** needle, but the incidence of complications is high.

Fine needle aspiration cytology. Recently, fine needle aspiration cytology (FNAC) has gained favour in which the aspirate of a nodule obtained by a 25-gauge needle on a 10 ml syringe is evaluated. Interpretation is not easy, and should be made only by a trained cytologist. In the case of follicular lesions the technique cannot distinguish between benign and malignant lesions since no information is available about capsular and vascular invasion.

CONGENITAL ANOMALIES OF THE THYROID

The thyroid arises as a bud from the foramen caecum and descends to its final position in the neck. Some residual thyroid tissue may be found along the course of the thyroglossal tract. Very rarely the whole gland is ectopic.

Lingual thyroid. Most or all of the thyroid may be located at the back of the tongue at the foramen caecum, where it forms a swelling which may cause dysphagia, impairment of speech, respiratory obstruction or haemorrhage. It may be treated by L-thyroxine, when it usually becomes smaller. If it does not, it may have to be removed. Before such an operation the neck must be isotope-scanned for the presence of thyroid tissue, because in 70% of cases there is no thyroid tissue at the normal site. In such a case removal of the lingual thyroid will result in myxoedema. The removed thyroid is sliced, and some of the slices implanted into the muscles of the neck, in view of the rich blood supply of muscular tissue.

Thyroglossal cyst. A small segment of the thyroglossal tract may persist and produce a cyst, which is called a thyroglossal cyst. It is commonly located just below the hyoid bone (Fig. 1). Because it is attached to the foramen caecum of the tongue *it moves upwards not only on swallowing but also on protrusion of the tongue.* A thyroglossal cyst should be *treated* by excision, because it very commonly becomes infected. If the chances of recurrence are to be minimized, the central portion of the body of the hyoid must be removed with the cyst, as the tract is inti-

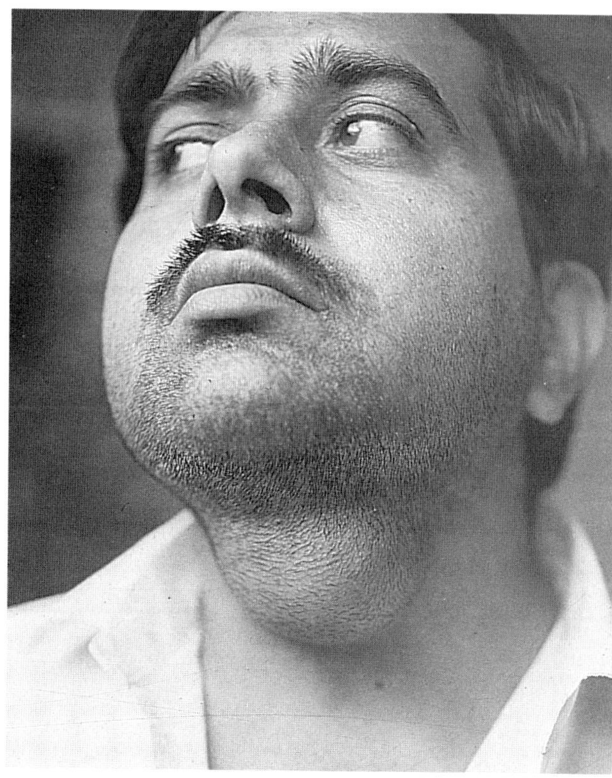

Fig. 1 Thyroglossal cyst, located just below hyoid bone.

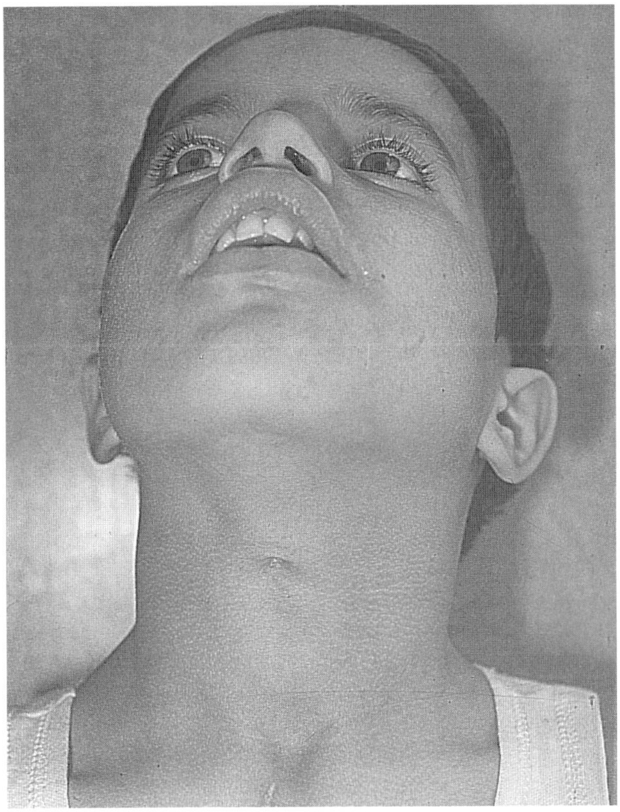

Fig. 2 Thyroglossal fisula. The upper margin is crescentic.

mately related to the hyoid. Further, the dissection must be carried upwards to the base of the tongue. An infected cyst may be mistaken for a simple abscess and incised, in which case a thyroglossal fistula often results. Before removing what appears to be a thyroglossal cyst, the surgeon must make sure by isotope scanning that thyroid tissue is present at the normal site. Sometimes this is ectopically placed thyroid tissue instead of a cyst, and the child may be rendered athyreotic by its removal.

Thyroglossal fistula. A thyroglossal fistula arises when a thyroglossal cyst becomes infected and bursts, or is inadequately removed. As the track proceeds upwards, characteristically its upper margin is sharp and crescentic (Fig. 2). It discharges mucus and becomes repeatedly inflamed. The thyroglossal tract is closely related to the body of the hyoid; therefore, when a cyst or fistula is excised, the body of the hyoid must be removed, in order to avoid a recurrence.

'Lateral aberrant thyroid'. In the past, if thyroid tissue was found in the lateral part of the neck it was considered to be an ectopically placed (or 'aberrant') thyroid. We know now that these are instances of metastases in the cervical lymph nodes from a carcinoma of the thyroid which is too small to be palpable.

HYPOTHYROIDISM

Hypothyroidism is defined as the failure of the thyroid gland to maintain an adequate plasma level of hormone. It is important for the surgeon due to the following three reasons:

1. Removal of most of the thyroid, or putting it out of action by radioactive iodine, is an important cause of hypothyroidism.
2. The clinical features of hypothyroidism may mimic different surgical illnesses.
3. It is important to recognize the hypothyroid state in the pre-operative patient, because major surgery in a grossly hypothyroid patient is associated with an increased mortality rate.

Aetiology. Hypothyroidism may result from one of the following:

1. Aplasia of the thyroid.
2. Replacement of the gland by a non-functional goitre or autoimmune thyroiditis.
3. Hypopituitarism.
4. Total or subtotal thyroidectomy.
5. Radioactive iodine therapy for hyperthyroidism.

Clinical features. Functional failure of the thyroid in the *newborn* is termed *cretinism.* This is not seen at birth, because during pregnancy the mother's thyroid hormones reach the foetus across the placenta; it becomes manifest later in infancy. The infant is markedly retarded mentally, and shows a poor growth pattern. The remaining features are similar to those in adults, as described below.

Spontaneous hypothyroidism in the *adult* is commonly due to lymphocytic thyroiditis, most patients being female. Whether hypothyroidism is spontaneous or follows an ablative procedure on the thyroid, its clinical features come on gradually. Its manifestations affect most systems. In mild cases only tiredness and an increase in weight may be present. In severe cases there is increasing fatigue and apathy. Mental and physical processes are slowed, and speech may be impaired. The skin is dry and thick; the hair becomes brittle and tends to fall out. The tongue is enlarged and fills the mouth. The voice is hoarse. Muscle cramps and headaches are common. The cardiac output is reduced, so that congestive heart failure may be present. The pulse is slow. Shortness of breath may be present. The bowels move sluggishly, so that constipation and abdominal distension are commonly seen. There is decreased libido in both men and women.

Investigations. Blood tests usually reveal the presence of anaemia. The ECG shows sinus bradycardia, diminished voltage and inverted or flattened T waves. The serum T_3 and T_4 levels are low, the serum TSH level being high. Serum cholesterol is usually raised above 300 mg/dl.

Treatment. The treatment of adult hypothyroidism is very effective, and aims at producing a normal metabolic state. L-thyroxine is most often used, in tablets containing 0.05 mg. To measure the effectiveness of treatment serum T_3, T_4 and TSH levels should be estimated. Treatment should be started with one tablet daily, and increased to 2 to 3 tablets gradually over a period of several weeks, to avoid cardiac problems arising due to a sudden increased metabolic demand on the myocardium.

HYPERTHYROIDISM

Hyperthyroidism refers to a spectrum of clinical manifestations which are due to excessive secretion of thyroid hormone. Three conditions are commonly associated with hyperthyroidism: Graves' disease (toxic diffuse goitre), toxic multinodular goitre, and toxic adenoma.

Pathology. *Graves' disease.* The cause of Graves' disease is not known. Generally this disorder is regarded as a systemic autoimmune disease in which hyperthyroidism, exophthalmos and a dermopathy called *pretibial myxoedema* are three parts of the same process. It is believed that the hyperthyroidism results from antibodies to the TSH receptors that bind in the region of the receptor and thus stimulate thyroid function. Contributory factors include heredity, female sex and emotional disturbances. Evidence supporting its recognition as an autoimmune process includes the presence of IgG, IgM and IgE in the thyroid, the lymphocytic infiltration of the gland, and the generalized lymphadenopathy often seen in Graves' disease. The thyroid of the patient with Graves' disease is moderately and diffusely enlarged, the surface being characteristically smooth. Microscopically the thyroid is hyperplastic, the epithelium is columnar and only a minimal amount of colloid is present. The nuclei may exhibit mitoses and the hyperplastic epithelium is thrown into papillary projections. There may be aggregates of lymphoid tissue, and the vascularity is greatly increased.

Toxic multinodular goitre. In this condition toxicity is usually superimposed on a multinodular goitre. Grossly, the gland contains multiple nodules many of which contain aggregates of irregular large cells and a scant amount of colloid. These areas function independently of stimulation by TSH, i.e. they are autonomously functioning nodules. The severity of hyperthyroidism is normally less than that associated with Graves' disease.

Toxic adenoma. The solitary toxic adenoma is a tumour. Like the multinodular toxic goitre it is capable of function independent of TSH, and the administration of exogenous thyroid fails to suppress the secretion of T_3 and T_4.

Clinical features. The age of onset is different in the three main pathological processes. Graves' disease most commonly becomes clinically apparent in young patients. Toxic adenoma occurs during the thirties or forties, while the thyrotoxicosis of toxic multinodular goitre becomes manifest after the age of fifty.

The patient *feels warmer* than other people in the same environment and becomes intolerant of heat. The excess heat resulting from the hypermetabolic state has to be dissipated; for this purpose there is increased *sweating*, which in turn results in increased *thirst* due to the fluid loss. As the body furnace is burning at a higher rate than normal there is *loss of weight* in spite of *increased appetite* and food intake; this feature is more marked in patients with Graves' disease than those with toxic multinodular goitre and toxic adenoma.

In contrast to the above, the cardiovascular manifestations of thyrotoxicosis are more prominent in the older patients with toxic multinodular goitres or toxic adenomas. They include tachycardia, frequent atrial fibrillation and congestive heart failure. Hyperthyroidism increases the force and rate of the heart beat, probably because of sensitization to adrenergic stimuli. Sleeping pulse rate is over 80 per minute. Palpitations are common. Due to peripheral vasodilatation the pulse pressure is increased. Atrial fibrillation may occur, specially among older patients.

The patient is excitable, restless, and emotionally unstable, often with insomnia. Muscle wasting and fatigue are common. The extended and abducted fingers show a fine tremor. The emotional and neurogenic signs are more marked in Graves' disease. The skin is warm and moist with facial flushing and perspiration. The hair is fine and readily falls off with combing. Menstrual periods are scanty.

Graves' disease. In Graves' disease goitre, thyrotoxicosis and exophthalmos occur together. A bruit is heard over the gland due to the extreme vascularity. The eye signs vary from minimal to severe, and include the following:

1. *Retraction of the upper eyelid.* If the lid is retracted the palpebral fissure is larger than normal. Further, normally the upper lid covers 1 to 2 mm of the cornea. If it does not, or if a strip of sclera is exposed, the lid is retracted.
2. *Exophthalmos.* It should be remembered that proptosis means protrusion of the eyeball; the word exophthalmos is generally used to mean proptosis due to thyrotoxicosis. To *detect* proptosis the examiner stands behind the seated patient and asks him to look downwards. The upper eyelid is drawn upwards and one looks to see if the cornea is bulging forwards. To *measure* proptosis the examiner sits on one side of the patient. He places a transparent ruler against the lateral orbital margin and reads off the distance the cornea is forwards of the orbital margin. He then repeats the same procedure on the opposite side and records the measurements.
3. *Supraorbital and infraorbital swelling.*
4. *Venous congestion and oedema.* This is a sign of severity, and has been described as *malignant exophthalmos.*

Toxic multinodular goitre. The thyroid contains many nodules, which have been present for a long time. Pressure effects on the trachea or oesophagus are more common than in Graves' disease. Exophthalmos is rare.

Toxic adenoma. There is a slowly growing mass in the neck. Rapid growth may be due to central necrosis and haemorrhage, when the signs of thyrotoxicity may show spontaneous remission. Exophthalmos is absent.

Investigations. In thyrotoxicosis T_3 and/or T_4 levels are elevated. The thyroidal radioiodine uptake is markedly elevated in Graves' disease, less markedly so in toxic multinodular goitre and toxic adenoma. In toxic adenoma the *isotope scan* demonstrates uptake of tracer in the area of the nodule, while the normal part of the gland is not visualized. If exogenous TSH is now given, the remaining part of the gland will take up the isotope.

Treatment. Hyperthyroidism can be treated by antithyroid drugs, radioactive iodine, or surgical excision of thyroid tissue. The method chosen depends upon the patient's age and general health, and the pathological process involved.

Antithyroid drugs. Most antithyroid drugs interfere with the organic binding of iodine in the thyroid and inhibit the coupling of iodotyrosines. They have no effect on the underlying cause of the disease. It takes these drugs about six weeks to restore a euthyroid state. The treatment is regulated by clinical observation and by noting the patient's pulse and weight. Most patients with Graves' disease are treated with antithyroid drugs in the hope that a natural remission will occur after the patient is rendered euthyroid. If treatment is continued for 6 months and then the drugs are stopped, only about 40 percent patients have long-lasting remissions.

The commonly used drug is carbimazole in the form of 5 mg tablets. The full adult dose is six tablets daily. Side effects include skin rash, fever and peripheral neuritis, serious complications being agranulocytosis and aplastic anaemia. If the white blood cell count falls significantly the drug must be stopped.

Radioactive iodine. In some centres radioactive iodine is considered as the treatment of choice for Graves' disease. The average dose is 8 to 10 mC of ^{131}I, which delivers approximately 6,000 rads. The advantage of radioiodine therapy lies in the avoidance of a surgical procedure with its attendant complications of recurrent laryngeal nerve paralysis or hypoparathyroidism. The disadvantages include the time required to control the disease, the incidence of permanent myxoedema, and the development of nodules. 80 to 98% patients show remission. Unfortunately, in the long term more than half the patients develop hypothyroidism due to overdosage.

The incidence of thyroid cancer or leukaemia is not increased by the use of radioiodine. At the same time the possibility of genetic abnormalities following radioiodine treatment is very remote. Most centres limit the use of radioiodine to women thirty-five years of age or older. Radioiodine should never be given to pregnant or lactating women because it crosses the placenta, is excreted in milk, and could destroy the foetal thyroid.

Surgical treatment. *Preoperative preparation.* Operation on a patient with hyperthyroidism cannot be carried out straightaway. First the patient must be rendered euthyroid:

1. Usually, *antithyroid drugs* are used for this purpose.
2. *Iodine* is then added to this regimen 8 to 10 days prior to the operation to decrease the vascularity of the gland.
3. Some surgeons add *thyroxine* to the regimen to prevent hypothyroidism and to decrease the size of the gland.
4. The beta-adrenergic blocker, *propranolol*, has added safety to the operation for Graves' disease. It reduces the pulse rate and the finger tremors, although the patient remains thyrotoxic. Some use propranolol alone for 5 to 7 days. But it is probably better to use antithyroid drugs along with propranolol.

Results of operation. Subtotal thyroidectomy provides rapid correction of the thyrotoxic state in over 95% of cases. The *advantages* of surgical therapy include prompt control of the disease and a lowered incidence of myxoedema as compared with radioiodine therapy. The important complications of thyroidectomy are recurrent laryngeal nerve paralysis and damage to the parathyroid glands resulting in tetany. In a few patients permanent hypothyroidism develops; in others hyperthyroidism recurs.

Selection of therapy. In young patients with *Graves' disease* antithyroid drugs are used initially. If prolonged drug therapy is required, or if recurrence of thyrotoxicosis follows the discontinuation of the drugs, thyroidectomy is used. Antithyroid drugs cross the placenta and may cause hypothyroidism and goitre in the foetus, so they cannot be used in pregnancy. If during pregnancy thyrotoxicosis is severe and cardiac symptoms herald cardiac failure later in pregnancy, subtotal thyroidectomy should be undertaken in the middle trimester, which is safe and effective. These drugs can be used in lactating mothers as their excretion into milk is at a level too low to cause hypothyroidism in the infant.

The preferred treatment for *toxic multinodular goitre* is surgical excision. Similarly, surgical resection of the hyperactive part of the thyroid gland in a case of *hyperfunctioning adenoma* is so straightforward that the other methods of treatment need not be seriously considered unless the patient is medically unfit for surgery.

Treatment of exophthalmos. The treatment of hyperthyroidism does not always improve the situation in respect of exophthalmos. Treatment is essentially symptomatic. The eyes should be protected against wind and sun. The patient should sleep in a sitting position to reduce venous congestion. If the oedema is severe the eyelids may be opposed by suturing them together (tarsorraphy) to prevent corneal ulceration. Steroid eye drops may help. If the intraorbital pressure threatens vision, the lateral bony wall of the orbit may be removed by operation to allow the orbital contents to expand (orbital decompression).

THYROIDITIS

Inflammatory processes of the thyroid may be acute, subacute or chronic. Chronic thyroiditis includes Hashimoto's disease and Riedel's thyroiditis.

Acute suppurative thyroiditis. This is a rare condition. It is essentially an abscess of the thyroid, which nearly always follows upon an acute upper respiratory tract infection. There is sudden severe pain with dysphagia, fever and chills. Treatment consists of incision and drainage.

Subacute thyroiditis (de Quervain's disease). This condition occurs at almost any age, being more common in women. It is probably not caused by a virus or by autoimmunity. The gland is adherent to the surrounding structures, but can be dissected free. There is infiltration by mononuclear cells, lymphocytes and neutrophils. Epithelioid type foreign body giant cells are present. There is swelling and pain, with fever and malaise. Needle biopsy helps establish the diagnosis. The acute pain can be alleviated by aspirin and a beta-blocker. If this fails, 20 to 30 mg of prednisolone daily for one month usually provides relief. Thyroxine may be required if hypothyroidism develops. Surgery is only required if the diagnosis is uncertain on fine-needle cytology.

Hashimoto's disease (Lymphadenoid goitre). Hashimoto's disease, or chronic lymphocytic thyroiditis, is the most common form of chronic thyroiditis. It is an autoimmune process in which the thyroid gland becomes sensitized to its own thyroglobulin and cell constituents. The serum contains antithyroid antibodies, which are either antimicrosomal or antithyroglobulin. The disease sometimes runs in a family where there is an increased incidence of Hashimoto's disease, goitre, spontaneous hypothyroidism and thyrotoxicosis.

Pathology. There is usually a symmetrical enlargement of the thyroid which is firm, and pale on section. Lymphoid tissue predominates. The epithelial cells are disrupted and the basement membrane fragmented. Gradually, the thyroid tissue may degenerate or be replaced by fibrous tissue.

Clinical features. Most patients are middle-aged women. The neck is enlarged with pain and tenderness in the region of the thyroid. There may be dyspnoea and dysphagia. Most patients are euthyroid or hypothyroid. Other autoimmune disorders, e.g. rheumatoid arthritis, haemolytic anaemia, may coexist with Hashimoto's disease.

Investigations. Early in the course of the disease thyroid function tests may occasionally indicate hyperfunction. Later, T_4 and T_3 are often abnormal. Diagnosis is confirmed by demonstrating high titres of thyroid antibodies in the serum. If the glandular enlargement is nodular or asymme-trical, large needle biopsy or needle aspiration with cytology may be necessary to rule out the diagnosis of carcinoma.

Treatment. If the thyroid is symmetrical and non-nodular, and if there are no symptoms of compression, the patient should be managed by suppressive doses of thyroxin if there is evidence of a goitre. Symptoms of pressure on the trachea and oesophagus are common and may be relieved by prednisolone 20 mg/day. If there is no goitre and the patient is euthyroid, no treatment is required. Surgical treatment, i.e. subtotal thyroidectomy, is required only if there are marked compression symptoms e.g. dysphagia, if a cancer is suspected, and for cosmetic reasons as in the case of a very large gland. Suppressive therapy with thyroid hormone should be continued postoperatively.

Riedel's thyroiditis. Riedel's thyroiditis is a rare chronic inflammatory disorder of the thyroid, often extending to the surrounding structures like fascia, muscles, trachea etc. Some workers regard it as a terminal stage of Hashimoto's disease. Microscopically, a few small follicles are seen, surrounded by dense fibrous tissue, which may constrict and narrow the trachea. When the lesion is only on one side, it is difficult to distinguish it from carcinoma. The disease mostly affects middle-aged persons, specially women. Tests may indicate the presence of hypothyroidism. Treatment consists of the administration of thyroid hormones. If symptoms of tracheal or oesophageal obstruction are present surgical intervention is required for their relief.

GOITRE

The dictionary defines goitre as any enlargement of the thyroid gland. However, in common usage the term is employed for benign enlargements of the gland. Toxic and inflammatory goitres have already been described. What remains to be discussed is the condition called simple goitre.

SIMPLE GOITRE

Aetiology. Simple goitre arises as follows: either due to a deficiency of iodine in the diet or a defect of synthesis of the thyroid hormones, the level of the circulating thyroid hormones falls. This results in increased secretion of thyroid stimulating hormone (TSH) by the anterior pituitary. TSH stimulates the thyroid gland which enlarges in size, and a goitre results. As just mentioned above, the factors leading to a fall in the levels of circulating thyroid hormones are two: deficiency of iodine in the diet, and defects of synthesis of thyroid hormones.

1. *Iodine deficiency.* In certain areas both food and water have a very low content of iodine. Usually these are mountainous regions, where rain water washes away the iodides from the soil. In the advanced countries iodine is added to table salt to remedy any possible deficiency of iodine in the diet, and this simple step has greatly reduced the incidence of deficiency goitre in certain regions where it used to be endemic.

2. *Defects of synthesis of thyroid hormones.* These may arise due to one of the following causes:

i. *Inherited defects of synthesis.* Sometimes many members of a family are seen to be suffering from goitre. If they come from a non-endemic area, they are usually suffering from an inherited defect of thyroid hormone synthesis. The metabolic defect may impair iodine accumulation, organification or coupling of iodotyrosine; or it may be related to a disorder affecting the serum iodoprotein. As the thyroid hormones are not synthesized in sufficient amounts, the inhibitory action of these hormones on the secretion of TSH is reduced. Increased secretion of TSH stimulates the thyroid so that a goitre results.

ii. *Goitrogens.* Certain chemicals block one or the other step in the synthesis of the thyroid hormones, and thus act as goitrogens. These include drugs such as para-aminosalicylic acid and the antithyroid drugs.

Evolution of a simple goitre. Due to iodine deficiency or a defect of synthesis of thyroid hormones persistent TSH stimulation occurs, and causes diffuse hyperplasia. All lobules are composed of active follicles, and iodine uptake is uniform. This is a *diffuse hyperplastic goitre* which may persist for a long time but is reversible if TSH stimulation ceases. Later, as a result of fluctuating TSH levels a mixed pattern develops, with areas of active and inactive nodules. Continual repetition of this process results in a *nodular goitre*. Most nodules are inactive, and active nodules are present only in the internodular tissue.

Diffuse goitre. Diffuse hyperplasia represents the first stages of the natural history of a simple goitre. Such a goitre usually appears at puberty when the accelerated metabolism results in an increased demand for iodine which outstrips the supply *(puberty goitre)*. If TSH stimulation ceases the goitre may regress, but can recur later at a time of stress. The goitre is soft and diffuse. A *colloid goitre* is a late stage of diffuse goitre, when many follicles are inactive and full of colloid; it is firm in consistency.

Multinodular goitre. Persistent but fluctuating TSH stimulation leads to progressive nodule formation. The nodules may be cellular or colloid, but cystic degeneration, haemorrhage, and even calcification may be seen. The *diagnosis* is easily made on finding multiple smooth, firm nodules in a patient who is euthyroid (Fig. 3). The goitre is painless and moves freely on swallowing. If a nodule appears suddenly and enlarges rapidly it may raise the suspicion of carcinoma; however, this is more often due to haemorrhage into a simple nodule.

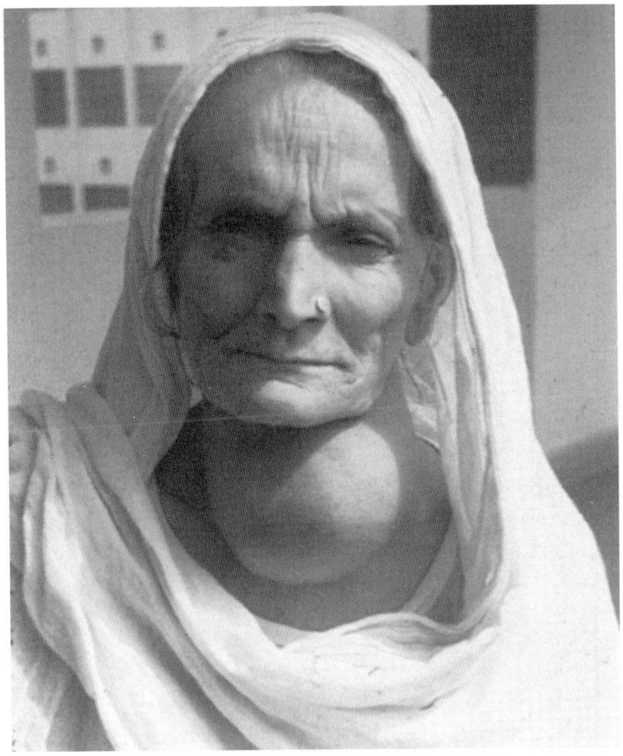

Fig. 3 Multinodular goitre in middle-aged woman.

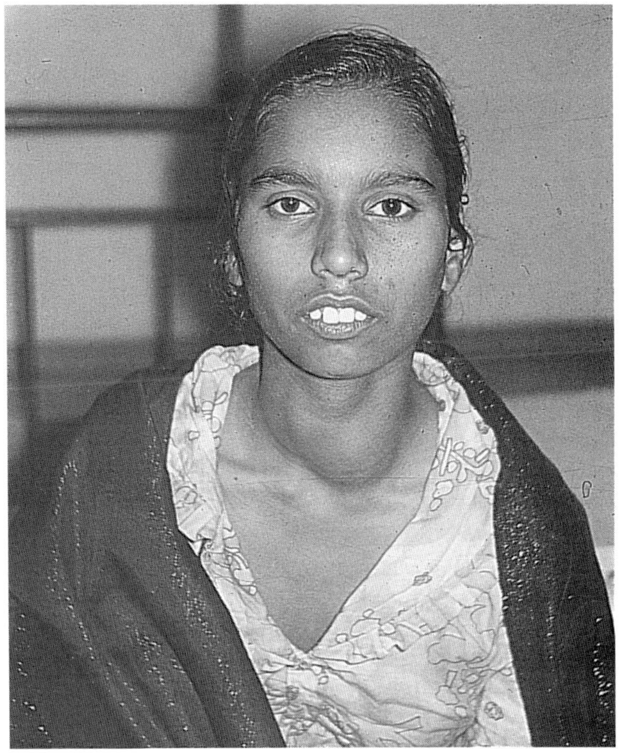

Fig. 4 Colloid nodule left lobe thyroid in young woman.

Investigations. *Thyroid function tests* should be performed to rule out mild hyperthyroidism. Estimation of *thyroid antibody titres* helps exclude Hashimoto's goitre. *Plain x-ray* of the neck should be taken to show up any tracheal deviation or compression, and any calcification in the thyroid.

Complications. The important complications to which a simple goitre is prone are three: pressure effects, toxic change and malignancy.

1. *Pressure effects.* The trachea may be obstructed due to gross lateral deviation or compression. Haemorrhage into a nodule may produce acute respiratory obstruction.
2. *Thyrotoxicosis.* A small number of patients with nodular goitres develop hyperthyroidism.
3. *Carcinoma*, commonly of the follicular type, also arises in a few cases.

Treatment. Adding 1 part of potassium iodide to 10,000 parts of table salt provides virtually complete *prophylaxis* against the development of simple goitre, and is universally employed in the advanced countries. In its early stages a *diffuse hyperplastic* goitre can be made to regress if thyroxine is given in maximum doses, i.e. 0.2 mg per day for several months. If regression does not occur thyroidectomy may be indicated for cosmetic reasons or pressure effects. On the other hand the pathological changes in a *nodular goitre* are irreversible. It should be treated by subtotal thyroidectomy because it is unsightly and uncomfortable; besides, it is prone to the complications of pressure effects, toxic change and malignancy. Resection aims at leaving about 8 gm of thyroid tissue on each side. The causative factors often persist after operation, and therefore a *recurrence* is quite likely unless further TSH stimulation is prevented. For this purpose 0.1 mg of thyroxine is given daily till after the menopause, or even better, for the rest of the patient's life.

THE CLINICALLY SOLITARY NODULE

A frequent and important clinical problem is seen when the thyroid is the seat of a single nodule. Such a nodule can be an adenoma, a carcinoma, or a colloid nodule in a multinodular goitre in which the other nodules are too small in size to be palpable. For the purpose of distinguishing between these lesions different *investigations* are carried out.

Clinical examination. A colloid nodule (Fig. 4) is usually firm in consistency. If it has degenerated into a cyst the consistency may be soft; however, if the cyst contains fluid under a good deal of tension the nodule may be tense. An adenoma is firm, whereas a carcinoma is usually hard to the feel. The remainder of the thyroid should be carefully palpated for the presence of other smaller nodules, which would show that this is really a multinodular goitre. The presence of fixity of the nodule, hoarseness of the voice, or enlarged hard lymph nodes in the lateral neck tends to label a nodule as malignant.

It should be remembered that the consistency of a cyst anywhere in the body depends upon the relationship between its capacity and the volume of fluid it contains. If it contains less fluid than its capacity it is soft, and in fact may be impalpable; if slightly more than its capacity, it is tense; if a lot more, it may even feel hard.

Radio-isotope scanning. A colloid nodule and a carcinoma are usually 'cold', i.e. they do not take up radioiodine. An adenoma is often 'warm', i.e. both the nodule and the surrounding thyroid take up the isotope. A toxic adenoma is 'hot'; not only does the adenoma take up the isotope, but the surrounding thyroid tissue does not. Here the normal thyroid tissue is inactive because the nodule is producing such high levels of thyroid hormone that TSH secretion is suppressed.

Ultrasound. An ultrasound examination can distinguish between a swelling which is solid and one which contains fluid, i.e. is cystic. When it is remembered that most cystic nodules in the thyroid are benign and most solid nodules neoplastic, it will become obvious that ultrasound examination has a role to play in the differential diagnosis of a solitary nodule. At the same time, ultrasound examination helps demonstrate the presence of additional small nodules if any such are present, which shows that the case is one of a multinodular goitre. In that case the possibility of a malignancy becomes quite remote.

Needle biopsy. Two methods of needle biopsy are in use:

1. *Tru-cut needle biopsy.* This large needle brings out a core of tissue suitable for histological examination; however, the method is associated with a significant number of complications such as bleeding, tracheal damage, and recurrent laryngeal nerve palsy.
2. *Fine needle aspiration cytology (FNAC).* This method is simple and quick to perform in the outpatients department, and in skilled hands has a high diagnostic accuracy. However, the specimen should only be examined by someone who has had specialized training in the method. It can distinguish between colloid nodules, thyroiditis, papillary, medullary and anaplastic carcinoma, and lymphoma. It cannot distinguish between a follicular adenoma and a follicular carcinoma, as this distinction does not depend upon cytology but on capsular and vascular invasion.

Treatment. A solitary *toxic* nodule is never malignant, it is a toxic adenoma; it can be treated by either radioiodine or surgical excision. A euthyroid *warm* nodule is either a functioning adenoma or a simple nodule. Rarely, it may be a well-differentiated carcinoma; therefore it should be excised. A euthyroid *cold* nodule can be a carcinoma; therefore it should be excised by total lobectomy. Incisional biopsy should never be carried out as it could result in seeding of malignant cells.

TUMOURS OF THE THYROID

BENIGN TUMOURS

The common benign tumour of the thyroid is a follicular adenoma, which presents as a slowly growing nodule. When solitary nodules removed at operation are examined microscopically, 80 percent of the specimens prove to be benign, while 20 percent are malignant. *Follicular adenoma* can be distinguished from a follicular carcinoma only on histological examination, by demonstrating that there is no invasion of the capsule or the pericapsular blood vessels. Therefore, treatment should consist of wide excision, which in this case means total lobectomy. On the other hand when a tumour has a *papillary* structure it is nearly always malignant, even though of a very low grade; a pure papillary adenoma probably does not exist.

Treatment. When a solitary nodule of the thyroid shows up on ultrasound examination as a solid lesion, it is highly likely to be a neoplasm, whether benign or malignant. In such a case the best treatment is lobectomy. Ideally, the specimen should be examined by frozen section while the patient is still under anaesthesia. If it proves to be an adenoma nothing further needs to be done.

MALIGNANT TUMOURS

The common malignant tumours of the thyroid are all carcinomas. Papillary, follicullar and anaplastic carcinomas arise from the follicular cells, while medullary carcinoma is derived from parafollicular cells. In addition, lymphomas and metastatic carcinomas are seen from time to time.

Papillary carcinoma. Papillary and follicular carcinomas are referred to as the differentiated thyroid cancers. Papillary carcinoma is the most common thyroid malignancy, accounting for two-thirds of all thyroid carcinomas. The peak age incidence occurs in the third and fourth decades of life, three-fourths of the patients being women.

Pathology. Papillary carcinoma contains columnar epithelium arranged in papillary projections and characteristic pale, empty nuclei called Orphan Annie nuclei. The tumour may contain localized deposits of calcium arranged in concentric layers *(psammoma bodies).* Papillary carcinoma is the most slowly growing of thyroid cancers, but has a tendency to become more malignant with advancing age. The tumour is very frequently multicentric in origin, and there is some evidence that its growth is dependent on TSH stimulation. Some of these tumours contain both papillary and follicular elements. However, if any papillary structure is present the tumour behaves as a papillary carcinoma.

Clinical features. The lesion usually presents as an asymptomatic mass in the thyroid or as a solid swelling in a lymph node draining the thyroid.

Fixation of the thyroid, signs of pressure on adjacent structures, and metastases are all evidence of advanced disease.

Investigations. An x-ray of the neck may show calcium flecks suggesting psammoma bodies. Isotope scan demonstrates a lack of iodine uptake. An ultrasound scan shows a solid lesion. A needle aspiration is usually diagnostic.

Treatment. The treatment of choice for a papillary carcinoma of the thyroid is surgery. However, there is some disagreement about the extent of the resection required. The author subscribes to the view that while considering surgical treatment, papillary carcinomas are best divided into two groups:

1. *Minimal or occult papillary carcinoma.* This term refers to a small papillary tumour, less than 1 cm in diameter and without invasion through the thyroid capsule or lymph node metastases, and usually found in the specimen in a young person when thyroidectomy has been done for another benign condition. In such a case lobectomy is sufficient.
2. *Standard treatment.* For tumours larger than 1 cm in diameter, a near-total or total thyroidectomy should be carried out. Usually the best course to follow is to excise the mass completely by lobectomy, and submit the excised

lobe to frozen section examination. If the lesion is reported to be benign, or smaller than 1 cm with no capsular invasion, nothing more needs to be done; otherwise a near-total or total thyroidectomy is carried out.

Decision between lobectomy and total thyroidectomy can be arrived at by a scoring system devised to identify low- and high-risk patients based on four variables: age, grade, extent, and size (AGES); a higher score on each indicates a poorer prognosis and the need for more radical surgery.

The *advantages* of carrying out a total thyroidectomy are the following:

1. Papillary carcinoma is very often multicentric; therefore the likelihood of eradicating the disease is much greater after total thyroidectomy.
2. The best method of follow-up for metastases is by repeated isotope scans. If some functioning thyroid tissue is present, metastases do not show up. Therefore total thyroidectomy facilitates follow-up for metastases, and their treatment by radioiodine.
3. If after total thyroidectomy a measureable amount of thyroglobulin is detected in the serum it means that metastatic disease is present, and requires localization by isotope scanning and treatment by radioiodine.

About the lymph nodes. Any abnormal lymph nodes in the tracheo-oesophageal groove should be removed. A neck dissection should be carried out only if the lateral neck nodes are involved with tumour. To determine this, a lymph node from the jugular chain should be removed for biopsy using the frozen section technique.

Follow-up. 1. After operations for differentiated thyroid cancers, it is standard practice to place all patients on *thyroid hormone for life* to suppress serum TSH levels, and to follow them up at regular intervals. T_3 in a dose of 80 microgram is usually appropriate. T_3 is preferred over T^4 because it need be stopped for only 1 week before scanning. T_4 has to be discontinued for 1 month and during this time mild hypothyroidism may occur.

2. The *measurement of serum thyroglobulin* is of value in the follow-up for detecting metastatic disease after surgery for differentiated thyroid cancer. It is a good example of a 'tumour marker'. A sensitive radioimmunoassay for thyroglobulin has recently become available. It provides a more convenient means of follow-up than scanning with radioiodine, as thyroid suppression therapy does not have to be stopped. However, if a rise in the level occurs a scan should be carried out to confirm and localize the metastatic disease.

3. Radiotherapy and chemotherapy are described along with follicular carcinoma.

Prognosis. If the disease is limited to the thyroid and regional lymph nodes, it carries one of the most favourable prognoses of all forms of cancer, with 5-year survivals of 90%, scarcely reduced at 10 years. Patients with extrathyroidal disease i.e. trachea or oesophagus, do not fare so well.

Follicular carcinoma. Follicular carcinoma of the thyroid occurs at a somewhat later age, with a peak incidence in the fifth decade, again being three times more common in women.

Pathology. Grossly, the tumour appears encapsulated. The follicles are crowded with cells, there being hardly any colloid. Capsular and vascular invasion are prominent features. The tumour is much less often multicentric than papillary carcinoma; however its malignant potential exceeds that of the latter tumour. Spread to the regional lymph nodes occurs in only a few cases, while haematogenous spread to distant sites such as bone, lung and liver predominates and occurs early.

Clinical features. The common presentation is as a solitary nodule in the thyroid, though sometimes there is a long history of goitre with recent change in the gland. Although carrying a better prognosis than most cancers, it is much more aggressive and dangerous than papillary carcinoma. Regional lymph nodes are seldom enlarged, but distant metastases are frequent. The metastases usually possess the ability to concentrate iodine.

Treatment. For the treatment of a follicular carcinoma of the thyroid, some favour hemithyroidectomy with removal of the isthmus but others, including the author, favour total or near-total thyroidectomy; not because of multicentricity, but rather to facilitate later scanning of the body with radioiodine and treatment with ^{123}I if metastases are found. The usual method is to withhold thyroxine after thyroidectomy for 3 to 6 weeks so that the patient becomes hypothyroid. The increased TSH secretion makes the secondaries hungry for iodine and therefore more likely to be identified. Since lymph node metastases are uncommon, neck dissection is rarely required. Overall, the *survival rate* of follicular tumours is about 70%, being about 45% if invasiveness is present, and as high as 85% if the tumour is not invasive.

Other methods of treatment for differentiated tumours.

Radioiodine therapy. After thyroidectomy for a differentiated carcinoma a total body scan should be carried out to locate any metastases. If 30 mC of radioiodine are now given, this will ablate most small remnants of normal thyroid in the neck. In order to destroy metastases a dose of 150 mC is commonly employed.

External irradiation therapy. This is used when thyroid cancer has invaded the trachea or oesophagus, or for the treatment of metastatic disease that no longer takes up radioiodine.

Chemotherapy. Widely metastatic lesions that no longer take up radioiodine can be treated with moderate success with systemic chemotherapy. Adriamycin has been the single most successful agent.

Medullary carcinoma. Medullary carcinoma is composed of C cells. These cells are derived from the neural crest, and are part of the APUD series of polypeptide-secreting cells. They secrete calcitonin, which lowers the serum calcium by inhibiting bone resorption. The tumour sometimes runs in a family, being inherited as an autosomal dominant. It spreads both via the lymphatics and through the bloodstream.

Clinical features. Patients present with a single nodule or with multiple nodules. In addition, these tumours may present with very distinct symptoms. Diarrhoea is a very common complaint. It may be due to 5-hydroxytryptamine or prostaglandin produced by the tumour. Medullary carcinoma can occur in combination with phaeochromocytoma and hyperparathyroidism in the syndrome known as multiple endocrine neoplasia (MEN type IIa). If the tumour occurs with neuromas involving the lips and tongue the syndrome is called MEN type IIb. As would be expected these tumours are not hormone-dependent and do not take up radioiodine. Calcitonin is a good marker for this tumour; therefore close relatives of the patient should be screened by determining their serum calcitonin levels. At the same time, the progress of the tumour can be monitored after surgery by serial estimations of serum calcitonin.

Treatment. Total thyroidectomy is the procedure of choice in view of the high incidence of multicentric lesions in both familial and sporadic disease. The upper poles and the lymph nodes in the primary lymphatic area should be completely resected. Lymph nodes in the secondary drainage areas should be sampled, and if positive removed by neck dissection. Before operation, a coexisting phaeochromocytoma or parathyroid tumour should be excluded, as failure to attend to these tumours first may be catastrophic.

Anaplastic carcinoma. In these tumours local infiltration is an early feature, with spread both by the lymphatics and the blood stream. They affect predominantly the older age group. Anaplastic tumours are very lethal, and survival beyond four years is unusual. There is rapid progressive swelling with voice changes due to involvement of the recurrent laryngeal nerves and stridor from tracheal compression. Whenever possible an attempt should be made to decompress the trachea by surgery to relieve respiratory obstruction. External radiotherapy is normally used in addition although the tumour is rarely very sensitive. Chemotherapy has little place in treatment.

SURGERY OF THE THYROID

The common operations carried out on the thyroid include subtotal or total lobectomy on one or both sides.

Exposure. Most operations on the thyroid are carried out through a transverse collar incision. If a skin crease is present at approximately this site, the incision should be made through it. If a nodule is to be removed from only one side, the skin incision should still be extended equally on either side, otherwise the asymmetrical scar is more noticeable. The platysma muscle is divided with the skin. The upper flap is now dissected upwards to the thyroid cartilage and the lower one downwards to the suprasternal notch. The deep fascia is divided vertically in the midline, separating the strap muscles. If more exposure is required, the strap muscles can be divided; in such a case the anterior jugular veins also require ligation (Fig. 5).

Control of blood supply. Each lobe in turn is now delivered outside, and the blood vessels supplying it ligated. At the upper pole of the lobe the superior thyroid artery is ligated and divided. In the proximal part of its course this artery is accompanied by the external branch of the superior laryngeal nerve; therefore it is ligated low down, close to the thyroid, to avoid injury to the nerve, which results in loss of the characteristic quality (timbre) of the voice. At

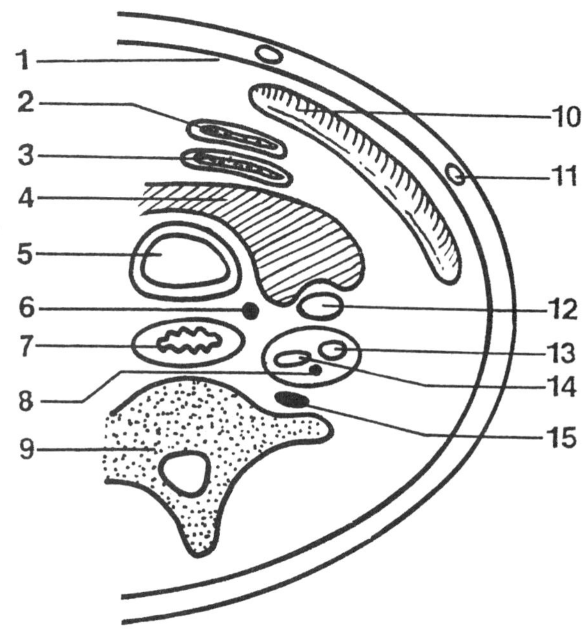

Fig. 5 Transverse section through neck at level of thyroid isthmus. 1. anterior jugular vein, 2. sternohyoid muscle, 3. sternothyroid muscle, 4. thyroid isthmus, 5. trachea, 6. recurrent laryngeal nerve, 7. oesophagus, 8. vagus nerve, 9. vertebral body, 10. sternomastoid muscle, 11. external jugular vein, 12. parathyroid gland, 13. carotid artery, 14. internal jugular vein, 15. sympathetic chain.

the middle of the outer border of the lobe, the middle thyroid vein enters the internal jugular vein. It is next ligated and divided, and allows a more complete delivery of the lobe. The inferior thyroid artery is now located, running across from behind the carotid sheath to the thyroid lobe. When it is traced towards the thyroid the recurrent laryngeal nerve comes into view, which runs upwards either through or behind the branches of the artery. The artery is ligated in continuity to reduce the blood supply to the lobe. If, instead, branches of the artery are ligated after they have given off supply to the parathyroid glands, postoperative parathyroid deficiency is prevented. Finally, the inferior thyroid veins are ligated and divided at the lower pole of the thyroid.

Resection. The blood supply having been controlled, the desired amount of the lobe is now removed, being sectioned off with a knife or scissors. In a *subtotal lobectomy* three to six grams of thyroid tissue is left behind on either side. This confers two incidental benefits: firstly, it protects the recurrent laryngeal nerve from injury; secondly, this part of the lobe contains the parathyroid glands, so they are protected from inadvertent removal. Bleeding points on the cut surface of the lobe are next ligated or coagulated by diathermy. The cut surface may now be sutured over.

In *total lobectomy* the whole lobe is removed, care being taken to avoid injury to the recurrent laryngeal nerve. If both lobes are being removed completely, tetany very commonly results. Therefore, one or more parathyroids are dissected out of the posterior border of the thyroid lobe, sliced, and implanted in the neck muscles, whose rich blood supply often ensures survival and function of the grafted parathyroid tissue.

In a *near-total thyroidectomy* a small amount of thyroid is left on the contralateral side to protect the parathyroid glands and recurrent nerve.

Postoperative complications. 1. *Haemorrhage.* A ligature on the superior thyroid artery may slip; alternatively, bleeding may take place from a thyroid remnant or a thyroid vein. If the blood has already compressed the trachea and produced dyspnoea the sutures should be removed in the ward to relieve the pressure, before taking the patient to the theatre for evacuation of the haematoma, followed by visualization and control of the bleeding point.

2. *Respiratory obstruction.* The most common cause of respiratory obstruction is laryngeal oedema, which itself may be due either to a haematoma or trauma to the larynx by anaesthetic intubation. If evacuation of the haematoma does not immediately relieve the obstruction, an endotracheal tube should be passed at once and may require to be left in place for a few days.

3. *Recurrent laryngeal nerve paralysis.* This may be transient or permanent. In unilateral injury the voice is husky. Bilateral injury is much more serious because both cords can assume a medial position and cause airway obstruction. Often tracheostomy is required.

4. *Thyroid insufficiency.* This can develop after a subtotal or total thyroidectomy. It comes on imperceptibly and may be difficult to recognize.

5. *Parathyroid insufficiency.* This is rarely the result of removal of all the parathyroid glands, but more commonly due to disruption of their blood supply. It can be minimized by ligating the branches of the inferior thyroid artery on the thyroid capsule distal to their supply of the parathyroid glands. Symptoms include circumoral numbness and tingling in the fingers and toes. The serum calcium level should be measured daily for a few days. In patients with symptoms 1g (10 ml of 10%) calcium gluconate should be given i.v. over 10 minutes, followed by several grams in each liter of i.v. solution. Oral calcium should also be started (2 to 4 g calcium carbonate daily).

6. *Thyrotoxic crisis.* This is an acute exacerbation of hyperthyroidism, and occurs if a thyrotoxic patient has been inadequately prepared for operation. Apart from signs and symptoms of thyrotoxicosis, there may be vomiting, diarrhoea, dehydration, fever, disorientation and rarely mania. There is severe tachycardia and sometimes heart failure. Treatment consists of intravenous fluids, ice-packs, oxygen, diuretics for cardiac failure, digoxin for uncontrolled atrial fibrillation, sedation, and intravenous hydrocortisone. Specific treatment is by carbamizole 15 mg, Lugol's iodine 8 drops and propranolol 40 mg, given 6 hourly.

49 Parathyroids and adrenals

Parathyroid glands

HYPOPARATHYROIDISM

Hypoparathyroidism is defined as the condition caused by greatly reduced function of the parathyroid glands, or by their removal. It is manifested clinically by tetany, which consists of cramps in the hands and feet, convulsions, and sometimes stridor. The common causes of hypoparathyroidism include the following:

1. Temporary hypoparathyroidism may be seen after subtotal thyroidectomy, when some of the parathyroid glands have been removed, or their blood supply compromised. Symptoms usually appear on the second or third postoperative day, and often clear up in a few days or weeks.
2. Mild forms of hypoparathyroidism may also be seen during the long-term follow-up of cases after thyroidectomy.
3. Permanent hypoparathyroidism is commonly seen after total thyroidectomy for cancer.
4. Tetany in the first few days of life may be seen in an infant born of a mother suffering from undiagnosed hypoparathyroidism.
5. Profound hypocalcaemia (not due to hypoparathyroidism) may be seen in some severe bone diseases where the calcium tends to be deposited in the bone. This is made worse when the patient has some degree of renal disease that itself tends to lower the serum calcium level.

Clinical features. The first symptoms produced by a lowered serum calcium level are tingling in the face, fingers and toes. In extreme cases cramps in the hands and feet are very painful. The extended fingers are flexed at their metacarpophalangeal joints, with the thumb strongly adducted. The toes are plantar flexed and the ankle joints extended *(carpo-pedal spasm)*. Tonic and clonic convulsions of the respiratory muscles and laryngeal stridor cause great distress, and may prove fatal. In chronic hypoparathyroidism cataracts and mental changes may occur. In mild cases of hypocalcaemia, tetany may be precipitated by one of the following tests:

1. *Trousseau's sign.* A sphygmomanometer cuff applied to the arm and inflated above the systolic pressure for about two minutes produces carpo-pedal spasm.
2. *Chvostek's sign.* Tapping over the branches of the facial nerve at the angle of the jaw produces twitching of the corners of the mouth, the alae of the nose, and the eyelids.

Treatment. In *acute* cases the slow intravenous injection of 10 to 20 ml of a 10% solution of calcium gluconate rapidly relieves the symptoms. This should be repeated until the patient's serum calcium level becomes stabilized. For *long-term* management the absorption of calcium is enhanced by oral administration of the most active metabolite of vitamin-D, namely dihydoxycholecalciferol. This substance accelerates the active absorption of calcium and phosphorus, raising the calcium levels to normal within a few days.

HYPERPARATHYROIDISM

Hyperparathyroidism, or excessive secretion of parathyroid hormone, occurs in three different forms.

Primary hyperparathyroidism. The cause of this condition is commonly a parathyroid adenoma, sometimes hyperplasia of the parathyroids, and rarely a parathyroid carcinoma. Unlike secondary hyperparathyroidism, the excessive parathyroid secretion here is not a response to a lowered serum calcium concentration; it is an unstimulated and inappropriately high level, due to an autonomous tumour or hyperplasia.

Secondary hyperparathyroidism. In this condition the excessive secretion of the parathyroid occurs in response to a low serum calcium concentration; this in turn may be due either to insufficient absorption of calcium from the gut in one of the malabsorption syndromes, or excessive urinary excretion of calcium in chronic renal failure. All four parathyroid glands are involved.

Tertiary hyperparathyroidism. This is a further stage of reactive hyperplasia, where the parathyroids become autonomous, as they no longer respond to physiological stimuli.

PRIMARY HYPERPARATHYROIDISM

Clinical features. Primary hyperparathyroidism is a disorder involving autonomous parathyroid hormone secretion. It presents clinically as hypercalcaemia or the sequelae of long-standing hypercalcaemia. The condition occurs twice as often in women as in men, and its incidence peaks in the sixth decade. The mode of presentation varies a great deal:

1. There may be *no symptoms*; in the advanced countries the most common presentation is the detection of unsuspected hypercalcaemia by routine biochemical scanning employing multichannel chemical analyzers.
2. There may be *non-specific symptoms*, e.g. polyuria, thirst, anorexia, weight loss, and muscle weakness. If such symptoms cannot be explained, the serum calcium level should be determined.
3. There may be generalized decalcification of *bones*, along with cysts (the 'osteitis fibrosa cystica' of the past). Early radiographic changes appear in the phalanges, consisting of subperiosteal erosions and osteoporosis. Therefore, if the condition is suspected the phalanges are x-rayed.
4. *Kidney stones* may be present. Hyperparathyroidism must be considered in every case of renal calculus, specially in the case of recurrent stones.
5. *Dyspepsia* may be present, due to a peptic ulcer or pancreatitis. These two conditions are commonly seen along

with hyperparathyroidism, although the association has not been explained.

6. *Psychiatric cases* may have hyperparathyroidism as the underlying cause. There may be tiredness, listlessness and personality changes. The clinician should remain on his guard, in order not to miss the correct diagnosis.

7. *Hypercalcaemic crisis.* If the serum calcium level rises above 16 mg/dl, nausea and abdominal pain can occur, followed by severe vomiting, dehydration, oliguria, and finally coma. This is sometimes called *acute hyperparathyroidism* or *parathyroid crisis*, but since it occurs during hypercalcaemia from any cause (for example in advanced breast cancer), it is best to refer to it as a hypercalcaemic crisis. Treatment should be with saline (to rehydrate) and furosemide (to help excrete the calcium), followed by early operation to correct the hyperparathyroid state. Patients whose hypercalcaemia is not due to hyperparathyroidism should be treated by a medical regimen to lower the serum calcium concentration.

On *physical examination* nothing abnormal may be found, except for any pathological fractures or bony swellings.

Investigations. *Plasma calcium* (normal 2.35–2.55 mmol/l) and *phosphorus* (normal 1.0–1.5 mmol/l) are estimated. *Plasma albumin* should be estimated at the same time (normal 35–50g/l). Albumin is the main calcium binding protein in the plasma so alterations in the albumin level have to be taken into account and the plasma calcium corrected accordingly. *Immunoradiometric assay* (IRMA) is carried out for parathyroid hormone (PTH) (normal 0.9–5.4 pmol/l). *Abdominal x-rays* may show renal calculi or nephrocalcinosis. *High-definition x-rays of the hand* may show subperiosteal erosions in the middle or terminal phalanges.

Hydrocortisone suppression test. If steroids (hydrocortisone 40 mg thrice daily) are given for 10 days, normally the plasma calcium level is suppressed, but not so in hyperparathyroidism.

The following tests are next carried out to rule out different causes of secondary hyperparathyroidism:

Plasma electrophoresis is carried out to exclude myeloma, and *serum TSH* and T_3 levels are determined to exclude thyrotoxicosis. *Biopsy* is performed to rule out sarcoidosis.

If primary hyperparathyroidism is confirmed, the following tests help in localization of the adenoma:

Ultrasound, though it fails to detect small tumours.

CT scan. Again, very high resolution is required. MRI may prove more sensitive.

Radioactive subtraction scan. This method of isotope scanning is quite interesting. Technetium is taken up by the thyroid, while thallium is taken up both by the thyroid and the parathyroids. Technetium 99m is first given and a scan carried out to outline the thyroid. Next, thallium 201 is administered which is taken up by both thyroid and parathyroids, and another scan is performed. A computer now subtracts the digital figures representing the thyroid image from the those of the thyroid plus parathyroids. The enlarged parathyroid remains as a 'hot spot'.

Barium swallow may show indentation of the oesophagus by an adenoma.

Catheterization of the parathyroid veins to measure parathormone is usually reserved for cases where previous operation has failed to localize the adenoma.

Treatment. The only corrective treatment is surgical removal of the overactive gland or glands. In symptomatic patients the indication for operation is clear cut. However, patients in whom hypercalcaemia has been discovered incidentally, e.g. during routine screening, are often asymptomatic and the decision to proceed with operation is more difficult. All agree that with renal disease or bone involvement surgery is indicated, as there is no medical treatment. If the plasma calcium is mildly raised: most researchers feel that if mild symptoms are present which are probably due to hypercalcaemia, parathyroidectomy should be carried out. Those who are asymptomatic should receive careful follow-up; if renal, bony or other symptoms appear, surgical treatment should be undertaken.

Adenomas, either single or multiple, are removed. If all four glands are hyperplastic, three and a half glands are removed, leaving half a gland with intact blood supply. If it is desired to avoid repeated potentially difficult explorations of the neck, parathyroid tissue can be successfully autotransplanted into the muscles of the forearm in the form of eight fragments of 1 cu mm each.

Parathyroid surgery should be performed only by surgeons with both proper training and experience.

Prognosis. With successful surgery, bones recalcify and pseudotumours resolve. Kidney stones do not disappear, but the incidence of recurrence after surgical removal is reduced and deterioration in renal function prevented. Psychiatric patients often show a remarkable recovery.

Adrenal glands

ADRENAL MEDULLA

TUMOURS

These include the following:

1. Tumours of the sympathetic neurones:
   i. Ganglioneuroma.
   ii. Neuroblastoma.
2. Tumour of chromaffin cells, namely phaeochromocytoma.

Ganglioneuroma. This tumour can occur at any age. It is symptomless, and can slowly grow to a large size. Only a small percentage occur in the adrenal medulla; the remainder arise anywhere along the sympathetic chain. If this tumour is removed early, a cure can be expected.

Neuroblastoma. A neuroblastoma of the adrenal medulla arises in infants and children. It is a reddish-grey tumour that is highly malignant. It grows rapidly to a large size, filling nearly the whole abdomen, and although arising on one side, extends across the midline. At this stage it can be confused with a Wilms' tumour (nephroblastoma), which is the other common large-sized abdominal tumour of infancy. The nodular feel of the neuroblastoma may help the distinction, because the Wilms' tumour has a smooth surface.

Unusual biological behaviour. Occasionally, a neuroblastoma exhibits rather curious behaviour. Sometimes a baby is brought when his tumour is so advanced that only a piece is removed for biopsy. However, the tumour undergoes *spontaneous remission*, so much so that even the secondaries disappear. Again, if the case is borderline between ganglioneuroma and neuroblastoma, and large doses of folic acid are given, the tumour sometimes becomes *converted into a ganglioneuroma* and the prognosis is improved.

Investigation. ***Imaging.*** *Ultrasonography* distinguishes neuroblastoma (solid, extrarenal) from cystic lesions and renal tumours. *X-ray* detection of calcification in the tumour suggests neuroblastoma. Intravenous urography shows displacement rather than distortion of the pelvicalyceal system. A skeletal survey and chest x-ray are essential to detect possible metastases. *CT* gives good anatomical data about the tumour. *MRI* provides the same, as well as evidence of vascular involvement and extension into the spinal cord.

Laboratory tests. *m-iodobenzyl guanidine* (MIBG) resembles adrenaline, and is specifically taken up by neurectodermal tumours. Labelled with ^{123}I it is used for localizing the primary tumour as well as for detecting residual and metastatic disease. *Monoclonal antibodies* to neuroblastoma are available and can be radiolabelled for similar purposes.

Neuroblastomas produce high levels of *catecholamines* and their metabolites:

1. A vanilmandelic acid spot test is used for screening.
2. The metabolites can be quantified by analysis of a 24-hour urine collection.
3. The higher the ratio of vanilmandelic acid to homovanilic acid the better the prognosis.

Staging. A staging system for neuroblastoma is presented in Table 1.

Treatment. The recommended treatment regimes for neuroblastoma in the different stages are given in Table 2.

Prognosis depends upon the factors presented in Table 3.

Phaeochromocytoma. Phaeochromocytomas are tumours of the adrenal medulla and related chromaffin tissues elsewhere in the body that release epinephrine, norepinephrine, or both, resulting in episodic or intermittent hypertension, and other symptoms of catecholamine secretion. They occur in two forms. Firstly, they occur *sporadically* as isolated tumours in patients with no other disease. Secondly, they are seen *as part of a multiple endocrine neoplasia syndrome* (MEN-II), in which the other neoplasms include medullary carcinoma of the thyroid, neurofibromas, ganglioneuromas, and hyperparathyroidism.

Pathology. Phaeochromocytomas are reddish-brown vascular tumours. They feel firm but may be multicystic, and necrotic areas are common. Although the tumour is benign, the veins and the capsule may be invaded.

Clinical features. The clinical findings in cases of phaeochromocytoma are very variable. Therefore it is recommended that every new case of hypertension should be investigated to exclude phaeochromocytoma as the cause. In actual fact, however, this tumour makes up only 0.5% of all the cases of hypertension.

The classic symptoms are those one would expect from an injection of epinephrine. They include *episodic* hypertension, pallor followed by flushing, palpitations, headache, excessive perspiration, nervousness and anxiety. In about half the cases, phaeochromocytomas cause *sustained* hypertension with or without evidence of excessive catecholamine secretion. The usual signs include tachycardia, retinopathy, emotional lability and weight loss. The clinical findings may mimic hyperthyroidism. Excessive secretion of epinephrine raises the blood glucose level and therefore may be confused with diabetes mellitus.

Table 1 Staging of neuroblastoma.

Stage I	Confined to organ of origin and totally excised
Stage II	Extends beyond organ but not across midline
Stage III	Extends across midline
Stage IV	Distant metastases
Stage IVs	Primary tumour localized; disseminated only to liver, skin or marrow.

Table 2 Treatment regimens for neuroblastoma in the different stages.

I:	Total excision alone
II:	Total excision + – chemo and/or radiotherapy
III:	Resectable tumours: excision + chemo + radiotherapy. Unresectable tumours: cytoreduction with chemo and radiotherapy, followed by excision of shrunken tumour
IV:	Combination chemotherapy. If response, excise residual tumour
IVs:	Excision of primary tumour
Note:	Rapidly enlarging liver may embarrass respiration. Treat: i. By low dose irradiation, or ii. By enlarging abdominal cavity temporarily by putting silastic patch in abdominal wall

Table 3 Prognostic factors in neuroblastoma.

Factors	Good prognosis	Poor prognosis
Age	<1 year	>1 year
Stage	I and II (all ages) III & IVs (if <1 Year)	III (if >1 year) IV (all ages)
DNA content	Euploidy	Hyperploidy
Histology	Differentiated	Undifferentiated
Urinary catecholamine metabolites	Low HVA:VMA	High HVA:VMA

Investigations. *Biochemical tests.* Urinary vanilylmandelic acid (VMA) determination is helpful for screening, VMA being a breakdown product of the catecholamines. If the result is positive, urinary assay for the individual catecholamines, epinephrine and norepinephrine is indicated. Direct measurement of elevated epinephrine and norepinephrine levels in the blood or urine is the key to diagnosis. In the past certain chemicals were injected to induce a hypertensive attack, which was diagnostic of a phaeochromocytoma. However, they have mostly been abandoned, as these tests were hazardous.

Localization of the tumour. A good *plain x-ray* may show the soft tissue shadow of a phaeochromocytoma, along with displacement of the kidney downwards. *CT scan* and *MRI* are very useful; they give good localization and are non-invasive.

Isotope scanning also helps localize the tumour. *Selective sampling of venous blood* from the right and left renal veins for the presence of increased quantities of catecholamines helps indicate the presence of this tumour, and identify the side on which it is located.

Arteriography can precipitate a hypertensive attack, and should be attempted only if the blood pressure has already been controlled medically.

Differential diagnosis. The differential diagnosis of phaeochromocytoma includes the different causes of hypertension. Apart from that, hyperthyroidism, acute attacks of anxiety, and carcinoid syndrome have to be kept in mind.

Complications. The complications of phaeochromocytoma are usually the sequelae of hypertension i.e. stroke, renal failure, myocardial infarction and cardiac decompensation.

Treatment. *Medical.* Once the biochemical diagnosis is established, treatment with alpha-adrenergic blocking agents should be started. The aim of treatment is to control the blood pressure and protect the patient from the danger of a severe hypertensive attack with its potential complications. Phenoxybenzamine is the usual drug employed for this purpose. Propranolol, a beta-adrenergic blocking agent, is useful when cardiac arrhythmias are present, but should only be given after the patient has received an alpha-blocker, otherwise a hypertensive crisis may occur.

Surgical. The definitive treatment of phaeochromocytoma is excision. The tumour is usually approached transabdominally. An arterial catheter and continuous ECG should be employed, for constant monitoring of the arterial pressure and heart action.

Phentolamine or nitroprusside and propranolol should be immediately available to treat sudden hypertension or cardiac arrhythmias that often occur when the tumour is manipulated. The surgeon should try to ligate the adrenal veins early in the procedure to avoid these crises. The results of surgery for the usual benign tumours are very gratifying, though mild to moderate hypertension usually persists.

THE ADRENAL CORTEX

HYPOCORTICISM

Adrenocortical insufficiency may be acute or chronic.

Acute hypocorticism. Acute adrenocortical insufficiency arises due to massive bilateral adrenal haemorrhage. The common situations in which it occurs include the following:

1. In the newborn, after a long and difficult labour.
2. In cases of fulminating septicaemia, commonly meningococcal, but occasionally streptococcal, staphylococcal or pneumococcal.
3. After major and extensive surgery, specially in cases suffering from intra-abdominal sepsis, pneumonia, coagulation defects and cancer.

Clinical features. The blood pressure falls precipitously, and the patient goes into a severe state of shock. Other evidence of acute adrenal failure is seen in the form of vomiting, diarrhoea and mental confusion. In cases of septicaemia, rigors and hyperpyrexia may be seen, along with petechial haemorrhages and purpuric patches. Eosinophilia is very suggestive, but the most useful laboratory finding is a low plasma cortisol.

Treatment. Treatment consists of the intravenous administration of hydrocortisone hemisuccinate. 100 mg is first given very rapidly in 500 ml of isotonic saline, and is repeated in about an hour. If there is a response, it should be continued in a dose of 50 mg every 6 hours. When the patient's condition is stabilized, treatment with a synthetic oral steroid should be substituted. In cases with septicaemia, appropriate antibiotic therapy must be immediately started by the intravenous route.

Chronic hypocorticism. (Addison's disease). This condition occurs due to adrenocortical deficiency from progressive destruction of first the cortex and then the medulla of the adrenal glands. The most common cause is supposed to be an autoimmune disease, other causes being tuberculosis, metastatic carcinoma and amyloidosis.

Clinical features. Addison's disease is most often seen in young adults. The leading features are muscular weakness and a low blood pressure. Increased pigmentation is seen at points of pressure and at the flexion creases. The mucous membrane of the mouth becomes pigmented. Episodes of acute adrenal insufficiency occur from time to time.

Treatment. The treatment is medical. Most patients need 20 to 30 mg of cortisone daily in divided doses, along with 0.05 mg fludrocortisone as mineralocorticoid replacement. If an excess of the drugs is given there is hypertension, hyperkalaemia and oedema; if enough is not given there is fatigue and hypotension. By the use of cortisone, the patient's life expectancy is greatly increased.

HYPERCORTICISM

Cushing's syndrome. ***Aetiology.*** Cushing's syndrome consists of a set of symptoms and signs which is caused by excessive hydrocortisone concentrations. The causes of the syndrome include the following conditions:

1. Most often, Cushing's syndrome results from the long-term administration of corticosteroids, in the treatment of different illnesses specially rheumatoid arthritis, and in patients receiving transplants, where steroids are given to suppress the rejection of the transplant.
2. The next most common cause of the syndrome is Cushing's disease, which is produced as follows: a basophil

adenoma of the anterior pituitary secretes an excess of adrenocorticotrophic hormone (ACTH). This leads to hyperplasia of the adrenal cortex and hypersecretion of hydrocortisone (cortisol) resulting in the signs and symptoms of Cushing's syndrome.

3. Cushing's syndrome can be caused by an adrenocortical adenoma or carcinoma, which secretes hydrocortisone independently of ACTH control.

4. Rarely, certain non-adrenal neoplasms may secrete ACTH leading to Cushing's syndrome.

Clinical features. Cushing's syndrome is most often seen in young females, in whom there is an excessive deposition of fat in certain unusual situations. The face becomes rounded like a full moon, the abdomen becomes protuberant, the neck is thick, and the supraclavicular fossae are obliterated. The arms and legs are thin, and the patient complains of increasing weakness. As the corticosteroids inhibit fibrous tissue, the skin becomes inelastic and feels like tissue-paper. Purple striae are seen on the abdomen, and the patient bruises easily. There is increased growth of hair, and acne is common. Amenorrhoea is frequent and in the male, impotence.

Due to a negative calcium balance severe osteoporosis occurs, and pathological fractures commonly result. Mild glycosuria is often seen and hypertension is frequent, often resulting in congestive cardiac failure. In more than half the cases a psychosis eventually supervenes. Cushing's syndrome is rare in children; when it occurs, an adrenal tumour is usually the cause.

A condition similar to Cushing's syndrome is the *adrenogenital syndrome*, which is caused by an excessive secretion of adrenal androgens, and commences in females shortly after puberty. The onset of amenorrhoea is followed by excessive growth of hair on the face, acne, atrophy of the breasts, and muscular development, with deepening of the voice and enlargement of the clitoris.

Investigations. Diagnostic testing for Cushing's syndrome is divided into two stages:

1. Firstly, patients with suspected hypercorticism undergo tests to *confirm the diagnosis:*

i. The demonstration of increased *urinary excretion of corticosteroids* in a 24 hour period is of more value than the presence of increased levels of these *steroids in the plasma.*

ii. If dexamethasone, a synthetic steroid, is administered, ACTH release is blocked, and in normal subjects the level of hydrocortisone in the plasma falls; not so in patients with Cushing's syndrome. This is the basis of the *dexamethasone suppression test.* Utilizing both the 24-hour urinary cortisol excretion and the dexamethasone suppression test together increases the accuracy of testing compared with one test alone.

2. Further tests are now carried out to *determine the primary pathology:*

i. The *plasma ACTH level* is raised or normal in pituitary pathology or ectopic ACTH secretion. Patients with adrenal pathology have undetectable ACTH levels due to suppression through the negative feedback mechanism.

ii. *ACTH stimulation test.* Intravenous administration of ACTH to patients with adrenal cortical hyperplasia produces a greater rise in the plasma hydrocortisone level than in normal persons. On the other hand in patients with adrenocortical adenomas, cortisol secretion is autonomous, and does not rise after ACTH is administered.

Treatment. If a *basophil adenoma* of the pituitary is the cause of the syndrome, *pituitary adenectomy* using microsurgical techniques is the treatment of choice. This method has replaced *irradiation* of the pituitary, where a major disadvantage is the long interval between initiation of therapy and the clinical response, often 18 months or even longer.

In the case of an *adrenal adenoma* unilateral *adrenalectomy* is the treatment of choice. With adrenal carcinoma, radical *resection* of the tumour should be carried out where feasible. Postoperative adjunctive radiotherapy and cytotoxic chemotherapy appear to improve survival.

50 Skin

Naevi. *Definition.* A naevus is a circumscribed stable malformation of the skin which is not due to external causes and is therefore presumed to be of hereditary origin. It is a hamartomatous malformation of the skin (A hamartoma is a benign tumour-like nodule composed of an overgrowth of mature cells that normally occur in the part, but with one element predominating).

Naevi may be composed of epidermal or dermal elements. *Epidermal* naevi are wart-like papules which may form linear plaques. They are asymptomatic and have little effect on the general health. *Connective tissue* naevi are firm, flesh-coloured papules. They are harmless and are excised for cosmetic reasons.

Haemangiomas. Haemangiomas are proliferations of vascular elements (Fig. 1). Their endothelium-lined vascular spaces are commonly capillary-sized, but large 'cavernous' spaces are also found. The most common types of haemangiomas include strawberry and cavernous haemangiomas:

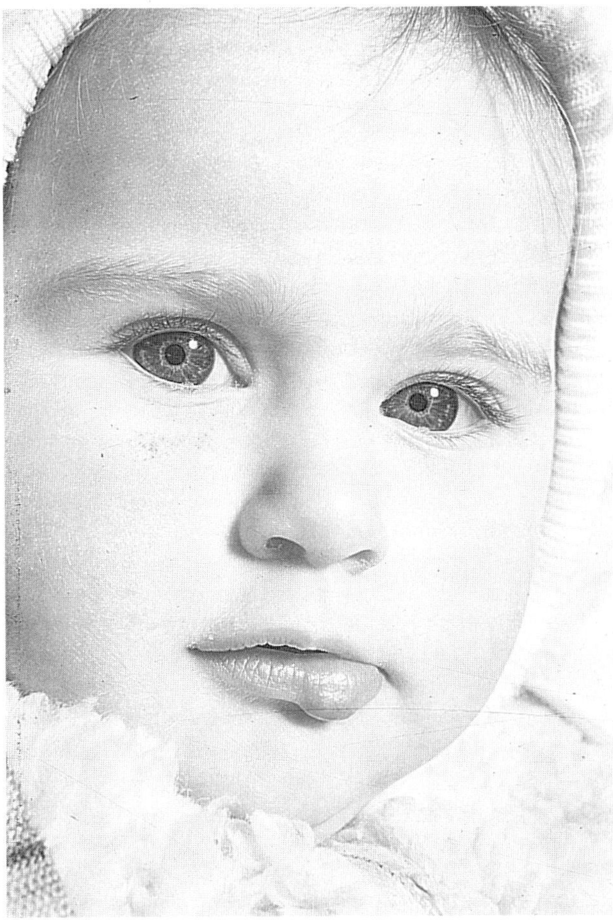

Fig. 1 Haemangioma lower lip.

Strawberry haemangiomas (Plate III–II) may be present at birth, but more commonly appear during the first few weeks of life. They are lobular, bright red nodules with a spongy consistency, so that blood can be compressed out of them. The surface is studded with small capillary tufts so that the lesion resembles a strawberry. These lesions seldom require treatment, because the vast majority involute spontaneously by the age of about 6 years. However, treatment may be required for lesions situated on the eyelids, nose or lips, where they cause functional impairment. Rapidly growing strawberry haemangiomas are usually first treated by corticosteroids, which may stimulate gradual involution.

Cavernous haemangiomas also may present at birth and grow rapidly during the first few months of life, after which they involute spontaneously. They are situated just beneath the skin and appear as soft, bluish masses. A typical strawberry haemangioma may form the cutaneous component of a cavernous haemangioma.

Emptying sign. In infants, in the case of every soft swelling, the possibility of haemangioma should be excluded by testing the swelling for the 'emptying' sign, which is a hallmark of an haemangioma. Firm, continuous pressure should be applied to see if the swelling empties. The importance of carrying out the test is this: most haemangiomas in infants, after enlarging for some time, regress spontaneously over a period of months. Therefore, specially if they are located in the vicinity of important structures which could be damaged by the dissection, they should be left well alone, and will regress with time.

Platelet-trapping haemangioma. A problem can arise if a haemangioma is very large, because the blood flows through its spaces sluggishly and platelets get trapped in the mass. When this happens on a massive scale, the thrombocytopenia results in a bleeding tendency. When this bleeding takes place in the haemangioma itself the mass continues to enlarge, and specially if located in the vicinity of the trachea, may produce respiratory obstruction. Such a condition is called a platelet-trapping haemangioma.

Cysts. *Epidermal (sebaceous) cysts.* These cysts, which were incorrectly called sebaceous cysts in the past, are the most common cysts of the skin. The most frequent sites are the scalp, face and back. They may be solitary or multiple, and present as 0.5 to 3 cm spherical, slightly compressible intradermal masses. A follicular orifice, the 'punctum', usually connects the cyst to the skin surface at the dome of the cyst (Fig. 2). The wall consists of stratified squamous epithelium. Desquamated keratin cells are shed into the cavity of the cyst, forming a cheesy white material. Infection can lead to fibrosis of the surrounding dermis and make the cyst difficult to dissect.

Pigmented lesions. ***Benign.*** These include benign and dysplastic naevi.

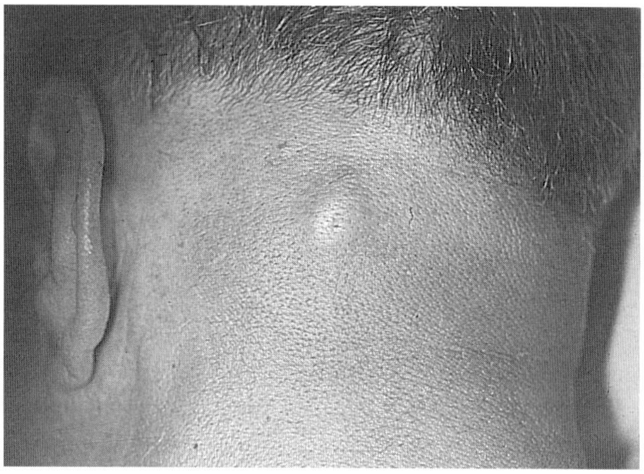

Fig. 2 Sebaceous cyst back of neck.

Benign naevi include junctional, compound and blue naevi, haemangiomas and subungual haematomas. They differ from dysplastic naevi as follows: they are usually less than 6 mm in diameter, have a uniform colour throughout, and possess a sharp, clear-cut border.

Dysplastic naevi are larger in size, contain a mixture of light brown and black within the same naevus, and have irregular borders. *Dysplastic naevi are markers of increased risk for, or even precursors to, cutaneous melanoma.*

TUMOURS

Premalignant. ***Keratoacanthoma.*** These tumours appear suddenly and grow rapidly, achieving a diameter of several centimeters within a few weeks. They are benign and typically regress spontaneously within one year. However, the behaviour of large keratoacanthomas is more like that of squamous cell carcinomas, with locally destructive growth and the potential for invasion. The tumour is domed with a central crater. Histologically it resembles a squamous cell carcinoma, and differentiation between the two may be difficult. However, unlike the latter tumour its base is flat and it does not show invasion of the deeper dermis. Therefore, the biopsy should extend into the subcutaneous fat so as to include this deeper portion of the tumour. Surgical excision is the treatment of choice.

Malignant. ***Squamous cell carcinoma.*** After basal cell carcinoma this is the most common malignant tumour of the skin. In white-skinned people it arises most often due to chronic damage by sunlight, most patients being elderly. It also develops:

1. At mucocutaneous interfaces as a result of the use of tobacco or papilloma virus infection.
2. At sites treated with radiation.
3. In the scars of burns.
4. In chronic ulcers of the skin.

Tumours caused by sunlight rarely metastasize and usually require only local excision; those due to other factors are aggressive and metastasize frequently. These tumours occur more often in immunosuppressed patients, specially following organ transplantation. The tumour presents as a nodule or plaque, which may ulcerate. In white-skinned patients the lesions are typically pink or flesh-coloured; in those with darker complexions they may be hypopigmented or hyperpigmented.

Squamous cell carcinomas should be *treated* by excision with a 1 cm margin, if possible, and the fact that the margins are not involved by tumour confirmed by histological examination. As far as the regional lymph nodes are concerned:

1. They should be excised only if clinically palpable (therapeutic lymph node dissection).
2. However, lesions arising in chronic wounds behave more aggressively and are more likely to spread to regional lymph nodes. In these cases lymph nodes should be excised even if not palpable (prophylactic lymph node dissection).

Alternatives to surgical therapy include radiation and topical applications of 5-fluorouracil; these should be employed in patients unfit or unwilling for surgery. Distant metastases indicate a poor prognosis; only 13 percent of patients are alive after 10 years.

Basal cell carcinoma. Basal cell carcinomas contain cells that resemble the basal cell layers of the epidermis. They are locally destructive but rarely metastasize. They are common in males over the age of 40 years and occur mostly on the upper and central parts of the face. Starting as a translucent papule the tumour may assume one of several forms. The *noduloulcerative* type is the most common. When large such a lesion is often called a 'rodent ulcer'. *Pigmented* basal cell carcinomas need to be distinguished by biopsy from melanoma. *Superficial* basal cell cancers form red, scaly lesions difficult to distinguish from other skin conditions. Basal cell carcinomas are slow growing, and patients often neglect these lesions for years. Metastasis and death are extremely rare, but the tumours cause extensive local destruction.

Nodular lesions smaller than 2 mm can be *treated* by dermatologists with curettage and electrodesiccation or laser vaporization. However, a drawback to these procedures is that no pathological specimen can be obtained to confirm the clinical diagnosis. Larger tumours, tumours that invade bone or surrounding structures, and more aggressive types, are best treated by surgical excision with an 8 mm margin of normal tissue. Histological confirmation that the margins do not contain tumour is required. If the patient is unwilling or unfit for surgery, radiation may be employed.

Cutaneous melanoma. Cutaneous melanoma is malignancy of the pigment producing cell, the melanocyte, which is normally located in the basal layer of the epidermis. It is common in light-skinned caucasians. Patients used to present late and die rapidly of the disease. However, since the early signs of the disease have been publicized, the 5 year survival rates have more than doubled. The most frequent site for cutaneous melanoma is the upper back in men and the lower leg as well as upper back in women. Table 1 lists the risk factors in decreasing order of importance; the highest risk is associated with a persistently changing mole*. Increase in size and change in colour are the two most common characteristics of early cutaneous melanoma.

---

* *Mole* A naevus. The term is also applied loosely to any blemish of the skin.

Table 1 Risk factors for cutaneous melanoma (in decreasing order of importance).

Mole exhibiting persistent changes
Dysplastic naevus in patient with family history of melanoma
Family history of melanoma
Dysplastic naevus, no family history
Personal history of melanoma
Caucasian patient
Immunocompromised individual
Excess exposure to sunlight

Biopsy. Total excisional biopsy with narrow margins is the procedure of choice for the diagnosis of cutaneous melanoma; this provides the entire specimen for histopathological examination and also provides definitive therapy for benign lesions. Where total excisional biopsy is not easily accomplished, removal of a partial biopsy specimen is a reasonable course of action. Either punch (trephine) or incisional biopsy can be used. When a partial biopsy is performed, biopsy from the most raised portion is usually sufficient for diagnosis. In flat lesions biopsy of the darkest portion produces a representative specimen.

Prognosis. The thickness of the primary tumour in millimetres is the single most important prognostic factor in patients with no clinical evidence of disease elsewhere. Apart from this, increased numbers of mitoses, the presence of an ulcer, and the presence of microscopic satellites are associated with a poor prognosis. Thus, early recognition followed by prompt surgery offers the best chance for cure.

Treatment. Classical treatment consisted of excision of the tumour with 5 cm surgical margins. It has recently been shown that in the case of tumours 1 mm or less in thickness 1 cm margins are adequate, while in thicker tumours 3 cm margins are required; these latter usually require a graft or a flap to resurface the wound.

Lymph node dissection. Tumours thinner than 1 mm rarely have nodal metastases, so that elective nodal dissection is not considered necessary. Tumours thicker than 4 mm have systemic metastases, hence node dissection does not improve their prognosis. Studies are being conducted to determine whether or not melanomas of a thickness of 1.5 to 4 mm benefit from lymph node dissection. Until the results are available, elective nodal dissection in these patients should be carried out at the discretion of the surgeon, after discussion with the patient.

Limb perfusion. At specialized centres perfusion of the affected extremity with phenylalanine mustard at elevated temperatures has produced good control of in-transit lesions and satellite lesions. This is accepted as a palliative measure. However, its benefit as an adjuvant in the treatment of primary extremity melanomas has not been established.

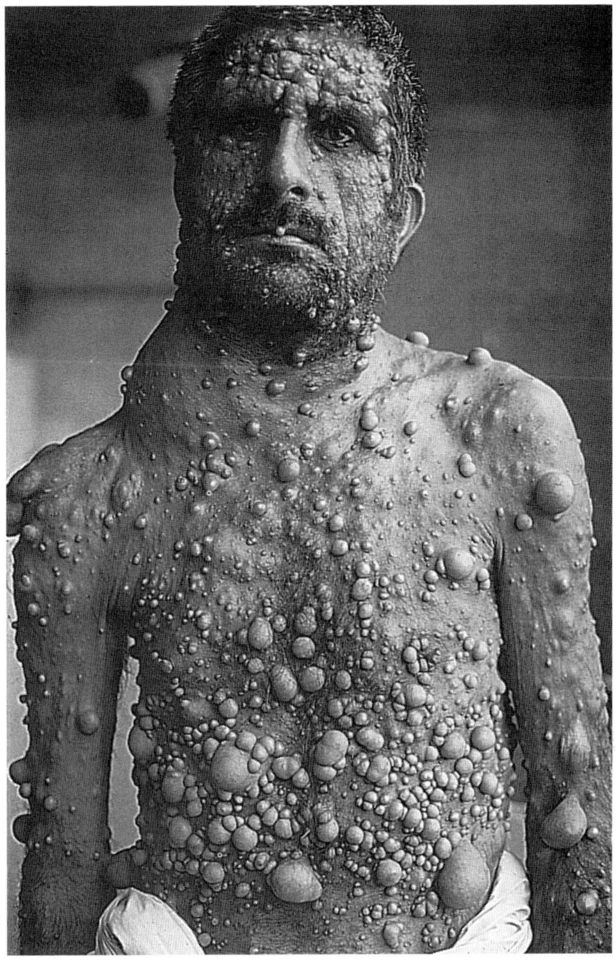

Fig. 3 Neurofibromatosis.

In the presence of *disseminated disease* a systemic approach is appropriate, the response to chemotherapy being greatest in the case of tumours in the skin, lymph nodes and lungs.

Neurofibromatosis is an inherited disorder which is transmitted in an autosomal dominant manner. Two types are seen. Neurofibromatosis type 1 occurs approximately once in every 4000 births. Its common manifestations include multiple cutaneous neurofibromas (Fig. 3), cafe au lait spots*, freckles in the axillae and groins, and nodules of the iris. Neurofibromatosis type 2 is less common (1 in 100000 births). It is manifested by multiple intracranial and spinal tumours, specially bilateral acoustic neuromas.

* *Cafe au lait* (Fr.) coffee with milk. Cafe au lait spots: pigmented macules of a light brown colour, as in neurofibromatosis and Albright's syndrome.

Answers to photoquiz

1. Cystic hygroma neck in newborn. Note the large size of the swelling, which is lobulated.

2. Accessory auricles in infant.

3. Cancrum oris: ganrene of lips and cheeks has resulted from thrombosis of labial arteries. A high fever accompanied by a boil developed on the 3rd day of life. The boil extended and the lips became black. The baby died from the toxaemia.

4. Baby thriving after repair of oesophageal atresia and tracheo-oesophageal fistula on the day of birth. Notice the anterior end of the thoracotomy scar and the scar of the temporary gastrostomy.

5. Neurilemmomma (nerve sheath tumour) neck with numerous branches reaching upto chin, occiput, mediastinum and posterior triangle, removed intact through a submandibular incision.

6. Case of major exomphalos. Abdominal wall could not come together; therefore a synthetic mesh has been stitched to the defect to accomodate abdominal contents without excessive pressure on inferior vena cava and diaphragm. Successive rows of sutures will produce gradual contraction of the mesh as the abdominal cavity enlarges. Ultimately the mesh will be detached and the abdominal wall repaired by mass closure.

7. Congenital diaphragmatic hernia through pleuroperitoneal canal (foramen of Bochdalek). The whole of the small intestine is lying in the left pleural cavity, having pushed the heart markedly to the right and compressing the right lung. The baby was blue, cold and cyanosed. Successful repair through a laparotomy.

8. 'Invertogram' showing gas rising up to reach very close to the small metal piece over the anal dimple. Thus, the anorectal anomaly is of the low type, the gas having reached well below the line joining the pubis and the coccyx.

9. 'Minerva' type jacket of plaster of Paris applied. The young girl had a severe postburn contracture front of neck excised and split-skin grafted. The jacket has been applied for a few weeks to prevent contraction of the scar and recurrence of the contracture.

10. Maxillectomy has been carried out for a carcinoma of the maxilla. Through the open mouth the cavity left behind by the removal of the maxilla and half of the palate can be seen.

11. Pilonidal sinus. Hair can be seen peeping through one of the sinuses.

12. Case of road traffic accident, resulting in midthigh amputation and loss of skin from flexor surface of forearm and elbow. *To show what granulation tissue looks like.* In this case the wound is clean and ready for resurfacing with split-skin grafts.

13. Fibrous polyp anal canal.

14. Hydatid cyst removed from lung and opened out, showing daughter cysts.

15. Kidney and grossly dilated pelvis displayed at operation.

16. Kidney and pelvis (shown in 15 above) removed by nephrectomy and opened out. The pelvis is reduced to a mere fibrous bag.

17. Cystogram showing very gross benign enlargement of the prostate.

18. Prostate shown in the cystogram in 17 above removed at open 'prostatectomy'.

19. Strawberry haemangioma face of an infant, with an underlying cavernous haemangioma which is producing a swelling in the subcutaneous tissue. The central portion of each of the two masses is pale due to commencing endarteritis obliterans which is likely to cause its shrinkage within a few months. As it is not located on the eyelids, etc. it would be best left alone to involute in time.

20. Large meningocele over lumbar spine of newborn infant.

21. Low type anorectal anomaly. Underneath, the anal canal is fully formed. Excessive fusion of the skin in the midline has resulted in beads of meconium along the perineal raphe.

22. Large number of seeds, buttons, screws, etc. removed at laparotomy from the duodenum of an infant suffering from congenital duodenal stenosis, who presented with recurrent vomiting. This also shows the type of objects babies will swallow.

23. Theirsch's type skin grafts applied to raw area forearm, remaining after healing of lacerated wound with skin loss.

24. Mesenteric cyst, shown along with the segment of small intestine carrying it, and treated by resection of the loop of gut.

25. Third degree piles at 3, 7 and 11 o'clock. As is usual, the largest pile is at 11 o'clock. Note the secondary piles between the main piles. Note also the rim of raised skin all round, the 'external piles'.

26. Three raw areas left behind after removal of piles at operation.

27. Fibrolipomatosis (Dercum's disease). The subcutaneous swellings are more numerous than usual. One such swelling on the forearm has been removed for biopsy, so that the diagnosis is beyond any shadow of doubt. The other swellings then need not be removed unless any one starts growing or is otherwise troublesome.

28. Fistula-in-ano, showing external opening.

29. Complete prolapse of rectum, many inches in length, in 2 year old boy. Suitable by treatment by submucosal sclerosing injection.

30. Complete prolapse of rectum in an adult. Will re-

quire operative treatment.

31. Paronychia, with pus under the skin around the whole nail fold.

32. Arteriogram axillary artery showing false aneurysm resulting from lateral tear of artery during blunt trauma. The aneurysm was treated by excision and repair of the artery.

33. Large amoebic abscess in boy, lifting the abdominal wall and causing emaciation due to the toxaemia.

34. Facies of moribund patient ('facies hippocratica'). This 60 year old man had an untreated strangulated inguinal hernia of 15 days' duration! He died a few hours after the photograph due to multiple organ dysfunction syndrome from sepsis resulting from peritonitis.

35. Dry gangrene skin of upper arm resulting from thrombosis of vessels under skin after subcutaneous injection of drug meant for intramuscular injection. After the dead skin separated, split-skin grafts were applied.

36. Single internal pile prolapsed out of the anal canal. Note accompanying external skin tags.

Index

PLATE I

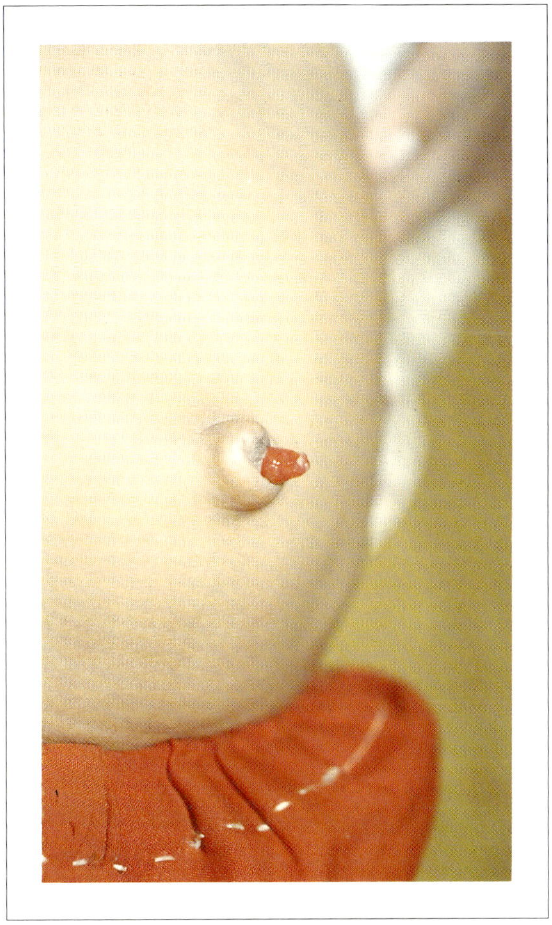

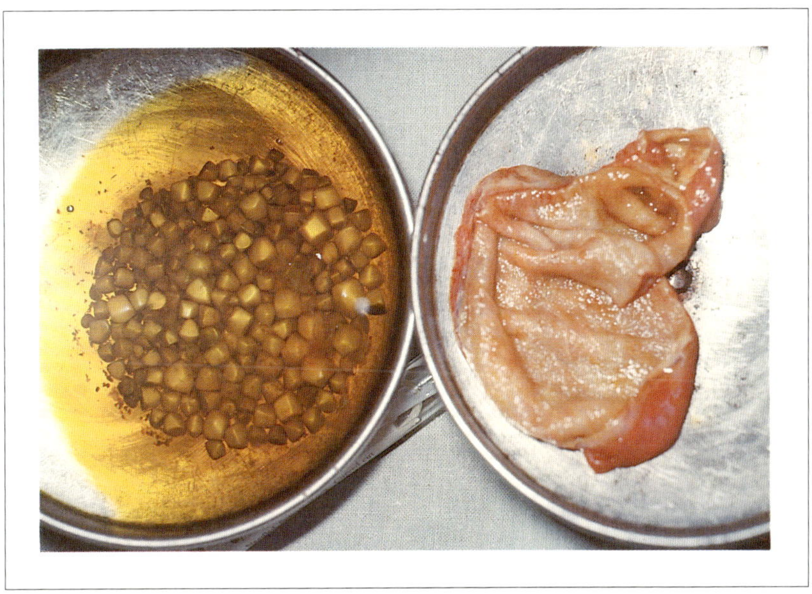

I. 'Raspberry' tumour, so called because of its resemblance to a raspberry, and representing the persistent umbilical end of the vitellointestinal duct.
II. Gallbladder with a large number of small faceted mixed stones and clear bile. The wall of the gallbladder is not thickened.

PLATE Ia **Photoquiz** (Answers before Index)

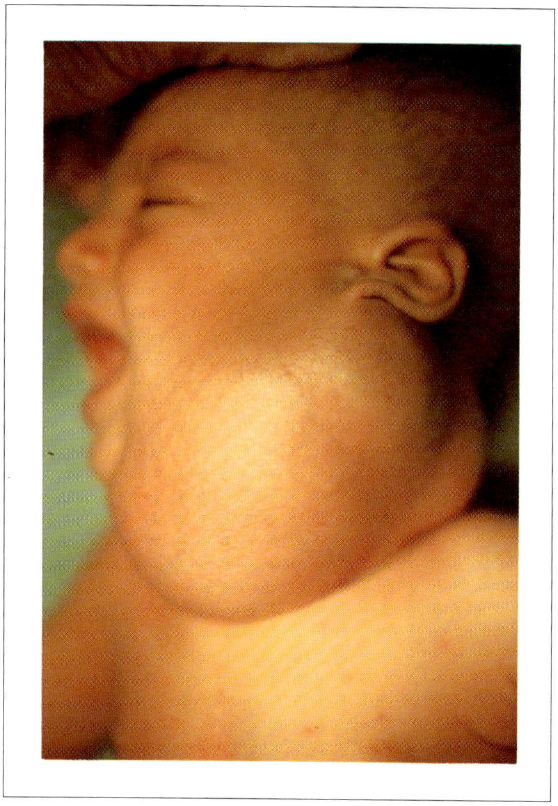

1

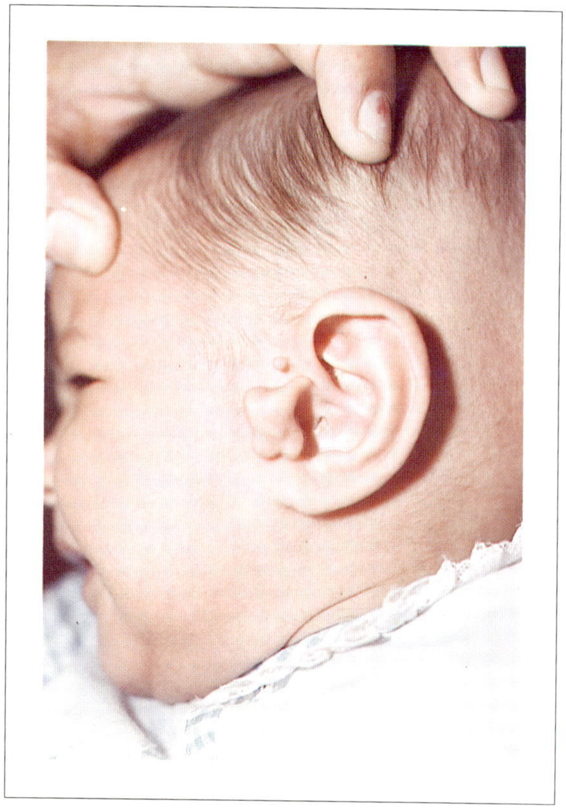

2

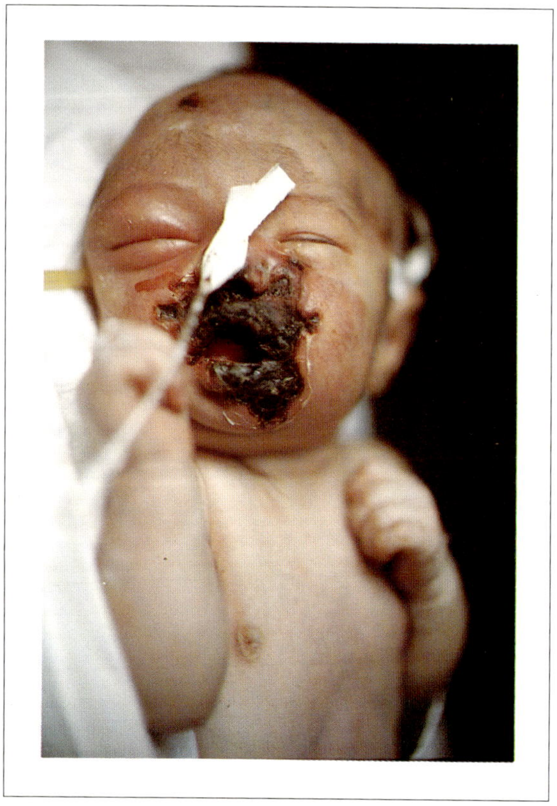

3

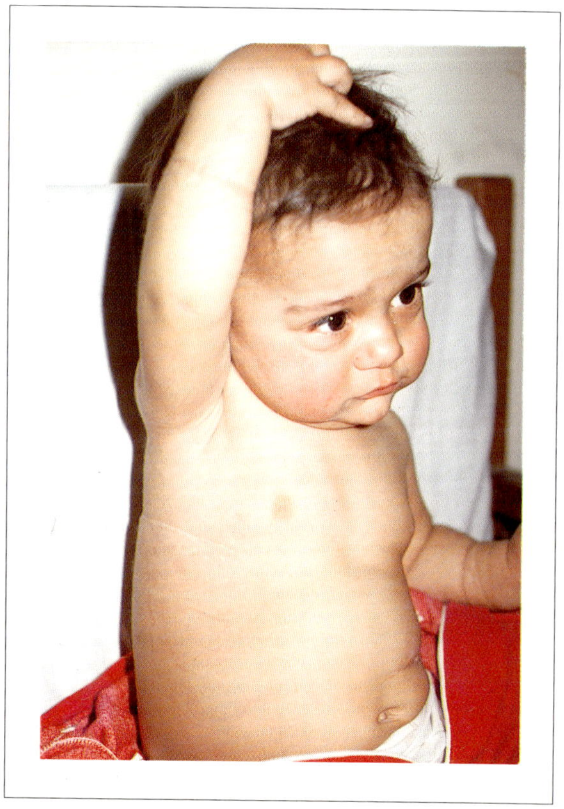

4

PLATE II

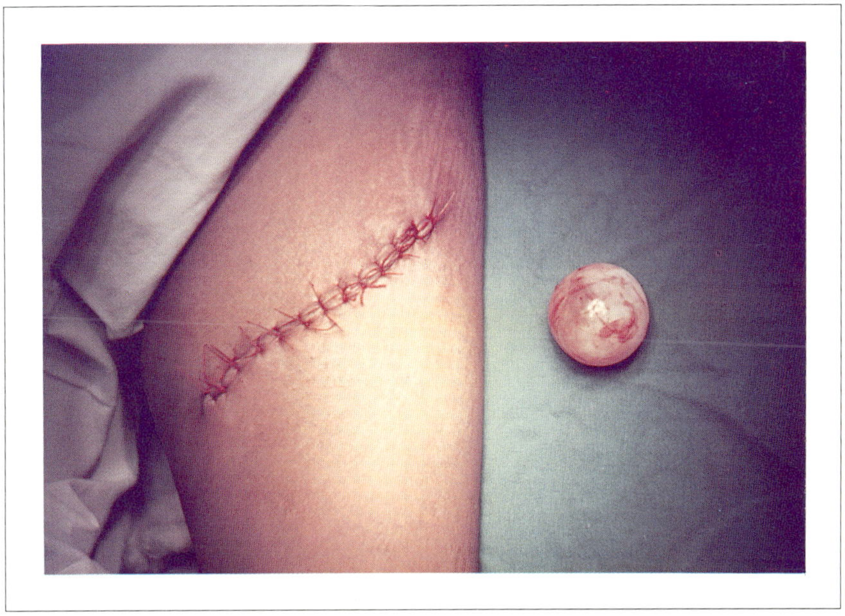

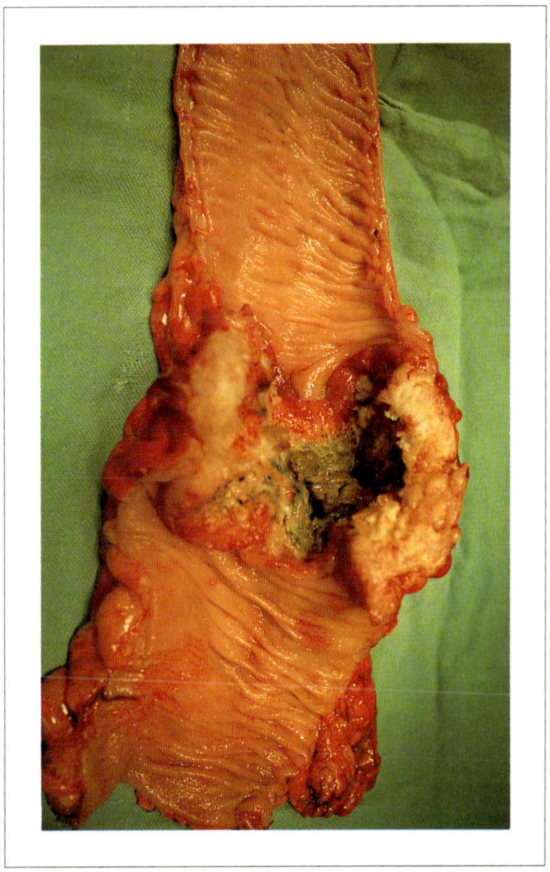

I. Hydatid cyst removed from thigh of adolescent girl, showing that a hydatid cyst can occur anywhere. The preoperative diagnosis was fibroma, as the mass was quite firm.
II. Malignant ulcer rectum due to a carcinoma. The ulcer has gone through all the coats of the rectum. Note the raised, everted edge which is characteristic of neoplastic ulcers.

PLATE IIa Photoquiz (Answers before Index)

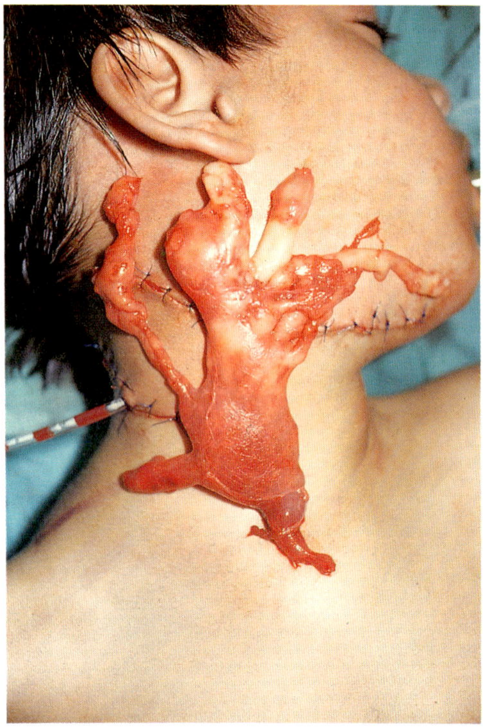

5

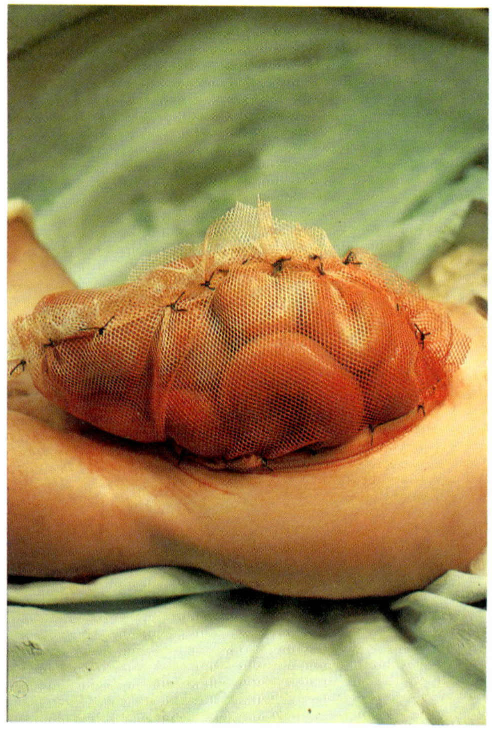

6

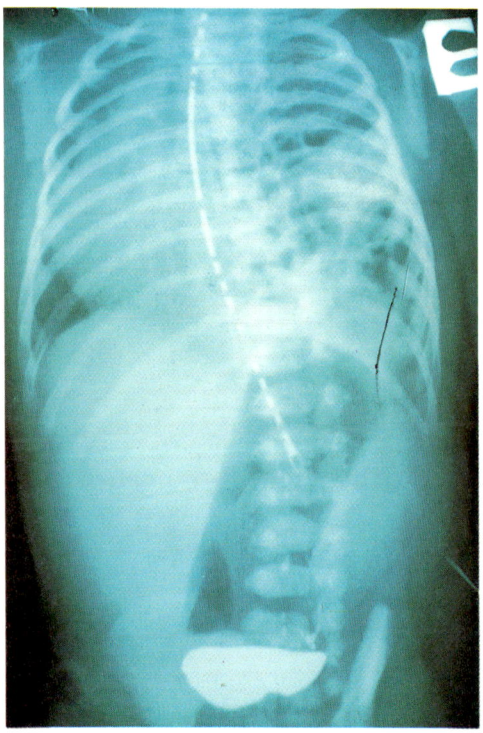

7

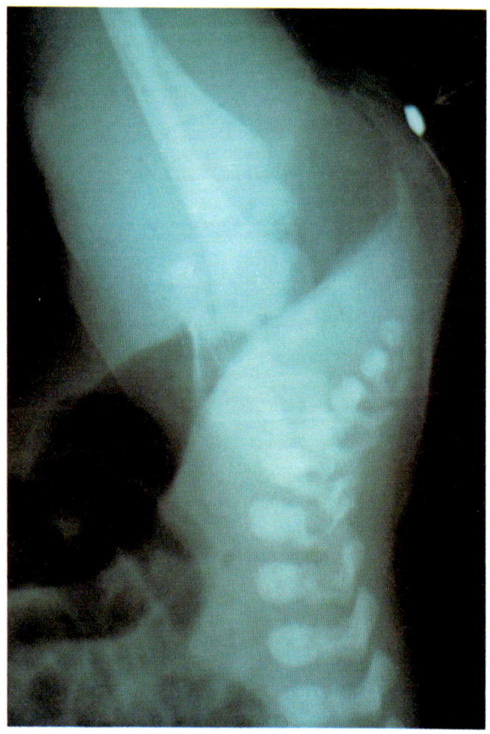

8

PLATE III

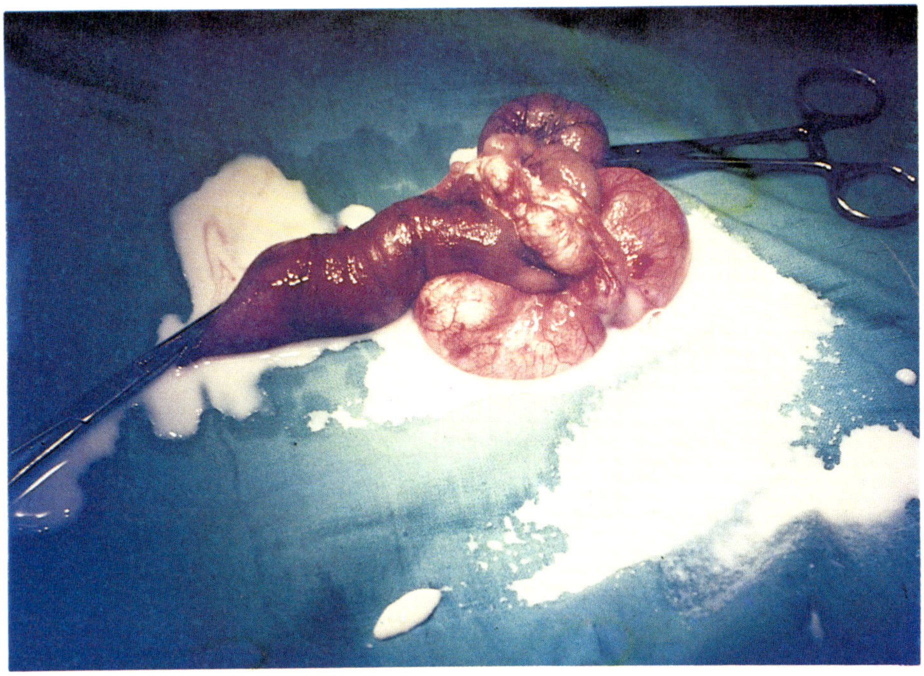

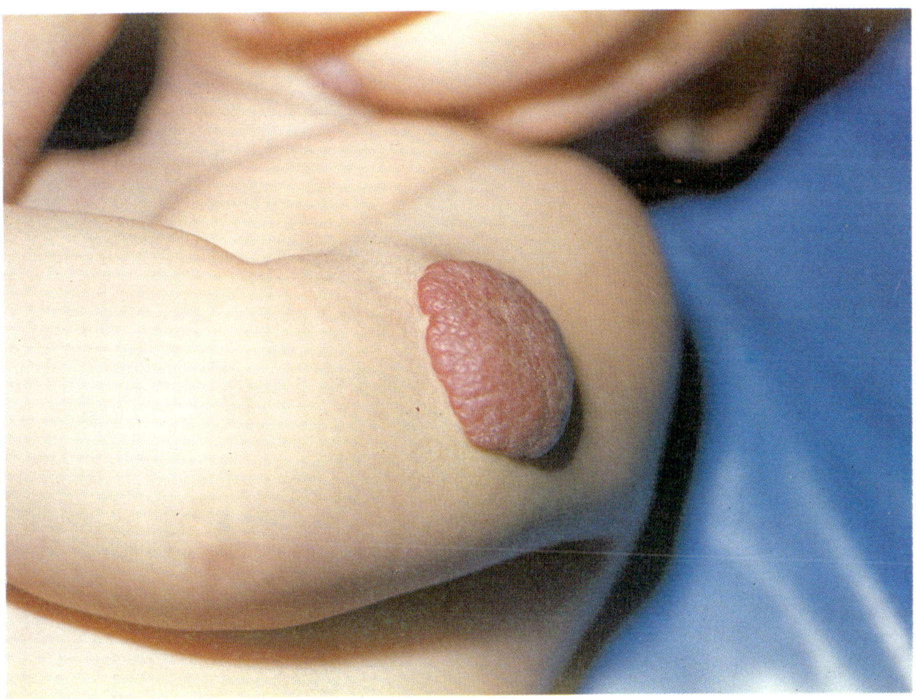

I. Chylolymphatic cyst, with 'milk' spilt due to rupture of the cyst. Due to the intimate relationship of the cyst with the small intestine, a segment of gut usually has to be removed with the cyst.
II. 'Strawberry' haemangioma, so named because of its resemblance to a strawberry. The mass regresses spontaneously by the age of one or two years, so excision can be postponed with benefit.

PLATE IIIa Photoquiz (Answers before Index)

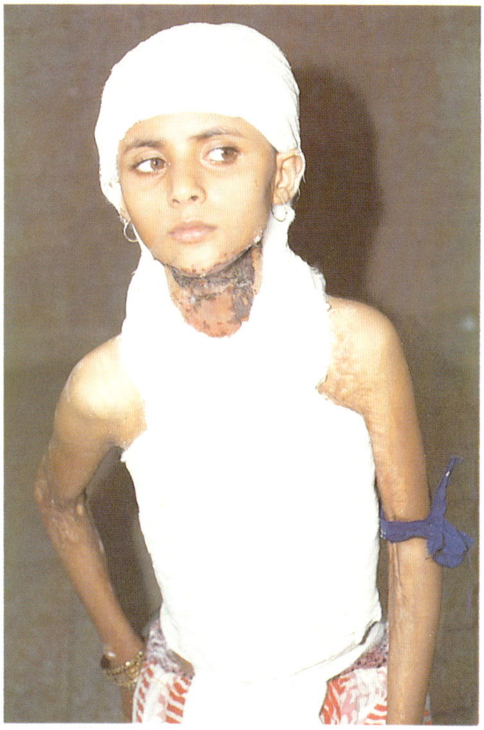

9

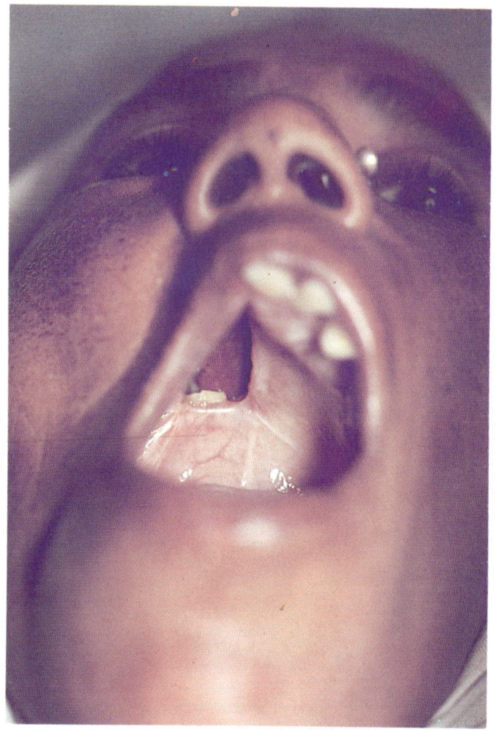

10

11

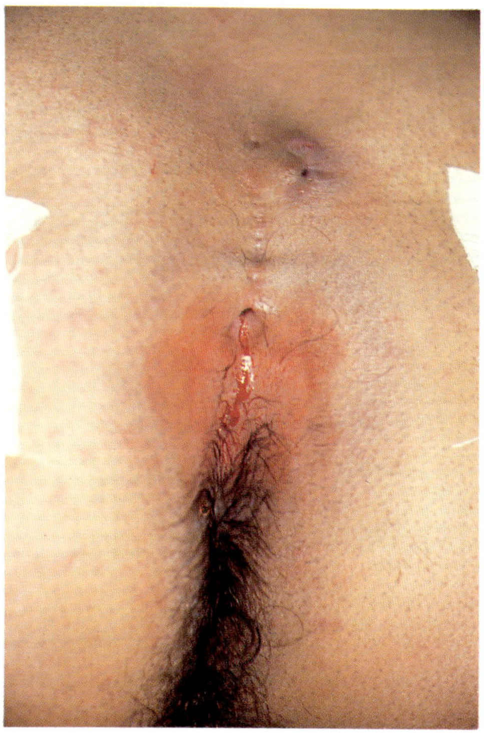

12

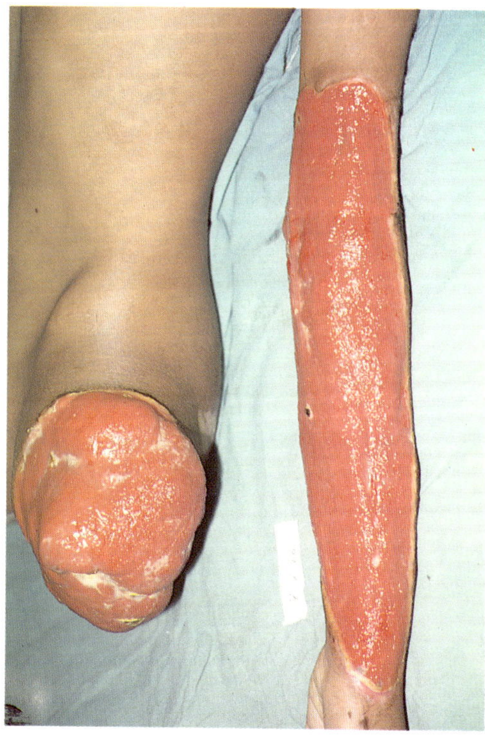

PLATE IV

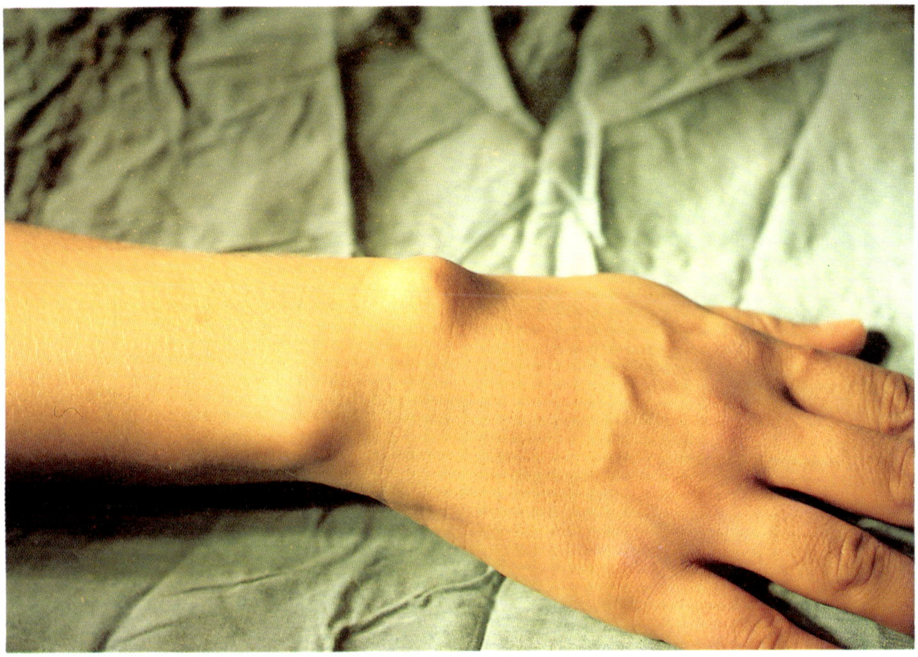

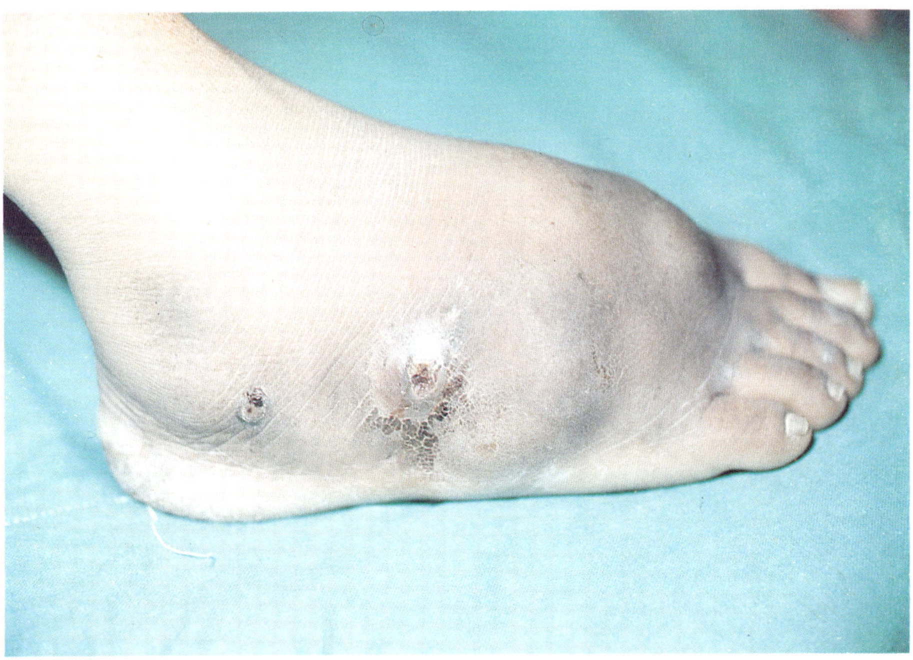

I. 'Ganglion' wrist, at its usual location over the *radial* part of the back of the wrist.
II. Actinomycosis foot. Note the swelling of the whole foot and the numerous sinuses.

PLATE IVa Photoquiz (Answers before Index)

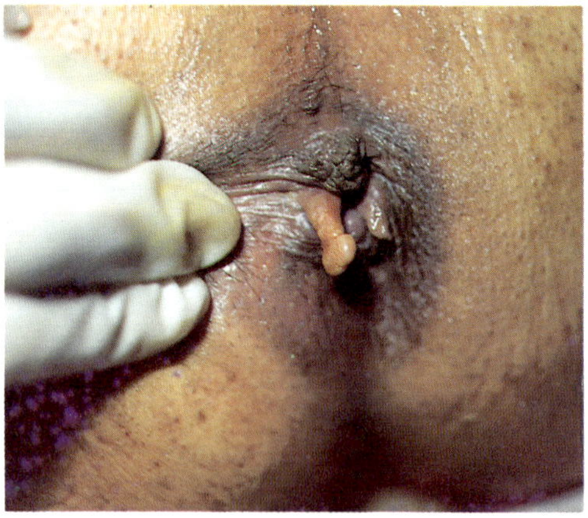

13

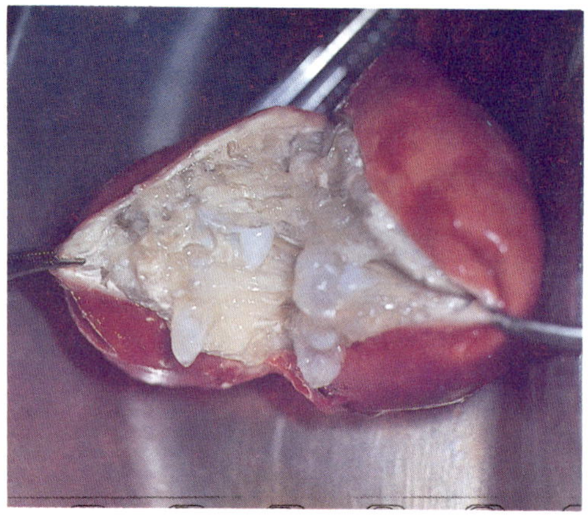

14

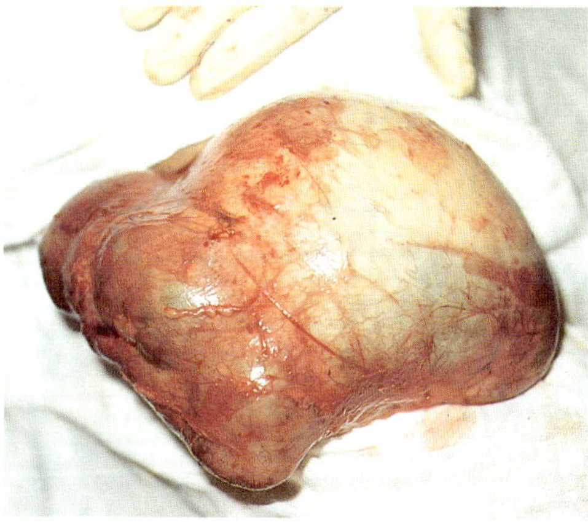

15

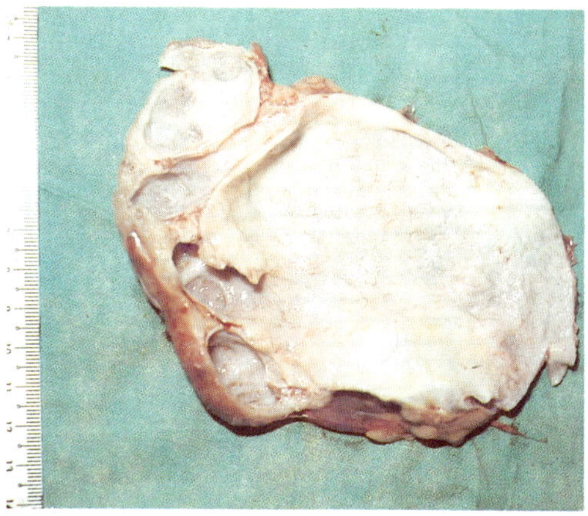

16

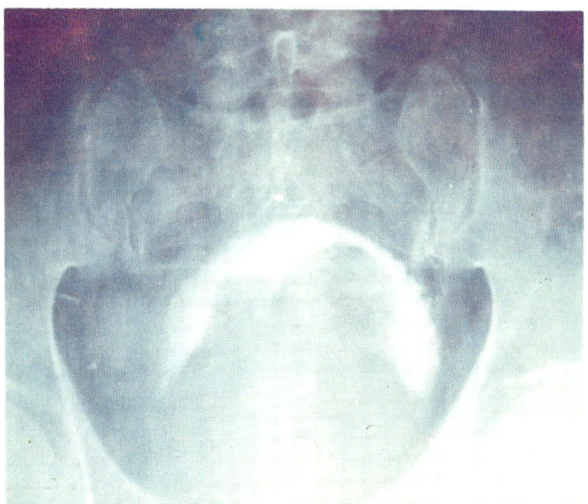

17

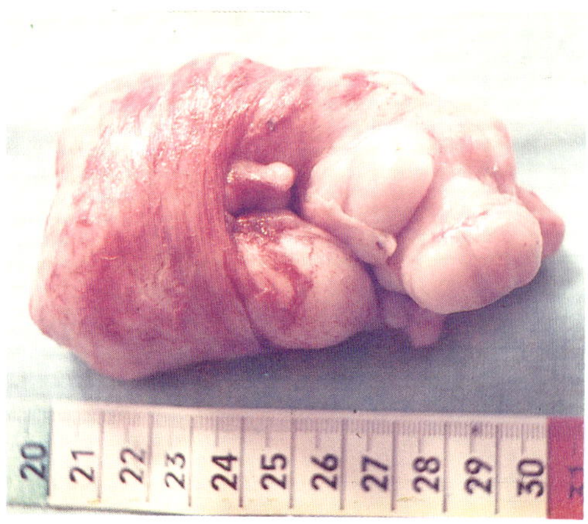

18

PLATE V

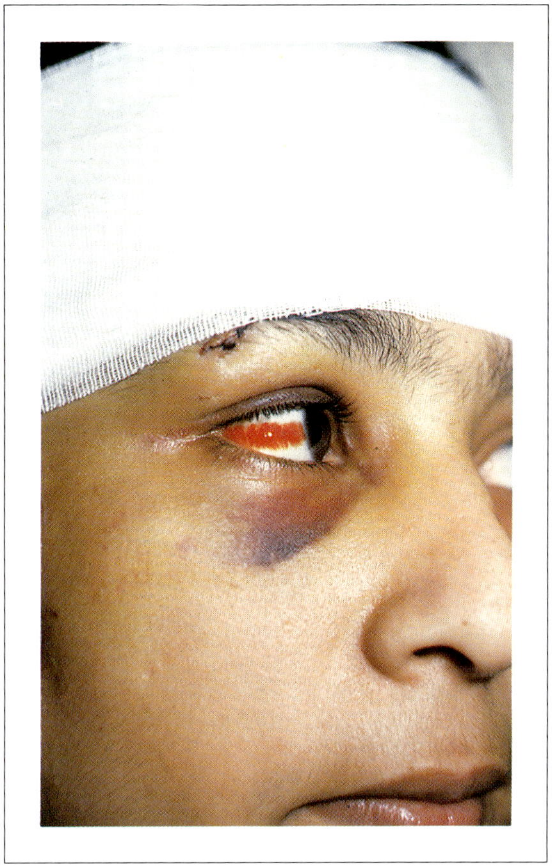

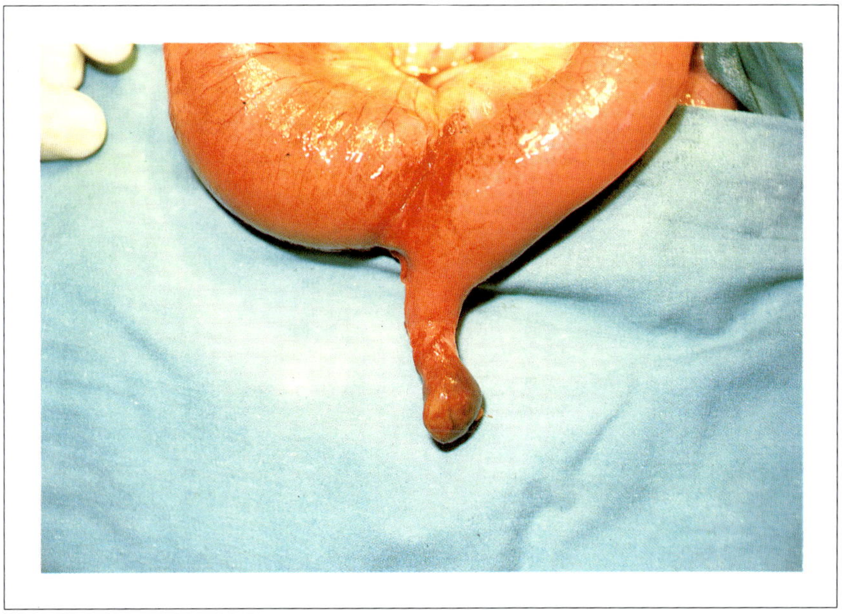

I. Fracture base of skull, showing red blood under conjunctiva whose posterior limit cannot be seen, purple blood confined within orbital margin, black bruise on cheek, and lacerated wound eyebrow, covered by bandage.
II. Meckel's diverticulum arising from antimesenteric border of small intestine. Suitable for excision without resection of a segment of small gut.

PLATE Va Photoquiz (Answers before Index)

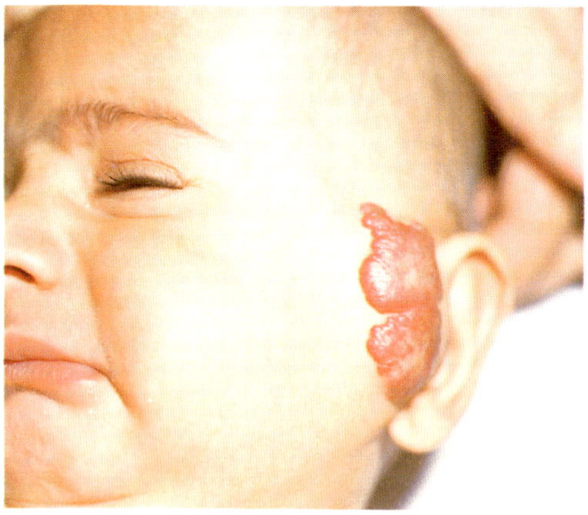

19

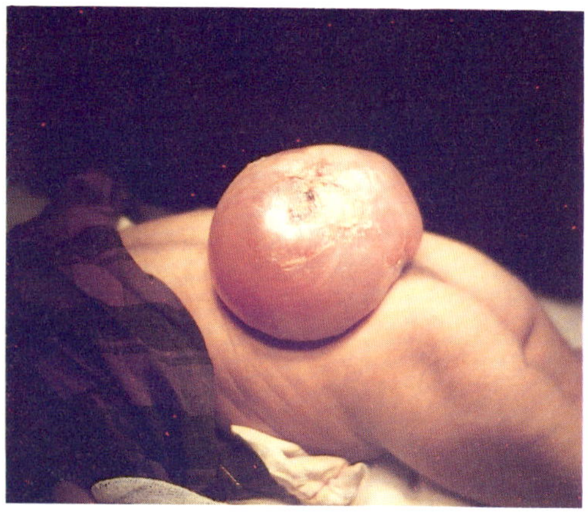

20

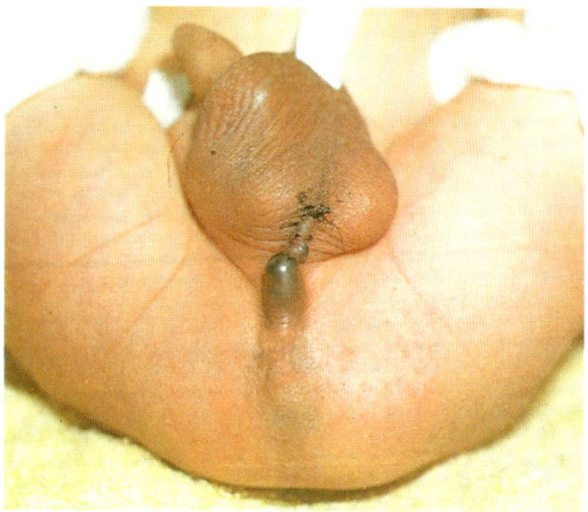

21

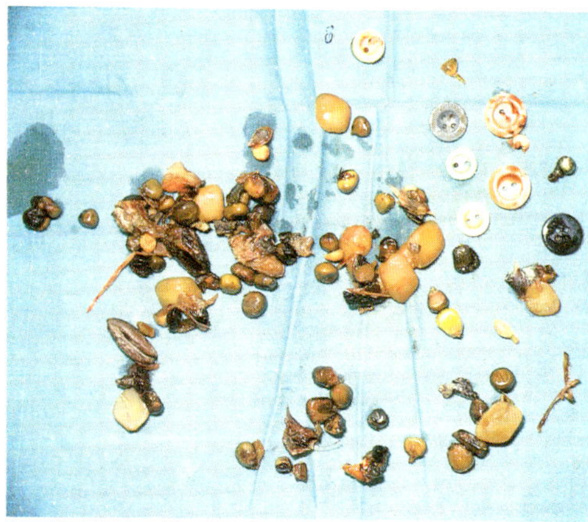

22

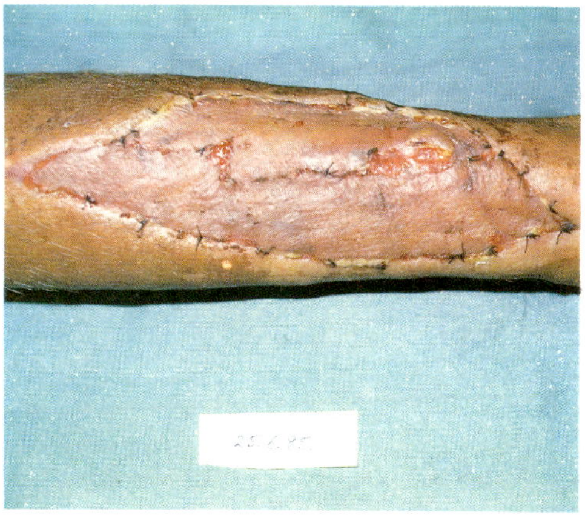

23

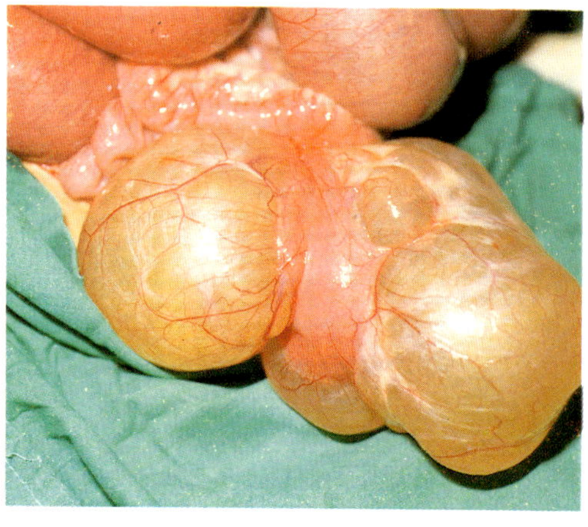

24

PLATE VI

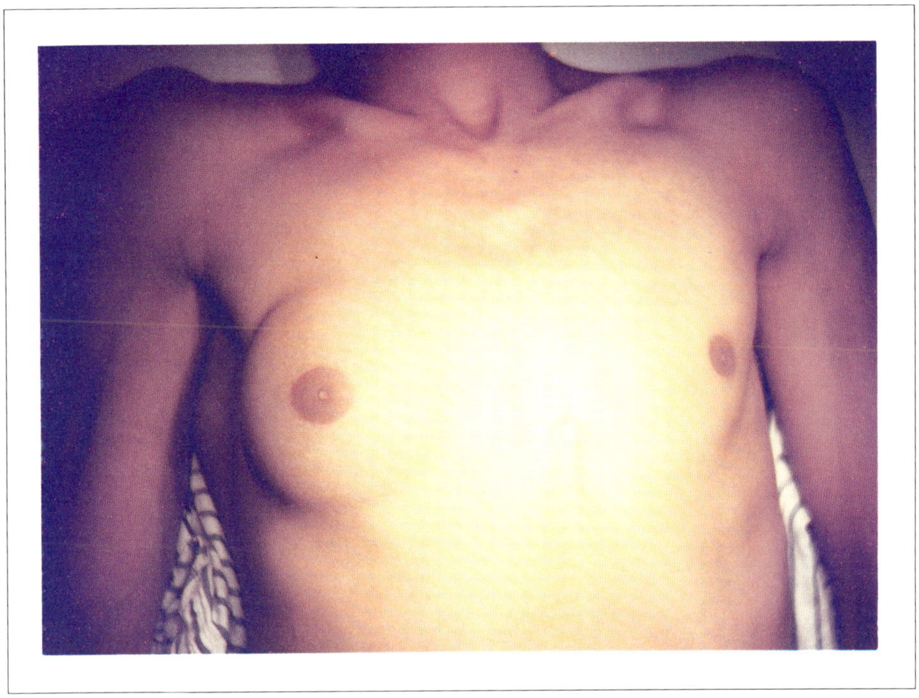

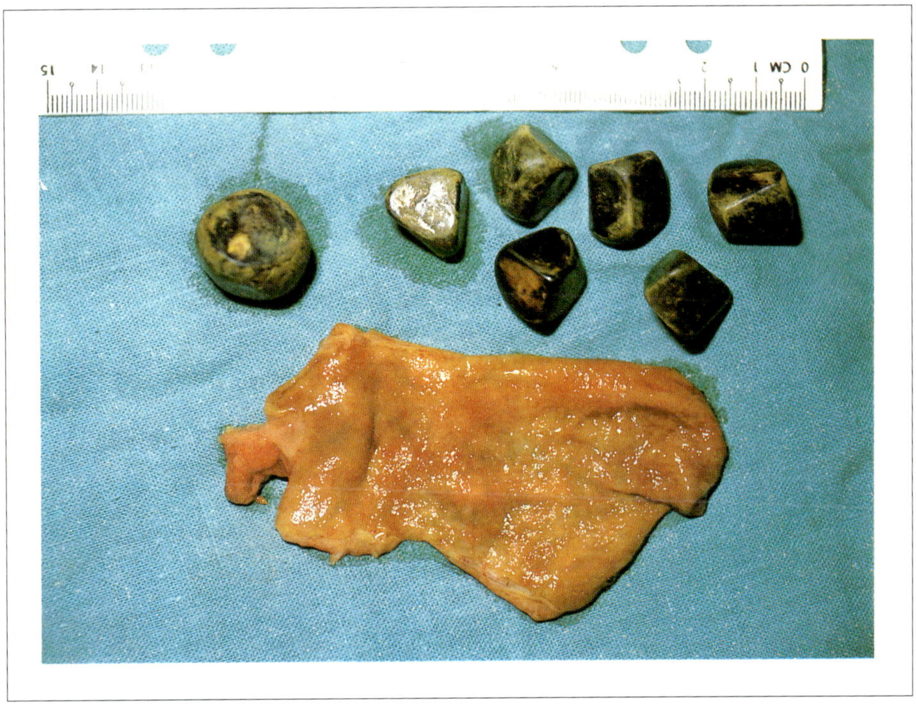

I. Gynaecomastia. When unilateral as in this case, it is not necessary to investigate for the presence of hormonal imbalance. If such a condition had been present, the gynaecomastia would have been bilateral.
II. Gallbladder with a few large faceted gallstones. The gallbladder wall is only moderately thickened.

PLATE VIa Photoquiz (Answers before Index)

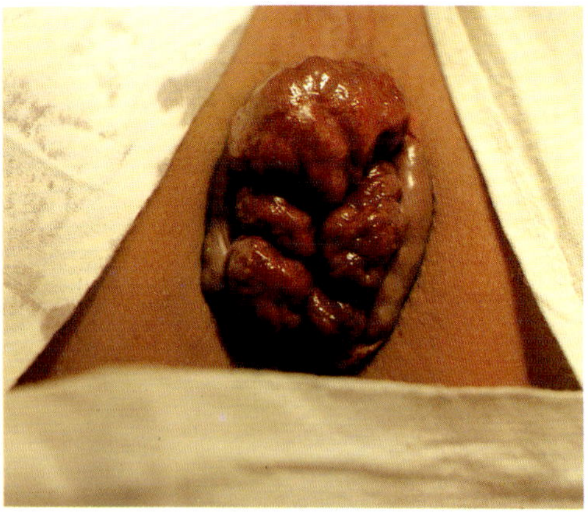

25

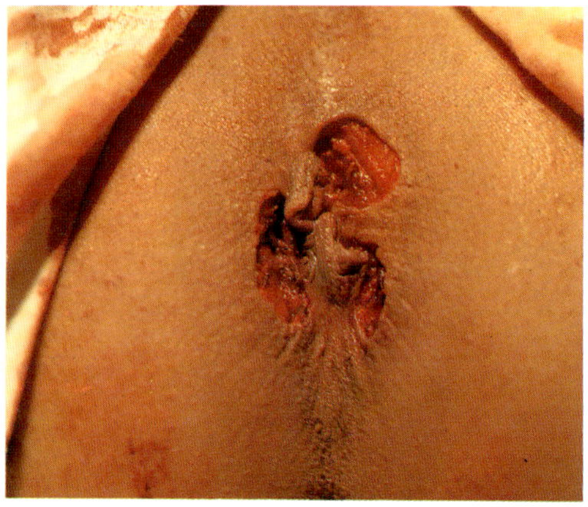

26

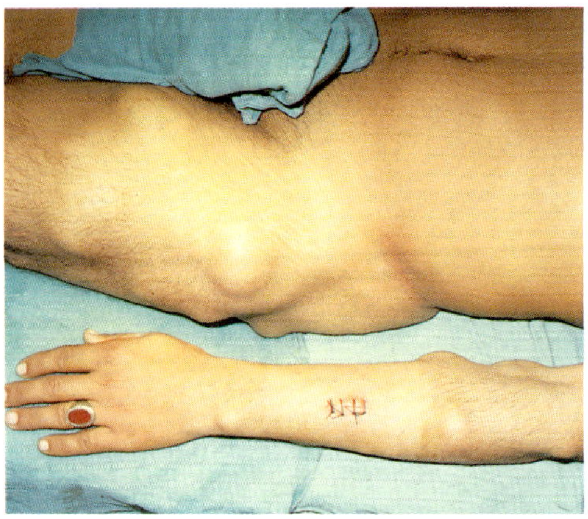

27

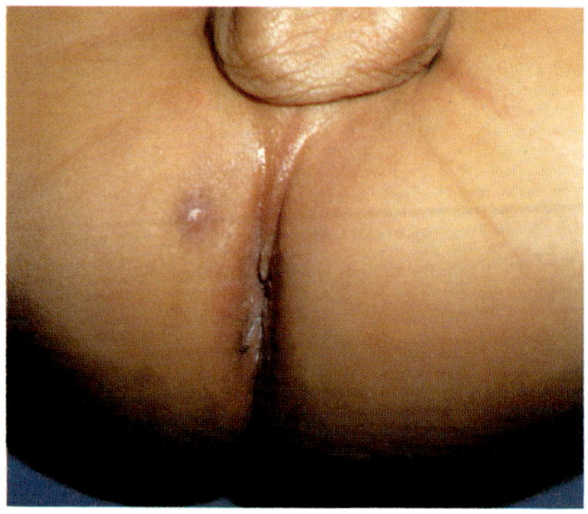

28

29

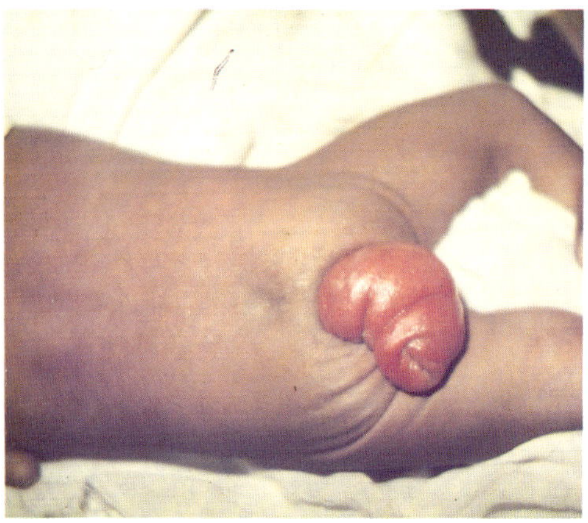

30

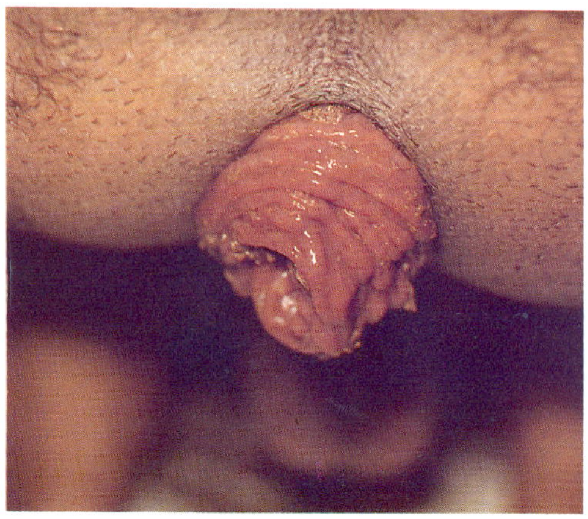

PLATE VII

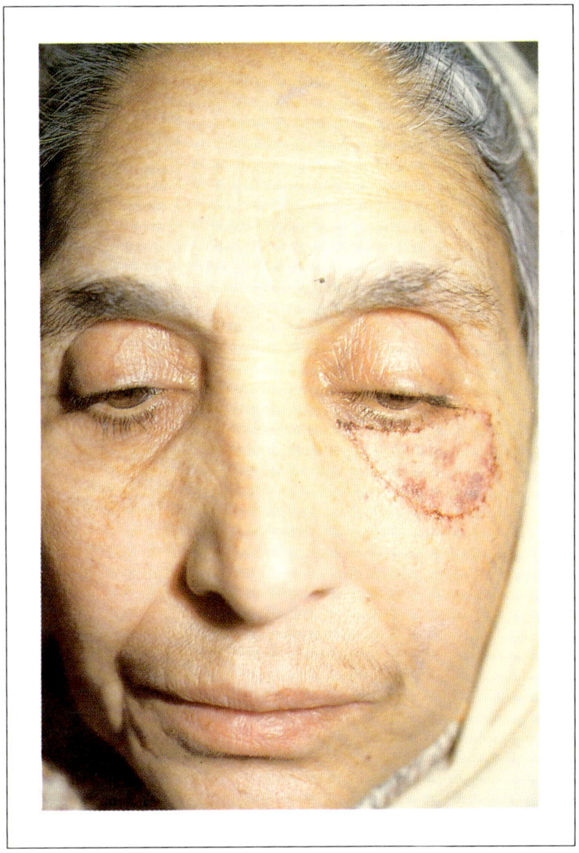

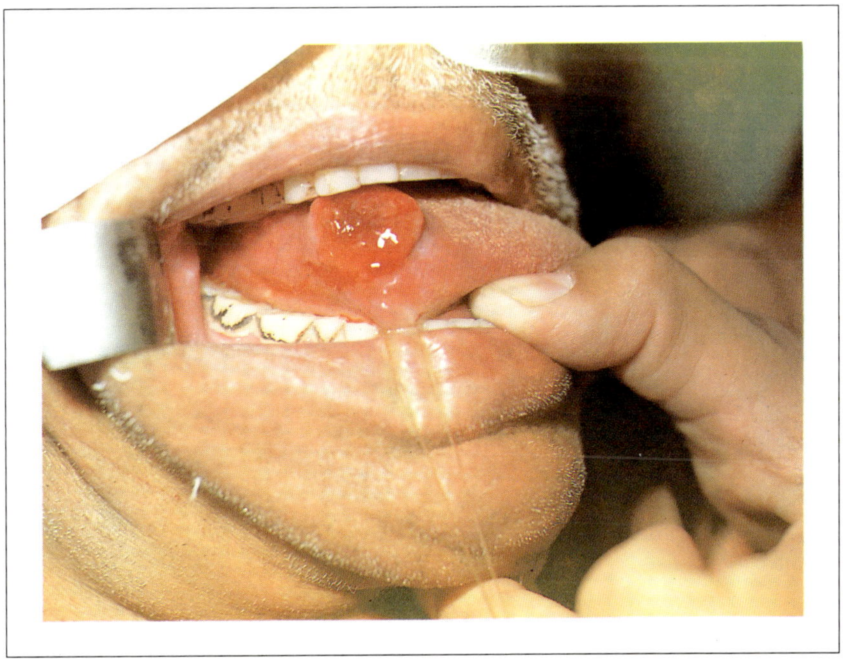

I. Basal cell carcinoma excised and full-thickness retroauricular skin graft applied to resurface defect. Immediately after removal of sutures.
II. Ulcer tongue due to squamous cell carcinoma. Note raised, rolled out margin of ulcer.

PLATE VIIa Photoquiz (Answers before Index)

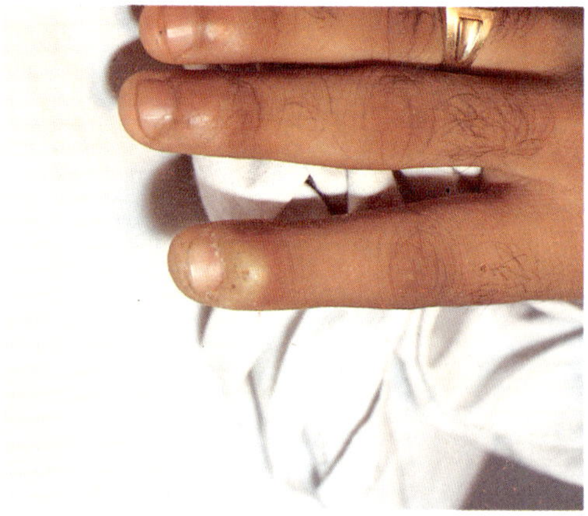

31

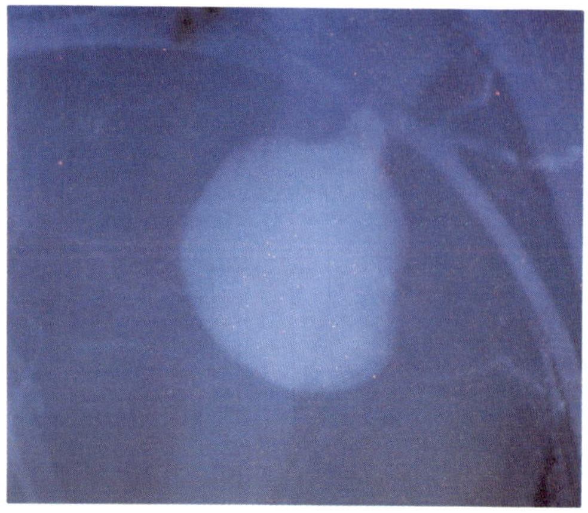

32

33

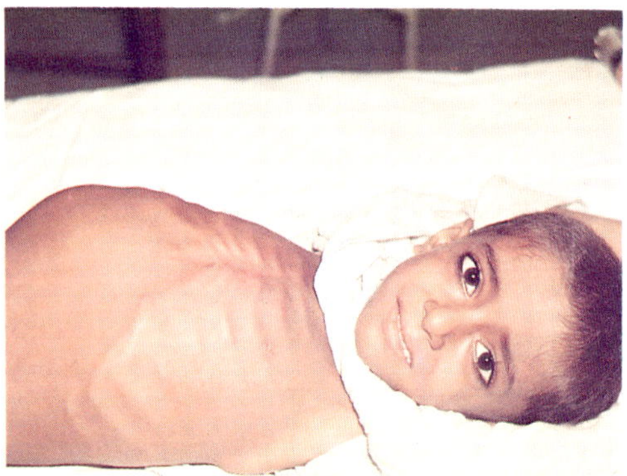

34

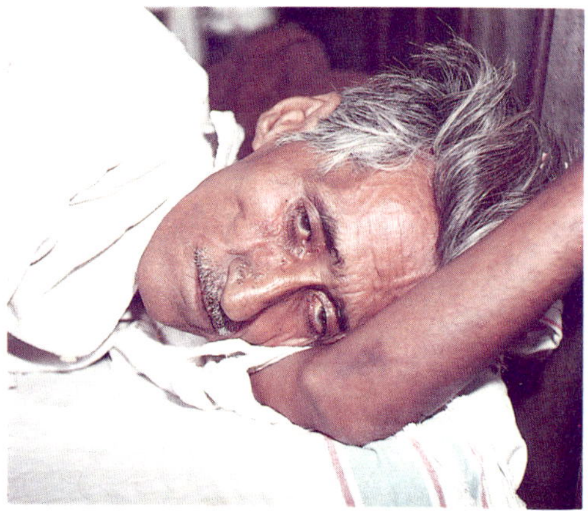

PLATE VIII

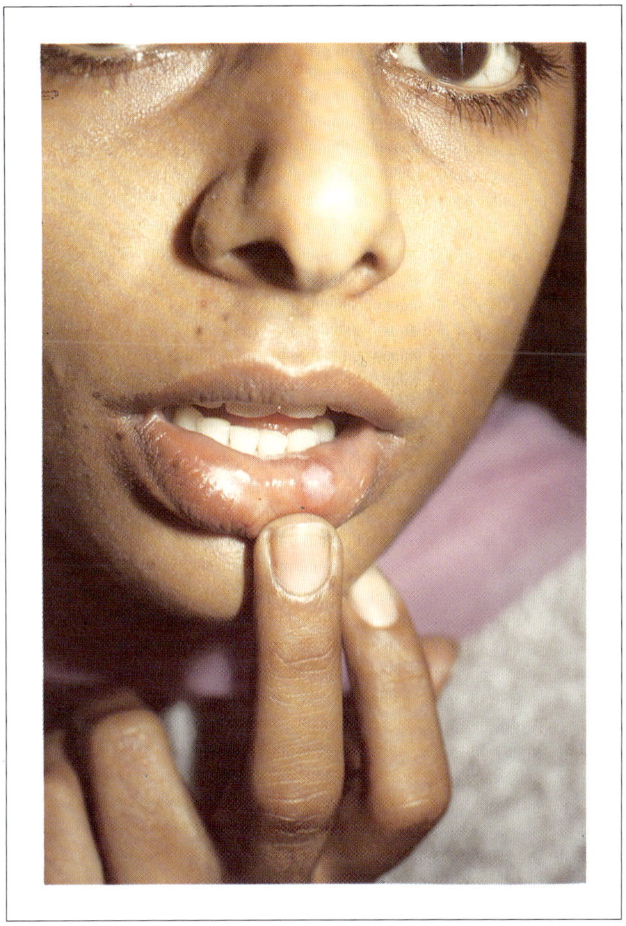

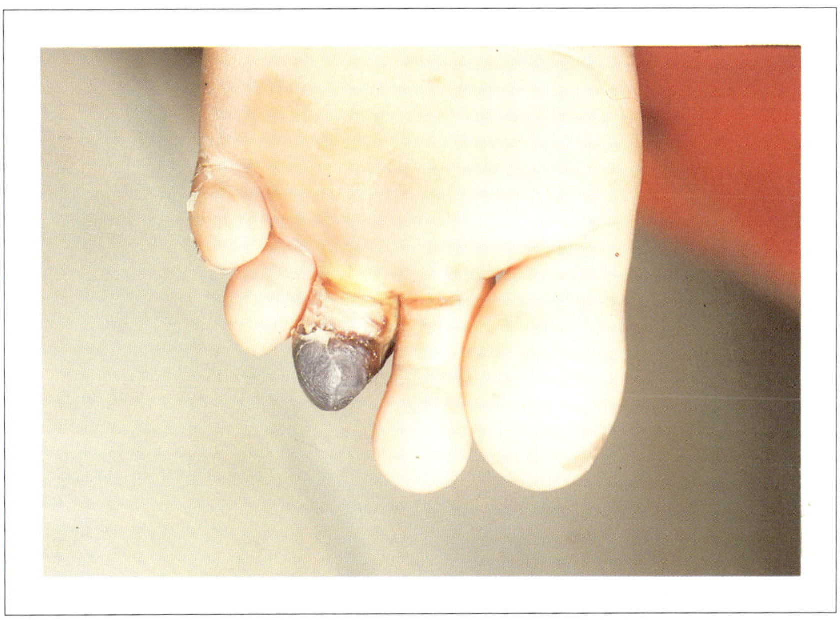

I. Mucous cyst lower lip.
II. Dry gangrene toe. The affected part of the toe is black, dry and shrivelled.

PLATE VIIIa Photoquiz (Answers before Index)

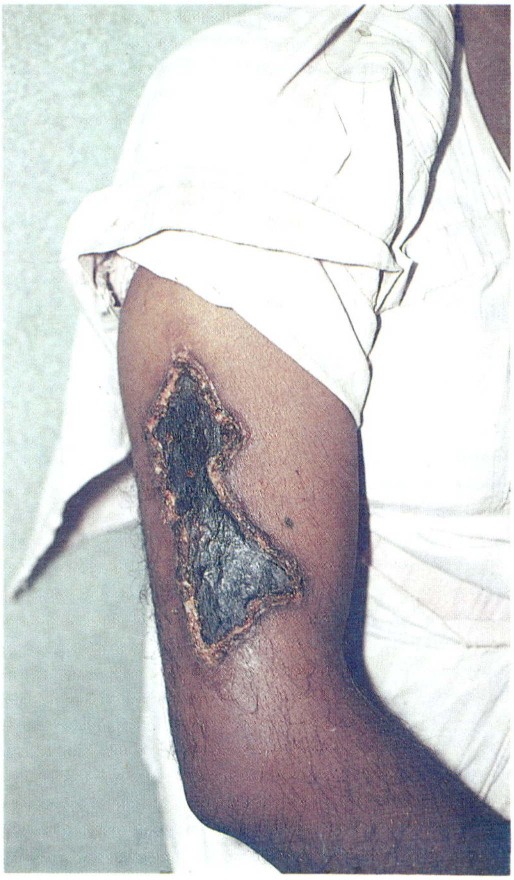

35

36

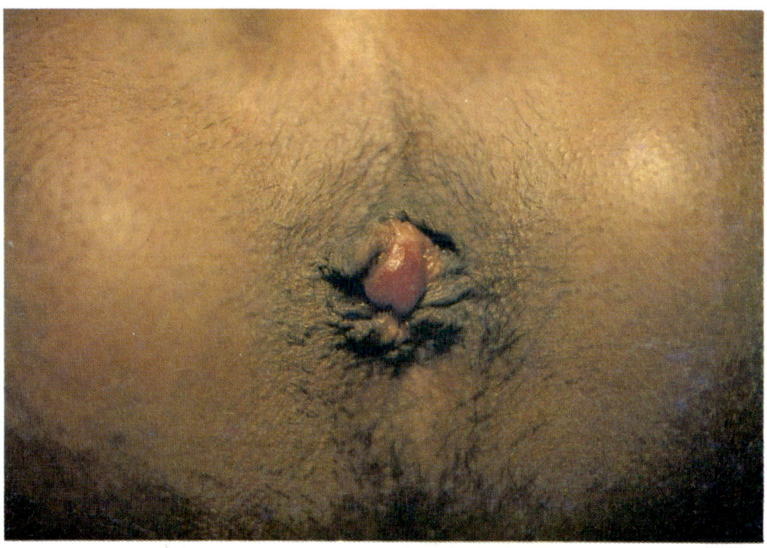